APPLIED PHARMACOLOGY

APPLIED PHARMACOLOGY

Stan K. Bardal, BSc (Pharm), MBA, PhD

Senior Instructor
Division of Medical Sciences
University of Victoria
Victoria, British Columbia
and
Instructor, Anesthesiology
Pharmacology and Therapeutics and Island Medical Program
University of British Columbia
Vancouver, British Columbia
Canada

Jason E. Waechter, BSc, MD, FRCP(C)

Clinical Assistant Professor
Departments of Critical Care and Anesthesiology
University of Calgary
Calgary, Alberta
Canada

Douglas S. Martin, PhD

Professor, Basic Biomedical Sciences
Sanford School of Medicine
University of South Dakota
Vermillion, South Dakota
United States

ELSEVIER
SAUNDERS

3251 Riverport Lane
St. Louis, Missouri 63043

APPLIED PHARMACOLOGY

ISBN: 978-1-4377-0310-8

Library of Congress Cataloging-in-Publication Data

Bardal, Stan K.
  Applied pharmacology / Stan K. Bardal, Jason E. Waechter, Douglas S. Martin.
     p. ; cm.
  Includes index.
  ISBN 978-1-4377-0310-8 (pbk. : alk. paper) 1. Clinical pharmacology—Textbooks. I. Waechter,
Jason E. II. Martin, Douglas S. III. Title.
  [DNLM: 1. Pharmacology, Clinical. QV 38]
  RM301.28.B365 2011
  615'.1—dc22

                                                                            2010026131

Acquisitions Editors: Kate Dimock, Madelene Hyde
Developmental Editor: Barbara Cicalese
Publishing Services Manager: Patricia Tannian
Team Manager: Radhika Pallamparthy
Senior Project Manager: Sarah Wunderly
Project Manager: Joanna Dhanabalan
Design Direction: Steven Stave

Printed in China

Last digit is the print number: 9 8 7 6 5 4 3 2 1

This work is dedicated to my family,
most notably my father, Konrad, for his continued support throughout the years;
my wife, Jen, for her love and understanding;
and my son Kalman, my inspiration for all future endeavors.
Stan Bardal

To my fiancée, Andrea Neilson
Jason Waechter

To my wife, Joanne, and children, Darren and Karissa, thank you for your love, and patience,
without which my career in pharmacology would not have been possible.
Thank you to Dr. Robert McNeill, a mentor and friend, who guided me into pharmacology.
Doug Martin

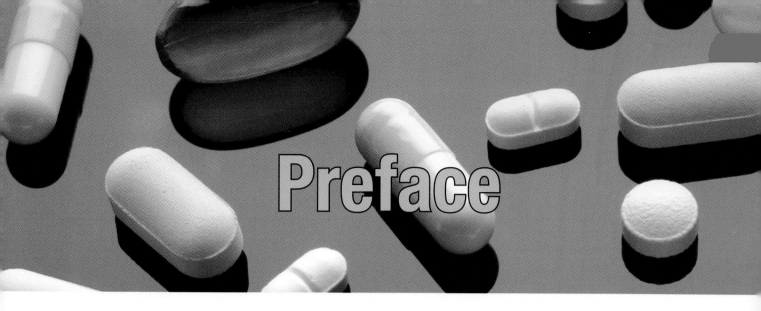

Preface

This textbook is designed to provide a concise yet comprehensive review of pharmacology, with an emphasis on information that is useful for clinicians in training or in practice. With its emphasis on basic science and clinical pharmacology, as well as evidence-based practice, this book is intended to be used from the beginning of students' training through their clinical years and beyond.

The book is divided into two sections. The **Introduction** covers basic pharmacologic principles such as pharmacodynamics, pharmacokinetics, autonomic pharmacology, and toxicology, as well as a number of more clinically oriented topics such as drug interactions, impact of age on pharmacology, drug discovery and evaluation, pharmacogenetics, herbal medicines, and addiction.

The **Drug Classes section** is divided into individual drug classes, which are grouped into larger sections, typically reflective of the body system (e.g., cardiovascular, pulmonary) or indication (e.g., psychiatry, infectious diseases) for which the drug is most commonly used. Each drug chapter follows a similar template as outlined below:

TITLE (DRUG NAME OR CLASS)
Description
■ Brief description of the drug or class of drug

Prototype and Common Drugs
■ Most important drug names
■ Nomenclature is boldfaced, if applicable (e.g., **-olol** for beta blockers)

MOA (Mechanism of Action)
■ Physiology and biochemical action of the drug or drug class
■ How and why the effects of the drug occur

Mechanisms of Resistance

Pharmacokinetics
■ Major pharmacokinetic issues with the drug class or a given drug. This is not intended to be comprehensive but will cover the most important issues a practioner might face when prescribing a given drug, including the route of metabolism, clinically important drug interactions, and issues pertaining to administration.
▲ If the half-life is at an extreme or an exception, it will be listed
▲ If the drug has a narrow therapeutic index or is potentially toxic, elimination will be described
▲ If the drug has special routes of administration, these will be described

Indications
■ Clinical conditions for which the drug is used

Contraindications
■ Situations for which the drug **should not** (*relative* contraindication) or **must not** (*absolute* contraindication) be used

Side Effects
■ Side effects of the drug or drug class
■ Explanations of why side effects occur, when mechanisms are known

Important Notes
■ Additional information that is considered to be essential for effective prescribing

Advanced
▲ Details that pertain to pharmacokinetics, pharmacodynamics, drug interactions, pharmacogenetics, or other drug-specific details
▲ Clinical details, including rare diseases, complicated mechanisms, theoretical concerns, or other details

Evidence
■ The focus is on recent, high-quality, systematic reviews. If such reviews are not available, evidence will not be included.
■ The actions of the drug or drug class must be isolatable in the systematic review; therefore indications such as cancer,

in which combination therapy is used, will have a smaller amount of available evidence.

- Treatment of infectious diseases, which is typically dictated by temporal and regional susceptibility patterns, will also have less available evidence.

FYI

- Notes of interest to help the reader remember or understand other information

FACULTY RESOURCES

An image collection and test bank are available for your use when teaching via Evolve. Contact your local sales representative for more information, or go directly to the Evolve website to request access: http://evolve.elsevier.com.

ACKNOWLEDGMENTS

The authors would like to acknowledge the dedication and support of Elsevier to this project, most notably the work of Kate Dimock, Madelene Hyde, and Barbara Cicalese.

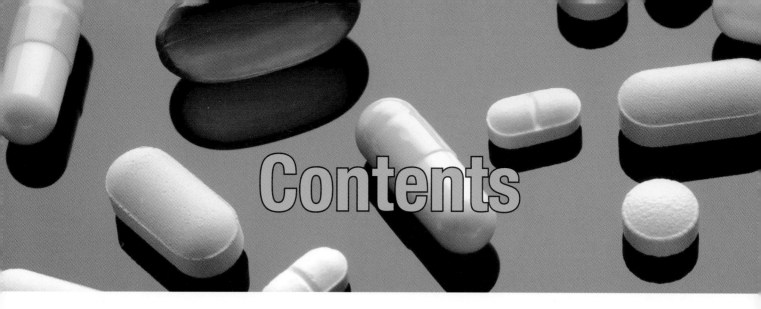

Contents

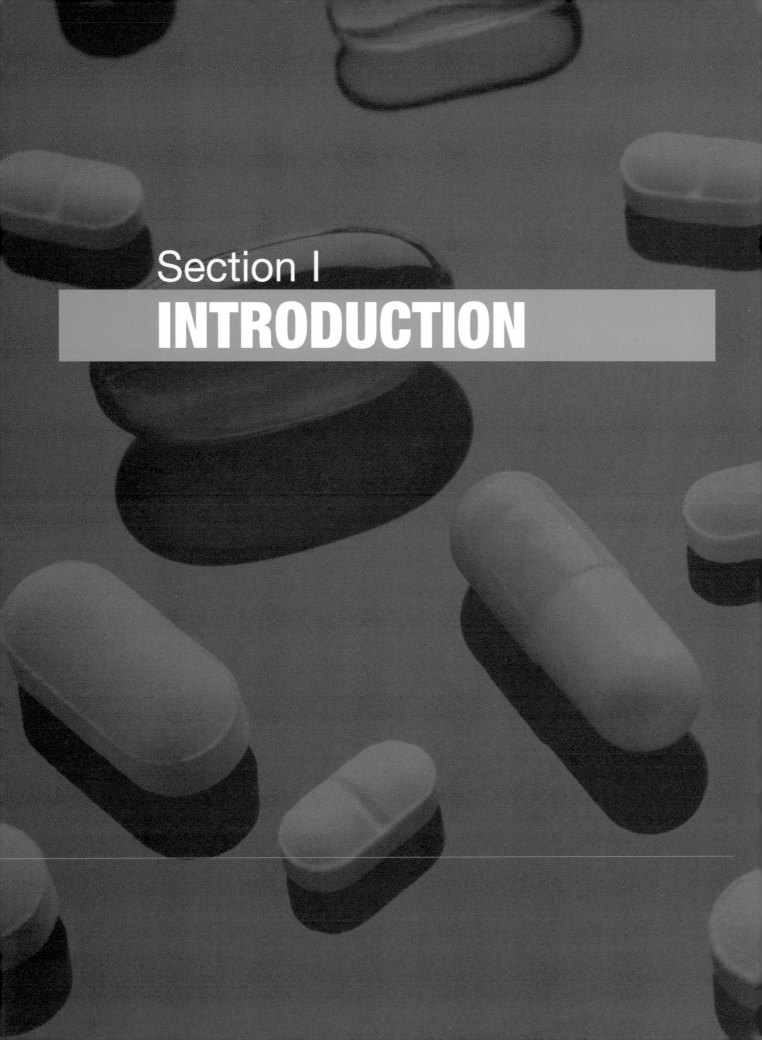

Section I
INTRODUCTION

Chapter 1

Basic Principles and Pharmacodynamics

The term *pharmacology* is derived from the Greek words *pharmakon*, meaning drug, and *logos*, meaning rational discussion or study. Thus pharmacology is the rational discussion or study of drugs and their interactions with the body. Classically there are two major divisions of pharmacology: pharmacodynamics and pharmacokinetics. Pharmacodynamics is the study of actions of drugs on the body—what effects a drug has on the patient, including mechanisms of action, beneficial and adverse effects of the drug, and the drug's clinical applications. Pharmacokinetics is the inverse: the study of actions of the body on drugs—the absorption, distribution, storage, and elimination of a drug. An emergent third division is pharmacogenomics: the study of how genetic makeup affects pharmacodynamics and pharmacokinetics and thus affects drug selection and application to individual patients.

There is no precise uniformly accepted definition for the term *drug*. However, it is commonly accepted that a drug is any exogenous non-nutritive substance that affects bodily function. Drugs may influence bodily functions via several general mechanisms, including physical interactions (e.g., antacids), by affecting enzymatic activity (e.g., increasing or decreasing), or by binding to molecular structures on or in the cell that affect cellular function (e.g., antihistamines).

DRUG NOMENCLATURE

Several names refer to the same drug, which can be a source of confusion for students and practitioners alike.

Chemical Name

The chemical name is based on a drug's chemical and molecular constituents and structure. Chemical names are precise but complex and cumbersome and therefore are seldom used in medical practice.

Generic Name (Nonproprietary, Approved)

The generic name (also called *nonproprietary* or *approved*) is assigned by the manufacturer after approval by the regulatory body in the country of origin (e.g., United States Adopted Names Council; the [Invented] Name Review Group [NRG] of the European Medicines Agency [EMEA]). Each drug has only one generic name, which bears some common feature of other drugs in the same class (e.g., the ending *-artan* for most members of the angiotensin receptor type 1 antagonists). Once assigned and approved, the generic name is in the public domain and is commonly used.

Generic names will be used in this textbook.

Trade, Brand, or Proprietary Name

The trade name is assigned by the manufacturer. It is copyrighted and therefore can be used commercially only by the originating pharmaceutical company.

When patent protection expires, the drug can be manufactured and marketed by many companies, and thus a drug can have many trade names.

■ **Clinical Connection:** Drugs can have many different names. For example, a prototypical calcium channel blocker of the dihydropyridine class has the chemical name *3,5-dimethyl 2,6-dimethyl-4-(2-nitrophenyl)-1,4-dihydropyridine-3,5-dicarboxylate*, the generic name *nifedipine*, and is available in the United States under several trade names including Adalat, Nifedical, and Procardia. Although marketing emphasizes trade names, the use of generic drug names is encouraged in practice to reduce prescribing errors and offers the opportunity for substitutions if appropriate.

DRUG-RECEPTOR INTERACTIONS

Although some notable exceptions exist, a fundamental principle of pharmacology is that drugs must interact with a molecular target to exert an effect. Drug interaction with molecular targets is the initiating event in a multistep process that ultimately alters tissue function. For the purposes of current discussion, the target will be referred to as a *receptor*. An in-depth discussion of molecular targets and a description of these processes will be presented later in this chapter (see the discussion of molecular mechanisms of drug action). Let us first consider the relationship between drug binding to its target receptors and the ultimate response of the tissue.

At its most fundamental level, the interaction of drug and receptor follows the **law of mass action**. The law of mass action dictates that:

- ▲ The combination of drug (also called **ligand**) and receptor depends on the concentrations of each
- ▲ The amount of drug-receptor complex formed determines the magnitude of the response
- ▲ A minimum number of drug receptor complexes must be formed for a response to be initiated (**threshold**)
- ▲ As drug concentration increases, the number of drug-receptor complexes increases and drug effect increases
- ▲ A point will be reached at which all receptors are bound to drug, and therefore no further drug-receptor complexes can be formed and the response does not increase any further (**saturation**)

Law of Mass Action Applied to Drugs

$$\text{Drug} + \text{Receptor} \rightleftharpoons \text{Drug-Receptor Complex} \rightarrow \text{Effect}$$

Although the amount of drug receptor-complex formed is proportional to the concentrations of drug and receptor, this relationship is not linear but is in fact parabolic (Figure 1-1, A).

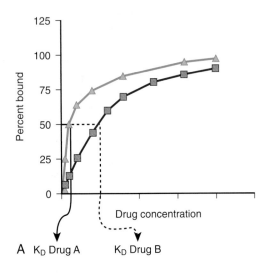

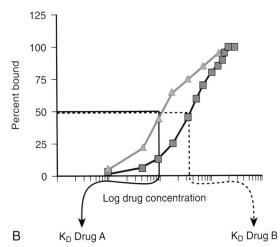

Figure 1-1. Drug receptor occupancy curves: law of mass action. **A,** Linear scale. **B,** Logarithmic scale.

Accordingly, this relationship is most often diagrammed on a semilogarithmic graph to linearize the relationship and encompass the large range of concentrations typical of the drug-receptor relationship (Figure 1-1, B).

Factors Affecting Drug-Target Interactions

Two basic properties of the drug-receptor interaction contribute importantly to drug responses: the ability of the drug to bind to its receptor, and the ability of the drug to alter the activity of its receptor.

Drug Binding

At the molecular level, a number of factors contribute to the interaction between drug and receptor and control the strength, duration, and type of the drug-receptor interaction. Collectively these factors dictate the strength with which the drug forms a complex with its receptor, also known as the *affinity*:

- ■ **Size and shape** of the drug molecule
- ■ **Types, number, and spatial arrangement** of drug binding sites (stereochemistry)
- ■ **Intermolecular forces** between drug and binding sites
  - ▲ Van der Waals forces = weak bonds and transient reversible effects
  - ▲ Hydrogen bonds = intermediate bonds and transient reversible effects
  - ▲ Covalent bonds = strong bonds and long-lasting or irreversible effects

It is important to recognize that, in most cases, binding of drug to target molecules involves weaker bonds. Accordingly, the drug-receptor complex is not static, but rather there is continuous association and dissociation of the drug with the receptor as long as drug is present. A measure of the relative ease with which the association and dissociation reactions occur is the equilibrium **dissociation constant** (K_D). Each drug-receptor combination will have a characteristic K_D value. Drugs with *high affinity* for a given receptor display a *small value* for K_D, and vice versa. In Figure 1-1, *A* and *B*, Drug A has a higher affinity for the receptor than Drug B. K_D also represents the concentration of drug needed to **bind 50% of the total receptor** population. These concepts are important in the study of basic pharmacologic data regarding different compounds with affinity for the same receptor. In general, drugs with lower K_D values will require lower concentrations to achieve sufficient receptor occupancy to exert an effect.

Selectivity of Drug Responses

Another important and desirable facet of pharmacologic responses is selectivity of drug action, determined by **drug molecules exhibiting preferential affinity for receptors**, as follows:

- ■ The cell will respond only to the spectrum of drugs that exhibit affinity for the receptors expressed by the cell.
- ■ The greater the extent to which a drug molecule exhibits high affinity for only one receptor, the more selective will be the drug's actions, with lower potential for side effects.

■ The higher the affinity and efficacy of a given drug, the smaller the amount of drug necessary to activate a critical mass of drug receptors to effect a tissue response, and the lower the potential for nonselective actions.

It is important to note that **selectivity of drug action** is a key concept. Few drugs are entirely specific for one receptor. Rather, drugs exhibit selectivity toward different receptors based on their relative affinities. Thus, selectivity is also relative. As the concentration of a drug increases, the drug will combine with receptors for which it has lower affinity and may generate off-target effects.

■ **Clinical Connection:** β-Adrenergic receptor antagonists are effective drugs for a number of cardiovascular disorders. Some β-adrenergic receptor antagonists are selective for β₁-adrenergic receptors to limit the potential for bronchoconstriction caused by blocking β₂-adrenergic receptors. However, even β₁-selective antagonists must be used cautiously in asthmatic patients, particularly at higher doses, to avoid further impairment of airway function in these patients.

Tissue Distribution of Receptors

■ Only those tissues possessing receptors will respond to the drug.

■ The more restricted the distribution of drug receptor, the more selective will be the effects of drugs that interact with that receptor.

■ **Clinical Connection:** Knowledge of receptor subtypes and their regional distribution can assist in drug selection. A useful example is the use of α-adrenergic receptor antagonists for the treatment of urinary retention secondary to prostatic hypertrophy. Nonselective α-adrenergic antagonists are not routinely used to treat urinary retention in men with prostatic hypertrophy, because although they block α receptors in the prostate and improve urine flow, they also block α receptors in blood vessels and cause hypotension. The prostate expresses primarily α₁B-adrenergic receptors, whereas blood vessels express other subtypes. Consequently, drugs such as tamsulosin that are selective for the α₁B subtype expressed primarily in the prostate are much more useful in the treatment of prostatic hypertrophy.

Activation of the Molecular Target

The relationship between the drug-receptor binding event and the ultimate biologic effect is complex. Quite often in experimental settings, the K_D (concentration causing 50% receptor occupancy) does not correspond to a 50% **maximal response** from the test tissue or organism. In fact, in many cases half-maximal tissue responses are obtained at drug concentrations below the K_D, suggesting that amplification of drug response occurs. Amplification of drug responses is discussed in a later section. This observation suggests that other factors, in addition to affinity and receptor occupancy, determine the strength of response. Accordingly, an additional modifier termed **intrinsic activity** was proposed. Intrinsic activity indicates the ability of receptor-bound drug to activate the receptor and initiate downstream events, leading to

an effect. Drugs are categorized based on their intrinsic activity at a given receptor:

■ **Agonists** (sometimes called *full agonists*) produce maximum activation of the receptor and elicit a maximum response from the tissue. They are assigned an intrinsic activity of 1.

■ **Antagonists** bind but produce no activation of the receptor and therefore block responses from the tissue. They are assigned an intrinsic activity of 0.

■ **Partial agonists** exhibit intrinsic activity between 0 and 1. Partial agonists produce weaker activation of the receptor than full agonists or the endogenous ligand. Partial agonists produce only partial activation of the receptor and its downstream signaling events. The clinical effect of a partial agonist will depend on its intrinsic activity and the concentration of the endogenous ligand. If concentrations of the endogenous ligand are really low, then a partial agonist will increase receptor activation, functioning as a weak agonist. In contrast, if concentrations of endogenous ligand are high, the partial agonist will compete for receptors and bind to a certain proportion of receptors previously bound by endogenous ligand. Because the partial agonist produces weaker activation of the receptor than endogenous ligand, the net effect will be less cumulative receptor activation. This will produce inhibition of the response mediated by the endogenous ligand, and the partial agonist will act as a weak antagonist.

■ **Inverse agonists** inhibit rather than activate the receptor. This phenomenon is evident with receptors that exhibit baseline (ongoing or constitutive) activity in the **absence of agonist binding.** In these cases, binding of the inverse agonist **reduces** the baseline activity of the receptor, which in turn elicits an effect opposite that of binding of the agonist. Inverse agonists and antagonists will elicit similar effects because both types of drugs will reverse the effects of endogenous ligands. Many clinically used antagonists may in fact be inverse agonists. Inverse agonists may assume particular **clinical importance** in disease states in which constitutive activity of receptors plays an important role. Increasing evidence suggests that a number of diseases are a result of **gain of function** mutations at the receptor that result in constitutive activity of the receptor in the absence of agonist.

■ **Clinical Connection:** Drugs that act as inverse agonists may have important clinical applications for diseases in which receptors are activated in the absence of **endogenous agonist.** One example is in cancer chemotherapy. In a number of human cancers, mutations of the epidermal growth factor receptor cause the receptor to be active in the absence of epidermal growth factor. In this setting, a traditional antagonist would be of no benefit. However, drugs that act as inverse agonists at the epidermal growth factor would suppress receptor activation and reduce the growth signaling via this pathway. Epidermal growth factor inverse agonists are being studied as cancer chemotherapy drugs.

Thus, the ultimate action of a drug will depend on both its affinity and its intrinsic activity. It is important to remember that **affinity and intrinsic activity are distinct properties.** A weak partial agonist, which by definition activates a receptor only minimally, may have very high affinity for a receptor. In this case the drug will be able to effectively compete for the receptor and will usually out-compete the endogenous agonist for receptor occupancy and inhibit the endogenous response.

Quantifying Drug-Target Interactions: Dose-Response Relationships

Ultimately, to make informed clinical decisions regarding drug treatment, it is necessary to understand the relationship between the amount of drug given and the anticipated effect in the patient. This relationship is described quantitatively by the dose-response curve. There are two basic types of dose-response curves—**graded** and **quantal**—and each provides useful information for therapeutic decisions.

Graded Dose-Response Curves

- Measure an effect that is continuous such that, in theory, any value is possible in a given range (0% through 100%).
- Have a sigmoidal shape similar to the drug receptor occupancy curves shown in Figure 1-2, because the biologic response to a drug is determined by the interaction of a drug with a receptor or molecular target.
- Exhibit a dose beyond which no further response is achieved (maximal effect; E_{max}). E_{max} is a measure of the pharmacologic efficacy of the drug.
- Show the dose that produces 50% of the E_{max} (**ED$_{50}$**).
- ED$_{50}$ is an index of the potency of the drug.
- Agonists with higher potency will have lower ED$_{50}$ values.

The ED$_{50}$ and E_{max} are useful parameters to assess drugs. In Figure 1-2, A, Drug A is more potent than Drug B or Drug C, whereas Drugs B and C have equal potency. Potency is sometimes used **incorrectly** as a measure of therapeutic effectiveness. In fact, in most cases potency is secondary to E_{max} in drug selection. However, in situations in which the absorption of drug is very poor, such that only small quantities of the drug reach the target, potency can be a critical consideration. Drugs with higher E_{max} values have higher pharmacologic **efficacy**.

In Figure 1-2, A, Drug B has the greatest efficacy, followed by Drug C, whereas Drug A, despite being the most potent, has the least efficacy. Drug C is equipotent with Drug B but has less efficacy. Thus, potency and efficacy can vary independently. It is important not to confuse the pharmacologic usage of *efficacy* with the more general usage. Pharmacologic **efficacy is a measure of the strength of effect** produced by the maximum dose of drug. By definition, *antagonists* do not activate their receptors after binding and therefore have an intrinsic activity and efficacy of 0. Nevertheless, an antagonist may be very clinically "efficacious" or beneficial because it blocks activation of the receptor by endogenous agonist.

These variables can be useful in determining how much of a drug to administer. For example, knowledge of the ED$_{50}$ concentration for blood pressure lowering can be used to determine the dose of antihypertensive agent to administer to achieve a certain magnitude of blood pressure reduction. However, the astute clinician recognizes that ED$_{50}$ values are

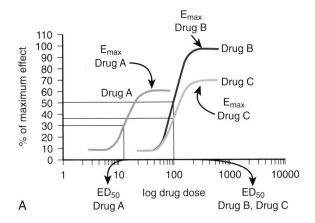

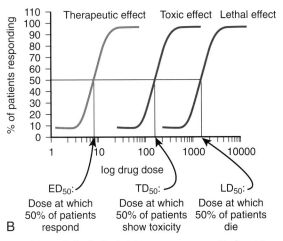

Figure 1-2. **A,** Graded dose-response curve. **B,** Quantal dose-response curve.

derived from the average of a great many patients and thus should be used only as initial guidelines. Because of interindividual **variability**, each patient may respond in ways that differ from the average. The second type of dose-response curves, quantal dose-response curves, provide an estimate of this variability.

Quantal Dose-Response Curves

Quantal dose-response curves do the following:

- Quantify responses for variables that are **all or none** (e.g., seizure or no seizure).
- Describe the relationship between drug dosage and the frequency with which a biologic effect occurs. For example, in individuals administered an anticonvulsant medication, the **percentage of individuals** not experiencing a convulsive episode at any given dose is plotted in cumulative fashion (Figure 1-2, B).
- Represent a **cumulative frequency distribution** for a given response.
  - ▲ Provide an **ED$_{50}$** value that reflects the dose of drug that **produces a response in 50% of the population** (also called the *median effective dose*).
  - ▲ Provide an **E_{max}** value that is the dose at which **all of the patients** respond to the drug.

▲ Provide an **estimate of the variability in response** of the patient population to the drug. A **steep slope** indicates that all the patients respond in a narrow range of doses, whereas a **shallow slope** indicates considerable variability in the ability of the drug to elicit a response in the patient population.

▲ Can be constructed for a graded or continuous response by choosing a target magnitude of response (e.g., blood pressure reduction of 20 mm Hg) and plotting the proportion of patients that achieves this magnitude of response at each increase in dosage. This type of information can be useful in determining a starting dosage to achieve a given level of effect

▲ Can be plotted for **therapeutic, toxic,** and **lethal effects** to obtain:

- **TD_{50}** (median toxic dose), is the dose that produces toxic effects in 50% of the patient population.
- **LD_{50}** (median lethal dose), the dose at which 50% of patients die
- Comparison of these parameters can provide an estimate of the relative safety of treatment.
- **Therapeutic index (TI)** or therapeutic ratio is the **ratio of the LD_{50} and ED_{50}. Large values** of TI are desirable because they indicate that the doses that produce death are much greater than those that produce a therapeutic effect.
- **Therapeutic window** is a loosely defined term that generally refers to the **range of doses** that produce therapeutic effects with minimal toxic effects. It can be viewed as the lack of overlap between the quantal dose-response curves for therapeutic and toxic or lethal effects. There are several indices of the degree of this overlap.
- **Certain safety factor:** The certain safety factor is the dose of drug that produces a lethal effect in 1% of the population (LD_1) divided by the dose that produces a therapeutic effect in 99% of the population (ED_{99}) (LD_1/ED_{99}).
- **Protective index:** The protective index is calculated as the dose for an undesirable effect in 50% of patients (TD_{50}) divided by the ED_{50} for the desired effect (TD_{50}/ED_{50}).
- For both the certain safety factor and the protective index, large values signify that there is little overlap between the therapeutic and toxic or lethal effects of the drug, and thus there is a relatively large margin of safety for its use.

Antagonism as a Mechanism of Drug Action

Although stimulation of molecular targets is a major mode of drug action, **inhibition of stimulation** by endogenous ligands is perhaps an even more important mechanism. In many disease states, excessive activation or sensitivity of endogenous physiologic pathways (e.g., bronchial hyperreactivity in asthma) occurs, and effective pharmacologic therapy acts to inhibit these pathways. The ways in which drugs act as antagonists can be classified into several general mechanisms, including the following:

Chemical (Physical) Antagonists

Chemical antagonists do **not** act at the receptor level, but rather there is a chemical or physical interaction between the drug and the endogenous target substance. A routinely used example is antacid used in the treatment of heartburn. Most antacids are basic magnesium, aluminum, or calcium salts that react with and neutralize gastric acid.

Physiologic (Functional) Antagonists

- Physiologic antagonists represent another type of antagonism in which the antagonist does **not** interact directly with the actions of the agonist at its molecular target.
- The agonist and antagonist each act on **different molecular targets,** but the responses elicited by these interactions are diametrically opposed and negate each other.
- Epinephrine and histamine are good examples of physiologic antagonists. Histamine is a vasodilator and bronchoconstrictor. Histamine release in anaphylactic reactions can cause hypotension and respiratory compromise. Epinephrine supports blood pressure and causes bronchodilation but does not act through the histamine receptor. Thus, epinephrine is given as acute treatment for anaphylactic reactions in part because it is a physiologic antagonist to histamine.

Pharmacokinetic Antagonists

- One drug attenuates the action of another drug by **decreasing its concentration** at the site of action.
- This may occur through changes in absorption, distribution, metabolism, or excretion.
- An example is activated charcoal used in acute treatment of poisonings. Ingestion of activated charcoal binds drug in the intestine and reduces or prevents its absorption.

Pharmacologic Antagonists

The majority of antagonists used as drug therapy are pharmacologic antagonists that act by **directly interfering** with an agonist's ability to activate its molecular target. The antagonist prevents agonist binding or agonist activation of the receptor and inhibits the biologic effects generated by the agonist. The interaction between antagonist and agonist can take several forms, including competitive reversible, competitive irreversible, and noncompetitive antagonism.

$$\text{Agonist} + \text{Antagonist} + \text{Receptor} \rightleftharpoons$$
$$\text{Agonist-Receptor Complex} \rightarrow \text{Agonist Effect}$$
$$\text{Antagonist-Receptor Complex} \rightarrow \text{No Agonist Effect}$$

- **Competitive reversible** antagonism (also called *competitive surmountable* antagonism)
  - ▲ The antagonist competes directly for the target receptor with the agonist molecule. These interactions will follow the **law of mass action** and the same general principles described earlier, with the added facet that now two drugs are competing for receptor occupancy.

▲ Because there is a fixed number of receptors (at least in the short term), each antagonist-receptor complex formed removes receptor molecules from the mass action equation and **reduces the likelihood** of formation of an agonist-receptor complex.

▲ Owing to the constant competition for receptors, the **concentrations and affinities** for both the agonist and antagonist drugs will determine the **overall balance** of the mass action equation.

▲ As the **concentration** of antagonist increases, the number of antagonist-receptor complexes increases and the number of agonist-receptor complexes decreases. Therefore the agonist effect decreases. Figure 1-3, *A* shows a graded dose-response curve for increasing concentrations of antagonist in the presence of a fixed concentration of agonist. The concentration of antagonist that reduces the agonist response to 50% of maximum is the IC_{50}, one index for quantifying antagonist effectiveness.

Note that IC_{50} values vary with agonist starting concentration.

▲ The greater the **affinity** of the antagonist, the greater the number of antagonist-receptor complexes formed at any given concentration of antagonist.

▲ The agonist-antagonist relationship can also be depicted on agonist dose-response curves. Figure 1-3, *B* illustrates graded agonist dose-response curves in the absence (control) and presence of increasing doses of antagonist.

▲ Addition of antagonist causes a reduction of agonist-driven response at any concentration of the agonist. It is important to note, however, that as the agonist concentration is increased, response increases because of greater competition for the receptors by the agonist. Ultimately, an agonist concentration will be reached, at which all of the receptors needed to elicit a maximal response are occupied by agonist and a maximal effect will be elicited.

▲ There is a rightward displacement of the agonist dose-response curve in the presence of a competitive reversible antagonist, but E_{max} is not affected.

▲ Increasing the concentration of antagonist produces a greater rightward displacement of the agonist dose-response curve, and the ED_{50} value for the agonist increases progressively. However, a maximal effect can always be reached by increasing the dose of agonist. The rightward parallel displacement of the agonist dose-response curves but with preserved E_{max} is characteristic of competitive reversible antagonism (see Figure 1-3).

▲ The magnitude of the rightward displacement of the agonist dose-response curve with increasing antagonist doses is an index of the affinity of the antagonist for the receptor and can be quantified by calculating a **dose ratio**, calculated as the ED_{50} in the presence of antagonist divided by the ED_{50} in the absence of antagonist. The dose ratio is used to calculate a pA_2 value, an index of the affinity of the antagonist.

▲ The pA_2 **scale** is an index of antagonist affinity for the receptor. The pA_2 is the negative logarithm of the dose of antagonist that necessitates a doubling of agonist dose—in other words, a dose ratio of 2.

▲ A lower pA_2 signifies greater antagonist affinity with greater effects at lower doses.

■ **Competitive irreversible** antagonism (also called *competitive insurmountable antagonism*) (in older literature these are also labeled as *noncompetitive antagonists*)

▲ The antagonist competes directly with the agonist for receptor binding as described previously. However, the binding forces between the antagonist and receptor are so strong that the antagonist-receptor complex is virtually irreversible.

▲ The net effect is that the total number of receptors available to the agonist is permanently reduced (at least until new receptor is synthesized).

▲ An important characteristic of this type of antagonism that distinguishes it from competitive reversible antagonism is that E_{max} **is reduced** (Figure 1-4).

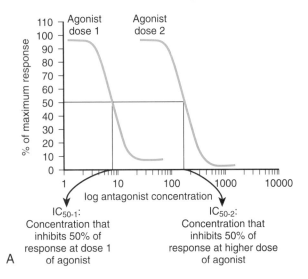

A

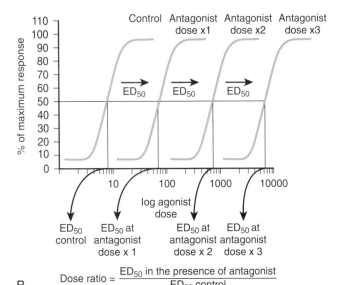

B

$$\text{Dose ratio} = \frac{ED_{50} \text{ in the presence of antagonist}}{ED_{50} \text{ control}}$$

Figure 1-3. A, Competitive reversible antagonism. **B,** Effect of competitive antagonist on agonist dose-response curves; dose ratio.

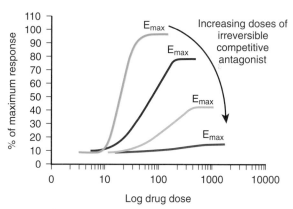

Figure 1-4. Competitive irreversible antagonism.

▲ A second distinguishing feature of this type of antagonist is that its effects will be constant irrespective of endogenous agonist levels. Thus fluctuations in the release of transmitter or hormone do not affect the response to this type of antagonist. This type of antagonist is useful clinically in situations in which endogenous agonist levels are unpredictable.

■ **Noncompetitive antagonism** (also called *allotropic* or *allosteric antagonism*)

▲ Noncompetitive antagonists do not directly compete with the agonist for binding at the same binding site but nevertheless impair the ability of an agonist to bind to or activate the receptor, and thus they prevent a response.

▲ An important characteristic of this type of antagonism is that both antagonist and agonist can be bound to the molecular target at the same time.

▲ Because agonists and antagonists bind at distinct sites, increasing concentrations of agonist do not out-compete or reverse the inhibitory action of the antagonist.

▲ Noncompetitive antagonism can occur through a number of mechanisms:

• Reduction in affinity of agonist binding site for the agonist

• Blockade of agonist-induced change in receptor

• Blockade of coupling of receptor to coupling or signaling mechanisms

▲ Noncompetitive antagonists will exert functional effects similar to those of competitive irreversible antagonists in that both types of antagonist will decrease the E_{max} or efficacy of the agonist.

▲ Because the agonist and antagonist act at different sites on the molecular target, increasing concentrations of agonist cannot overcome the inhibitory action of the antagonist. Thus, the effect of a noncompetitive antagonist will be independent of fluctuations in levels of the endogenous agonist, much like that of a competitive irreversible antagonist.

▲ A clinically relevant difference may be in the duration of action. Most allosteric antagonists combine reversibly with their binding site. Accordingly, discontinuation of the drug will result in a decrease in antagonist binding and effect. In contrast, as mentioned earlier, one of the

features of competitive irreversible antagonists is their prolonged duration of action.

■ **Clinical Connection:** Drugs that bind covalently to their molecular targets have the benefit of extended duration of action. Knowledge of this characteristic can influence clinical application of the drug. Acetylsalicylic acid (aspirin) irreversibly acetylates and inhibits the cyclooxygenase enzyme present in platelets and thereby inhibits platelet aggregation that contributes to coronary artery occlusion and myocardial infarcts. Although aspirin is cleared relatively quickly from the body, when used for its antiplatelet activity in patients with coronary artery disease, its administration is required only once a day because aspirin does not dissociate from its molecular target when plasma concentrations decrease.

MOLECULAR MECHANISMS MEDIATING DRUG ACTION

To this point we have considered the drug response as being elicited by agonist binding to and activating a receptor. In fact, there are many intervening steps between drug binding or receptor activation and the ultimate tissue response. In many cases this is because the drug is not able to interact directly with the cellular mechanisms eliciting the response. Instead, the drug must rely on intermediaries to relay (transduce) the drug signal to the cellular communication (second messenger signaling) and effector systems that ultimately cause the response. In addition, these transduction and signaling mechanisms are also integral in integrating convergent inputs to the cell and to modulation of drug responses by cells. In the preceding discussion, we used the general concept of receptor as the molecular target for drug action. In reality, there are many different types of molecular targets mediating drug responses. Knowledge of the different types of molecular targets and their associated transduction and signaling mechanisms aids in understanding drug action and the factors that modify drug responses.

Drug Targets

Drugs alter the activity or prevent the activation of a target molecule in some way. Although the term *drug receptor* is used generally to indicate the initial site of drug action, these molecular targets are composed of the following broad types.

Receptors

In the strictest pharmacologic sense, receptors are molecular entities that evolved specifically to bind certain substances, with the purpose of cellular communication (e.g., cardiac β-adrenergic receptors). The concept of the receptor was introduced at the end of the nineteenth century (Langley, 1878) and beginning of the twentieth century (Ehrlich, 1909). This in turn spurred considerable and ongoing research into the nature of the interaction between drugs and receptors.

General Sites

General sites may not have specifically evolved as communication mechanisms and thus may or may not adhere to all pharmacodynamic principles discussed earlier (e.g., intrinsic activity). Nevertheless, in a general sense these **can act as receptors** for drug action. Examples of general sites mediating drug action include the following:

- Components in key signaling or metabolic pathways
- Ion channels or transporters found in the cell membrane
- Intracellular or extracellular enzymes
- Structural components

Unidentified Targets

Finally, the molecular targets for some drugs have not been completely elucidated yet. An example would be the target for inhaled general anesthetics.

Receptor Coupling and Transduction Mechanisms

In pharmacology, *transduction* refers to the conversion of the information contained in the drug molecule (e.g., size, shape) into a signal that can be recognized and acted on by the cell. This process of receptor coupling, or transduction, is critically important to generating the ultimate biologic response. Transduction events are also important mechanisms contributing to the sensitivity of tissues to most drugs. Only minute amounts of drug are generally necessary to initiate or inhibit a response, because transduction mechanisms greatly amplify the signal generated by the drug-target complex. Transduction generally involves a sequence of events that represent opportunities for interaction between different drug signals, for the cell to modulate the initial signal produced by the drug (feedback), and for future drug development. Indeed, many currently used drugs do not interact directly with endogenous substances or their receptors but rather interact with transduction events to cause their actions.

Extracellular Transduction Mechanisms

A number of dugs act outside of the cell to affect cellular function. Generally, these types of drugs act via the following:

- **Extracellular enzymes.** Drugs acting via this mechanism alter the activity of extracellular enzymes involved in the synthesis or degradation of endogenous signaling molecules. These drugs affect the levels of endogenous compounds that then alter cellular function by acting on their receptors. Examples of clinical utility for this mechanism include:
  - ▲ Angiotensin-converting enzyme (ACE) inhibitors, which prevent the formation of angiotensin II and are used in the treatment of hypertension
  - ▲ Inhibition of acetylcholinesterase, which results in increased levels of acetylcholine for the treatment of:
    - • Neuromuscular disorders
    - • Glaucoma
  - ▲ **Clinical Connection**: Myasthenia gravis is an autoimmune disorder that targets the acetylcholine receptor. Loss of these receptors at the neuromuscular junction leads to muscle weakness. Edrophonium, a drug that inhibits the extracellular enzyme (cholinesterase) that degrades acetylcholine, can be used to confirm the diagnosis of myasthenia gravis. Injection of edrophonium produces a short-lived increase in acetylcholine at the neuromuscular junction and an improvement in muscle strength in patients with myasthenia gravis.

- **Direct interaction** with endogenous molecules to affect their ability to reach their sites of action. The clearest example of this type of mechanism is the use of monoclonal antibodies to directly target endogenous signaling molecules. An example of this application is the use of a monoclonal antibody to the cytokine tumor necrosis factor α (TNF-α) (adalimumab) in the treatment of certain autoimmune disorders. Administration of adalimumab binds TNF-α and prevents the cytokine from reaching and activating its receptor.

Transmembrane Transduction Mechanisms

In many cases, the drug or endogenous ligand is a hydrophilic substance that cannot easily cross the plasma membrane of the cell and binds to receptors or other targets embedded in the plasma membrane. Accordingly, mechanisms are needed to transduce or relay the drug signal across the plasma membrane. It is possible to cluster these coupling and transduction mechanisms into several general groups (sometimes called *superfamilies*).

- **G protein–coupled receptors (GPCRs).** GPCRs, also called *seven transmembrane pass receptors*, are a large class of receptors that mediate the majority of endogenous transmitter and hormone driven responses (Figure 1-5).
  - ▲ **G proteins** are trimeric macromolecules that consist of α, β, and γ subunits.
  - ▲ Ligand activation of the receptor causes the GPCR to interact with G proteins.
    - • G_α is activated by binding of **guanosine-5'-triphosphate** (**GTP**) and dissociation of the G_α-GTP complex from the receptor and from its companion βγ subunits.
    - • Activated G_α-GTP complex then activates downstream effector systems (e.g., adenylate cyclase) to initiate a cascade of cellular events (e.g., cyclic

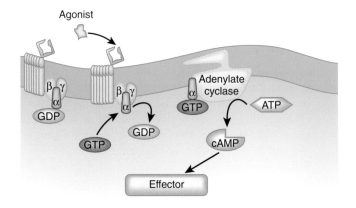

Figure 1-5. G protein–coupled receptors.

adenosine monophosphate [cAMP] production) that lead to activation of the effector system and the biologic response.

- G_α subunit has intrinsic **GTPase** activity and eventually hydrolyzes GTP to guanosine diphosphate (GDP), which represents a termination signal for this receptor transduction mechanism.
- G proteins exist in as many as 23 isoforms coupled to different signaling paths. The type(s) of G protein coupled to the receptor determines the response to receptor activation.
- Individual cells may contain receptors coupled to many G proteins.
- The ultimate biologic response to activation of a receptor will be the integrated action of G protein action.
- Approximately 30% of all clinically used drugs interact with GPCR.

■ **Receptor-coupled enzymes.** Receptor-coupled enzymes bypass the G protein coupling mechanism and link directly to cellular communication cascades. The receptor is directly coupled in some way to kinase enzymatic activity within the cell. Ligand binding stimulates the kinase enzymatic activity, which then initiates and amplifies intracellular signals and feedback responses by changing the phosphorylation status of cellular proteins. As shown in Figure 1-6, these mechanisms can be grouped into four general types that include receptors:

- ▲ With integral tyrosine kinase (TK) activity
- ▲ That recruit TK to the receptor and activate the enzyme
- ▲ Coupled to serine threonine kinases
- ▲ With guanylate cyclase activity that generate a second messenger, cyclic guanosine monophosphate (cGMP)

  The receptor-coupled enzymes phosphorylate intracellular proteins at tyrosine (Tyr), serine (Ser), or threonine (Thr) residues to change protein function. Alternatively, cGMP generated by guanylate cyclase activates downstream enzymes (effector in Figure 1-6) that change the phosphorylation status of proteins to alter their function. Receptors with TK activity and guanylate cyclase activity are currently the most clinically useful. Examples of these two receptor-linked enzymes include the following:

- ▲ Receptors with integral TK activity
  - Characteristic of hormones linked to metabolism, growth, and differentiation, such as insulin and epidermal growth factor
  - Examples of clinical utility include:
    ○ Insulin therapy in diabetic patients
    ○ Trastuzumab (monoclonal antibody to HER2 receptor) for treatment of breast cancer
- ▲ Receptors coupled to **guanylate cyclase**
  - Generate cGMP
  - Characteristic of natriuretic peptide receptors
  - Example of clinical utility includes:
    ○ Agonists at these receptors are used in the treatment of heart failure. A recombinant form of brain natriuretic peptide (nesiritide) is used to reduce pulmonary congestion in acute decompensated heart failure because of the drug's potent vasodilator properties.

■ **Transmembrane ion channels.** Transmembrane ion channels allow the passage of ions from one side of a membrane to another. Channels can exist in the open, closed, or inactive state, which represent different conformations of the channel protein. As shown in Figure 1-7, drugs may affect the function of these channels by directly opening or closing the channel (ligand gated channels), by influencing the voltage-dependent characteristics of the channels (voltage gated channels) and the amount of time the channel spends in a given state, or by generating second messengers that subsequently open or close the channel (second messenger gated). Common examples of functions governed by ion channels include the following:

- ▲ Electrophysiology of cardiac and skeletal muscle
- ▲ Neurotransmission

  There are several subtypes of ion channels, based on the ways that drugs or endogenous substances regulate the channels (see Figure 1-7).

- ▲ **Ligand gated ion channels or receptor-operated channels.** These ion channels possess a receptor for an endogenous ligand to which the drug can bind. They are composed of a multimeric protein complex that constitutes both the receptor and the ion channel. Agonist activation opens the channel, and antagonists close or inactivate the channel. Examples include the following:
  - Cholinergic receptors located in skeletal muscle bind nicotine, resulting in opening of sodium channels, initiation of an action potential in the muscle, and finally muscle contraction. Neuromuscular (paralyzing) drugs antagonize this nicotinic receptor, thereby preventing muscle contraction.

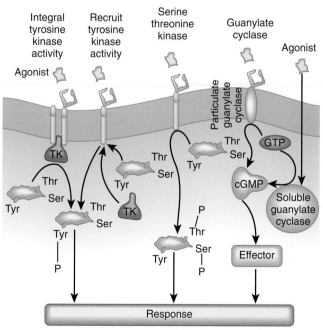

Figure 1-6. Receptor-coupled enzymes.

**Ligand or receptor
operated channel**

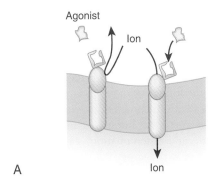

A

Voltage gated

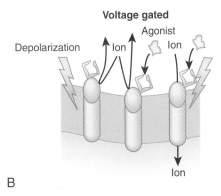

B

Second messenger gated

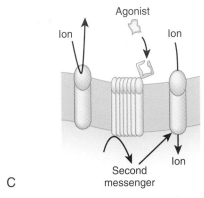

C

Figure 1-7. Receptor-coupled transmembrane ion channels. **A,** Ligand gated or receptor-operated channel. **B,** Voltage gated channel. **C,** Second messenger gated channel.

- γ-Aminobutyric acid (GABA) A receptors are *inhibitory* receptors in the brain. Drugs that stimulate GABA$_A$ receptors open chloride channels, causing hyperpolarization (making the cell more negative) and reducing the probability of an action potential being produced, thereby turning *off* the target neuron. Drugs that treat anxiety and sleep disorders are clinical examples of these types of drugs.

▲ **Voltage gated ion channels.** These ion channels change conformation (open, closed, or inactive) in response to changes in membrane voltage. Drug binding to the channel alters the response of the channel to changes in membrane voltage such that the open, closed, or inacti-

vate state may be lengthened or shortened. An example is a local anesthetic agent that binds to sodium channels that are responsive to the arrival of an action potential. Local anesthetics lock the channels in the inactive state, thereby rendering them temporarily nonresponsive to future action potentials and thereby block transmission of pain signals.

▲ **Second messenger gated ion channels.** These ion channels respond directly or indirectly to second messenger molecules (see second messenger section, later, for details). Drug binding to receptor elaborates a second messenger that in turn affects channel function. Examples of clinical utility include the following:

- Drugs that block the hyperpolarization cyclic nucleotide gated channel (HCN or *funny* channel) in the sinoatrial node and thereby reduce heart rate. This class of drug represents a new approach to the treatment of angina.

Membrane-Bound Transporters

Membrane-bound transporters control movement of substances between intracellular and extracellular space and therefore control a wide range of physiologic functions. Consequently drugs that act at membrane-bound transporters have a wide range of utility including the following:

- Treatment of heart failure (digitalis inhibition of sodium potassium ATPase).
- Diuretics. The loop diuretics, a major class of diuretic agents, inhibit the sodium, potassium, two chloride cotransporter in the thick ascending limb of the loop of Henle, promoting loss of sodium and water in the urine.
- Antidepressants. Selective serotonin inhibitors, a major class of antidepressant medication, block the reuptake of serotonin into neurons.
- Gastrointestinal disorders (e.g., peptic ulcer). Proton pump inhibitors slow the secretion of hydrogen ions into the stomach and reduce gastric acidity.

Intracellular Transduction Mechanisms

A number of drugs bind to their primary site of action after being transported or diffusing into the intracellular space of the cell. Once inside the cell these receptors may be coupled to a number of transduction mechanisms, including transcriptional regulation, second messenger generation, and structural mechanisms.

Intracellular Receptors

Lipophilic drugs passively cross the cell membrane and thus do not require cell membrane receptors. As shown in Figure 1-8, one target for these drugs is an intracellular receptor that activates transcriptional pathways. In this mechanism, the agonist receptor complex diffuses to DNA, where it binds to DNA binding elements. Via this mechanism drugs act directly or through recruitment of coactivators or co-repressors, which increase or decrease transcription of RNA to ultimately change protein expression. This process is referred to as *ligand gated transcriptional regulation.* In many cases these drugs effect

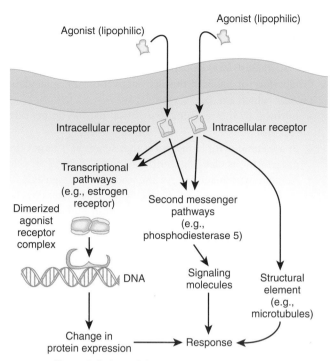

Figure 1-8. Intracellular receptor-coupling mechanisms.

long-term changes by affecting gene transcription. Receptors using this coupling mechanism include:

■ Sex hormones: estrogen, androgens
■ Glucocorticoids
■ Mineralocorticoids
■ Thyroid or retinoid receptor family
■ Vitamin D receptors

Responses to these types of drug may be tissue dependent based on differential recruitment of coactivators or co-repressors. For example, selective estrogen receptor modulators (SERMs) acting on the same receptor may behave as an agonist in bone and as an antagonist in breast tissue (e.g., raloxifene).

Examples of ligand gated transcription regulation with clinical utility include:

▲ Replacement therapy (e.g., at menopause)
▲ Contraception
▲ Treatment of osteoporosis (via vitamin D)
▲ Treatment of breast cancer with SERMs
▲ **Clinical Connection:** Tamoxifen and raloxifene are selective estrogen receptor modulators. Tamoxifen and raloxifene act as antagonists in breast tissue and are useful in the treatment of breast cancer. However, use of tamoxifen is complicated by estrogen receptor agonist activity in the uterus, where the drug triggers an increased risk for uterine cancer. Raloxifene, despite combining to the same receptor, does not exhibit agonist activity in the uterus, and therefore its use is not complicated by concerns about uterine cancer.

Intracellular Enzymes

Some drugs directly target intracellular enzymes, such as phosphodiesterase (PDE), that control second messenger pathways (see Figure 1-8) and thereby alter the concentrations of intracellular signaling molecules, which then effects a cellular response. As greater understanding of intracellular signaling is achieved, it is likely that more drugs using this mode of action will be developed. Often there are multiple levels of intracellular signaling molecules downstream from the enzyme being targeted. A common example of the utility of this approach is PDE5 inhibition, to prevent the breakdown of cGMP, which results in increased vasodilation. This approach is useful in the treatment of erectile dysfunction because of the ability to somewhat selectively target blood vessels in the penis.

Structural Mechanisms

Drugs can also target structural components of cells (e.g., the cytoskeleton or microtubules) to affect their function (see Figure 1-8). Examples of clinical utility include the following:

■ Vinca alkaloids (e.g., vincristine) disrupt microtubule formation and arrest cell division and are used in cancer chemotherapy.
■ DNA cross-linking agents (e.g., cisplatin) that inhibit DNA replication and transcription are also used in cancer chemotherapy.

In addition to activation of receptors, drugs may also target postreceptor events in second messenger cascades. For example, some drugs used in the treatment of heart failure inhibit the degradation of cAMP by blocking the PDE enzymes responsible for degradation of cAMP. Similarly, cGMP is an important second messenger molecule. Drugs used in the treatment of erectile dysfunction act by inhibiting PDE5, which is responsible for cGMP degradation. The phospholipase C (PLC), inositol trisphosphate (IP3), diacylglycerol (DAG) pathway is involved in many cellular processes. Drugs under development as antineoplastic agents target this pathway.

Second Messenger Systems

After formation of the drug-receptor complex and activation of a coupling mechanism (e.g., G proteins), the drug signal is transmitted to the final effector system of the cell. In many cases the transduction or coupling mechanism is linked to the final effector system via an intermediate cell signaling (second messenger) system. Drugs may also target enzymes or other processes regulating the concentrations of intracellular second messengers. This represents an important mode of drug action. In addition, it opens the possibility for synergistic or antagonist interactions among drugs that act at different sites in the same pathway. These interactions may enhance therapeutic effects or lead to adverse effects. The field of cell signaling is extremely dynamic, with new signaling molecules or new functions for established molecules discovered on a seemingly daily basis. Therefore, it is not possible to discuss the intricacies of all second messenger systems linked to clinically relevant drug actions. Nevertheless, several pathways serve as good illustrations of the involvement of cell signaling mechanisms as mediators of drug responses and as targets for future drug development. Figure 1-9 illustrates three of the best understood second messenger systems.

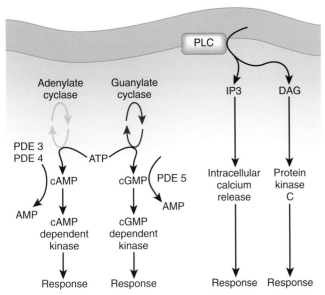

Figure 1-9. Second messenger systems.

Cyclic Adenosine Monophosphate Pathway

- cAMP is generated by activity of adenylate cyclase.
- Adenylate cyclase is modulated by activated G_α-GTP complexes in either a stimulatory ($G_{\alpha s}$-GTP) or inhibitory ($G_{\alpha i}$-GTP) fashion.
- Multiple isoforms of adenylate cyclase show isoform-specific interactions with G_α-GTP and tissue-specific distribution.
- Agonists activating adenylate cyclase may elicit differential responses in different target tissues.
- cAMP signaling can proceed through:
  - ▲ cAMP-dependent protein kinases triggering phosphorylation of effector molecules (e.g., cardiac voltage gated calcium channel) to elicit short-term effects
  - ▲ cAMP-dependent protein kinases triggering phosphorylation of cAMP response element binding protein (CREB), which subsequently affects gene transcription to effect long-term responses
  - ▲ Direct interaction of cAMP with effectors such as the hyperpolarization-activated cyclic nucleotide gated (HCN) channel that are present in cardiac pacemaker cells
- PDEs play a critical role in cAMP signaling by degrading cAMP and serve to shut off signaling via this pathway. Many isoforms of PDE exist, some of which are specific for cAMP and/or show selective tissue distributions.
  - ▲ PDE3 inhibitors are used in the treatment of heart failure.
  - ▲ PDE4 inhibitors are used in the treatment of chronic obstructive pulmonary disease.

Clinical Connection: Knowledge of coupling and second messenger systems can help in understanding drug action. Clinical use of β-adrenergic antagonists is associated with two apparently disparate effects. In the short term, β antagonists reduce cardiac function by blocking the formation of cAMP and signaling to the cardiac calcium channel. However, when used chronically in heart failure patients, β antagonists actually improve cardiac function, presumably via their long-term actions on gene transcription.

Cyclic Guanosine Monophosphate

- Production of cGMP through activation of guanylate cyclase, which can be:
  - ▲ Intrinsic to the receptor (e.g., atrial natriuretic peptide receptor)
  - ▲ In a soluble cytoplasmic form that serves as a target for gaseous molecules (e.g., nitric oxide)
  - ▲ Activation of guanylate cyclase leads to increased cGMP as a second messenger molecule that activates downstream cGMP-dependent kinases to cause phosphorylation of effector systems. An important effector system is the contractile apparatus of vascular smooth muscle, where cGMP phosphorylation leads to vasodilation.
  - ▲ PDEs also play a critical role as an off switch for this pathway. Accordingly, PDE inhibitors are used to interact with this signaling pathway. The development of drugs that selectively inhibit PDE5 (e.g., sildenafil), which is selective for cGMP, revolutionized the treatment of erectile dysfunction by improving penile blood flow.

Phospholipase C, Inositol 1,4,5 Trisphosphate (IP3), Diacylglycerol (DAG)

- Phospholipase catabolizes membrane phospholipids to release IP3 and DAG.
- IP3 serves as a second messenger controlling intracellular calcium release.
- DAG activates the protein kinase C (PKC) family of enzymes.
  Activation may be isoform and tissue specific.
  - ▲ The IP3-DAG-PKC pathway is very widespread and linked to many functions. This signaling mechanism is coupled to receptors for some of the major homeostatic pathways, including α-adrenergic receptors, serotonin receptors, angiotensin receptors, acetylcholine receptors, and prostaglandins, to name but a few. The widespread nature of this pathway makes it very important but also very difficult to manipulate to achieve selective therapeutic actions with minimal side effects. Nevertheless, this is an area of ongoing research, and isoform-specific inhibitors of PKC are in development for clinical applications. Enzastaurin, a selective PKC-β isoform inhibitor, is in clinical trials as an antineoplastic agent.

Many more second messenger systems and signaling modalities exist and participate in drug responses. Improved understanding of this facet of pharmacology will point to greater opportunities for development of new drug targets.

- **Clinical Connection:** Knowledge of coupling and second messenger systems can help in understanding drug interactions. Nitrates used in the treatment of coronary ischemia stimulate guanylate cyclase to produce cGMP. PDE5 inhibitors used in the treatment of erectile dysfunction inhibit the breakdown of cGMP. Concurrent use of these two drugs can lead to excessive levels of cGMP, which in turn

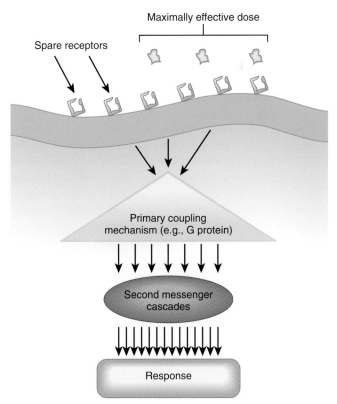

Maximally effective dose

Spare receptors

Primary coupling
mechanism (e.g., G protein)

Second messenger
cascades

Response

Figure 1-10. Amplification of drug responses.

cause excessive vasodilation and potentially dangerous reductions in blood pressure. Consequently, patients are warned to not use PDE5 inhibitors if they are on nitrate therapy for angina.

Amplification of Drug Responses

Amplification is an important component of pharmacologic responses. A great deal of amplification occurs in pharmacologic pathways, such that only a minute quantity of drug (often in the picomolar or femtomolar range) is capable of eliciting biologic responses. In general, only minute concentrations of neurotransmitters, hormones, or exogenously administered drugs need reach the molecular target to initiate a biologic response. This exquisite sensitivity of tissues to drugs results in large part from amplification of the original signal provided by the drug molecule. Amplification can occur at several points in the drug-receptor coupling and signaling systems (Figure 1-10).

■ Receptor
  ▲ Increases or decreases in receptor expression will increase or decrease, respectively, tissue sensitivity to the agonist because of the law of mass action.
  ▲ Many tissues express more receptors than are necessary to elicit a full response (spare receptors). This concept is called **spare receptors** or **receptor reserve.**
  ▲ The presence of spare receptors or receptor reserve provides a mechanism to drive the mass balance equation governing interaction of drug and receptor toward the formation of drug-receptor complexes.

  ▲ Spare receptors greatly increase a tissue's sensitivity to agonist and decrease a tissue's sensitivity to antagonists.
■ G proteins
  ▲ G_α-GTP remains active until the intrinsic GTPase activity of the G_α subunit hydrolyzes GTP.
  ▲ The G_α-GTP complex may be considerably longer lived than the original drug receptor activation step, which generates multiple intracellular signaling molecules for each drug-receptor complex, leading to enhanced activation of downstream molecules.
■ Second messengers
  ▲ Once activated, each signaling cascade enzyme can produce multiple copies of signaling molecules for each signal generated from the primary coupling mechanism.
  The net result is progressive amplification of the drug signal until the final effector system elicits a biologic response. Collectively, these mechanisms endow pharmacologic pathways with tremendous sensitivity, such that in general only minute amount of drug are necessary at the receptor to produce an effect.

Factors Modifying Drug Responses

The principles governing drug responses in overall terms were described earlier. It is important for clinicians to recognize that many of the parameters that have been discussed (e.g., ED_{50}) were derived from population averages. However, in practice there is considerable variability in responsiveness to drugs among individuals. Drug responsiveness may also vary in the same patient over time or with disease progression. Therefore each patient will likely respond in a distinct manner. Variability in responsiveness may be an intrinsic feature of the patient, may be related to the disease process, or may occur in response to repeated administration of the drug. Multiple mechanisms may be involved, including:

■ Changes in the amount of drug at the intended molecular target
  ▲ Polymorphisms in drug absorption, distribution, or metabolism are major causes of interindividual variability.
  ▲ Prolonged drug administration can alter these variables.
    • Prolonged use of phenobarbital as an anticonvulsant medication is known to up-regulate (i.e., increase) the enzymes responsible for the drug's degradation.
  ▲ Disease processes can alter drug absorption, distribution, and metabolism.
    • Absorption of heart failure medication can be slowed by intestinal edema caused by progression of heart failure.
■ Changes in the drug receptor itself
  ▲ Different patients express differing numbers or composition of receptors (receptor polymorphisms), leading to differences in affinity or efficacy of the drugs they bind (see Chapter 6, on pharmacogenomics).
  ▲ Chronic drug administration, disease, or age can alter drug receptor numbers and function.
    • Receptor internalization, receptor degradation, and changes in transcription and translation may

contribute to reduction in the quantity of receptor molecules on the cell surface (receptor down-regulation).

- Myasthenia gravis—a disease characterized by muscle weakness—involves, in part, down-regulation of nicotinic cholinergic receptors in the neuromuscular endplate.

■ Changes in coupling or signaling mechanisms

▲ Activation of signaling pathways can result in feedback modification of the receptor or upstream signaling molecules to decrease their effectiveness.

- For example, kinase phosphorylation of the β-adrenergic receptor subsequent to its activation recruits and activates cAMP phosphodiesterase, which in turn degrades cAMP, a primary signaling molecule in this pathway.

Tachyphylaxis or **desensitization** refers to the relatively rapid (minutes, hours) changes in drug responsiveness caused by repeated drug administration.

Tolerance generally refers to reductions in responsiveness that occur over a longer time frame (days or longer) caused by prolonged drug administration.

Homologous desensitization or tolerance is specific to one receptor type or drug class.

Heterologous desensitization or tolerance affects many receptor types or drugs.

■ **Clinical Connection:** Nitrates are used extensively in the treatment of coronary ischemia. Continuous administration of nitrates is known to produce a reduction in drug response. In some patients, this can occur in as little as 24 hours. Accordingly, the drug regimen for patients taking nitrates includes a daily nitrate-free period or *drug holiday* of approximately 8 hours each day. Such intermittent administration prevents the development of nitrate tolerance.

Website

American Society for Experimental Therapeutics: http://aspet.org/pharmacology_resources/#Databases.

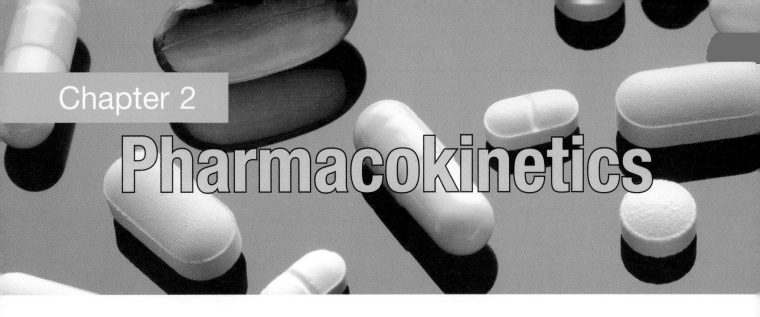

Chapter 2

Pharmacokinetics

For a drug to exert an effect, it must reach its intended molecular target. Conversely, removal of drug from its intended site of action is an important factor in terminating drug action. Pharmacokinetics is the study of the variables that affect drug delivery to, and removal from, its site of action. Pharmacokinetics includes the study of **absorption, distribution, storage, and elimination** of drugs. Elimination of drugs consists of biotransformation (metabolism), in which the drug's chemical properties are altered by the body, and/or excretion of the drug, in which the drug (or its metabolites) are removed from the body. Pharmacokinetics is influenced by the properties of the drug itself, the properties of the body, and the actions of the body on the drug. The pharmacokinetic behavior of drugs is a dynamic balance among drug absorption, distribution, sequestration in tissues, biotransformation, and excretion. The summation of these processes will determine the plasma drug concentrations at any point in time. An understanding of these processes is helpful in the determination of drug dosage and administration protocols.

BASIC CONCEPTS
Drug Transfer

Drugs must traverse a number of barriers to be absorbed, distributed, and eliminated. Major mechanisms are described in the following paragraphs.

Passive Diffusion

Passive diffusion is proportional to the **concentration gradient** of drug between two adjacent compartments, the **thickness of the barrier,** and the drug's **ability to dissolve** into the barrier separating the two compartments. These barriers are generally lipid membranes. Therefore the degree of **ionization** and the **lipid solubility** will affect passive drug transfer.

Active Transport

Active transport is mediated by a very large family of transporters collectively referred to as **ATP binding cassette transporters** (or ABC transporters). These transporters rely on adenosine triphosphate (ATP) as a source of energy to transport drug molecules across biologic membranes. There are several important features of this mechanism, including saturability, structural selectivity, and ATP dependence.

Saturability

In contrast to passive diffusion, these carriers often exhibit a concentration beyond which no further increase in transport occurs.

Structural Selectivity

These transporters exhibit a varying degree of structural selectivity for drugs and endogenous molecules. Structurally similar molecules will compete for binding at these transporters. This is an important mechanism of drug interaction.

ATP Dependence

- *ATP dependence* refers to the ability to move drugs against a concentration gradient.
- Examples of the ATP binding cassette group of transporters include the multidrug resistance transporters (MDR transporters) such as P-glycoprotein (Pgp, MDR1 or ABCB1).
  - P-glycoprotein is an efflux transporter that transports drugs out of cell to the extracellular space.
  - P-glycoprotein is found in a number of locations, including the gut and the blood-brain barrier.
  - P-glycoprotein plays an important role in drug pharmacokinetics and in drug interactions.
    - In the intestine, P-glycoprotein substrates that diffuse into intestinal epithelial cells are pumped back into the intestinal lumen, reducing their absorption. P-glycoprotein is also found in the endothelial cells of the blood brain barrier. Substances that diffuse into these cells and are substrates for P-glycoprotein can be transported back out into the blood, limiting their penetration into the brain.
    - Drugs that inhibit P-glycoprotein increase the absorption of P-glycoprotein substrates.
    - Drugs or disease conditions that induce P-glycoprotein decrease absorption of P-glycoprotein substrates.

Facilitated Transport

Facilitated transport is mediated by another large family of transporters collectively referred to as the **human solute-linked carrier** (SLC) family. This group of transporters is similar to the ABC transporters with the exception that they **do not directly bind and hydrolyze ATP** as a source of energy. Examples of this type of transporter include the **organic ion transporter** in the renal tubules that is responsible for secretion of some diuretics into the renal tubule, their site of action.

Drug Properties

The general chemical properties of a drug can greatly influence its pharmacokinetics. For a drug to be absorbed and distributed to its site of action or its site of elimination, it must be liberated from its formulation, it must dissolve in aqueous solutions, and at the same time it must be able to cross several hydrophobic barriers (e.g., plasma membrane).

Drug Formulations (Table 2-1)

- **Solid** formulations (e.g., tablets, capsules, suppositories) must **disintegrate** to release the drug. Disintegration of the dosage form may be compromised under certain conditions (e.g., dry mouth caused by aging, disease, or concurrent drug treatment slows dissolution of nitroglycerin tablets). On the other hand, drugs may be specifically formulated to allow disintegration only in certain sections of the gastrointestinal (GI) tract (e.g., enteric-coated tablets disintegrate in the small intestine), for the purpose of **protecting the drug from destruction** by gastric acid of the stomach (e.g., erythromycin) or **protecting the stomach from an irritant drug** (e.g., enteric-coated aspirin). Tablets and capsules may also be formulated to **slowly release drugs** (controlled-release, extended-release, or sustained-release formulations) and prolong their duration of action. Sustained-release formulations are particularly useful for drugs that have very short durations of action (see Table 2-1).

- **Semisolid** formulations include creams, ointments, and pastes. These formulations are generally for topical application to the skin and require liberation and diffusion of the drug across the skin.

- **Liquid** formulations may be suspensions or solutions, which do not require disintegration of the formulation and thus are generally absorbed more readily than solid formulations. Suspensions or solutions are also advantageous for patients who cannot swallow tablets or capsules. Drugs in **suspension are not dissolved** in the liquid vehicle. Therefore, the drug must first dissolve before it can be absorbed. Drugs in **solution are already dissolved.** Consequently, solutions are generally absorbed more rapidly than suspensions. Drug solutions may also be administered directly into the bloodstream.

- **Polymer** formulations are a special category of solid formulations that incorporate the drug into a matrix that then gradually releases the drug over a prolonged period of time or at specific locations. Examples include **transdermal patches** and **drug-eluting stents.** Novel polymer-based formulations for intravenous (IV) delivery are also being designed.

Drug Chemistry

The physical and chemical properties of a drug will influence its ability to traverse biologic membranes and to be dissolved and transported in biologic fluids.

TABLE 2-1. Pharmacokinetic Characteristics of Different Drug Formulations		
Drug Formulations	**Examples**	**General Pharmacokinetic Characteristics**
Solids	Tablets Capsules Powders Suppositories	For absorption: Solid must disintegrate to release drug Drug must dissolve into solution. For a drug intended for the sublingual or buccal route of administration, disintegration of solid may be an issue in patients with drymouth (e.g., elderly). Slow disintegration may be designed into the drug formulation to produce extended-release formulations. Solid formulations may be designed to disintegrate only at certain pH levels to protect the stomach from the drug (e.g., enteric-coated aspirin).
Semisolids	Ointments Creams Pastes	For absorption: Drug must be liberated from the formulation Drug must dissolve into solution. Drugs can be applied for local or systemic action. For systemic action, drug must diffuse across skin or mucous membranes.
Liquids	Suspensions Solutions	Drug in suspension must dissolve into solution. Drug in solution is already dissolved. Solutions are generally absorbed more quickly than suspensions. Suspensions and solutions are useful for patients who cannot swallow tablets or capsules. Solutions can be administered directly into the bloodstream.
Polymers	Transdermal patches Drug-eluting stents	Drug is impregnated into a polymer matrix. Drug diffuses out of the matrix, across a membrane to the site of action. Duration of action is controlled by rate of release of the drug from the polymer. With transdermal patches, the drug must diffuse through the skin to enter the circulation. With drug-eluting stents, the polymer is coated onto the mesh of the stent. Drug diffuses out of polymer directly into surrounding tissue.

- **Molecular size and shape.** Smaller molecules are absorbed more readily. Drug shape affects affinity of the drug for carrier molecules or other binding sites such as plasma proteins or tissue. Drugs of similar structure may exhibit competition for such binding sites, which can affect their pharmacokinetics.
- **State of ionization.** The **nonionized** form of drugs is **more lipid permeable** and therefore better able to diffuse across biologic barriers. The pK_a is a characteristic of the drug and reflects the pH at which the drug will be **equally partitioned between the ionized and nonionized** forms.
- **The lipid-water partition coefficient** is an index of lipid solubility. Drugs with **higher lipid-water partition coefficients** will cross biologic membranes more quickly.

Effect of pH

Most drugs are **weak acids or bases** and, as such, in solution show varying degrees of dissociation into their ionized and nonionized forms. The distribution between ionized and nonionized forms will be **determined by the pK_a of the drug and the pH of the solution** in which the drug is dissolved.

- For drugs that are **weak acids,** the following equation applies, where HA = drug with proton, which is therefore **nonionized.** H$^+$ = proton, and A$^-$ is the **ionized** drug.

$$HA \rightleftharpoons H^+ + A^-$$

- Under **basic conditions, weak acids are ionized** to a greater extent (because the basic environment will shift the reaction to the right).
- Under **acidic conditions, weak acids are nonionized** to a greater extent (because the acidic environment will shift the reaction to the left).
- The greater the difference between the pH and the pK_a, the greater the degree of ionization or nonionization.
- The relationship between the pH of the drug's environment and the degree of its ionization is determined by the **Henderson-Hasselbalch** equation:

Henderson-Hasselbalch Equation Applied to **Acidic** Drugs

$$Log \frac{[HA]}{[A^-]} = pK_a - pH$$

- For drugs that are **weak bases,** the **reverse is true** compared with weak acids: HB$^+$ = drug with proton, which is therefore **ionized.** H$^+$ = proton, and B is the **nonionized** drug.

$$HB^+ \rightleftharpoons H^+ + B$$

- Under **basic conditions, weak bases are nonionized** to a greater extent (because the basic environment will shift the reaction to the right).
- Under **acidic conditions, weak bases are ionized** to a greater extent (because the acidic environment will shift the reaction to the left).
- Again, the greater the difference between the pH and the pK_a, the greater the degree of **ionization or nonionization.**

- The relationship between the pH of the drug's environment and the degree of its ionization is determined by the Henderson-Hasselbalch equation:

Henderson-Hasselbalch Equation Applied to **Basic** Drugs

$$Log \frac{[BH^+]}{[B]} = pK_a - pH$$

The **practical implications** are as follows: The ionized form of the drug may become *stranded* in certain locations. This effect, referred to as **ion trapping** or **pH trapping,** occurs when drugs accumulate in a certain body compartment because they can diffuse **into** this area, but then become ionized owing to the prevailing pH and are **unable to diffuse out** of this location. An example, shown in Figure 2-1, is the trapping of basic drugs (e.g., morphine, pK_a 7.9) in the stomach. The drug is approximately 50% nonionized in the plasma (pH approximately 7.4) because it is in an environment with a pH close to its pK_a. In the stomach (pH approximately 2), the drug is highly ionized (approximately 200,000×), it cannot diffuse across the cells lining the stomach, and the drug molecules are *trapped* in the stomach.

The concepts of acidic and basic drugs and their relative ionization at different pH values can be used clinically. For example, **acidification of the urine** is used to increase the elimination of amphetamine, a basic drug with pK_a approximately 9.8. Rendering the urine acidic increases the amount of amphetamine in the ionized state, preventing its reabsorption from the urine into the bloodstream. Conversely, alkalinization of the urine is used to increase the excretion of acetylsalicylic acid (aspirin), an acidic drug. Increasing the pH of urine above the pK_a of acetylsalicylic acid increases the proportion of the drug in the ionized state by about 10,000 times. The ionized form of the drug is not able to be reabsorbed across the renal tubule into the bloodstream. Moreover, the low concentration of the non-ionized form in the renal tubule compared with that in the blood favors diffusion of the non-ionized drug into the renal tubules (see Figure 2-2).

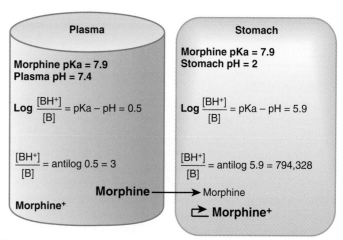

Figure 2-1. Effect of pH on drug ionization: ion trapping or pH trapping.

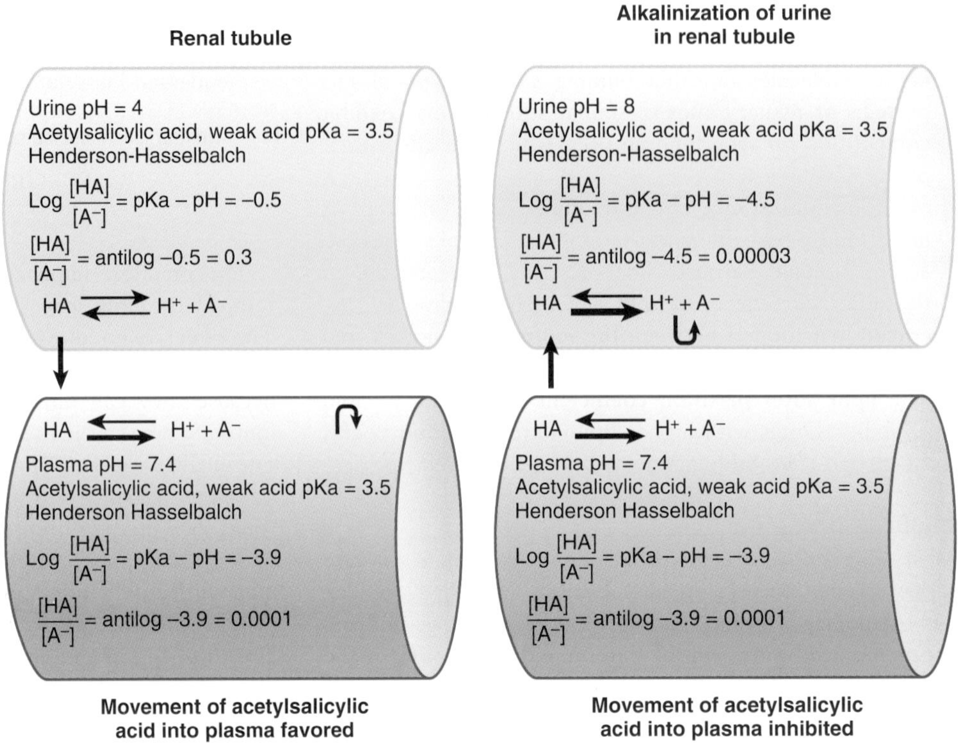

Renal tubule
Urine pH = 4
Acetylsalicylic acid, weak acid pKa = 3.5
Henderson-Hasselbalch
Log [HA]/[A⁻] = pKa – pH = –0.5
[HA]/[A⁻] = antilog –0.5 = 0.3
HA ⇌ H+ + A–
HA ⇌ H+ + A–
Plasma pH = 7.4
Acetylsalicylic acid, weak acid pKa = 3.5
Henderson Hasselbalch
Log [HA]/[A⁻] = pKa – pH = –3.9
[HA]/[A⁻] = antilog –3.9 = 0.0001
Movement of acetylsalicylic acid into plasma favored
Alkalinization of urine in renal tubule
Urine pH = 8
Acetylsalicylic acid, weak acid pKa = 3.5
Henderson-Hasselbalch
Log [HA]/[A⁻] = pKa – pH = –4.5
[HA]/[A⁻] = antilog –4.5 = 0.00003
HA ⇌ H+ + A–
HA ⇌ H+ + A–
Plasma pH = 7.4
Acetylsalicylic acid, weak acid pKa = 3.5
Henderson Hasselbalch
Log [HA]/[A⁻] = pKa – pH = –3.9
[HA]/[A⁻] = antilog –3.9 = 0.0001
Movement of acetylsalicylic acid into plasma inhibited

Figure 2-2. Application of pH trapping to renal drug elimination.

Oral administration
Gut lumen
Gut epithelial cell
Portal circulation
Hepatic metabolism
Systemic circulation
Bioavailability = 30%
Gut lumen
P glycoprotein

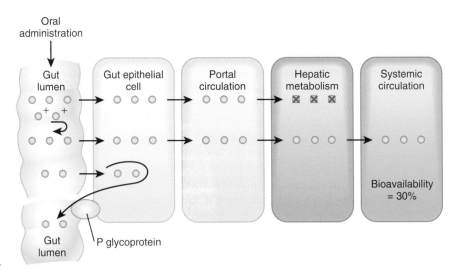

Figure 2-3. Factors affecting bioavailability of drugs.

ABSORPTION

In general, for a drug to reach its intended target, the drug must be present in the bloodstream (an exception is application of drug for local effects such as local anesthesia). Thus, *absorption of drugs* refers to the amount of drug reaching the general circulation from its site of administration. The fraction of drug reaching the systemic circulation is expressed as the **bioavailability.** The concept of bioavailability is important in practice because the clinician can use routes of administration that maximize bioavailability. In addition, changes in bioavailability resulting from genetic variation, disease, or drug interactions are a frequent cause of **loss of drug effectiveness,** because of a decrease in bioavailability, or, conversely **drug toxicity,** because of an increase in bioavailability.

$$\text{Bioavailability (F)} = \frac{\text{Amount of active drug in general circulation}}{\text{Amount of drug administered}}$$

Bioavailability will be influenced by any factors that impede the active drug from reaching the systemic circulation (Figure 2-3). These include diffusion across physiologic barriers, the effect of transporters that prevent accumulation of drug in the blood, and metabolism of the drug before it reaches the systemic circulation. For example, after oral administration, a drug may have low bioavailability if:

- ▲ The drug is highly ionized at gut pH (does not readily cross lipid barrier).
- ▲ The drug is actively transported from the epithelial cell cytoplasm back into the gut lumen by drug transporters such as P-glycoprotein (e.g., cyclosporine).
- ▲ The drug is extensively metabolized during its passage through the liver.

Factors that alter a drug's ability to cross biologic membranes, its interaction with pumping mechanisms, or its metabolism will affect drug bioavailability, drug effect, and drug toxicity.

Oral bioavailability of some drugs (e.g., nitroglycerin) can be reduced so severely by these mechanisms that this route of administration is not practical, requiring the use of alternate routes of administration that bypass the major barriers to bioavailability.

Routes of Administration

Routes of administration greatly affect bioavailability by changing the number of biologic barriers a drug must cross or by changing the exposure of drug to pumping and metabolic mechanisms.

Enteral Administration

Enteral administration involves absorption of the drug via the GI tract and includes oral, gastric or duodenal (e.g., feeding tube), and rectal administration

- ■ **Oral (PO)** administration is the most frequently used route of administration because of its simplicity and convenience, which improve patient compliance. Bioavailability of drugs administered orally **varies greatly**. This route is effective for drugs with moderate to high *oral bioavailability* and for drugs of varying pK_a because gut pH varies considerably along the length of the GI tract. Administration via this route is less desirable for drugs that are irritating to the GI tract or when the patient is vomiting or unable to swallow. Drugs given orally must be **acid stable** or protected from gastric acid (e.g., by enteric coatings). Additional factors influencing absorption of orally administered drugs include the following:
  - ▲ **Gastric emptying time.** For most drugs the greatest absorption occurs in the small intestine owing to its large surface. More rapid gastric emptying facilitates their absorption because the drug is delivered to the small intestine more quickly. Conversely, factors that slow gastric emptying (e.g., food, anticholinergic drugs) generally slow absorption.
  - ▲ **Intestinal motility.** Increases in intestinal motility (e.g., diarrhea) may move drugs through the intestine too rapidly to permit effective absorption.
  - ▲ **Food.** In addition to affecting gastric emptying time, food may reduce the absorption of some drugs (e.g., tetracycline) owing to physical interactions with the drug (e.g., chelation). Alternatively, absorption of some

drugs (e.g., clarithromycin) is improved by administration with food.
  - ▲ **Intestinal metabolism and transport.** The intestinal wall has extensive metabolic processes and transport mechanisms (e.g., P-glycoprotein) that affect absorption of drugs given via the oral route.
  - ▲ **Hepatic metabolism.** Orally administered drugs are absorbed into the portal circulation and carried directly to the liver. The liver has extensive metabolic processes that can affect drug bioavailability.
- ■ **Rectal** administration via suppositories to produce a systemic effect is useful in situations in which the patient is unable to take medication orally (e.g., is unconscious, vomiting, convulsing). Drugs are absorbed through the rectal mucosa. Because of the anatomy of the venous drainage of the rectum, approximately **50% of the dose bypasses the portal circulation,** which is an advantage if the drug has low oral bioavailability. On the other hand, drug absorption via this route is **incomplete and erratic,** in part because of variability in drug dissociation from the suppository. Rectal administration is also used for local topical effects (e.g., antiinflammatory drugs in the treatment of colitis).
- ■ **Sublingual** (under the tongue) or **buccal** (between gum and cheek) administration is advantageous for drugs that have low oral availability because venous drainage from the mouth bypasses the liver. Drugs must be **lipophilic** and are absorbed rapidly. Buccal formulations can provide extended-release options to provide long-lasting effects.

Parenteral Administration

Parenteral administration refers to any routes of administration that do not involve drug absorption via the GI tract (*par* = around, *enteral* = gastrointestinal), including the IV, intramuscular (IM), subcutaneous (SC or SQ), and transdermal routes. Reasons for choosing a parenteral route over the oral route include drugs with low oral bioavailability, patients who are unable to take the drug by mouth (e.g., it irritates the GI tract), the need for immediate effect (e.g., emergency situations), or the desire to control the rate of absorption and duration of effect.

- ■ **IV** administration is the most reliable method for delivering drug to the systemic circulation because it bypasses many of the absorption barriers, efflux pumps, and metabolic mechanisms. In fact, by definition, **bioavailability of drugs is 100% by IV injection** because the drug is administered directly into the vascular space. It is also one of the preferred routes of administration to rapidly achieve therapeutically effective drug concentrations. IV infusions may be used to achieve a constant level of drug in the bloodstream. Drugs must be in aqueous solution or very fine suspensions to avoid the possibility of embolism. Caution must be used with drugs or drug combinations with the propensity to form precipitates.
- ■ **IM** administration of drugs in aqueous solution results in rapid absorption of drug in most cases. Drug absorption is **dependent on muscle blood flow** and thus is influenced by

factors that alter blood flow to the muscle (e.g., exercise). It is also possible to achieve a slower, more constant absorption and effect of drug by altering the drug vehicle. **Depot IM injections** use drug formulation to slowly release drug at the site of injection.

- **SC** administration is used for drugs that have low oral bioavailability (e.g., insulin). In addition, the rate of absorption can be manipulated by using different formulations of the drug (e.g., fast-acting versus slow-acting insulin preparations). This route is not appropriate for solutions that are irritating to tissue because these may produce necrosis and sloughing of the skin.
- **Transdermal** administration is administration through the skin. The drug must be **highly lipophilic**. Drugs may be applied as ointments or in special matrices (e.g., transdermal patches). Absorption via this route is slow but conducive to producing long-lasting effects. Special slow-release matrices in some transdermal patches can maintain steady drug concentrations that approach those of constant IV infusion.
- **Inhalational** administration can be used. The lungs serve as an effective route of administration of drugs. The pulmonary alveoli represent a large surface and a minimal barrier to diffusion. The lungs also receive the total cardiac output as blood flow. Thus, absorption from the lungs can be **very rapid and complete**. Drugs must be nonirritating and gaseous or very fine aerosols. The intended effects may be **systemic** (e.g., inhaled general anesthetics) or **local** (e.g., bronchodilators in the treatment of asthma).
- **Topical** administration involves application of the drug primarily to elicit local effects **at the site of application** and to avoid systemic effects. Examples include drugs administered to the eye, the nasal mucosa, or the skin. Generally drugs are formulated to be **less lipophilic** to reduce systemic absorption.
- **Intrathecal** administration penetrates the subarachnoid space to allow access of the drug to the **cerebrospinal fluid** of the spinal cord. This approach is used to circumvent the blood-brain barrier. Intrathecal administration is used to produce spinal anesthesia and in pain management and, in select cases, to administer cancer therapy.

DRUG DISTRIBUTION

After absorption into the bloodstream, drugs are distributed to the tissues via blood flow and diffusion and/or filtration across the capillary membranes of various tissues. Because the circulatory system is the main distribution mechanism and it is a readily accessible body compartment, **plasma concentrations are used as an index** of tissue concentrations in determining pharmacokinetics of drugs and in clinical management of drug therapy.

Initial Drug Distribution

- Initial distribution is determined by **cardiac output** and **regional** blood flow.
  - ▲ Drugs are initially distributed to tissues with the **highest blood flow** (e.g., brain, lungs, kidney, and liver).

- ▲ Tissues with lower blood flow (e.g., fat) receive drugs later.
- Distribution to some tissue compartments is restricted by barriers.
  - ▲ The **blood-brain barrier** restricts distribution of hydrophilic drugs into the brain.

Drug Redistribution

- After the initial distribution to high–blood flow tissues, drugs **redistribute** to those tissues for which they have affinity.
- Drugs may **sequester** in tissues for which they have affinity. These tissues may then act as a sink for the drug and increase its apparent volume of distribution (see later). In addition, as plasma concentrations of drug fall, the tissue releases drug back into the circulation, thus prolonging the duration of action of the drug.

Effect of Drug Binding on Distribution

In addition to specific molecular targets, drugs show varying degrees of binding to different components in body compartments. These binding sites are not specific sites linked to coupling mechanisms. However, this type of binding can play an important role in a drug's pharmacokinetic profile and in drug interactions.

Plasma Protein Binding

- Plasma proteins, such as **albumin, α-glycoprotein,** and **steroid hormone binding globulins,** exhibit affinity for a number of drugs.
- Binding to plasma protein is generally reversible and determined by the concentration of drug, the affinity of the protein for the drug, and the number of binding sites available.
- Plasma protein binding **greatly reduces** the amount of drug free in the plasma.
- Only free drug in the plasma is able to diffuse to its molecular site of action. Thus plasma protein binding can greatly reduce the concentration of drug at the sites of action and necessitate larger doses.
- For highly protein-bound drugs, a **small change in plasma protein binding** can lead to a large change in the proportion of free drug in the plasma and may lead to toxicity.
  - ▲ For a drug that is 99% bound to plasma protein, only 1% is free in the plasma. Reduction of plasma protein binding to 98% results in a **doubling** of free drug and drug effect.
- Changes in plasma protein binding can occur as a result of:
  - ▲ Disease
  - ▲ Competition between drugs for the same binding site
  - ▲ Saturation of binding sites

Tissue Binding

- Similarly to binding to plasma proteins, drugs may also bind to individual components of tissues.
- Binding to tissues results in sequestration of drug in the tissue.

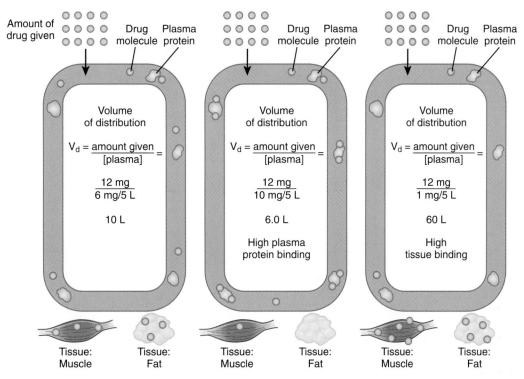

Figure 2-4. Volume of distribution.

- Tissue bindings sites:
  - ▲ **Increase** the apparent volume of distribution.
  - ▲ Represent potential sites for drug interactions.
  - ▲ Result in sequestration of drug in the tissue.
  - ▲ May **release the drug back** into the circulation as the plasma concentration falls. Thus tissue binding may represent a reservoir of drug that can extend the duration of action of the drug.

Volume of Distribution

The volume of distribution represents the **theoretical volume** in liters (therefore also called *apparent volume of distribution*) into which a drug is dissolved to produce the plasma concentration observed at steady state. Volume of distribution is calculated as the quotient of the amount of drug administered and the steady state plasma concentration (Figure 2-4).

$$\text{Volume of distribution } (V_d) = \frac{\text{Amount of drug given} = Dose}{\text{Steady state plasma concentration } (Plasma_{ss})}$$

- V_d will be affected by **drug binding** to different physiologic compartments.
- V_d can be used to infer some characteristics of drug distribution.
- V_d is largely determined by the chemical characteristic of the drug and its ability to interact with various tissue compartments.
  - ▲ V_d in excess of total body water (approximately 42 L) indicates that drug is being sequestered in a tissue compartment.

- Lipophilic drugs (e.g., thiopental) tend to sequester in fat.
- Some drugs bind with high affinity to certain tissues. Digoxin tends to bind to protein in skeletal muscle.
- Water-soluble drugs have a V_d that approximates the total extracellular water (approximately 14 L).
- Drugs that bind extensively to **plasma proteins** generally have a relatively small volume of distribution (e.g., 7 to 8 L) because these drugs will be highly restricted to the plasma.
- Changes in V_d influence drug plasma concentrations and may necessitate changes in dosage or result in toxicity. For example, loss of skeletal muscle mass with aging or disease (heart failure) requires a reduction in the dose of digoxin, a drug that is highly bound to skeletal muscle protein. The dose of digoxin is often adjusted to lean body mass.

DRUG ELIMINATION

Drugs are eliminated from the body via two basic mechanisms: **biotransformation** (metabolism) and **excretion**. These processes are initiated as soon as the drug reaches the systemic circulation. Accordingly, elimination mechanisms also contribute to the plasma concentration profile of drugs.

Biotransformation (Metabolism)

Many drugs are **lipophilic** molecules that resist excretion via the kidney or gut because they can readily diffuse back into the circulation. Biotransformation is an essential step in eliminating these drugs by **converting them to more polar water-soluble** compounds. There are several different biotransformation pathways that drug molecules may follow (Figure 2-5). Biotransformation:

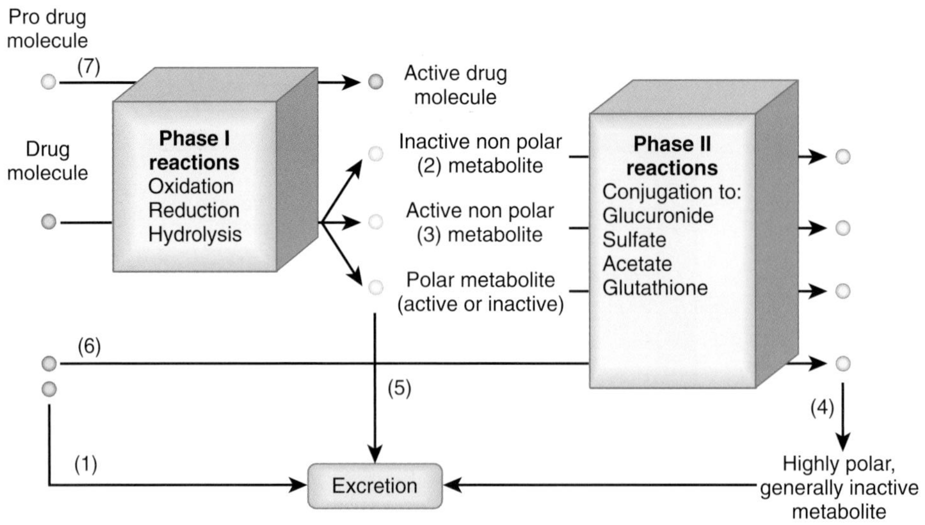

Figure 2-5. Drug biotransformation pathways.

- May convert drugs to **inactive** metabolites, thus terminating their actions
- May convert drugs to **active** metabolites that may have the same or different beneficial actions as the parent drug
- May convert inactive drug molecules (prodrugs) to active drugs
- May convert drugs to reactive intermediates that exert toxic effects
- Occurs in many tissues including the **kidney, gut,** and **lungs,** but for most drugs the **liver** is the major site of biotransformation
- Factors affecting drug biotransformation include the following:
  - ▲ Interactions with **other drugs** or dietary substances
  - ▲ **Aging,** generally associated with a decrease in drug biotransformation
  - ▲ Disease, especially **liver disease,** which may reduce drug biotransformation
  - ▲ **Genetic polymorphisms** affecting biotransformation, which can result in loss of effectiveness or toxicity of a number of drugs

Two major processes contribute to biotransformation of drugs.

Phase I Reactions

Phase I reactions are also called *oxidation-reduction reactions* or *handle reactions.*

- These reactions uncover or add a reactive group to the drug molecule through **oxidation, reduction,** or **hydrolysis.**
- They make the drug molecule **more polar** and more reactive, which **facilitates excretion** or **further biotransformation** of the drug through phase II reactions.

Oxidation

Oxidation accounts for a large proportion of drug metabolism.

- It is mediated primarily by **mixed function oxygenases** (monooxygenases; microsomal mixed function oxidases) located in endoplasmic reticulum, which include the following:

  - ▲ Cytochrome P-450 (CYP) family of enzymes
  - ▲ Flavin monooxygenase family of enzymes
  - ▲ Hydrolytic enzymes (e.g., epoxide hydrolase)
- The cytochrome P-450 family accounts for **over 80%** of drug oxidation. In this group of enzymes:
  - ▲ CYPs account for **over 80%** of drug oxidation.
  - ▲ Isoform **family** is indicated by a numeral (e.g., CYP3).
  - ▲ Isoform **subfamily** is indicated by capital letter (e.g., CYP3A).
  - ▲ **Specific isoform** is denoted by a numeral (e.g., CYP3A4).
  - ▲ CYP1, CYP2, and CYP3 families account for most drug metabolism.
  - ▲ CYPs are *not* substrate selective, meaning that many different drugs may be metabolized by one or more CYP isoforms, although there is generally one isoform that accounts for the majority of a given drug's biotransformation.
  - ▲ Interaction at CYPs is an important pharmacokinetic mechanism that can affect clinical use of drugs. Knowledge of CYP isoforms involved in metabolism of drugs and the type of interaction can guide clinical selection of drugs and explain adverse drug interactions. Interactions may take the form of competition, inhibition, or induction.
    - **Competition** between drugs that are substrates for the same CYP isoform, which may inhibit the biotransformation of each
    - **Inhibition** of CYP isoforms by dietary substances or other drugs, which is a major mechanism of drug toxicity
    - **Inhibition** of CYP activity will:
      - ○ Generally **increase plasma concentrations of substrate drugs,** drug effect, and potentially drug toxicity
      - ○ **Decrease plasma concentrations of active drug and drug effect of prodrugs** that rely on biotransformation to an active form (e.g., codeine must be metabolized to morphine for analgesic effect)
      - ○ Often result from interaction between **grapefruit juice** and many drugs because compounds in grape-

fruit juice inhibit CYP3A4 and greatly increase bio-availability of drugs metabolized by CYP3A4

- **Induction**, a process by which expression and activity of the CYP enzyme are **increased**, such that other drugs are more extensively metabolized
- **Induction** of CYP activity will:
  ○ Generally decrease plasma concentrations of drugs and reduce their effectiveness
  ○ Generally increase the active form of prodrugs and increase their effect, possibly leading to toxicity
  ○ Increase reactive intermediates of drug metabolism that may contribute to drug toxicity (e.g., metabolism of acetaminophen biotransformation leads to formation of reactive intermediate associated with liver damage)

■ Examples of clinically important CYP isoforms include the following:
  ▲ CYP1A2
    - CYP1A2 is induced by smoking.
    - Smokers require higher doses of drugs that are CYP1A2 substrates.
  ▲ CYP2D6
    - CYP2D6 exhibits genetic polymorphism.
    - Approximately 10% of patients show reduced CYP2D6 expression and increased plasma concentrations of drugs that are CYP2D6 substrates.
    - Important for metabolism of:
      ○ Antidepressants
      ○ Antipsychotics
      ○ Some narcotics (e.g., codeine)
  ▲ CYP2C9
    - CYP2C9 is important for metabolism of anticoagulants such as warfarin.
    - Antifungal drugs are potent inhibitors.
  ▲ CYP3A4
    - CYP3A4 is the most abundant hepatic CYP (approximately 30% total).
    - It has significant expression in the intestine.
    - It is involved in metabolism of a wide spectrum of drugs.
    - It accounts for metabolism of approximately 50% of commonly used drugs, including:
      ○ Antidepressants
      ○ Tricyclic antidepressants
      ○ Selective serotonin reuptake inhibitors
      ○ Cancer chemotherapy drugs
      ○ Macrolide antibiotics
      ○ Statins
      ○ Calcium channel blockers
      ○ Drugs for treatment of erectile dysfunction
      ○ Some oral contraceptives
      ○ Some analgesics
    - CYP34A is involved in many drug interactions; it is inhibited by:
      ○ Antidepressants
      ○ Antifungals
      ○ Macrolide antibiotics

○ For example, azole antifungals (e.g., ketoconazole) and macrolide antibiotics (e.g., erythromycin) inhibit CYP3A4, which may lead to accumulation of drugs that are CYP3A4 substrates (e.g., verapamil).

■ Non-CYP forms of oxidation also contribute to drug oxidation. Notable examples are the conversion of ethanol to acetaldehyde via **alcohol dehydrogenase**, and **monoamine oxidase**, which is responsible for biotransformation of catecholamines.

Reduction

Reduction quantitatively accounts for a much smaller proportion of drug metabolism; however, it is involved in biotransformation of some common drugs with low therapeutic indices. One example is nitroglycerin, a drug used in the treatment of angina.

Hydrolysis

Hydrolysis is mediated by enzymes such as **hydrolases** and **esterases**. Examples include the following:

■ Epoxide hydrolase is responsible for the degradation of highly reactive epoxide intermediates formed by CYP biotransformation. Thus epoxide hydrolases play an important protective role.

■ Cholinesterases degrade acetylcholine.

Phase II Reactions

Phase II reactions are also called *conjugation reactions.*

■ These reactions add a polar group, such as **glucuronide, glutathione, acetate,** or **sulfate,** to the drug molecule.

■ They **increase the water solubility** of compounds to facilitate excretion.

■ Generally they inactivate **the drug** but in some cases can produce active metabolites (e.g., conversion of procainamide to *N*-acetylprocainamide).

■ Conjugation reactions can occur:
  ▲ Directly with the parent drug molecule *or*
  ▲ With a reactive intermediate generated by phase I reactions. In this case, conjugation reactions may play an important role in **neutralizing reactive intermediates**. For example, phase I metabolism of acetaminophen generates a reactive intermediate capable of producing liver damage. Generally, liver damage does not occur because the reactive intermediate is rapidly conjugated to glutathione. However, under conditions in which cellular glutathione levels are depleted or excessive doses of acetaminophen lead to such high levels of reactive intermediate that glutathione conjugation is overwhelmed, acetaminophen will cause liver damage.

■ Phase II reactions are also subject to **genetic polymorphisms. Acetylation** capacity is an important polymorphism. Approximately 40% to 50% of the population exhibits slow acetylation capacity (*slow acetylators*). In these patients, drugs that are biotransformed through acetylation (e.g., hydralazine, isoniazid, procainamide) exhibit slowed metabolism. Dosages of such drugs must be adjusted downward to account for slowed biotransformation in affected patients.

Drug Excretion

Drug excretion refers to the removal of drug **from the body**. Generally, only **hydrophilic** molecules are excreted effectively. Accordingly, drugs may be excreted as unchanged parent molecules if they are sufficiently hydrophilic. Lipophilic drugs must be biotransformed to hydrophilic drug metabolites to be excreted. Drug may be excreted via a number of routes, such as the **kidney** or in **bile, sweat,** and **breast milk**. The **lungs** are an excretion route by which volatile lipophilic substances (e.g., inhaled general anesthetics) can be excreted. Changes in excretion rates will affect the plasma concentration of drugs and their metabolites and thus play an important role in the design of drug regimens.

Renal Excretion

Renal excretion is quantitatively the **most important** route of excretion for most drugs and drug metabolites. Renal excre-

tion involves three processes: **glomerular filtration, tubular secretion,** and/or **tubular reabsorption** (Figure 2-6). The sum of these processes determines the extent of net renal drug excretion.

- **Glomerular filtration**
  - ▲ The kidney filters approximately 180 L of fluid per day; thus there is a large capacity for drug excretion via this route.
  - ▲ The glomerular barrier restricts passage of plasma proteins, red blood cells, and other large blood constituents. Accordingly, **drugs that are bound** to these blood elements will not be effectively filtered.
  - ▲ Free drug in the plasma will be carried by bulk flow through the glomerulus into the renal tubules.
  - ▲ Factors influencing the amount of drug excreted by filtration include the following:
    - **Renal blood flow** influences the rate of delivery of drug to the kidney.
    - **Glomerular filtration rate** can be affected by disease or age. Glomerular filtration rate decreases by approx-

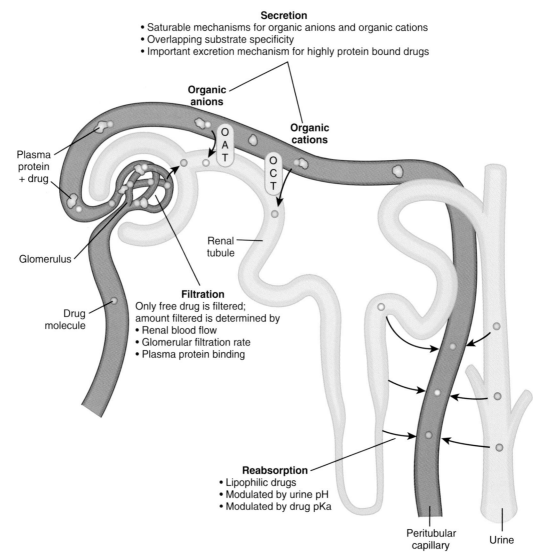

Secretion
- Saturable mechanisms for organic anions and organic cations
- Overlapping substrate specificity
- Important excretion mechanism for highly protein bound drugs

Organic anions

Organic cations

O A T

O C T

Plasma protein + drug

Renal tubule

Glomerulus

Drug molecule

Filtration
Only free drug is filtered;
amount filtered is determined by
- Renal blood flow
- Glomerular filtration rate
- Plasma protein binding

Reabsorption
- Lipophilic drugs
- Modulated by urine pH
- Modulated by drug pKa

Peritubular capillary

Urine

Figure 2-6. Renal mechanisms in drug excretion.

imately 1% per year and may be significantly compromised in elderly patients. The decline in glomerular filtration rate is accelerated by disease states such as diabetes. For drugs that are eliminated by glomerular filtration, dosages are often adjusted based on the patient's glomerular filtration rate.

■ **Tubular secretion**
  ▲ Secretory mechanisms in the renal tubules **actively transport** endogenous substances and drug molecules from the plasma in peritubular capillaries to the **tubular lumen.**
  ▲ Although quite diverse in some characteristics, the tubular transporters can be classified into two major groups: the **organic anion transporter** (OAT) and the **organic cation transporter** (OCT) families.
  ▲ Members of the OAT and OCT families belong to the larger superfamilies of ATP binding cassette (ABC) transporters and the solute carrier proteins (SLCs).
  ▲ Tubular transporters exhibit:
    • **Saturability.** Transporters reach a maximum rate of excretion, after which further increases in drug concentration do not cause further increases in secretion.
    • **Overlapping substrate specificities.** Multiple compounds may be transported via the same mechanism.
      ○ Compounds may compete for the same transporter.
      ○ Compounds may inhibit transporters.
      ○ Competition at, or inhibition of, the transporter results in decreased excretion and increases in plasma concentrations of substrate drugs.
  ▲ Tubular secretion is:
    • Especially important for drugs that are **highly plasma protein bound,** because these drugs are not excreted effectively by glomerular filtration.
    • Important in delivering some drugs, such as diuretics, to their site of action in the renal tubule.
    • **Not affected** by the degree to which a drug binds to plasma proteins.
    • Manipulated clinically via the use of inhibitors to extend the duration of action and increase the plasma concentration of drugs that are rapidly excreted by tubular secretion. For example, the drug probenecid blocks the OAT transporter responsible for secretion of some penicillin and cephalosporin antibiotics into the renal tubule. Probenecid can be prescribed along with antibiotics in the penicillin and cephalosporin families to prolong their duration of action.
    • Reduced in neonates, infants, and the elderly.
    • Affected by **genetic polymorphisms** in the OAT and OCT family of transporters.
■ **Tubular reabsorption**
  ▲ Once in the renal tubule, the **nonionized** form of the drug is able to diffuse across the tubular membrane and **reenter the plasma.**
  ▲ As water is reabsorbed along the renal tubule the tubular drug concentration increases, providing a concentration gradient favoring drug reabsorption.
  ▲ Manipulation of the **pH of the tubular fluid** can be used to enhance or inhibit tubular reabsorption according to the Henderson-Hasselbalch relationship. Acidification of urine can be used to decrease reabsorption of weak bases by increasing the proportion of drug in the ionized form. Conversely, alkalinization of urine can be used to increase the renal excretion of acidic drugs because a greater proportion of the drug is in the ionized form.

Biliary Excretion

Biliary excretion involves active secretion of drug molecules or their metabolites from hepatocytes into the bile. The bile then transports the drugs to the gut, where the drugs are excreted. The transport process is similar to those described for renal tubular secretion. The efficiency of biliary excretion is **quite variable.** Although many drugs may reach the gut through this route, deconjugating enzymes in the gut and the gut pH cause many drugs to assume nonpolar lipophilic forms that then are promptly **reabsorbed by diffusion into the plasma.** This process is referred to as **enterohepatic cycling.** Drugs that undergo extensive enterohepatic cycling generally have long durations of action.

Pulmonary Excretion

Pulmonary excretion is important for gaseous lipophilic substances. The gaseous general anesthetics are the most common example. Drug diffuses from the plasma into the alveolar space and is excreted during expiration.

Excretion via Breast Milk

Breast milk is a quantitatively relatively **minor route** of drug excretion. Nevertheless, it is clinically important for breast-feeding mothers and their infants. The baby will ingest drugs excreted in the breast milk. Moreover, breast milk has a lower pH than plasma. Accordingly, **basic drugs** will be concentrated in the breast milk through the phenomenon of **ion (pH) trapping.** A number of drugs can reach clinically significant concentrations in the breast milk and thereby affect nursing babies.

CLINICAL PHARMACOKINETICS

The ultimate goal of pharmacotherapy is to produce drug concentrations at the site of action that exert beneficial effects with minimal adverse effects. In most cases, drug concentrations at the site of action are **not known directly** but are inferred from plasma concentrations. Clinical pharmacokinetics uses mathematical modeling to predict the plasma drug concentration to better manage pharmacotherapy. This is particularly important for drugs with **low therapeutic indices,** where even minor changes in pharmacokinetics could lead to toxicity. Knowledge of pharmacokinetic variables is not quite as critical for (safer) drugs with large therapeutic windows, because toxic concentrations far exceed effective concentrations. Nevertheless, a general grasp of pharmacokinetic principles is invaluable in understanding dosages, dosing intervals, and duration of drug action.

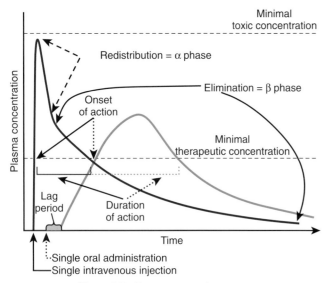

Figure 2-7. Plasma concentration curves.

Plasma Concentration Curves

Plasma concentration curves depict the plasma concentration of drugs over time (Figure 2-7). These curves are useful in illustrating several important principles. Although the different phases of the plasma drug profile will be discussed sequentially, it is important to note that the processes of absorption, distribution, and elimination occur simultaneously. As soon as a drug reaches the systemic circulation (absorption), it is also being distributed and eliminated.

■ Plasma concentrations that exceed the **minimally therapeutic concentration** will exert a pharmacologic effect. The point at which plasma concentrations exceed this level represents the **onset of action** of the drug. The **duration of action** of the drug is the time over which the plasma concentrations exceed the minimally therapeutic concentration. Plasma concentrations that exceed the minimally toxic concentration will produce toxic effects. An important goal of pharmacotherapy is to maintain plasma concentrations between the minimally therapeutic and minimally toxic concentrations.

■ IV administration delivers drug directly to the systemic circulation. If given as a **single bolus injection**, drugs will reach their **peak concentration** immediately. Subsequently, plasma concentrations will decrease rapidly as drug is **distributed** to various tissues. This is the so-called **alpha (α) or redistribution phase**. The plasma concentration profile then enters a phase of **slower monoexponential decay** that reflects predominantly **elimination** of the drug and is called the **beta (β) or elimination phase**. Plasma sampling for drug-monitoring purposes is generally performed in the β phase, because plasma concentrations in this stage are deemed to be representative of the drug concentrations at the site of action.

■ **Oral** or other nonvascular routes of administration result in a **delayed** peak plasma concentration.
  ▲ The **rate of absorption and bioavailability** of the drug determine the magnitude and time of peak drug concen-

tration. Slower absorption will result in reduced peak concentration and increased time to peak concentration.
  ▲ The *area under* the plasma concentration *curve* (AUC) reflects the total amount of drug absorbed.
  ▲ Distribution also affects this plasma profile, but the effects are not as evident because absorption and distribution occur at the same time.

The Drug Elimination or β Phase

Although drug elimination via biotransformation and excretion begin as soon as the drug reaches the circulation, as absorption and distribution end, elimination dominates the latter stages of the plasma concentration profile.

Elimination Kinetics

Drug elimination is the summation of the processes described earlier. Drug elimination proceeds in two types of time dependent patterns: **first-order** kinetics and **zero-order** kinetics.

First-Order Kinetics

When drug elimination proceeds by first-order kinetics, **a constant proportion or fraction of drug is eliminated per unit time** (e.g., 25%/hr). As a result, plasma drug concentrations decline **exponentially**. This occurs because the elimination mechanisms adjust their activity to the prevailing drug concentration. When drug concentrations increase, elimination mechanisms can accept more drug. Conversely, when plasma concentrations decline, the elimination mechanisms process less drug. **Important**: as long as elimination proceeds **by first-order kinetics the fraction of drug eliminated per unit time remains constant regardless of the starting concentration.** An example is shown in Figure 2-8. In this example 50% of the drug is eliminated in 1 hour. One hour after the

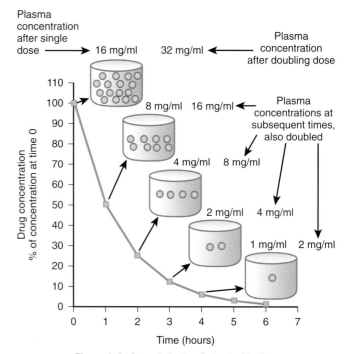

Figure 2-8. Drug elimination: first-order kinetics.

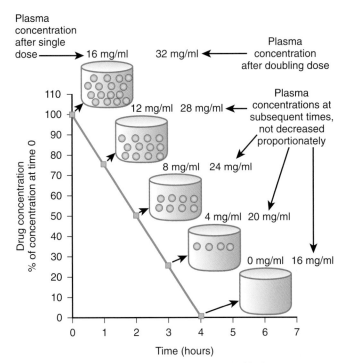

Figure 2-9. Drug elimination: zero-order kinetics.

peak concentration of 16 mg/mL, the drug concentration is 8 mg/mL. After 1 additional hour, the plasma concentration has been reduced to 50% of 8 mg/mL, and so on for each additional hour. An important feature of first-order kinetics is that the *proportion* of drug eliminated is independent of the starting concentration. If the dose of drug was doubled and peak concentration reached 32 mg/mL, 50% of the drug would still be eliminated each hour. The constant proportionality of first-order elimination allows relatively accurate prediction of plasma concentrations over time. Doubling of the dose results in a doubling of plasma concentrations at any time point. As a result, for drugs that are eliminated by first-order kinetics:

- The time to eliminate the drug is **independent** of dose.
- Increasing dose or frequency of administration produces predictable rises in plasma concentrations.

Zero-Order Kinetics

Zero-order kinetics is also called *saturation kinetics*. In this case, elimination mechanisms become **saturated** and unable to process more drug when drug concentrations rise. Consequently, for drugs that are eliminated by zero-order kinetics, a *constant amount* of drug is eliminated per unit time (e.g., 5 mg/hr) regardless of drug plasma concentration. Plasma concentrations decline in **linear fashion** (Figure 2-9). As a result, a progressively smaller proportion of drug is eliminated as plasma concentrations increase. In other words, the proportion of drug eliminated depends on the starting concentration. Zero-order kinetics makes prediction of drug concentrations over time problematic. In the example shown in Figure 2-9, 4 mg/mL of drug is eliminated per hour. In the case of a dose that produced a starting concentration of 16 mg/mL, plasma concentrations will have declined to 4 mg/mL in 3 hours.

However if the dose is doubled to achieve initial plasma concentrations of 32 mg/mL, after 3 hours plasma concentrations would be 20 mg/mL or 5 times higher than the lower dose at a comparable time, a much greater level than we would have predicted by doubling the dose. Thus, the effects of changing dosage can be quite unpredictable for drugs that are eliminated by zero-order kinetics. For drugs that are eliminated by zero-order kinetics:

- The time to completely eliminate the drug is **dependent** on dose. This make repetitive administration complicated.
- Increasing dose or frequency of administration can produce unpredictable increases in plasma concentrations.

The majority of drugs are eliminated by first-order kinetics. For drugs that exhibit first-order kinetics, the β phase is used to obtain several important parameters (Figure 2-10).

Elimination Rate Constant (k_{el}, k_e)

First-order kinetics dictate that plasma concentrations fall exponentially during the elimination phase. It is typical to plot these data on a semilogarithmic scale to linearize the plasma concentration time curve. The slope of this curve is the elimination rate constant (k_{el}). The elimination rate constant describes the fraction of drug eliminated per unit of time or the rate at which plasma concentrations will decline during the elimination phase. For example (see Figure 2-10), **if 25% of a drug were eliminated per hour, then k_{el} would be 0.25/hr.** The value for k_{el} is estimated as the slope of the elimination phase of the plasma concentration curve. Note that **k_{el} is independent of the dose or starting concentration** for drugs that follow first-order kinetics. As long as elimination mechanisms are not saturated, in our example, 25% of the starting concentration will be eliminated per hour whether the starting concentration (dose) is 10 units or 100 units. **The elimination rate constant (proportion per unit time) can be used to calculate the time necessary to eliminate a certain proportion of drug (inverse of rate constant). Clinically, a very useful time interval is the time necessary to reduce drug concentration by one half—in other words, the half-life.**

- Half-life ($t_{1/2}$) is the time for plasma concentrations to decline to one half their starting value. Half-life is calculated as:

$$t_{1/2} = \frac{0.693}{k_{el}}$$

where 0.693 is a constant derived from the natural log (ln) (because the decay is exponential for first-order kinetics) of the ratio of drug concentration at the beginning and end of one half-life, which by definition is 2 (100%/50%) (ln 2 = 0.693).

- Thus the half-life is **inversely related** to the elimination rate constant because $t_{1/2}$ estimates the time needed to eliminate a specific proportion (50%) of drug. This makes the $t_{1/2}$ a **very useful parameter** that can be used to estimate the:
  - ▲ Time for the drug to be completely eliminated from the body. **Four to five half-lives** are necessary to reduce drug concentration by 95% to 97%.

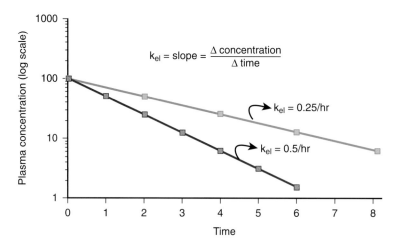

$$k_{el} = slope = \frac{\Delta\ concentration}{\Delta\ time}$$

$$k_{el} = 0.25/hr$$

$$k_{el} = 0.5/hr$$

For exponential elimination: concentration at anytime = concentration at time 0 $\times\ e^{-kel \times time}$
Half life = time concentration to decrease to one half of original concentration

$$\frac{concentration}{concentration\ t = 0} = \frac{1}{2} = e^{-kel \times time}$$

$$Ln\ \frac{1}{2} = \frac{1}{k_{el} \times time} \longrightarrow In\ 2 = k_{el} \times time \longrightarrow 0.693 = k_{el} \times time$$

Figure 2-10. Elimination rate constant for first-order kinetics.

$$\frac{0.693}{k_{el}} = time = half\ life$$

▲ Duration of action of the drug. The longer the half-life of the drug, the longer the plasma concentration of the drug will remain above the minimally effective concentration.

▲ Time to achieve steady state. On continuous or repeated administration, approximately **4 to 5 half-lives are required to reach steady state.**

▲ Appropriate dosage interval to achieve steady state concentrations.

■ Because the half-life is derived from the k_{el}, **half-life is also independent of dosage,** as long as the drug is eliminated by first-order kinetics. In contrast, for drugs that exhibit zero-order kinetics (saturable elimination), half-life generally increases with dosage because a constant amount (not proportion) of drug is eliminated.

Clearance

Clearance is another index of the ability of the body to eliminate drug. Rather than describing the amount of drug eliminated, **clearance describes the *volume of plasma* from which drug would be totally removed per unit time.** Clearance can be visualized as the circulation consisting of units or packets of blood containing a given concentration of drug. Clearance removes all of the drug from a certain unit of plasma in a given period of time (Figure 2-11). Although somewhat difficult conceptually, clearance is very valuable practically. Having an idea of how much plasma is cleared of drug over time allows estimation of how much drug must be given to maintain a constant plasma concentration.

■ Clearance is expressed in units of **volume and time** (e.g., milliliters per minute). Because clearance is removal of drug from the circulation, clearance is related to the **elimination**

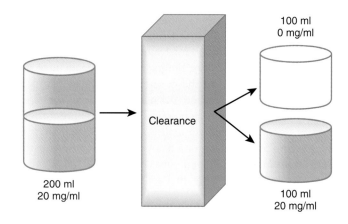

100 ml
0 mg/ml

Clearance

200 ml
20 mg/ml

100 ml
20 mg/ml

$$Clearance = V_d \times k_{el} \qquad Clearance = \frac{0.693 \times V_d}{t_{1/2}}$$

Continuous administration $\rightarrow$ Dosing rate = $\dfrac{Clearance \times \begin{array}{c} steady\ state \\ plasma\ concentration \end{array}}{Bioavailability}$

Intermittent administration $\rightarrow$ Dosing interval = $\dfrac{Dose \times bioavailability}{\begin{array}{c} Average\ plasma \\ concentration \end{array} \times clearance}$

Figure 2-11. Clearance and drug administration.

rate constant and the **apparent volume** into which the drug is dissolved:

$$Clearance = V_d \times k_{el}$$

■ Clearance is **inversely related to half-life.** Intuitively, the higher the clearance, the shorter the half-life and vice versa. Mathematically, clearance can be determined as follows:

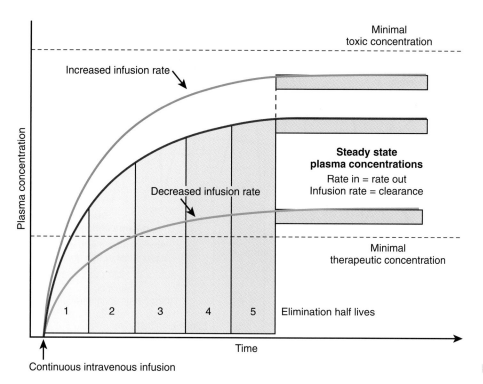

Figure 2-12. Continuous drug administration.

$$\text{Clearance} = \frac{0.693 \times V_d}{t_{1/2}} \text{ or } \mathbf{t_{1/2}} = \frac{0.693 \times V_d}{\text{Clearance}}$$

■ Clearance can be used to calculate the rate at which drug must be added to the circulation to **maintain the steady state plasma concentration** or, in other words, the dosage rate. If you know what is going out, you can administer the same amount *going in*, and theoretically the plasma concentration should remain constant.

Administration Protocols

If a single administration of drug is given, plasma concentrations will rise to a peak and then fall to zero if another dose is not given. The challenge then is to design a protocol to maintain therapeutic drug concentrations, to avoid toxic drug concentrations, and to minimize fluctuations away from the desired drug concentration between administrations.

Continuous Administration

The most effective way to achieve a desired steady state drug concentration with minimal fluctuations is to administer the drug as a continuous infusion. Figure 2-12 illustrates that plasma drug concentrations begin to rise with the onset of an IV infusion because drug is continually delivered directly into the circulation. As plasma concentrations begin to increase with onset of the infusion, drug elimination will also begin to occur. Thus, simultaneously, drug is being added to the circulation and drug is being taken away. Plasma drug concentrations will continue to rise as long as the rate of drug delivery exceeds the rate of drug elimination until a point is reached at which the clearance of the drug from plasma is equal to the delivery of new drug into the plasma. At this point the **rate of drug delivery equals the rate of elimination**, and steady

state has been achieved. This balance between drug in and drug out, or steady state, will be achieved in four to five half-lives. A change in the infusion rate will result in a change in the steady state plasma concentrations; however, the time to reach steady state will still be four to five half-lives. Plasma drug concentrations will remain stable unless the rate of infusion or the clearance is altered in some way (e.g., by induction of metabolic enzymes).

■ For direct administration into the circulation (e.g., IV route), the dosing rate is calculated as follows:

$$\text{Dosage rate} = \text{Clearance} \times \text{Steady state plasma concentration}$$

■ Rearranging this, the **steady state plasma concentration** can be estimated as a ratio of delivery over removal rate, or:

$$\text{Steady state plasma concentration} = \frac{\text{Dosage rate}}{\text{Clearance}}$$

■ For other routes of administration, it is important to take into account the bioavailability of the drug. Accordingly, dosage rate is then calculated as follows:

$$\text{Dosage rate} = \text{Clearance} \times \frac{\text{Steady state plasma concentration}}{\text{Bioavailability}}$$

Intermittent Administration

Although there are many examples in which continuous administration of drug is practiced, drugs are usually administered on an intermittent basis. Intermittent administration will result in much **greater fluctuations** in plasma drug concentrations. Plasma concentrations will rise in the absorptive phase to reach a peak and then decrease in the redistribution and elimination phases to reach a trough concentration until

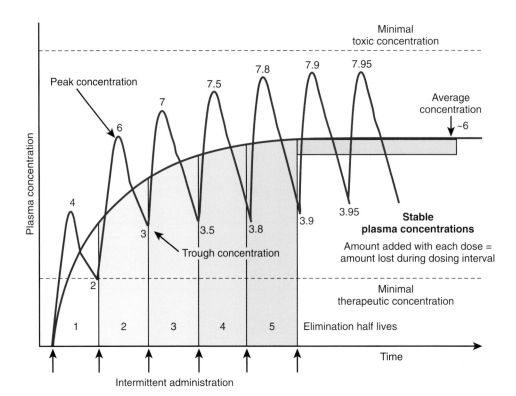

Figure 2-13. Intermittent drug administration.

the next dose is given (Figure 2-13). In keeping with the general principle discussed earlier, **stable average plasma drug concentrations** will be reached when **the amount of drug added in the next dose equals the amount eliminated during the interval between doses.** For drugs that obey first-order kinetics, stable average drug concentrations will be achieved in 4 to 5 half-lives. Thus, the clinician must estimate a dose and administration interval to attain the desired steady state concentration of drug while once again minimizing the fluctuations in drug concentrations to **avoid potential toxicity or lack of efficacy.** An additional factor to consider is patient compliance. It would be possible to closely approximate a continuous infusion and very steady plasma concentrations using very small doses administered very frequently. However, most patients would not readily accept such a regimen. Thus dosage schedules should also be designed to provide **convenient intervals** to promote patient compliance. For intermittent dosage regimens:

- The plasma concentration of drug is constantly changing, rising to a **peak** value sometime after absorption and falling to a **trough** value immediately before the next dose.
- Accordingly, **steady state concentrations** are never truly achieved. Instead an average drug concentration between the peak and trough concentration is achieved.
- Average drug concentrations will be determined by the size of the dose, the time between each dose (dosage interval), the bioavailability, and the clearance of the drug.

$$\text{Average plasma concentration} = \frac{\text{Dose} \times \text{Bioavailability}}{\text{Dosage interval} \times \text{Clearance}}$$

- Intuitively, as **bioavailability** and **dose** increase, so should the average concentration of drug in the plasma. Con-

versely as the **interval** between doses increases, the average concentration should decrease. Similarly, as **clearance** of drug increases, for any given dose and dosage interval, the average concentration should decrease.

- In many cases, only a limited number of dosage strengths are available based on what is manufactured (only certain strengths of tablets are available). Thus, the clinician can adjust the dosage interval. Rearranging the previous equation, the **dosage interval** can be calculated as follows:

$$\text{Dosage interval} = \frac{\text{Dose} \times \text{Bioavailability}}{\text{Average plasma concentration} \times \text{Clearance}}$$

- It is important to note that dose and dosage interval, the two variables most readily controlled by the physician, will affect the average drug concentration in the plasma and therefore the time to reach a therapeutic concentration. However, dose and dosage interval do **not** affect the time to reach a stable average concentration.
- The **time to reach a stable average concentration** will be determined by **clearance** and **half-life.** As described earlier, **4 to 5 half-lives** will be required to reach a stable average drug concentration regardless of the dose or dosage interval. In practice:
  - ▲ For a drug with a $t_{1/2}$ of 5 hours, stable average plasma concentrations will be obtained in about a day (20 to 25 hours).
  - ▲ Administering a drug at a **dosage interval equal to the drug's $t_{1/2}$** will result in **peak** drug concentration of approximately **twice that of trough** concentrations, or a twofold variation of concentrations between doses. Unless the drug has a low therapeutic index, this is generally an acceptable fluctuation in drug concentrations.

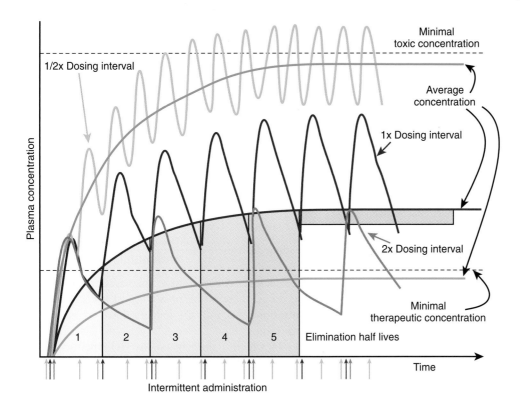

Figure 2-14. Effect of altering dosage intervals.

▲ Figure 2-14 illustrates the effect of altering dosage intervals on a drug that is eliminated by first-order kinetics. Note that in all cases the initial dose produces approximately equivalent plasma concentrations. However, plasma concentrations at subsequent doses differ greatly based on how much time is available for drug elimination during the dosage interval. Halving the dosage interval (purple curve) approximately doubles the average plasma concentration. Peak concentrations of drug exceed the minimal toxic concentrations and may be associated with adverse effects. Conversely, when the dosage interval is doubled (yellow curve), the peak concentrations initially exceed the minimal therapeutic concentrations but fall below that level during the dosage interval. The average plasma concentration also falls below therapeutic levels, and the drug is not effective. In both cases, the time to achieve stable average concentrations is approximately 4 to 5 half-lives.

▲ If the drug has a very **high therapeutic index,** much larger variations may be acceptable to **allow longer dosage intervals.** Some penicillin-like antibiotics have a very large therapeutic index but short half-lives (1 to 2 hours). A dosage interval near the half-life would clearly be inconvenient. Therefore very **large doses** of drug are given at dosage intervals that may be much **greater than the half-life.** In such cases the plasma concentrations peak at very high levels, and the majority of drug (>95%) is eliminated before the next dose. However, plasma concentrations remain above the minimal therapeutic concentrations for the better part of the dosage interval owing to the high initial concentrations. For example,

ampicillin (half-life 1.8 hours) is given orally at dose of 500 mg, 4 times per day.

▲ If the drug has a very **low therapeutic index,** large variations in plasma concentrations could be dangerous. Therefore doses and dosage intervals are designed to maintain effective average concentrations with slight differences between peak and trough concentrations. This is generally achieved by using very **short dosage intervals.**

▲ Basic pharmacokinetic principles can also predict the **effect of changes in dosage** or **in dosage interval** that occur during maintenance therapy. An increase or decrease in dosage will be associated with changes in peak, trough, and average plasma concentrations. An increase in dosage will cause peak concentrations to increase progressively with each dose until elimination mechanisms match the new increment in plasma concentrations at each administration. Conversely, with a reduction in dosage, trough concentration will progressively decrease until elimination matches the new, lower amount of drug added to the circulation at each administration. In both cases, peak, trough, and average plasma concentrations will stabilize over the course of 4 to 5 half-lives (Figure 2-15).

Loading Doses

In some circumstances, it is desirable to raise plasma concentrations above therapeutic levels **rapidly.**

■ Loading doses are useful in emergency situations in which it is important to achieve a drug effect as soon as possible—for example, the administration of an anticonvulsant

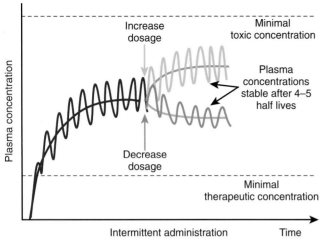

Figure 2-15. Effect of altering dosage after steady state is achieved.

medication during a seizure. In these cases the drug would be given directly into the circulation to eliminate the time needed for absorption.

■ Loading doses are also useful for drugs that have a **very long half-life**. In these cases the normal maintenance doses are generally small to avoid excessive accumulation of the drug. Consequently, plasma concentrations will rise very slowly on initiation of therapy. Therefore one or two larger loading doses may be given to increase plasma concentrations to therapeutic levels in a reasonable amount of time. These are then followed by the normal maintenance doses.

■ The primary determinants of the **size of the loading dose** are the **volume of distribution** and the **desired plasma concentration**. In addition, if the drug is not given directly into the circulation, the bioavailability of the drug must be accounted for. Accordingly,

$$\text{Loading dose} = \frac{\text{Desired plasma concentration} \times \text{Volume of distribution}}{\text{Bioavailability}}$$

■ Because plasma concentration increases rapidly with loading doses, there is the possibility of exceeding **toxic concentrations**. Accordingly, loading doses are calculated conservatively.

■ In cases in which a drug has a **low therapeutic index**, loading doses may be **divided** and given as multiple doses to avoid exceeding toxic concentrations.

Chapter 3

Autonomic Pharmacology

The autonomic nervous system (ANS) is so named because it is autonomous; it **functions independently** of the *conscious* or somatic nervous system. For example, you do not need to consciously tell your heart to beat faster when you exercise or your digestive tract to increase activity after eating. However, the ANS can be influenced by conscious thought; a classic example was demonstrated by the experiment on Pavlov's dog, which salivated at the sound of a bell because the bell had been rung before every meal, so the dog had learned to associate the bell with meals.

To understand autonomic function, and by extension to understand how to manipulate the ANS, you will need to understand how the two types of the ANS coexist and function, how each system exerts its effects, and finally what pharmacologic mechanisms exist to increase or decrease each component of the ANS. *Memorization of the receptors, their distribution, and their effects is mandatory* for achieving this goal and will enable you to accurately predict effects and side effects of drugs (Table 3-1).

The ANS has two parts:
▲ The sympathetic nervous system (SNS)
  • The SNS is the *fight-or-flight* response. The term *sympathetic* means supportive, and the SNS is designed to **support survival** during times of stress.
▲ The parasympathetic nervous system (PNS)
  • The PNS *usually* causes the opposite effect from that of the SNS. *Para* means *beside*, and the parasympathetic system works alongside the sympathetic system to help keep it in balance.

As a primer to help you remember the fight-or-flight response, consider a caveman who requires an intact SNS to stay alive. While he is fighting with (or maybe running away from) a saber-toothed tiger, what physiologic effects would promote his survival?
▲ Dilated eyes to see better
▲ Quiet digestive processes to save energy (dry mouth and inactive digestive tract)
▲ Availability and liberation of energy (glucose production)

▲ Increased cardiac performance (faster heart rate, faster conduction, stronger contractions)
▲ Increased respiratory performance (dry, dilated airways)
▲ Sweating to cool off
▲ Piloerection to make the hair on the arms stand up and make one look bigger
▲ Bladder control

The PNS, to keep everything in balance, would therefore oppose all these effects. If you remember the flight-or-fight response and think of the opposite of the fight-or-flight response, you will remember the majority of the important ANS functions.

AUTONOMIC ANATOMY

Parasympathetic nerves are arranged in a *craniosacral* distribution. They:
▲ Follow **cranial nerves** III, VII, IX, and X (X is the vagus nerve)
▲ The vagus nerve is the most important parasympathetic nerve.
▲ Also follow **splanchnic nerves**, which arise from sacral nerves

The sympathetic nerves primarily arise from the **thoracic** and **lumbar** spinal roots.

Therefore the parasympathetics anatomically originate from the *top* and *bottom* of the brain and spinal cord, and the sympathetics are *in the middle* of the spinal cord.

Ganglia and Neurotransmitters

For both the sympathetic and parasympathetic systems, the autonomic nerves exit the brain or spinal cord and then enter a *relay station* called a **ganglion**. The function of the ganglia is to transfer (and sometimes modify) the signals from the **presynaptic** neuron to the **postsynaptic** neuron. The neurotransmitter for **both** the SNS and PNS *ganglia* is **acetylcholine (ACh)**.

The **postsynaptic** neuron then innervates an organ. If the neuron is a *sympathetic* neuron, then the neurotransmitter will

TABLE 3-1. Autonomic Receptors: Function and Distribution

Receptor	Function	Distribution
Sympathetic		
α₁	**Constriction** of smooth muscles	Blood vessels and piloerectors *in skin* (vasoconstriction and goose bumps) Sphincters (bladder, gastrointestinal [GI]) Uterus and prostate (contraction) Eye (contraction of the *radial* muscle = pupillary dilation/mydriasis)
α₂	*Inhibition* of sympathetic autonomic ganglia (decreases the sympathetic nervous system [SNS])	**Presynaptic ganglionic neurons** GI tract (less important pharmacologically, included for completeness)
β₁	**Increase cardiac performance** and liberation of energy	**Heart,** the most important for β₁; (increased heart rate, contractility, conduction speed) Fat cells (release fat for energy via lipolysis) Kidney (release renin to conserve water)
β₂	**Relaxation** of smooth muscles and liberation of energy	Lungs (bronchodilation) Blood vessels *in muscles* (vasodilation) Uterus (uterine relaxation) GI (intestinal relaxation) Bladder (bladder relaxation) Liver (to liberate glucose via glycogenolysis)
Parasympathetic		
N (Nicotinic)	"Nerve to nerve" and "nerve to muscle" communication	Sympathetic and parasympathetic ganglia Neuromuscular junction (NMJ)
M (Muscarinic)	To oppose most sympathetic actions at the level of the organs	Lung (bronchoconstriction) Heart (slower rate, decreased conduction, decreased contractility) *Sphincters* of GI and bladder (relax) Bladder (constriction) GI (intestinal contraction) Eye (contraction of the *circular* muscle = pupillary constriction or meiosis) Eye (contraction of the *ciliary* muscle = focus for near vision) Glands: lacrimal, salivary, bronchial (secretion)

Special Notes

There is no *parasympathetic* innervation of blood vessels.

Sweat glands are innervated by *sympathetic* nerves, but paradoxically use *M receptors*.

Sexual arousal is parasympathetic, but orgasm is sympathetic.

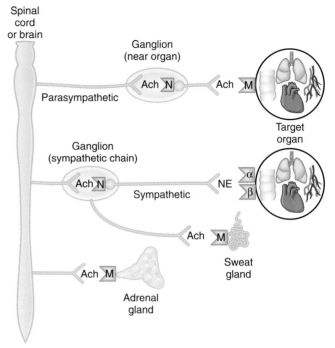

Figure 3-1. Ganglia and neurotransmitters.

be **norepinephrine (NE)**. If the neuron is a *parasympathetic* neuron, then the neurotransmitter will be **acetylcholine**.

The *parasympathetic* ganglia are located **close to the organs** that they innervate. Some examples include the **ciliary, pterygopalatine, submandibular, otic,** and **pelvic** ganglia.

This is in contrast to *sympathetic* ganglia, which are located in the **sympathetic chain** that runs alongside the spinal column and are located at a distance from the organs. They are described as the "**paravertebral (beside)** and **prevertebral (in front of)** sympathetic chains, depending on their physical relationship to the vertebral column (Figure 3-1).

ACh is the "**preganglionic** nerve to **postganglionic** nerve" transmitter in the ganglia for *both* the sympathetic and parasympathetic systems. Only special drugs manipulate the ganglia. It would be logical to assume that drugs that influence ACh would have a strong influence on ganglia, but they do not.

ACh is the "**postganglionic** nerve to organ" neurotransmitter for the parasympathetic system, and NE is the transmitter for the sympathetic system. It is important to understand this difference, because drugs that focus on ACh will manipulate the parasympathetic system, whereas drugs that manipulate effects related to NE will manipulate the sympathetic system.

Special Cases

The *sympathetic* innervation of the adrenal gland is direct from the spinal cord and uses ACh as the neurotransmitter. The adrenal gland functions as a *special form of ganglion* that secretes epinephrine directly into the bloodstream.

Another special case is the innervation of sweat glands. They are sympathetically innervated, but the postsynaptic nerve releases ACh instead of NE.

Autonomic Receptors

ACh binds to **muscarinic** and **nicotinic** receptors, abbreviated **M** and **N**.

▲ M receptors are on **organs** that receive parasympathetic innervations.

▲ N receptors are in ANS **ganglia** and function as *nerve to nerve* neurotransmitters. N receptors are also important in *nerve to muscle* communication (the **neuromuscular junction**).

NE (and epinephrine) bind to **alpha** and **beta** receptors (α and β). Another name for epinephrine is *adrenaline*, so these receptors are also commonly referred to as *adrenergic receptors*.

Subtypes of these receptors exist, such as M_1, M_2, M_3, α_1, α_2, β_1, and β_2. Even more subtype classifications exist than are listed here, but not all of them are clinically important.

The receptor types that are **clinically important** include M, N, α_1, α_2, β_1, and β_2. *You must know the distribution and function of these receptors in the body to understand and predict the effects of drugs that influence the ANS* (see Table 3-1).

Important, autonomic receptors also exist in many parts of the body but function in a way *unrelated to the ANS*. Some examples include:

▲ Nicotine receptors in the addiction pathway

▲ Adrenergic receptors in the brain, related to mood

▲ Muscarinic receptors in the brain, involved in Parkinson's disease and related movement disorders

Manipulating the Autonomic Nervous System

The ANS consists of two systems: the SNS and the PNS. Most of the time, each system is opposing the other. Therefore to change this balance, we can strengthen one system or weaken the other.

■ ↑ Parasympathetic:
  ▲ Increase stimulation of the M receptors
    • Give an agonist (**vagotonic**: the vagus nerve is the primary PNS nerve, hence the name "vago").
    • Inhibit the breakdown or removal of endogenous (the body's own) ACh.
■ ↓ Parasympathetic:
  ▲ Decrease M receptor stimulation
    • Give an antagonist (**vagolytic**).
■ ↑ Sympathetic:
  ▲ Increase stimulation of the α and β receptors via:
    • Administration of an agonist (**sympathomimetic**) that stimulates these receptors
    • Inhibition of the breakdown or removal of endogenous NE or epinephrine
    • Inhibition of synaptic NE reuptake by the presynaptic cell, leading to increased NE in the synaptic cleft
■ ↓ Sympathetic:
  ▲ Decrease stimulation of the α and β receptors
    • Give an antagonist (**sympatholytic**) that blocks these receptors.
    • Give a drug to *turn down* the ganglion (relay station).

Ganglionic Pharmacology

An additional mechanism of manipulating the ANS is through drugs that affect the autonomic ganglia. They can be ganglionic stimulants or ganglionic blockers. Most of these drugs are no longer used clinically and are of *historical importance* only, because drugs that target the ganglia usually have a broad range of effects and therefore many side effects; more directed, specifically acting drugs that do not act on the ganglia are now available and have replaced them. Some examples of these older ganglion-acting drugs include: guanethidine, hexamethonium, and mecamylamine.

Nicotine is a clinically important agent that influences activity of the autonomic ganglia. As would be suggested by the name, nicotine is an agonist of nicotine receptors and is best known as a component of tobacco products and for its role in addiction. The major action of nicotine consists initially of transient stimulation, followed by a more persistent depression of all autonomic ganglia. Effects of nicotine are similar to increasing the effects of the SNS, including increased blood pressure and heart rate. In addition, nicotine is strongly associated with the pathways in the brain responsible for reward and addiction.

PARASYMPATHETIC DRUGS
Handling of Acetylcholine

ACh is stored in vesicles in the terminal portions of the nerves. It is released when an action potential (AP) is conducted through the neuron. The presynaptic AP opens up Ca channels and allows Ca to enter the neuron. Ca causes binding of the ACh vesicles to the presynaptic membrane. ACh is then released into the synaptic cleft. In the synaptic cleft, ACh binds to M or N receptors (depending on the type of synapse and which receptors are present).

ACh has three fates once it has entered the synaptic cleft:

1. It is broken down by **acetylcholinesterase** (the most important of the three).
2. It is taken back (**reuptake**) into the **presynaptic** neuron.
3. It **diffuses** away out of the synaptic cleft.

Manipulating the Parasympathetic Nervous System

There are **three ways** to manipulate the PNS:

1. Administering a muscarinic **agonist** (increases PNS activity)
2. Administering a muscarinic **antagonist** (decreases PNS activity)
3. Administering a **cholinesterase inhibitor,** which results in an increase of ACh in the synaptic cleft (increases PNS activity)

Common muscarinic agonists include:

▲ Muscarine (the prototype, but not a clinically used drug)

▲ Pilocarpine

▲ Methacholine
▲ Bethanechol

Common muscarinic antagonists, which are also called **anticholinergics, antimuscarinics,** and **vagolytics,** include:

▲ Atropine (the prototype and *widely used clinically*)
▲ Others:
  • Benztropine
  • Glycopyrrolate
  • Ipratropium (inhaled only)
  • Tolteridine
  • Oxybutynin
  • Hyoscine
  • Scopolamine

Common cholinesterase inhibitors include:

▲ Neostigmine
▲ Physostigmine
▲ Edrophonium
▲ Echothiophate (eye drops only)
▲ Insecticides (malathion, parathion) and chemical warfare (sarin)

Effects of These Drugs

Instead of memorizing the effects of the individual drugs, it is better to **learn the distribution of the receptors of the SNS and PNS and then, by logic, determine what the effects of the drugs would be** (see Table 3-1). These drugs will have effects on the *desired* target organ but also have effects on other unintended target organs (which will cause side effects).

Main Clinical Uses of Muscarinic Agonists

■ Constrict the pupil
■ Promote salivation

Main Clinical Uses of Muscarinic Antagonists (Drug Names Given as Examples Only)

■ Dilating the pupil
■ Decreasing oral secretions (glycopyrrolate)
■ Increasing the heart rate (atropine)
■ Dilating bronchioles (ipratropium)
■ Treating incontinence and spasms of the bladder (tolteridine)
■ Relaxing gastrointestinal spasms
■ Treating movement disorders such as Parkinson's disease and tardive dyskinesia (benztropine)
■ Treating poisoning with insecticide or from chemical warfare (atropine)

Main Clinical Uses of Cholinesterase Inhibitors (Also Known as Anticholinesterases)

The primary indication for cholinesterase inhibitors is to increase levels of ACh in the **neuromuscular junction.** This increases muscle strength in conditions in which there is a problem with the nicotinic receptor on the muscle. Clinical uses include the following:

■ Treating myasthenia gravis
■ Reversing neuromuscular blocking drugs used for anesthesia

Some Drugs with (Unwanted) Anticholinergic Side Effects

■ Tricyclic antidepressants
■ Antihistamines
■ Antipsychotics

SYMPATHETIC DRUGS

The synthesis of adrenergics follows the pathway below (*adrenergic* means pertaining to systems that respond to adrenalin). Note that adrenalin and epinephrine are the same molecule, as are noradrenalin and NE:

$$\text{Tyrosine} \rightarrow \text{Dopamine} (+\text{OH}) \rightarrow \text{NE} (+\text{CH}_3) \rightarrow \text{Epinephrine}$$

▲ Note that the addition of the hydroxyl (OH) group is called *hydroxylation,* and the removal of the methyl (CH$_3$) group is called *demethylation.*
▲ The *nor* in *norepinephrine* refers to *no radical* (no CH$_3$ group), compared with epinephrine.

Manipulating the Sympathetic Nervous System

Manipulating the SNS is a little simpler than manipulating the PNS.

■ You can give an agonist:
  ▲ For α receptors
  ▲ For β receptors
■ You can give an antagonist:
  ▲ For α receptors
  ▲ For β receptors
■ *Fine print:* You can give drugs that prevent release of NE from presynaptic nerve endings with **ganglion blockers.** This will result in a decrease of ganglionic transmission and result in decreased SNS activity. However, these drugs are used less and less commonly because of side effects.
■ *Fine print #2:* Some drugs are inhibitors of enzymes that degrade adrenergic molecules. These drugs (catechol-O-methyltransferase [COMT] inhibitors and monoamine oxidase [MAO] inhibitors used for Parkinson's disease and depression) are designed to influence the adrenergic transmitter levels in the brain but are *not intended* to affect changes in the SNS. However, they can result in some systemic SNS changes.
■ Some adrenergic drugs are selective for a given receptor, but most of the drugs bind to and interact with **multiple receptors** (even if they are described as acting on only one receptor). For example, β$_1$ selective drugs will also bind β$_2$ receptors, and vice versa.

Adrenergic Agonists

■ Mixed receptor drugs (α and β agonists)
  ▲ Epinephrine
  ▲ Norepinephrine
  ▲ Dopamine
■ Pure α$_1$ agonists
  ▲ Phenylephrine
  ▲ Midodrine (an oral medication)
■ Pure β$_1$ agonists

▲ Isoproterenol
▲ Dobutamine

Adrenergic Antagonists
■ β-Blockers (β antagonists)
  ▲ -olol drugs (e.g., metoprolol)

■ α-Blockers (α_1 antagonists)
  ▲ Prazosin
  ▲ Phentolamine
  ▲ Phenoxybenzamine

See the related Chapter 3 Question Sets in Student Consult.

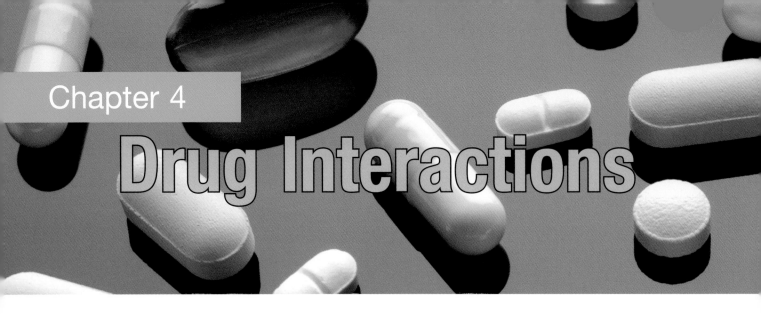

Chapter 4

Drug Interactions

Drug interactions are a frequent and preventable cause of drug-related adverse events. Interactions between drugs (*drug-drug* interactions) are particularly common, and as the number of conditions that can be treated with drug therapy increases, polypharmacy—the use of multiple medications in a single patient—will become commonplace.

Fortunately, not all drug interactions will harm the patient. If this were the case, it would severely limit our ability to prescribe a number of very useful drugs. In the following pages you will note that a number of very commonly prescribed drugs are involved in drug interactions. Understanding the mechanisms behind these interactions will help you develop a strategy for determining which interactions are manageable and which combinations should be avoided altogether.

MECHANISMS OF DRUG INTERACTIONS
Just as pharmacology is divided into two fundamental branches—pharmacokinetics and pharmacodynamics—the mechanisms of drug interactions can also be subdivided into these two branches. Note that there is a third type of interaction, a physical (chemical) interaction that may occur outside the body (*in vitro*). This last type involves direct interactions between drugs and is largely the concern of pharmacists.

Pharmacokinetic Interactions
Pharmacokinetic interactions can be subdivided into those involving absorption, distribution, metabolism, and excretion (ADME).

Absorption
A given drug may **directly** reduce the absorption of another drug through the following:
- Chelation
  - A chelator is an organic chemical that bonds with and removes free metal ions from solutions. Typically, the molecule being chelated will be a divalent cation (e.g., Ca^{+2}, Mg^{+2}, Fe^{+2}).
  - There are a few examples of agents that chelate drugs, reducing the absorption of both. The classic example

would be tetracycline, which is chelated by calcium. This can inhibit absorption of tetracycline, reducing its antibacterial activity, but perhaps more important, tetracycline can reduce the availability of calcium, which can have dramatic effects on the developing fetus.
- Binding
  - Drugs may also bind other drugs, although this is a relatively rare interaction. The classic example would be cholestyramine, a positively charged drug used to lower cholesterol. It lowers cholesterol by binding to negatively charged bile acids in the gut. Consequently, cholestyramine is also capable of binding other negatively charged drugs in the gut.
  - Note that cholestyramine is rarely used anymore, having been largely replaced by the *statins.*

A given drug may also **indirectly** reduce absorption of another drug, by altering the following:
- Gastric pH
  - Some drugs require a very acidic environment for their dissolution. Drugs that increase gastric pH can reduce the absorption of these agents.
- GI motility
  - Both drugs and food can alter gastrointestinal (GI) motility, enhancing or inhibiting the absorption of other agents.
    - The small intestine, with its large surface area, is a key area for drug absorption. Drugs such as anticholinergics, which reduce GI motility, may reduce the rate of absorption by delaying gastric emptying. Slowing the rate of absorption may have an impact on drugs that we want to work quickly, such as analgesics.
- Transport proteins, such as P-glycoprotein (Pgp) (Figure 4-1)
  - Pgp is one member of a superfamily of efflux transporters that are found in several regions of the body, including the GI tract and the blood-brain barrier. Pgp extrudes drug from the cell (i.e., pumps drug out of the cell).

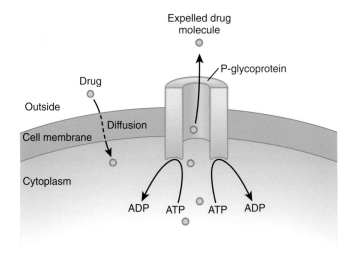

Figure 4-1. P-glycoprotein.

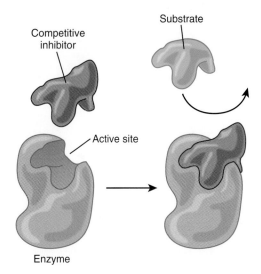

Figure 4-2. Competitive enzyme inhibition.

- In the cells lining the GI tract, these efflux pumps will therefore pump some of the drug that was going to be absorbed back into the GI tract, preventing a proportion of drug from being absorbed.
- Pgps have inhibitors and inducers:
  - ○ Pgp inhibition leads to retention of Pgp substrates. All things being equal, this would likely lead to increased absorption of the drug.
  - ○ Pgp induction leads to an increased number of Pgp pumps, leading to increased extrusion of Pgp substrates. All things being equal, this would likely lead to decreased absorption of the drug.

Distribution
Plasma Protein Binding

Recall details of plasma protein binding from the introductory chapter on pharmacokinetics. It is only the unbound portion of a drug that crosses cell membranes and is able to exert a pharmacologic effect.

Drugs compete with one another for binding to plasma proteins. If a given drug, drug A, displaces drug B from its binding site, this will increase the amount of drug B that is unbound and free to exert a pharmacologic effect.

Displacement from plasma proteins plays a **minimal role** in drug interactions. Aside from the fact that there are few reports of clinically significant interactions of this type, there are a couple of theoretical reasons why we would not expect to see displacement from plasma proteins causing major problems in the clinical setting:

- ▲ Free drug is also free to be metabolized and/or excreted from the body.
- ▲ Free drug distributes very rapidly into tissue, quickly reducing plasma levels.

Therefore for a clinically significant interaction to occur, the interacting agent must *also* interfere with the metabolism or excretion of a given drug.

Metabolism
Phase I Reactions

Cytochrome P-450 Enzymes Cytochrome P-450 (CYP450) enzymes are responsible for phase I (oxidative) metabolism of endogenous or exogenous substrates. See introductory chapter on pharmacokinetics for review.

CYP450 enzymes are categorized according to a number-letter-number system (e.g., CYP3A4). Thus 2C9 and 2C19 are more closely related than are 2C9 and 3A4. There are at least 40 CYP450 enzymes, although only a few are seen commonly, and it is only these that you need to be concerned with. The most common isozymes are 3A4, 2D6, 2C9 and 2C19, and 1A2.

Clinically significant drug interactions arise from either induction or inhibition of these enzymes.

Enzyme Inhibition Inhibition of a CYP450 enzyme will result in increased levels of a substrate (drug) that is metabolized by that enzyme. Inhibition may be either **competitive** or **allosteric**:

- ■ Competitive inhibition (Figure 4-2)
  - ▲ Two drugs are metabolized by the same enzyme system, and one of the drugs binds more readily to the enzyme, resulting in the inhibition of metabolism of the other drug.
  - ▲ Example: Erythromycin and atorvastatin are both metabolized by CYP3A4. Erythromycin is also a CYP3A4 inhibitor; therefore it inhibits the metabolism of atorvastatin.
- ■ Allosteric (noncompetitive) inhibition
  - ▲ A drug inhibits an enzyme that it itself is not metabolized by. This inhibition occurs at an allosteric site (i.e., not at the site where the substrates bind) (Figure 4-3).

Whether the inhibition is competitive or allosteric, if the enzyme is responsible for inactivating the drug in preparation for excretion from the body, then inhibiting this enzyme will lead to increased levels of active drug. All things being equal, this would likely result in increased biologic activity (or toxicity) of the drug.

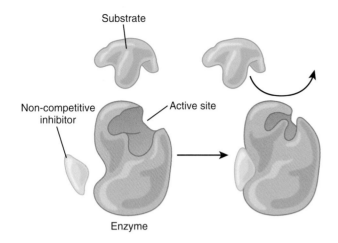

Figure 4-3. Noncompetitive (allosteric) enzyme inhibition.

Prodrugs require metabolic enzymes for transformation to an active (or more active) metabolite. In this case, an enzyme inhibitor would lead to a reduction in levels of active drug, in turn reducing the biologic activity of the drug. Few drugs are prodrugs; however, you should be aware of this *twist* on enzyme inhibition.

Enzyme Induction An inducer stimulates increased production of a CYP450 enzyme. This effect can be seen in days but often takes 2 to 3 weeks to be established. An inducer accelerates the metabolism of substrate (drug).

▲ If the drug is inactivated by that enzyme for the purpose of excretion, an inducer will result in reduced circulating levels of active drug. All things being equal, this will likely result in reduced biologic activity of the drug, perhaps leading to therapeutic failure.

▲ Most cases of induction are allosteric, although rarely a drug may also induce the enzyme system by which it is metabolized.

Now imagine a scenario in which a patient's condition has been stable on both a substrate (drug A) and another drug (drug B) that induces the metabolism of drug A.

▲ What would happen if the patient discontinued drug B?

• This is a classic example of why monitoring should not end once an interacting drug has been discontinued. This is particularly important if the dose of drug A was increased in order to accommodate the effects of the enzyme inducer. If the dose is not adjusted back down, the patient might experience toxicity from the elevated plasma levels.

Note the effect that enzyme induction will have on a prodrug. If its metabolism is accelerated, more prodrug will be activated, leading to an exaggerated effect, or the exact opposite of what would be seen with drugs that are not prodrugs. See Table 4-1 for a list of common substrates, inhibitors, and inducers of CYP450 enzymes.

Phase II Reactions

Details of Phase II reactions are available in the introductory chapter on pharmacokinetics. Phase II reactions are performed

TABLE 4-1. Common Substrates, Inhibitors, and Inducers of the Most Important CYP450 Drug-Metabolizing Enzymes

CYP450 Isoform	Substrates	Inhibitors	Inducers
CYP1A2	β-Blockers Tricyclic antidepressants	Grapefruit juice Quinolone antibiotics Amiodarone	Insulin Omeprazole Phenobarbital Phenytoin Smoking
CYP2D6	Antidepressants Antipsychotics β-Blockers Codeine	Antidepressants Cimetidine Antipsychotics Antihistamines	Carbamazepine Dexamethasone Phenobarbital Phenytoin
CYP2C9	Nonsteroidal antiinflammatory drugs Diuretics	Antifungal drugs Fluvastatin Isoniazid Lovastatin	Carbamazepine Phenobarbital Phenytoin
CYP3A4*	Anticancer drugs Antiarrhythmic drugs Benzodiazepines Calcium channel blockers Protease inhibitors	Antifungal drugs Calcium channel blockers Grapefruit juice Macrolide antibiotics Resveratrol (red wine) Tadalafil	Antidepressants Carbamazepine Corticosteroids Phenobarbital Phenytoin St. John's wort

*This is an abbreviated list, as CYP3A4 has many substrates. Metabolism of over 50% of drugs is thought to involve CYP3A4.

by a family of enzymes called uridine 5'-diphosphate glucuronosyltransferases. This enzyme system functions similar to the CYP450 system, with each enzyme having its own substrates, inhibitors, and inducers. The naming system is also the same alphanumeric system (e.g., 2B15).

■ The principles of inhibition and induction summarized earlier also apply to phase II reactions.

■ However, phase II reactions play a far less important role in drug interactions than the CYP450 enzyme system.

Other Metabolic Interactions

Enterohepatic recirculation involves the recycling of drug between the liver and gut.

Drugs are inactivated by glucuronidation in the liver. These glucuronides are delivered from the liver via the bile into the intestine, where they are hydrolyzed, releasing the active drug. Active drug can then be reabsorbed in a process known as *enterohepatic recirculation*. This recirculation prolongs the residence of active drug in the body. Drugs that interfere with enterohepatic recirculation will potentially reduce the activity of any drug that undergoes this process (Figure 4-4).

Bacteria in the gut play an important role in this hydrolysis of glucuronides. Antibiotics, particularly broad-spectrum antibiotics that kill off these bacteria, can interfere with the process of enterohepatic recirculation. Because the dosage of drugs such as oral contraceptives relies on enterohepatic recirculation to maintain therapeutic levels, an unexpected interruption in this process can lead to therapeutic failure. This is the explanation for the well-known interaction between **oral contraceptives** and **antibiotics**.

Monoamine oxidase (MAO) inhibitors (the *wine-cheese reaction*). MAO breaks down amines such as norepinephrine

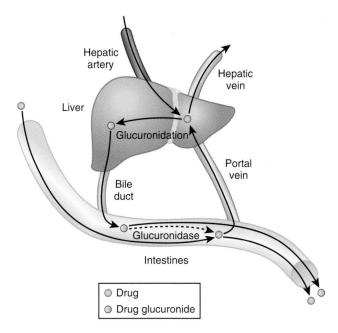

Figure 4-4. Enterohepatic recirculation.

(NE), dopamine (DA), and serotonin, as well as tyramine. Circulating tyramine releases NE.

Irreversible inhibitors of MAO were once commonly used as antidepressants. When a patient on an MAO inhibitor would ingest foods or beverages rich in tyramine, the patient would often experience a sudden and dangerous increase in blood pressure, sometimes leading to stroke or even death. Tyramine-rich foods tend to be aged, so this phenomenon became known as the *wine-cheese reaction.*

Excretion

In terms of excretion, we are most concerned with drugs that rely on the kidney for their elimination. As these drugs are not inactivated by the liver, inhibiting their excretion will prolong the residence of active drug in the body, potentially leading to an exaggerated (or prolonged) pharmacologic effect (Figure 4-5).

A drug can affect excretion of another drug in various ways:

▲ Filtration—by altering plasma protein binding
▲ Secretion—by inhibiting tubular secretion
▲ By altering reabsorption
▲ By altering urine pH

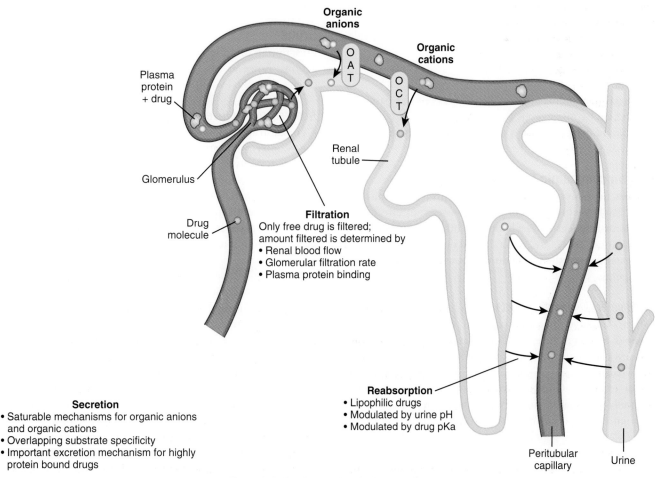

Figure 4-5. Renal mechanisms in drug excretion.

Filtration

Drugs that are bound to plasma proteins cannot be filtered (and excreted) by the kidney. Displacement of a drug will therefore facilitate its filtration and subsequent excretion.

As was the case with absorption and plasma protein binding, this plays a very **minor role** in drug interactions.

Secretion

A few drugs are actively secreted into renal tubules, leading to their excretion in the urine. One drug may inhibit the secretion of another drug, hence reducing its rate of excretion in the urine.

In some cases, this prolongation of effect can be beneficial to the patient. Probenecid is a drug that inhibits the renal tubular secretion of penicillin. By inhibiting the secretion of penicillin, probenecid actually prolongs the residence of penicillin in the body, allowing for longer intervals between doses.

Reabsorption

Reabsorption of one drug may also be enhanced by another. The kidney controls fluid balance by absorbing and excreting ions (for review, see Chapter 25).

Diuretics work by enhancing sodium (Na^+) excretion. As compensation for this reduction in fluid volume, your kidney will try to reabsorb Na^+. The kidney cannot differentiate between lithium (Li^+) and Na^+; therefore patients who are taking Li^+ and are volume depleted or lacking in Na^+ will retain both Na^+ and Li^+. To make things worse, Li^+ is toxic to the kidneys, so patients who retain Li^+ are prone to develop renal damage.

Urine pH

The excretion of drugs that are weak acids or weak bases may be affected by other drugs that change urinary pH. This is a toxicologic principle that is useful in overdose situations for eliminating a drug from the system.

Pharmacodynamic Interactions

Pharmacodynamic interactions are based on mechanisms of drugs having either an additive (or synergistic) effect or an antagonistic effect on each other. Unlike pharmacokinetic interactions, these are generally predictable based on an understanding of the mechanism(s) of action of the interacting agents.

Additive or Synergistic Effects

Often, additive pharmacologic interactions may seem obvious but nevertheless still occur as a result of either carelessness (on the part of patient or provider) or simple lack of knowledge.

■ For example, **Ginkgo biloba** is an herbal product commonly used as a "memory enhancer," and as such it is often taken by elderly patients. Among its many effects, *Ginkgo* inhibits platelet aggregation. **Warfarin** is an anticoagulant that is very commonly prescribed in the elderly, and combining the two agents can lead to increased bleeding.

■ Another example is the use of **alcohol** along with other central nervous system (CNS) depressants such as **benzodiazepines** (e.g., diazepam). This can be a particularly dangerous combination for those who are performing activities that require attention, such as driving.

Antagonistic Effects

Two drugs can oppose each other's actions. This typically occurs through competition for the **same receptor.**

■ A classic example of two drugs antagonizing the effects of each other is seen when an asthmatic is prescribed salbutamol, a β_2 agonist, along with nonselective β-blockers. Propranolol is a β-blocker (see Chapter 11) prescribed for many indications. It works as an antagonist at both β_1 and β_2 receptors.

■ Warfarin is an anticoagulant with a narrow margin of safety. Its anticoagulant effects are based on the fact that it is a vitamin K antagonist. Green leafy vegetables such as broccoli contain vitamin K, and therefore they antagonize the effects of warfarin.

CHARACTERISTICS OF DRUG INTERACTIONS

When considering drug interactions, it is important to understand that it is not just prescription drugs that interact with one another. The list of potentially interacting agents encompasses anything that can be ingested, whether drug, food, or other.

Drugs

Prescription **drugs** are the cause of the majority of drug interactions; however, there are some important drugs that are often overlooked when drug interactions are considered.

Nonprescription (Over-the-Counter) Drugs

A common and potentially dangerous assumption is that over-the-counter medications are safer than prescription drugs. Although safety is a consideration when regulatory agencies decide which drugs to approve for over-the-counter sale, there are numerous examples of over-the-counter agents that have the potential to cause harm. In many cases, these harmful effects are caused by drug interactions. Some examples of the more common interacting agents are listed in Table 4-2.

Illicit Drugs

Several drugs of abuse have clear potential for pharmacodynamic interactions. These interactions, and particularly pharmacokinetic interactions, have not been well characterized in the literature. For obvious reasons, few prospective studies have been performed assessing drug interactions with agents such as cocaine and cannabis.

Pharmacodynamic interactions generally demonstrate additive effects with either stimulants such as cocaine or depressants such as cannabis. For example, patients who are taking sedative-anxiolytics such as benzodiazepines would expect to encounter additional sedation if they are also taking cannabis.

In addition to the challenges in trying to characterize the nature and extent of interactions between illicit drugs and

	TABLE 4-2. Common Nonprescription Drugs That Are Involved in Drug Interactions		
Drug	**Common uses**	**Mechanism of Interaction**
Cimetidine	Antacid	CYP3A4 inhibitor
Omeprazole	Antacid	CYP2C19 inhibitor
St. John's wort	Antidepressant	CYP450 inducer Pgp inducer
Pseudoephedrine	Decongestant	Additive adrenergic effects
Antihistamines (various)	Allergy Upper respiratory tract infections	Additive anticholinergic effects
Ginkgo biloba	Memory enhancer	Additive antiplatelet effects

"conventional" agents is the stigma associated with the use of illegal substances. This almost ensures that, like over-the-counter agents, illicit drugs will continue to lurk in the shadows of a patient's drug profile, only revealing themselves when a serious problem arises.

Food

Food interactions are typically pharmacokinetic in origin. Most commonly, food can affect the absorption of drugs. The simplest example of this is when food delays gastric emptying, slowing down the passage of drug into the small intestine, the primary site for drug absorption. However, there are some notable pharmacodynamic drug interactions involving food. One of the most important examples of a food-drug interaction involves the anticoagulant warfarin and its interaction with green leafy vegetables, which contain vitamin K.

Alcohol

The role of alcohol in pharmacokinetic interactions changes depending on whether use is chronic or acute. Acutely, ethanol competitively inhibits CYP450 enzymes, whereas chronic use leads to CYP450 induction as the body tries to increase its ability to eliminate ethanol.

Environment

Cigarette smoking induces CYP450 enzymes.

ASSESSING THE CLINICAL IMPACT OF DRUG INTERACTIONS

The majority of drug interactions do not result in an absolute contraindication to the concomitant use of the two interacting agents. In fact, the spectrum of drug interactions represents a continuum from those that are actually clinically beneficial to those that may cause great harm, including death, to the patient.

Some considerations when attempting to predict the potential harm from a drug interaction include the following:

1. **The toxicity profile of the drug(s) in question**
   ▲ **Margin of safety**
     • Recall from the introductory pharmacodynamics chapter that the margin of safety is the difference

between the therapeutic and toxic doses of a drug. Drugs with a narrow margin of safety more easily reach toxic levels when they accumulate.
   ▲ **Nature of the toxicity**
     • Not all toxicities are created equal. The nature of the anticipated toxicity plays a key role in determining the potential clinical impact of a drug interaction, and, accordingly, whether the interaction represents a contraindication.
     • For example, the antihistamine terfenadine causes fatal arrhythmias once plasma levels become toxic, and drugs that cause elevation in the plasma levels of terfenadine would be contraindicated for use with terfenadine.

2. **Regimen**
A drug regimen consists of a dose, frequency, and duration, and each of these factors can contribute to the potential harm incurred from a drug interaction.
   ▲ **Dose**
     • There is typically a direct correlation between dose and plasma levels of a given drug. Therefore, the higher the dose of drug used, the more likely that a pharmacokinetic interaction leading to accumulation of that drug will cause a problem.
     ○ **Frequency**
       □ As noted earlier, the frequency with which a drug is administered will affect whether an interaction is manageable or not. This is particularly the case with interactions that are acute in nature, such as when two drugs interfere with each other's absorption. Simply separating the doses of these two drugs so that they do not interact with each other in the stomach can completely negate any interaction.
     ○ **Duration**
       □ Not all drugs are taken chronically. A drug interaction between a chronically administered agent and an acutely administered agent can have some distinct issues compared with interactions between two chronically administered agents.
       □ The advantage of a chronic-acute interaction is that the interaction is short-lived. The classic example is an interaction between a chronic agent and an antibiotic such as erythromycin. Depending on its margin of safety, a temporary interaction such as this might not last long enough to cause enough accumulation to push plasma levels into the toxic range.
       □ However, the disadvantage of these temporary interactions is that if dose adjustments are required, they also require a readjustment once the interacting agent has been discontinued. This may complicate drug regimens when patients have to undergo multiple, interrupted courses of therapy.

3. **The severity of the interaction**

Numerous drugs either induce or inhibit metabolizing enzymes; however, not all drug interactions result in dramatic drug accumulation or therapeutic failure. There are a few reasons why not every metabolic drug interaction results in disaster.

▲ A range of inhibition can occur. There are potent enzyme inhibitors and inducers, and relatively weak ones.

▲ Drugs may be metabolized by more than one enzyme. The effects of inhibiting one metabolic pathway may be mitigated somewhat by the use of a secondary pathway.

▲ Genetics likely play an important role. We are just beginning to understand how important a role, but we do know that the severity of the same drug interaction can vary widely among individuals. This is one of the reasons why severe drug interactions are sometimes not detected until a drug has been approved by regulatory agencies for widespread use.

4. **How frequently the interaction occurs**

▲ Related to the previous paragraphs, a given drug interaction may be clinically significant in one patient and have seemingly no effect on the next patient.

▲ Genetics (again) likely plays an important role here.

▲ Numerous other patient-related factors can also contribute, including other concomitant therapies, as well as the health status of the patient, age, diet, environmental factors, and so on.

Strategies for Mitigating Harm from Drug Interactions

The majority of harm that can occur from drug interactions is preventable; the key is knowledge.

1. **Reduce the use of nonessential prescriptions.**

▲ Patients are often prescribed drugs that they do not actually need. Prescribers should always set a therapeutic goal first before prescribing a medication, and consider nonpharmacologic options. For example, when a patient has been diagnosed with hypertension, consider lifestyle options first (diet, exercise) before moving to pharmacologic interventions.

2. **Ensure that the patient medication profile is complete, including nonprescription medications.**

▲ Numerous over-the-counter medications, including herbal products, interact with prescription drugs. Many jurisdictions do not officially record these agents in a patient's medication profile; thus unless the patient is interviewed about the nonprescription medications he or she is taking, these drugs will not be taken into account when drug interactions are assessed.

3. **Separate the administration of conflicting drugs.**

▲ In many cases, conflicting drugs can be used by the same patient. One of the strategies for minimizing harm in these patients is to separate doses of the conflicting drugs.

4. **When initiating therapy, start at lower doses and increase slowly, as needed.**

▲ The adage "start low and go slow" is based on the very simple principle that the lower the plasma levels of a given drug, the less likely problems are to arise from drug interactions that would increase the levels of that drug. A conservative approach such as this also allows the prescriber to assess whether an interaction is occurring and whether changes need to be made. Initiating therapy with a high dose reduces the margin of safety for that drug.

5. **Use the resources around you.**

▲ A list of some common resources is provided in the next section. A key point to remember is that given the large and ever-increasing number of drugs that interact with one another, it is impossible to memorize all of these interactions. Clinicians use resources, typically information technology, to identify interactions and in some cases to provide context around the clinical significance of the interaction.

RESOURCES

The Institute for Safe Medication Practices (ISMP) is an international nonprofit organization that educates the healthcare community and consumers about safe medication practices. The ISMP has several resources that are useful to healthcare providers, including safety newsletters that alert practitioners to recent safety issues arising from medications. Practitioners are also able to report adverse drug reactions that they have observed, using a simple online reporting system. Although the ISMP is not focused on drug interactions, it is a resource for up-to-date information on drug interactions that have significant impact on patient safety.

Other resources include the following:

1. Pharmacists.

2. Texts: Any general pharmacy reference will have information on drug interactions.

3. Computer programs.

The Epocrates drug database for personal digital assistants (PDAs) is free and contains a comprehensive tool for checking interactions: www.epocrates.com.

See the related Chapter 4 Case Studies in Student Consult.

Websites

www.hiv-druginteractions.org
www.ismp.org
www.epocrates.com

Chapter 5

Impact of Age on Pharmacology

There are four main stages of life, which have distinct characteristics with respect to the way that the body handles drugs: fetal, neonatal and infant, adult, and elderly. These differences are largely pharmacokinetic and reflect the averages in these populations. Note that variations among individuals within these populations also exist, and this topic will be addressed in the section on pharmacogenomics. The following summarizes the key considerations in the fetal, neonatal-infant, and elderly stages of life. The adult stage of life should be considered the reference with which all others are compared. The adult stage is considered normal, and the material covered in other sections of this textbook applies to that stage of life.

FETUS

A **teratogen** is defined as any agent that can cause malformations in a developing fetus.

The teratogenic effects of specific drugs are discussed throughout the drug chapters. The range of effects that a drug may have on the fetus spans from temporary effects after birth to death of the fetus, and everything in between.

The placenta separates the fetal and maternal circulations and is perfused by each. In addition to this and other important functions, the placenta serves as a protective barrier against the entry of drugs into the fetal circulation. However, despite this protective function, a number of drugs will still cross from the maternal to the fetal circulation. Several factors determine whether a drug will **cross the placenta:**

- ▲ Lipid solubility
  - As with other membranes, lipophilic drugs more readily cross the placenta. Even polar (hydrophilic) drugs can cross the placenta in small amounts, if their concentrations in the maternal circulation are high enough.
- ▲ Size of drug
  - The larger the drug, the less likely it is to cross the placenta. Therefore larger drugs, such as proteins, are less likely to cross. However, one cannot assume that large drugs will not cross, as the placenta does have

transporters that facilitate the transport of bulkier molecules.

- These transporters are typically used to transfer nutrients from the mother to the fetus and allow the fetus to transfer waste products of metabolism to the mother. Some of these transporters also facilitate transport of drugs, and in some cases, drugs can also inhibit the actions of these endogenous transporters. Examples of important substrates are listed in Box 5-1.
- ▲ Plasma protein binding
  - Drugs bound to plasma proteins may not cross as readily, given the added bulk, but this can be offset by drugs that are highly lipophilic, as these agents still appear to be able to cross readily despite being bound to plasma proteins.

The **placenta** itself contains some **drug-metabolizing enzymes,** and these enzymes may also help to detoxify drugs or in some instances may actually increase the toxicity of certain drugs. However, the relative importance of these metabolizing enzymes of the placenta to other metabolizing enzymes of either the mother or even the fetus is considered to be relatively minor.

Once a drug crosses the placenta, it enters the **fetal circulation,** and approximately half of it will flow through the liver. Drugs that normally undergo hepatic metabolism may also be metabolized by the fetus. It should be noted, however, that the metabolic capacity of the fetus and neonate differs from that of children and adults. In the fetus these differences result not only from a deficiency of CYP450 and other enzymes but also from the fact that much of the portal blood flow **bypasses** the fetal liver via the ductus venosus for up to 20 weeks of gestation.

The risk of a drug causing harm to the fetus is categorized using the system in Table 5-1, which is largely based on the evidence (or, most commonly, lack of evidence) of harm.

- ▲ Note that relatively **few** drugs are at the **extreme ends** of the spectrum (either safe or absolutely contraindicated); this is typically because of a lack of good

BOX 5-1. DRUGS TRANSPORTED ACROSS THE PLACENTA

Amphetamine	Ofloxacin
Cimetidine	Salicylates
Levofloxacin	Statins
Methotrexate	Valproate
Nicotine	Verapamil

TABLE 5-1. Risk Categories and Descriptions for Use of Drugs in Pregnancy

Risk Category	Description
A	Controlled studies in humans fail to demonstrate risk to the fetus in the first trimester or later trimesters, and the possibility of fetal harm appears remote.
B	Either animal reproduction studies have not demonstrated a fetal risk but there are no controlled studies in pregnant women, or animal reproduction studies have shown an adverse effect (other than a decrease in fertility) that was not confirmed in controlled studies in women in the first trimester (and there is no evidence of risk in later trimesters).
C	Either studies in animals have revealed adverse effects on the fetus (teratogenic or embryocidal or other) and there are no controlled studies in women, or studies in women and animals are not available. Drugs should be given only if the potential benefit justifies the potential risk to the fetus.
D	There is positive evidence of human fetal risk, but the benefits in pregnant women may be acceptable despite the risk (e.g., if the drug is needed in a life-threatening situation or for a serious disease for which safer drugs cannot be used or are ineffective).
X	Studies in animals or human beings have demonstrated fetal abnormalities or there is evidence of fetal risk based on human experience or both, and the risk of the use of the drug in pregnant women clearly outweighs any possible benefit. The drug is contraindicated in women who are or may become pregnant.

evidence. It is understandably difficult to conduct controlled trials in this population.

- The fact that **most drugs** fall in an intermediate area between *safe* and *unsafe* makes it difficult to decide whether a given drug should be used in pregnancy, and usually the decision depends on the **risk-to-benefit** assessment.
- In some cases, not taking the medication may be more harmful to the pregnant patient (and fetus) than taking a medication with questionable risk.
  - For example, many antiseizure medications are potential teratogens. However, withdrawing an antiseizure medication during pregnancy greatly increases the risk to the mother and the fetus.

Timing of exposure is also important and is correlated with the stages of fetal development (Figure 5-1).

- **First 14 days:** Typically this is *all or none*, meaning that exposure results in death of the embryo or has no effect.

The common feature of these two extremes is that they go undetected; if the embryo dies the patient does not realize she was ever pregnant.

- **Days 14-60 (organogenesis):** Exposure to teratogens at this stage may lead to death of the fetus or significant malformations affecting structure or function.
- **Day 61 onward:** Exposure does not typically result in major structural malformations unless blood supply has been disrupted. However, from this point onward the major concern is fetotoxicity.
  - **Fetotoxins,** rather than causing malformations, typically interfere with **function** of organs. Although this can have serious implications, including death, the one advantage of fetotoxicity is that it might be reversible in some cases. Malformations induced by teratogens are not reversible.
    - One example of fetotoxicity would be **angiotensin-converting enzyme (ACE) inhibitors,** which can cause renal failure in the fetus. This is because the fetus appears to be much more dependent on angiotensin II to maintain glomerular filtration.

Occasionally, drugs are actually targeted to the fetus. This is a growing area of research and therapeutics, but one of the early examples of this is the use of corticosteroids to facilitate lung maturation in fetuses that are expected to be born prematurely.

NEONATES, INFANTS, AND CHILDREN

Neonates, in particular, have several differences in their pharmacokinetics that may be of clinical significance. The neonatal period is typically defined as the time from birth to 4 weeks of age. The neonatal information that follows is typically for full-term births unless otherwise indicated. Preterm births require special considerations and will generally not be considered here.

Pharmacokinetics
Absorption

- Neonates typically have **reduced peristalsis,** although gastrointestinal (GI) motility can be unpredictable among neonates. Slowed peristalsis delays gastric emptying and drug absorption.
- Neonates have a **higher pH** in the stomach, beginning life with an essentially neutral pH and, after a period of instability, gradually developing more acidic levels until they reach adult values at around the age of 2. This increased pH can have several potential effects:
  - It may **reduce absorption** of those drugs that require an acidic pH for their dissolution. This might be another reason for avoiding the use of tablets as a dosage form in infants.
  - It may reduce absorption of drugs that become ionized at this higher pH. Remember that ionized (polar) drugs do not cross membranes as readily as nonionized drugs.
  - It may **enhance the absorption** of drugs that are unstable in an acidic environment.

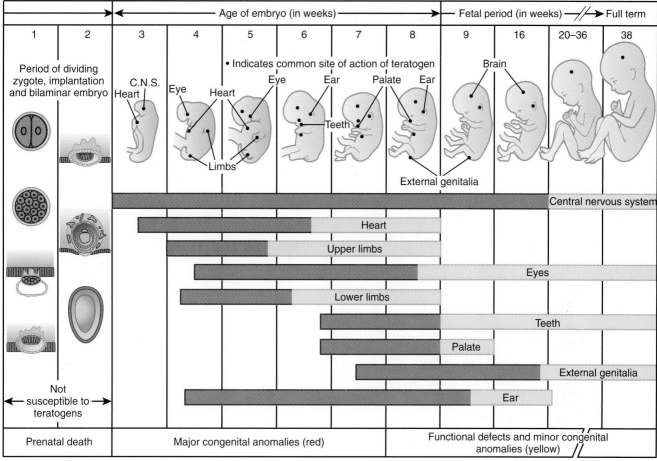

Figure 5-1. Critical periods in human development. Red color indicates highly sensitive periods when teratogens may induce major anomalies.

Red indicates highly sensitive periods when teratogens may induce major anomalies.

■ Absorption of **topically administered** drugs can be **enhanced** in the neonate and infant, as they have thin skin and a relatively large surface area.

Distribution

■ Neonates, in particular, are born "wet," with a much higher proportion of **total body water** than adults (80% versus 60%). This will affect the **volume of distribution** (V_d) of hydrophilic drugs.
  ▲ One example is the aminoglycoside gentamicin. Gentamicin is a hydrophilic drug and has a much larger V_d in neonates than in adults.
■ Neonates also have **lower levels of plasma proteins.** Remember that drugs bound to plasma proteins are unable to cross membranes and interact with their receptors. Drugs that bind plasma proteins will therefore have a much larger free fraction, and this may lead to enhanced pharmacologic effect and increased risk of toxicity.
■ Similarly, drugs may also **compete with bilirubin** for binding to plasma proteins. In the case of a neonate with jaundice, drugs may displace bilirubin from albumin. If this bilirubin reaches the brain, it may cause brain damage, a phenomenon known as **kernicterus.**

■ Blood flow to tissues varies greatly in the first few weeks of life, so the distribution of **intramuscular** injections will be unpredictable over this time.

Metabolism

■ Drug metabolism is impaired at birth and gradually increases with time. The neonate is not born with a full complement of **CYP450 enzymes** but gradually acquires these enzymes through the first few weeks and months of life.
■ Enzymes involved in **glucuronidation** take longer to develop, typically several months, and may not be fully operational for the first few years of life.
  ▲ Chloramphenicol and the "gray baby" syndrome is a classic example of the consequences of impaired glucuronidation in neonates. If dosage of this antibiotic is not appropriately determined, the drug can accumulate, leading to several serious outcomes (including a gray color) and potentially even death in the newborn.

Excretion

■ **Renal function** in infants is significantly reduced in the first year of life compared with that in adults. Full-term babies are born with only 30% of normal glomerular filtration rate, and in preterm babies this number is even lower.

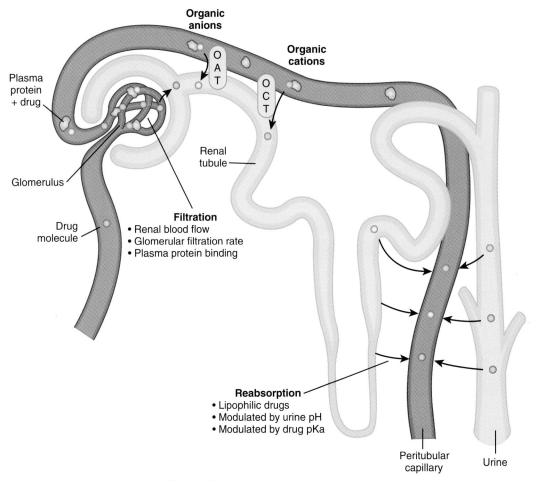

Figure 5-2. Renal mechanisms in drug excretion.

These differences can lead to dramatic increases in the elimination half-lives of drugs that rely on the kidneys for clearance.

▲ Gentamicin can again be used as an example. Gentamicin is primarily eliminated through renal excretion; therefore its elimination will be slower in neonates than in adults (Figure 5-2).

▲ Gentamicin is also a very toxic drug, with a narrow therapeutic index, so failing to adjust for these differences could easily lead to some very serious toxicities in the newborn.

■ Other renal functions, most notably **renal tubular secretion**, may also not be fully developed in the newborn. Active tubular renal secretion is another process, distinct from glomerular filtration, by which drugs are excreted by the kidneys. Secretion occurs via a number of different transporters in the proximal tubule of the nephron, and studies in animals suggest that these transporters may be deficient in the newborn.

■ Renal tubular secretion plays an important role in the excretion of several drugs, including penicillin and a number of diuretics.

Pharmacodynamics

Pharmacodynamic differences among neonates, infants, and adults have not been well studied. It is not known, for example, whether increased sensitivity to opioids in the newborn results from pharmacokinetic or pharmacodynamic differences or both.

Lactation

An important consideration when assessing the ability of neonates to eliminate drugs is exposure through breast milk. Data on the safety of drugs in breastfeeding mothers are generally inadequate, as are the data on pregnancy. Therefore it is important to understand some general principles about the **passage of drugs from the mother into breast milk**. These factors include the following:

- **Size of the drug molecule:** Smaller drugs are able to cross into milk more easily.
- **Lipophilicity:** The more lipophilic a drug, the more likely it is to pass into breast milk.
- **Percent of the drug ionized (based on pH of blood and milk):** Breast milk has a lower pH than plasma; therefore alkaline drugs, once they reach the milk, become ionized and are *trapped* in the breast milk.
- **Extent of plasma protein binding:** Drugs bound to plasma proteins are unable to cross membranes into the milk.

ELDERLY

The definition of *elderly* varies depending on the source but is often considered to be 65 years of age or older. It is also important to note the distinction between **biologic** and **chronologic age.** As the worldwide population ages, and with advances in preventative medicine, there will likely be an ever-widening biologic gap between patients of the same age, based on their lifestyle choices and genetics, among other considerations.

Pharmacokinetics

As with the very young, the impact of age on the very old is broken down here using the **ADME** system.

Absorption

- **Impaired GI motility and blood flow,** both common effects of aging, will impair absorption to an extent. As with infants, the elderly tend to have a higher gastric pH, and this may affect absorption in a manner similar to that described earlier.
- GI motility in general tends to be slowed, leading to **delayed gastric emptying.** This may reduce the rate of drug absorption, which may become clinically significant with drugs such as analgesics, in which delayed efficacy has an impact on the patient.

Distribution

- Humans tend to dry out with age, so the elderly have a **lower** proportion of **total body water** than adults. Conversely, the elderly have a **higher** proportion of body **fat.** This means that hydrophilic drugs have a higher plasma concentration, and lipophilic drugs have a lower concentration, than in adults.
- The elderly also tend to have **lower albumin levels.** However, they tend to have **higher α1-acid glycoprotein levels,** and the overall impact of **plasma protein binding** changes with age is **not** considered to be **clinically significant** in the healthy senior. However, in disease states, including liver failure, changes in plasma protein levels can be large enough to have clinical significance.

Metabolism

Compared with adults, the elderly have **impaired hepatic metabolic function** for some drugs. This is because of a combination of a reduction in liver mass, hepatic blood flow, and

---

BOX 5-2. DRUGS WITH AN AGE-RELATED DECREASE IN HEPATIC METABOLISM	
Alprazolam	Meperidine
Barbiturates	Nortriptyline
Clobazam	Propranolol
Diazepam	Quinidine
Flurazepam	Quinine
Imipramine	Theophylline

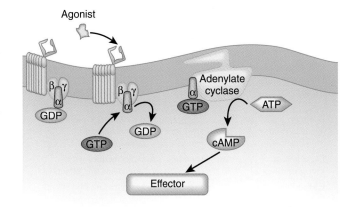

Figure 5-3. G protein–coupled receptors.

activity of phase 1 enzymes (Box 5-2). Drugs that are metabolized by phase 2 enzymes appear to be less affected by advancing age.

Excretion

- Declining renal function is a consistent but not universal consequence of the aging process. In many patients this **decline** in **renal function** begins in the early 20s and is a continuous process throughout life.
- It is important to note, however, that it appears that **not all patients** experience a clinically significant decline in renal function with age. Again, a distinction must be made between biologic and chronologic age.
- As in infants, this reduced renal function will prolong the elimination half-life of drugs that rely on the kidney for their clearance.

Pharmacodynamics

The influence of advancing age on **pharmacodynamics** has not been as comprehensively studied, probably an indication of the much greater complexity and variety of receptors involved. Studies have suggested **alterations in receptor density** or in second messenger activity in the elderly. Some notable examples include the following:

- **Reduced cardiac β receptor activity.** Although findings for receptor density have not been consistent, coupling of β_1

TABLE 5-2. List of Drugs That Are Inappropriate for Elderly Patients (Beers Criteria)

Drug	Class	Description of Concern
Indomethacin	NSAID	CNS side effects worse than other NSAIDs
Methocarbamol Cyclobenzaprine	Muscle relaxants	Anticholinergic side effects, sedation, weakness; questionable effectiveness
Flurazepam	BZD	Extended elimination $t_{1/2}$ in elderly (days), leading to falls
Amitriptyline	TCA	Strong anticholinergic and sedative
BZDs	BZDs	Increased sensitivity to BZDs requires lower dosage
Chlordiazepoxide Diazepam	BZDs	Prolonged elimination $t_{1/2}$ and therefore prolonged sedation, increasing risk of falls
Digoxin	—	Reduced renal clearance requires dosage adjustments
Dicyclomine Hyoscyamine	Antispasmodics	Anticholinergics with significant side effects
Chlorpheniramine Diphenhydramine Hydroxyzine Cyproheptadine	Antihistamines	Anticholinergic side effects
Barbiturates except phenobarbital	—	Cause more side effects than other sedatives or hypnotics in elderly
Ticlopidine	Antiplatelet	No more effective than aspirin but much more toxic
Naproxen Oxaprozin Piroxicam	NSAIDs (longer $t_{1/2}$ full dose)	Potential for GI bleeding, renal failure, hypertension, heart failure
Fluoxetine (daily)	SSRI	Long elimination $t_{1/2}$; excess CNS stimulation, sleep disturbances, agitation
Bisacodyl Cascara sagrada Neoloid	Stimulant laxatives	Long-term use may exacerbate bowel dysfunction
Nitrofurantoin	Antibiotic	Potential for renal impairment
Methyltestosterone	Steroid	Potential for prostatic hypertrophy and cardiac problems

BZD, Benzodiazepine; CNS, central nervous system; GI, gastrointestinal; NSAID, nonsteroidal antiinflammatory drug; $t_{1/2}$, half-life; TCA, tricyclic antidepressant.

adrenoceptors to G proteins appears to be impaired with age. Remember from the introductory pharmacodynamics chapter that G proteins mediate the cellular actions of a receptor (Figure 5-3).

- **Benzodiazepines.** Elderly people appear to be more sensitive to the central nervous system (CNS) effects of benzodiazepines, and although this has been attributed to pharmacokinetic changes with age, studies also suggest that the clinical impact of aging is greater than would be expected from changes in pharmacokinetics alone. It is therefore hypothesized that pharmacodynamic responses to these drugs may be altered.

SUMMARY AND CLINICAL CONTEXT

Perhaps the **most important factors** in determining the impact of age on drug efficacy and toxicity are **polypharmacy, health** of the patient, and **adherence** to therapy.

- Elderly patients are far more likely to be taking **multiple medications**, predisposing them to **drug interactions**.
- The elderly are far more likely to have **kidney** or **liver disease**, each of which would greatly accelerate the normal age-related reduction in the capacity of these organs to eliminate medications.
- The elderly are also far more likely to have cognitive deficits and are more likely to live alone, both of which would increase the risk of **nonadherence** to drug regimens.

The combination of all these limitations has increased focus on the issue of appropriate prescribing in the elderly. Lists of inappropriate drugs used in elderly patients have been generated and updated by several groups. One of the early lists consisted of the Beers criteria; some examples of the most harmful drugs from this list are in Table 5-2.

Chapter 6

Pharmacogenetics

The concept of interindividual variations in response to drug therapy is not new. The fact that some individuals will respond well, some will not respond, and still others will experience toxicity from a given drug has been an accepted part of medicine since the advent of widespread use of pharmaceuticals to treat human disease.

There are many reasons for this variability among patients, including factors such as age, gender, and health status. However, as we enter the era of personalized medicine, what has changed is the willingness to simply accept a *trial-and-error* approach to prescribing, rather than attempting to predict which drugs will be successful in a given patient. With the advent of the information and data collection age, clinicians have ready access to patient information such as laboratory values, concomitant medications, and medical conditions that may influence response to drug therapy. However, what is becoming increasingly obvious as all other factors are accounted for is that likely one of the most important predictors of an individual's response to drug therapy is, in fact, his or her genes.

THE PROMISE OF PERSONALIZED MEDICINE

Adverse events caused by drug therapy are a significant burden to the healthcare system and society in general. Many of these adverse events are preventable, a consequence of an individual's genetic makeup as described in the next sections. Personalized medicine certainly has a significant role to play in the avoidance of harm; however, the real promise of pharmacogenetics may be in **optimal prescribing**. From a health economics perspective, the use of personalized medicine may be one of the most effective ways to manage the seemingly intractable problem of rising drug costs and access to life-saving pharmaceuticals.

■ Take the example of a new anticancer drug, considered to be a breakthrough therapy for lung cancer. As a collection of diseases rooted in genetics, cancer has become one of the clearest examples of the potential for pharmacogenomics in predicting pharmacodynamics of a given drug in a given patient, as outlined in the following example.

■ An anticancer drug may be considered successful if 10% to 20% of patients respond to it. From a clinician's perspective and from the perspective of those 10% to 20% of patients, this is a success, but from a health economist's perspective, a $30,000-per-year drug that fails in 80% to 90% of patients is not cost-effective. If the annual cost for a new anticancer drug is going to be around $30,000 to $60,000, the only way to make these promising new drugs cost-effective is to administer them to only the 10% to 20% of patients who will benefit from them.

PHARMACOGENETICS AND PHARMACOGENOMICS

Pharmacogenetics and *pharmacogenomics* are often used interchangeably but do have distinct meanings. Although either term refers to the use of genetic information to guide therapeutic decision-making:

■ **Pharmacogenetics** focuses on the influence of **single genes** on drug response.
■ **Pharmacogenomics** takes a broader view of the influence of an **individual's entire genome** on his or her response to drug therapy.

One can consider *pharmacogenetics* to be the original term for this field, coined in the days when tools such as microarrays did not exist and the human genome had not been mapped. In those early days it seemed unlikely or impossible that an entire genome could be analyzed in an efficient enough manner to become a useful tool in everyday medicine. Now that we have the means and the knowledge to envision a genome-wide approach to everyday prescribing, the term *pharmacogenomics* is often used to refer to this field. Table 6-1 lists some of the terms commonly used in pharmacogenetics.

The most common basis for genetic variation, and thus the basis for a pharmacogenomic approach to drug therapy, is the **single nucleotide polymorphism**, or SNP (Figure 6-1). An SNP occurs when a **single nucleotide** is exchanged for another at a point in an individual's genome. It is estimated that the human genome consists of approximately 3 billion nucleotides, which in specific combinations form 25,000 to 40,000

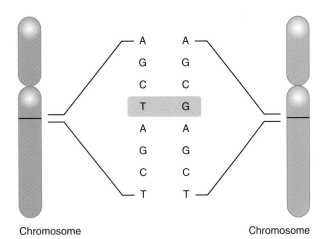

Figure 6-1. Single nucleotide polymorphism.

TABLE 6-1. Definitions of Some Common Terms Used in Pharmacogenetics	
Gene	A sequence of nucleotides that corresponds to a sequence of amino acids in an entire protein or part of a protein. Genes are typically found at a specific location on a chromosome.
Genome	The full genetic complement of an individual.
Allele	Any of the alternative forms of a gene at a particular locus. These alternative forms may or may not result in different phenotypes.
Null allele	A mutation in a gene that leads to a loss of function. Either the gene is not expressed at all (i.e., no protein or RNA) or the product is not functional.
Polymorphism	Variation in DNA sequence present at a specific locus within a population.
Genotype	The genetic makeup of an individual.
Phenotype	The observable physical or biochemical characteristics of an organism. Determined by genotype and environment.
Monogenic	Related to or controlled by a single gene
Polygenic	Related to or controlled by multiple genes. A polygenic trait is a phenotype that is determined by multiple genes rather than a single gene (*monogenic*).
Germ line	Cellular lineage; genetic information that is passed from one generation to the next.
Haplotype	A group of alleles of different genes on a single chromosome that are so closely linked that they are inherited as a unit.
Somatic cell	Any cell in the body, with the exception of those involved in reproduction.

genes and encode approximately 100,000 proteins (at last count). SNPs that occur in coding regions of the genome have the potential to influence protein expression by altering an amino acid within the protein.

▲ **Nonsynonymous coding** SNPs (cSNPs) or **missense** SNPs **change the identity** of an amino acid. Substitution of this amino acid may change the structure or function of the protein.

▲ **Synonymous** coding SNPs or sense SNPs **do not** change the identity of an amino acid and are not likely to affect the structure or function of the protein.

▲ **Nonsense** mutations are SNPs that lead to a **stop codon**. A stop codon will halt translation of nucleotides into a protein.

These variants are often indicated with an asterisk followed by a number indicating the specific mutation in that allele (e.g., CYP450 2D6*4). Certain alleles occur more commonly in some ethnic groups than in others. The impact of these SNPs on phenotypes and their subsequent clinical consequences can again be divided into the two fundamental branches of pharmacology: those that influence **pharmacokinetics** and those that influence **pharmacodynamics**.

PHARMACOKINETICS

The field of pharmacogenomics began with the observations of dramatic differences in the way that certain individuals metabolize drugs. This, along with the fact that adverse drug reactions (ADRs) were the first and most obvious application of pharmacogenomics, has meant that the influence of pharmacogenomics on pharmacokinetics has been much more extensively studied than the impact of pharmacogenomics on pharmacodynamics.

Until recently, the identification of genetically based aberrant metabolism would invariably begin with the observation of an ADR. An ADR can occur because of either higher- (more frequent) or lower-than-expected plasma levels of a given drug. A physician would note toxicities to therapeutic doses of a given drug and discover that plasma levels of that drug were much higher than expected. When other factors such as drug interactions or liver or renal disease were factored out, the clinician was left with genetics as the most viable option for explaining the unexpectedly high plasma levels.

▲ A classic example occurred with the antituberculosis drug isoniazid (Figure 6-2). Isoniazid is acetylated (metabolized) by *N*-acetyltransferase 2 (NAT2), and it was observed that some patients metabolized this drug slowly (i.e., were *slow metabolizers*), whereas others were *rapid metabolizers.*

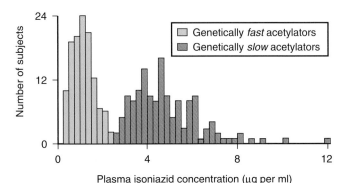

Figure 6-2. Influence of genetics on isoniazid metabolism. (Modified from Meyer UA: Pharmacogenetics: five decades of therapeutic lessons from genetic diversity, *Nat Rev Genet* 2004 5:669, 2004. Reprinted by permission from Macmillan Publishers.)

▲ The clinical consequence is that rapid metabolizers would have low plasma levels of the drug, increasing the potential for therapeutic failure, whereas slow metabolizers were predisposed to toxicities associated with the drug.

▲ This wide variation in response to isoniazid led researchers to speculate that genetics might be playing a role. Isoniazid became one of the first drugs to be identified as having a genetic component to its pharmacologic actions.

Further confirmation of a genetic role would come with the identification of other family members that share the same trait.

With regulatory bodies now either strongly suggesting or requiring that pharmacogenetic studies be submitted with new drug applications, the sequence of events noted earlier has been reversed. Once a new drug enters the market, the pharmacogenetic profile has typically already been characterized, and if an individual has undergone genotyping, many ADRs can be avoided, it is hoped, with adjustments to the drug regimen. The key is to be able to identify the polymorphisms in a given patient before initiation of therapy.

Phase I Reactions, CYP450, and Genetic Polymorphisms

The cytochrome P-450 superfamily of enzymes plays a key role in phase I drug biotransformation. The CYP450 family is itself a rather large collection of closely related enzymes, with a system of nomenclature that reflects these relationships—for example, CYP3A4 and CYP3A5 are more closely related than CYP3A4 and CYP2D6. However, with time it has become apparent that there is heterogeneity within these subfamilies and that this heterogeneity is genetically based.

An early example of genetic differences in CYP450 enzymes occurred with CYP2D6 and debrisoquine, an older sympatholytic once used for hypertension. A landmark study conducted in 1000 Swedish subjects clearly demonstrated the distinction between poor metabolizers, extensive metabolizers, and ultrarapid metabolizers in this population. CYP2D6 has since become a prime example of the impact of genetic polymorphisms on pharmacokinetics. Poor metabolizers have two null alleles of CYP2D6, the most frequent being *4, which occurs in 20% to 25% of Caucasians and is responsible for 79% to 90% of all poor metabolizers.

Conversely, ultrarapid metabolizers have a gene duplication or multiple duplications, meaning that they have excess enzyme.

▲ Figure 6-3 demonstrates how these phenotypes can influence the dosage of a drug, in this case the antidepressant nortriptyline. Note that most patients fall into the *extensive* or *intermediate* metabolizer category.

▲ It is the outliers, the poor metabolizers and the ultrarapid metabolizers, however, that require significant changes to the normal dose. Note that although there are fewer people with either of these phenotypes, poor metaboliz-

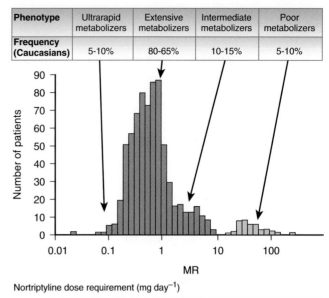

Phenotype	Ultrarapid metabolizers	Extensive metabolizers	Intermediate metabolizers	Poor metabolizers
Frequency (Caucasians)	5-10%	80-65%	10-15%	5-10%

Nortriptyline dose requirement (mg day^{-1})

>250–500	150–100	20–50

Nortriptyline (mg)

Figure 6-3. Influence of phenotype on dosing. (Modified from Meyer UA: Pharmacogenetics: five decades of therapeutic lessons from genetic diversity, *Nat Rev Genet* 2004 5:669, 2004. Reprinted by permission from Macmillan Publishers.)

ers and ultrarapid metabolizers are still present in 10% to 20% of this population.

The clinical impact of CYP450 polymorphisms varies among the various isoenzymes of this superfamily; the effects are summarized in the following sections.

CYP2D6

■ CYP2D6 is the CYP enzyme that is most associated with genetic polymorphisms. The frequency of polymorphisms varies greatly among ethnicities. For example, 5% to 10% of Caucasians are poor metabolizers, whereas only a small percentage (<1%) of Africans and Asians are poor metabolizers. Much of the phenotype in Caucasians is caused by the *4 null allele.

■ Table 6-2 illustrates how much the frequency of CYP2D6 ultrarapid metabolizers can vary within Europe. For example, 10% of Greek citizens are ultrarapid metabolizers, whereas only 1% of people from Finland have this phenotype.

■ CYP2D6 is most commonly associated with metabolism of antidepressants, including the tricyclics (e.g., nortriptyline), selective serotonin reuptake inhibitors (SSRIs) (e.g., paroxetine), and venlafaxine. Other notable drugs using this isozyme include β-blockers (e.g., metoprolol) and antipsychotics (e.g., risperidone). Other examples include the following.

▲ The conversion of **codeine to morphine** is also mediated by this isozyme, and ultrarapid metabolizers of CYP2D6 are prone to opioid toxicity owing to excess conversion of codeine to morphine.

▲ Similarly, CYP2D6 is responsible for conversion of **tamoxifen** to two active metabolites, and patients who

TABLE 6-2. Estimation of the Number of Ultrarapid CYP2D6 Metabolizers in Western Europe*

	Millions of Inhabitants	Frequency of UMs	Millions of UMs
Austria	8	0.04	0.32
Belgium	10	0.03	0.3
Denmark	5	0.01	0.05
England	60	0.03	1.8
Finland	5	0.01	0.05
France	60	0.04	2.4
Germany	82	0.04	3.28
Greece	10	0.1	1
Holland	15	0.03	0.45
Italy	57	0.1	5.7
Norway	5	0.01	0.05
Portugal	10	0.1	1
Spain	40	0.1	4
Sweden	9	0.01	0.09
Total	376		20.4

*Overall percentage in the population is 5.45%.

are poor metabolizers do not benefit as much from therapy with this anticancer agent.

CYP3A4

■ CYP3A4 is the isozyme that metabolizes the most drugs. Genetic testing has identified approximately 20 different variants and nearly 350 SNPs of the CYP3A4 gene. Polymorphisms in CYP3A4 appear to be more common in Caucasians than in Asians.

■ Although it is the CYP isozyme most commonly involved in drug metabolism, there are currently few CYP3A4 mutations identified that are considered to be of clinical importance.

CYP2C9

■ CYP2C9 is found on chromosome 10, close to CYP2C19 as well as 2C8 and 2C18. Several alleles have been implicated in abnormal metabolism, including *2 and *3, which are much more common in Caucasians (approximately 35%) compared with African and Asian ethnicities. These alleles are associated with impaired metabolism.

■ This isozyme is responsible for metabolizing a number of drugs with narrow therapeutic indexes, most notably warfarin. Other substrates of note include a number of oral hypoglycemics (e.g., glyburide), nonsteroidal antiinflammatory agents (NSAIDs) (ibuprofen and several others), cyclooxygenase-2 (COX-2) selective inhibitors, antiseizure medications (e.g., phenytoin), and angiotensin receptor blockers (e.g., losartan).

CYP2C19

■ The CYP2C19 isozyme has considerable genetic variation. The most common polymorphisms result in two null alleles, resulting in a phenotype of absent CYP2C19. This phenotype is most common in Asians (20%) and occurs in only 3% to 5% of Caucasians and Africans. The most common null alleles in Asians is *3 and in Caucasians is *2.

■ CYP2C19 is responsible for the metabolism of the proton pump inhibitors as well as a number of the tricyclic (e.g., amitriptyline) and SSRI (e.g., fluoxetine) antidepressants and benzodiazepines (e.g., diazepam).

■ There can be some advantages to being a poor metabolizer. Patients who are CYP2C19 poor metabolizers have experienced increased efficacy of proton pump inhibitors in Helicobacter pylori eradication.

CYP1A2

■ There is wide variation among individuals in CYP1A2 expression and activity. These differences are also marked among different ethnicities, with lower activity found in Asians and Africans compared with Caucasians. As of 2009, 15 variants of CYP1A2 have been identified, and 158 SNPs have been found.

■ This isozyme plays a role in biotransformation of some of the most widely used substances, including nicotine and caffeine, and it is the study of the latter that led to this isozyme being one of the earliest studied for pharmacogenetic differences. Important drugs metabolized by CYP1A2 include the antipsychotics olanzapine and clozapine, the cardiovascular drugs propranolol and verapamil, and acetaminophen. Genotypes conferring both enhanced and reduced metabolism of clozapine have been identified.

Phase II Reaction Polymorphisms

Phase II reactions are also prone to genetic polymorphisms, although phase II reactions are less important than CYP450 in metabolism. Therefore these polymorphisms also have less clinical significance than those involving CYP450.

PHARMACODYNAMICS

One of the most common ways that polymorphisms alter drug response is through mutations that alter the structure or even the presence of drug targets. Some examples include the following:

■ **Serotonin reuptake transporters in depression.** Patients with polymorphisms that lead to reduced expression of serotonin transporters may be more resistant to treatment with SSRIs. The problem with trying to draw a definitive link between this phenotype and treatment failure is the influence of other factors such as psychotherapy and even other genetic factors that may predispose the patient to treatment-resistant depression.

■ **β_2 receptors in asthma.** Polymorphisms in β_2 receptors can lead to either reduced or enhanced efficacy of β_2 agonists. One study found that children with a specific polymorphism leading to more rapid response had shorter stays in the ICU after an asthma attack.

Cancer is perhaps the most promising application for pharmacogenetics, particularly with respect to pharmacodynamics. As a disease that is rooted in genetics, polymorphisms that influence drug response are ubiquitous in cancer and contribute to the relatively low response rates to treatment after many decades of concerted effort in drug development.

It is not unusual to see response rates of 10% to 20% for *successful* cancer regimens, meaning that patients must endure considerable trial and error before an effective regimen is found. Unfortunately in many cases, these effective regimens are found too late. One of the promises of pharmacogenetics in cancer is that identification of polymorphisms may allow targeting of drug therapy to the correct patient.

- ▲ One recent success story occurred with a drug called gefitinib, for advanced non–small cell lung cancer. The response rate, measured by a significant reduction in tumor size, was only 10% in this difficult-to-treat population. However, it was also observed that women of Asian descent with no history of smoking responded particularly well to this drug.
- ▲ Eventually it was discovered that patients whose tumors had mutations in the epidermal growth factor receptor (EGFR), the target for gefitinib, responded to the drug with remarkable predictability, whereas patients who lacked these mutations rarely if ever responded to treatment.

Another promising feature of the interaction between pharmacodynamics and pharmacogenetics is in drug development. Again using cancer as an example, it is now possible to readily identify mutations in tumors that can then be used to direct the design of a given drug. For example, targeted therapies such as imatinib and dasatinib for **chronic myelogenous leukemia (CML)** have been designed with specific mutations in mind.

- ▲ CML is an ideal disease for personalized medicine, as it is caused by a single oncogene, known as *BCR-ABL*. *BCR-ABL* has a very specific marker that is part of the diagnostic process, and results in a gain of function (i.e., excess cell division).
- ▲ Imatinib was specifically designed to address this mutation. When it was discovered that cancers were mutating, resulting in loss of response to imatinib, another drug (dasatinib) was subsequently designed to specifically address patients with this new mutation, and so on.
- ▲ This use of pharmacogenetics has lead to CML being one of the most 'treatable' cancers, with >95% of patients responding to therapy, and possibility of a 100% response rate in the near future.

THE NEXT STEP: FROM GENETICS TO GENOMICS

One of the challenges with interpreting the influence of genetic polymorphisms on drug response is the interplay of multiple factors.

- ■ For example, warfarin levels are influenced by alterations in CYP450 expression, as described earlier, but another key polymorphism that influences warfarin response occurs in the enzyme vitamin K epoxide reductase (VKOR), which is the pharmacodynamic target for warfarin.
- ■ VKOR converts vitamin K to its reduced form, which is the form that activates several clotting factors in the coagulation cascade. Warfarin inhibits this enzyme, therefore inhibiting activation of clotting factors and inhibiting coagulation.
- ■ Depending on the VKOR phenotype of the patient, he or she may require either higher or lower doses of warfarin. Patients with low VKOR levels require lower doses, and patients with high VKOR expression need higher-than-average doses. This polymorphism is actually thought to have a greater role in determining variations in warfarin dosage than polymorphisms in CYP450.
- ■ Complications in determining clinical impact therefore arise when a patient has both the CYP450 and VKOR polymorphisms, particularly when they occur in opposing directions: one leading to an increased dose requirement, and one to a decreased requirement. In these cases, it would be difficult to predict whether there is no net effect (i.e., the two cancel each other out) or the net direction of effect.

Given the large number of patients with polymorphisms that affect pharmacokinetics, and a similarly large number with polymorphisms that affect pharmacodynamics, it is likely that the scenario just described will be identified frequently in the future. Addressing the impact of a patient's genome rather than a single genetic polymorphism on drug response requires tools that will manage this overwhelming amount of data for clinicians. Perhaps the most important tool that will allow the routine use of pharmacogenomic data is the microarray.

Detection of Genetic Polymorphisms

A **microarray** is a collection of immobilized single-stranded DNA fragments that contain a known nucleotide sequence that is used to identify and sequence DNA samples (Figure 6-4). Microarrays can be used in the analysis of gene expression. A microarray provides an automated means for

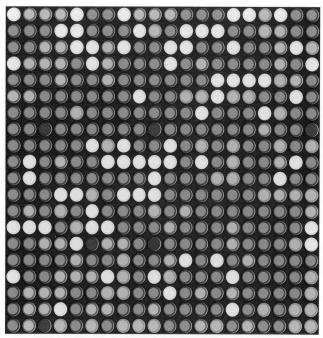

Figure 6-4. Microarray.

identifying genes in a given sample. For example, cancerous and healthy cells may be analyzed from a single patient in order to determine the differences in gene expression between these two types of cells.

- Tissue samples are collected from the patient, and mRNA is extracted from these cells.
- cDNA copies of the mRNA are made, and the cDNA is labeled with a fluorescent dye, one color (green) for one type of tissue, and another color (red) for the other tissue.
- Microarrays contain thousands of wells, each containing many identical copies of the same gene. Each well contains a different gene. The computer has a "map" of the microarray and knows which gene is contained in each well.
- The cDNA is then pipetted onto each well and hybridizes with its complementary DNA strands in the microarray. The cDNA from the samples that do not bind is washed away.
- The microarray is then placed into a scanner that identifies where each of the red and green samples have bound. In wells that have bound both samples, the color changes to yellow.
- Therefore an expression pattern can be determined, in which certain genes are expressed only in cancerous tissue whereas other genes are not expressed in cancerous tissue but are expressed in normal tissue. This information can then be used to identify genes that can be selectively targeted with drug therapy.

Microarrays have now made their way into the mainstream, with devices such as the AmpliChip. AmpliChip was the first pharmacogenetic test ever approved by the U.S. Food and Drug Administration (FDA). It is able to detect polymorphisms of the CYP2D6 and CYP2C19 enzymes, identifying the phenotype of the patient (e.g., ultrarapid metabolizers). The test can be ordered just like a standard blood test and is now available in many laboratories around the world. Results are available within a few days.

Similarly, microarrays can be used to identify genetic polymorphisms over an entire genome, comparing a patient's genome to a normal genome. Because microarrays are automated and work so quickly, they bring with them the potential to someday allow for routine, genome-wide screening, which might become part of the therapeutic decision-making process.

LIMITATIONS OF PHARMACOGENOMICS

The field of pharmacogenomics has grown incredibly fast within the past few years. This rapid growth has been accompanied by some skepticism, as well as concerns about where personalized medicine may take us as a society. Some of the issues include the following:

- **Access to therapy.** The ability to target new drug development to specific genes has lead to concerns over whether patients with unusual genotypes or phenotypes will be ignored in the process. Although this is a valid concern, a counterargument is that in the past, drugs that unintentionally targeted these rare genotypes likely did not make it to market, as they were unable to prove efficacy in a wide enough population.
- **Complexity.** The integration of pharmacogenetics as a regular aspect of the prescribing process will need information technology to make it feasible for busy clinicians. The advent of electronic medical records and electronic prescribing should facilitate this process, but there will be a significant knowledge gap between earlier generations and current clinicians who were trained in the genomics era.
- **Time and expense.** Even with the aid of information systems, pharmacogenetics will add another step to the prescribing process. Testing is also expensive at present, with a single test using AmpliChip technology costing around U.S. $1000. The advantage, however, is that the results can be used for a lifetime.
- **Much ado about nothing.** There are skeptics who believe that the role of personalized medicine has been exaggerated. They point to the litany of other considerations that play an equal or greater role in determining variability in drug response, including age, disease, and drug interactions.

RESOURCES FOR PHARMACOGENETIC INFORMATION

The U.S. National Institutes of Health (NIH) funds a Pharmacogenetics and Pharmacogenomics Knowledge Base, which is available at www.pharmgkb.org. The site offers pharmacogenetic data categorized by genes, pathways (e.g., renin-angiotensin-aldosterone system), SNPs, and drugs.

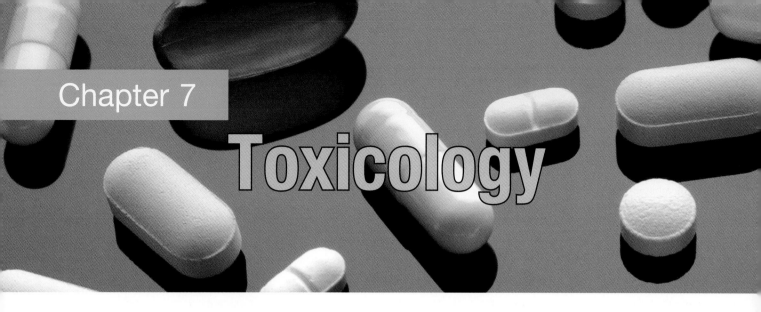

Chapter 7

Toxicology

The field of toxicology is a broad-based multidisciplinary science that examines the harmful effects of substances on living organisms, including humans. There are several major subdivisions of toxicology.

- **Descriptive** toxicology focuses on toxicity testing with the intent of defining the degree of risk associated with substances.
- **Environmental** toxicology involves the detection and understanding of environmental pollutants and their effects on humans and other organisms.
- **Forensic** toxicology is primarily concerned with detection and quantification of toxic substances for legal purposes.
- **Mechanistic** toxicology is focused on determining the mechanisms by which substances exert toxic effects.
- **Regulatory** toxicology uses toxicologic data to establish policies regarding exposure limits for toxic substances.
- **Medical or clinical** toxicology focuses on the diagnosis and treatment of toxic effects in humans.

This chapter focuses primarily on the concepts of medical toxicology. These concepts are similar in many respects, at least in principle, to those of pharmacodynamics and pharmacokinetics. This is not surprising, because any substance can be toxic under the appropriate conditions. Indeed, Paracelsus, an early toxicologist, stated, "All things are poison and nothing is without poison, only the dose permits something not to be poisonous." In fact, even water in excess can exert toxic effects (water intoxication) by disrupting electrolyte balance. Thus toxicity may be associated with therapeutic agents and nontherapeutic agents alike.

GENERAL PRINCIPLES
Terminology

Although toxicology has a long history, it is an evolving discipline, and consequently toxicologic terminology continues to evolve. There are ongoing efforts to standardize and codify toxicologic terminology (see Internet resources). The following are some useful definitions:

- **Poison** is any substance that may disrupt biologic function and potentially kill an organism.

- **Toxin,** by strict definition, is a poison of biologic origin that does not have the ability to replicate. However, the term *toxin* has been used more loosely. For example, *environmental toxin* has been used to describe toxic substances of nonbiologic origin.
- **Venom** is a toxin that is injected into the victim by some means (e.g., bee sting, snake bite).
- **Toxicant** is a general term that refers to any harmful substance and is generally interchangeable with *poison*.
- **Toxicodynamics** refers to the general concepts of pharmacodynamics (interaction with molecular targets and mechanisms of effects) as applied to interactions and mechanisms that generate toxic effects.
- **Toxicokinetics** refers to the general concepts of pharmacokinetics (absorption, distribution, biotransformation, and elimination) as applied to toxic substances.

General Mechanisms of Toxicity

Toxicity can be caused by both therapeutic and nontherapeutic substances. In terms of therapeutic drugs, toxicity may arise from a **direct extension** of the drug's primary action. For example, central nervous system (CNS) depression or coma may occur with excessive doses of barbiturates used in the treatment of epilepsy. The toxic effect may also be **unrelated to the primary therapeutic effect but related to the general pharmacology** of the drug (nonsteroidal antiinflammatory agents may increase edema in heart failure patients). The toxic effect may also have **no relationship to the therapeutic action of the drug** (ototoxicity induced by aminoglycoside antibiotics).

Detailed discussion of the mechanisms of toxicity is beyond the scope of this text. Nevertheless, it is useful to identify several general mechanisms by which toxic effects occur. These mechanisms can be classified as follows:

- ▲ **Physical.** The physical presence of the toxicant triggers reactions that are harmful (e.g., asbestos fibers in the lung).
- ▲ **Chemical.** Toxicants react chemically with the tissues or body fluids such as blood to produce harmful effects (e.g., strong acids or bases cause burns).

▲ **Pharmacologic.** Toxicants interact with endogenous pharmacologic pathways, resulting in inhibition or over-stimulation (e.g., botulinum toxin inhibits release of acetylcholine to cause paralysis).

▲ **Biochemical.** Toxicant reacts biochemically with cellular constituents to produce cellular damage (e.g., venom of many snakes contains phospholipases that destroy cell membranes).

▲ **Genomic (genotoxic).** Toxicant alters the genetic material of the cell, resulting in disruption of function. Genotoxic substances may be mutagenic or carcinogenic.

▲ **Mutagenic (carcinogenic).** Toxicants alter DNA structure or function sufficiently to cause mutations (benzene) or initiate and promote the development of cancers (polycyclic aromatic hydrocarbons such as benzo[a]pyrene, found in cigarette smoke).

▲ **Immunologic.** Toxicant may trigger an immune response that leads to cellular damage (e.g., penicillin-induced hemolytic anemia) or conversely suppresses the immune system, causing an increased susceptibility to infection (e.g., procainamide-induced agranulocytosis).

▲ **Teratogenic.** Toxicant alters fetal development, resulting in birth defects (e.g., phenytoin is associated with development of cleft lip).

Target Organs

Toxicity may be systemic, affecting the whole body, or it may be largely confined to select target organs, the so-called *toxic effect* organs. Some organs, such as the liver, brain, lungs, heart, and kidney, play a central role in poisonings (Figure 7-1). When toxicity is site specific, the word *toxic* is preceded by an indication of the specific target organ. Thus, *hepatotoxicity* refers to effects on the liver, *nephrotoxicity* refers to effects on the kidney, *ototoxicity* refers to effects on the auditory system, and so on. A number of factors interact to determine the susceptibility of organs to toxic effects. These include the organ's anatomic location, blood flow, metabolic processes and activity, affinity for the toxicant, and capacity for self-repair. Major toxic effect organs include the following:

■ **Liver.** The liver is exposed to a high concentration of toxic substances. Orally absorbed toxicants are **presented first** to the liver via the portal circulation. The liver also receives a large proportion of systemic blood flow. **Enterohepatic cycling** extends exposure to toxicants excreted through the bile. The **high metabolic activity** of the liver also results in the generation of reactive intermediates that may have toxic actions.

■ **Kidney.** The kidney receives a high proportion of the **cardiac output.** Many toxic substances are **excreted** by the kidney. These toxicants are **concentrated** in the urine as fluid is reabsorbed from the renal tubule.

■ **Heart.** The total blood volume passes through the heart. Thus it is exposed to all blood-borne toxicants.

■ **Lungs.** The lungs represent an extremely large surface area for interaction with toxicants, particularly those that are airborne. The total cardiac output passes through the lungs,

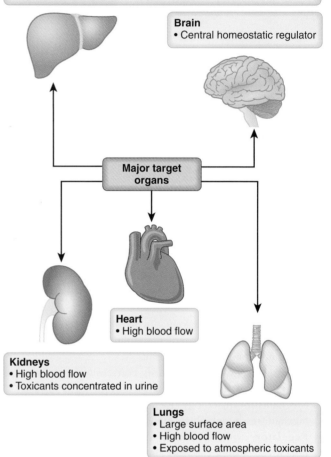

Figure 7-1. Major target organs.

so blood-borne toxicants are also distributed extensively to the lungs.

■ **Brain.** The brain is a critical target organ because of its central role in homeostasis. Thus toxicants that affect the brain may influence multiple systems and result in widespread systemic toxicity.

Risk Assessment

Poisoning remains a significant public health issue that affects up to approximately 5% of the population per year in industrialized countries. Many countries have established national poison control centers that can serve as valuable sources of information. The World Health Organization maintains a directory of these centers (see Websites).

Because virtually all substances are potentially toxic, key questions in toxicology are **how much risk** is associated with a particular substance and **under what conditions** does this risk become apparent? In addition, the level of acceptable risk will vary. In some circumstances, very toxic substances (e.g., anticancer drugs) are used therapeutically despite their known toxic effects because the benefits of such treatments outweigh

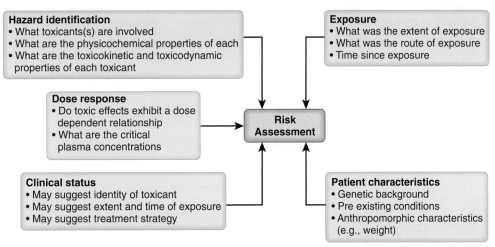

Figure 7-2. Risk assessment during management of toxic events.

the risks. Accordingly, risk assessment is a primary consideration in the management of toxic events (Figure 7-2).

Key factors contributing to risk assessment include the following:

▲ **Hazard identification.** What substances are involved and what are the adverse effects of each substance? Knowledge of the physicochemical properties, toxicokinetics, and toxicodynamics of the suspected toxicant(s) is invaluable in designing treatment strategies.

▲ **Dose response.** Is there a known dose response relationship for the toxic effects of the toxicant? Do toxic effects mirror plasma concentrations? At what dose (concentration) do toxic effects appear?

▲ **Exposure assessment.** Exposure assessment is a key process in determining the urgency and strategy for treatment of toxic events. Exposure assessment includes estimation of the following:

• **Degree of exposure.** An estimate of the degree of exposure is essential. This may be the dose of drug ingested, the concentration of chemical to which a patient was exposed, or some other measure (e.g., parts per million) of the amount of toxicant. Included in this assessment is whether the exposure was acute or chronic.

• **Route of exposure.** The route of exposure is an important determinant of both the extent and rate of absorption of the toxicant. For example, dermal exposure is generally associated with reduced rates and extent of absorption compared with oral ingestion or inhalation.

• **Time since exposure.** An estimate of the time since the exposure will be helpful in estimating the following:
  ○ Degree of absorption at presentation.
  ○ Usefulness of blood sampling. Blood sampling is useful for toxicants that exhibit a relationship between the plasma concentration and toxic effect(s). However, if the time of exposure has been long, it is most likely that plasma concentrations have reached a maximum value and are of lesser benefit compared with symptomatology in determining course of treatment.

○ Value of certain therapies. The time since exposure will dictate to a certain extent the appropriateness of treatment approaches. For example, if the time since initial exposure has been very long, then therapies aimed at inhibiting absorption may have only a minor influence on the course of poisoning.

▲ **Clinical status.** In many cases, information about the degree and time of exposure may be lacking. In such cases, careful determination of the clinical status of the patient coupled with knowledge of potential hazards can assist in determining the type of toxicant (e.g., recognition of anticholinergic effects of mushroom poisoning), the suspected time course, and the treatment protocol. In addition, recognition of compromised airway, circulatory, or neural function requires immediate supportive measures.

▲ **Patient characteristics.** The specific characteristics such as anthropomorphic characteristics, genetic background, and preexisting conditions of each patient also factor into risk assessment. Some (e.g., weight) may affect the course of poisoning indirectly, whereas others may have a more direct effect (e.g., alcoholism) by influencing the production or elimination of toxic substances. Genetic polymorphisms may affect absorption, biotransformation, or elimination of toxicants.

GENERAL STRATEGIES FOR MANAGEMENT OF TOXIC EVENTS

In some cases of poisonings, there are specific treatments or antidotes available that prevent, interrupt, or reverse the toxicity. In such cases, hazard identification and knowledge of the toxicodynamics of the toxicant are critically important for selection of the appropriate antidote or treatment. Antidotes or specific treatments may act via a number of mechanisms including the following:

■ **Antibodies** that neutralize toxicants or prevent their distribution to target organs (e.g., antivenin for snake bites)

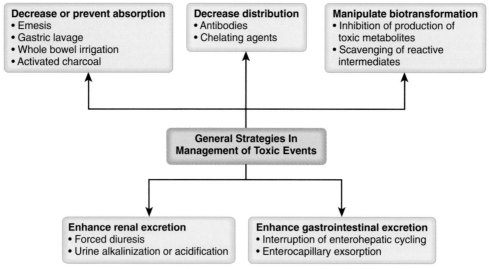

Figure 7-3. General strategies in management of toxic events.

- Compounds that **sequester** the toxicant, prevent its distribution, and promote its excretion (e.g., heavy metal chelators)
- Compounds that **scavenge** the toxicant to prevent its interaction with tissues (e.g., *N*-acetylcysteine [NAC] in acetaminophen poisoning)
- Pharmacologic **antagonists** that block receptors stimulated by the toxicant
- Pharmacologic **agonists** that stimulate receptors blocked by the toxicant
- Treatments that act **physiologically to oppose** the actions of the toxicant (e.g., pressor agents to reverse hypotension)
- **Enzyme inhibitors** that prevent the formation of toxic intermediates
- **Enzyme activators** that reverse enzymatic inhibition produced by toxicants

In addition to specific treatments, a number of generalized treatment strategies can be used in poisonings (Figure 7-3). These are toxicokinetic treatment strategies targeted at reducing or preventing the **absorption** of the toxicant, at reducing the **distribution** of the toxicant, at manipulating **biotransformation** to reduce formation of the toxicant, or at hastening **excretion** of the toxicant. These approaches rely heavily on the concepts of pharmacokinetics presented earlier, which will not be repeated here. These generalized approaches are very useful in situations in which there are no specific antidotes or the causative toxicant(s) and/or modes of action are not sufficiently well defined to allow application of a specific antidote.

Reduction or Prevention of Absorption

Because the majority of poisonings occur via **ingestion**, approaches to limit absorption via this route will be discussed here. Approaches to limit absorption via other routes are generally common sense approaches. For example, moving the patient to fresh air if the exposure route was inhalational or flushing the skin with water in the case of dermal exposure. Several options are available to reduce oral absorption of toxicant. Collectively, these approaches are sometimes referred to as **gastrointestinal (GI) decontamination.**

Forced Emesis

Vomiting can remove toxicants present in the stomach. This approach may be useful if there is reason to believe that there is toxicant remaining in the stomach. This may be the case if the time since exposure is relatively short or if gastric emptying has been delayed. In the past, a number of approaches have been used to induce emesis. However, most have been abandoned. The most frequent method in current use is ingestion of **syrup of ipecac.**

- **Mechanism of action**
  - ▲ Stimulation of sensory receptors in the GI tract
  - ▲ Stimulation of chemoreceptor zone in the CNS
- **Adverse effects**
  - ▲ Aspiration of vomitus into lungs
  - ▲ Physical damage due to the act of vomiting (e.g., gastric tears)
  - ▲ Impairment of other GI decontamination procedures since patient may continue to vomit for prolonged period
  - ▲ Electrolyte imbalance
- **Contraindications**
  - ▲ Ipecac should not be used with toxicants such as:
    - • Petroleum distillates (e.g., gasoline, furniture polish)
    - • Corrosives (strong acids, strong bases) (e.g., drain cleaner)
    - • CNS stimulants, because act of vomiting may trigger convulsions
  - ▲ Unless a secure (intubated) airway has been established, ipecac should not be used in the following patients:
    - • Those who are unconscious
    - • Those with impaired airway reflexes

▲ Anticipated use of other GI decontamination procedures, because emesis would remove the treatments from the GI tract

In the past, the use of ipecac to induce forced emesis was promoted for GI decontamination in both hospital and home settings. Recommendations from a number of poison control organizations now indicate a much **more conservative** use of ipecac because of the **potential for harm** and the relative **lack of evidence** for definitive benefits. Available data suggest that ipecac may be of use in the following situations:

▲ In prehospital settings when there are no contraindications for use

▲ When the ingested toxicant poses substantial risk

▲ If no alternative means of GI decontamination are available

▲ When ipecac can be administered within 30 minutes of toxicant ingestion

▲ When there will be a substantial delay (>60 minutes) in reaching treatment facilities

Gastric Lavage

Gastric lavage involves placing a tube through the mouth (orogastric) or through the nose (nasogastric) into the stomach. Toxicants are removed by flushing saline solutions into the stomach, followed by suction of gastric contents.

■ **Mechanism of action**
  ▲ Physical removal of toxicant
■ **Adverse effects**
  ▲ Aspiration of lavage into lungs
  ▲ Mechanical injury caused by placement of the gastric tube
  ▲ Endotracheal placement (into the trachea and thus into the lungs) of gastric tube
  ▲ Electrolyte imbalance
■ **Contraindications**
  ▲ Gastric lavage should not be used with toxicants such as the following:
    • Petroleum distillates (e.g., gasoline, furniture polish)
    • Corrosives (strong acids, strong bases) (e.g., drain cleaner)
    • CNS stimulants, because the act of vomiting may trigger convulsions
  ▲ Unless a secure (intubated) airway has been established, gastric lavage should not be used in the following patients:
    • Those who are unconscious
    • Those with impaired airway reflexes

Although in theory gastric lavage would seem to be the most direct way of removing a toxicant, the available **evidence does not support the routine use** of gastric lavage. Gastric lavage may be useful in cases in which there has been **very recent** ingestion (30 minutes to 1 hour) of a **life-threatening** toxicant.

Activated Charcoal

Activation of charcoal by oxidization increases its **adsorptive surface area.** The large surface area of charcoal is capable of

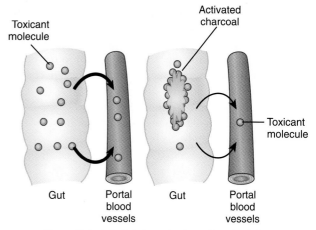

Figure 7-4. Activated charcoal reduces drug absorption.

adsorbing many toxicants, thus **sequestering** them in the gut. Because only free molecules are able to diffuse across membranes, reduction of the concentration of free toxicant in the gut by charcoal greatly reduces absorption into the bloodstream (Figure 7-4). This treatment is administered as a slurry of the activated charcoal powder.

■ **Mechanism of action**
  ▲ Toxicant molecules adsorbed to charcoal are not absorbed
  ▲ May increase elimination by decreasing free concentration of toxicant in gut
  ▲ May interrupt enterohepatic cycling
■ **Adverse effects**
  ▲ Vomiting, particularly with premade solutions containing sorbitol (seen in up to 40% of patients)
  ▲ Aspiration; charcoal can cause marked lung damage
  ▲ Reduced absorption of other drugs or antidotes
  ▲ Constipation
■ **Contraindications**
  ▲ Patients at risk for bowel perforation (e.g., ingestion of corrosives)
  ▲ Toxicants with significant potential for aspiration (e.g., petroleum distillates)
  ▲ Toxicants that are **not** adsorbed to charcoal
    • Alcohols
    • Iron
    • Highly polar molecules and salts
  ▲ Unless a secure (intubated) airway has been established, activated charcoal should not be used in the following patients:
    • Those who are unconscious
    • Those with impaired airway reflexes

Available data suggest that activated charcoal is effective at reducing the absorption of many toxicants. This treatment may be administered as **single-dose activated charcoal** (SDAC) or repeated as **multiple-dose activated charcoal** (MDAC). However, the efficacy of SDAC charcoal at preventing drug absorption is very time dependent and decreases rapidly with time from ingestion. SDAC is most effective if administered **within 60 minutes** of toxicant ingestion. MDAC is most frequently used in cases of poisoning with controlled-release substances, with the goal of binding toxicant as it is released from its formulation. In addition, MDAC also may be of benefit in increasing the elimination of toxicants. **Current recommendations** suggest that activated charcoal should be used in the following situations:

- ▲ When the toxicant is potentially fatal
- ▲ When no contraindications to its use are present
- ▲ If the toxicant binds to charcoal
- ▲ If the time since ingestion suggests toxicant is still present in the GI tract

Whole Bowel Irrigation and Cathartics

Whole bowel irrigation and cathartics are used to prevent the absorption of toxicants by increasing GI motility and passage of the GI contents, thereby **reducing the time** available for drug absorption. **Cathartics** use osmotic substances to draw fluid into the gut and **produce diarrhea**. The most commonly used cathartic is **sorbitol**. Available recommendations currently **discourage** the use of cathartics as sole therapy for poisonings because of the associated **dehydration and electrolyte disturbances**. Accordingly, cathartics will not be discussed further.

Whole bowel irrigation (also called *whole gut lavage*) is an evolution of the cathartic concept. This approach combines oral administration of **high–molecular-weight substances**, generally polyethylene glycol, with iso-osmolar electrolyte solutions (e.g., Golytely). This combination tends to prevent systemic electrolyte disturbances that complicate the use of cathartics alone. Large volumes of these solutions plus water are administered orally or by gastric tube.

- ■ **Mechanism of action**
  - ▲ Increased volume in GI tract promotes voiding
  - ▲ Administration is continued until rectal discharge is clear
- ■ **Adverse effects**
  - ▲ Nausea, vomiting
  - ▲ To date, systemic electrolyte disturbances have not been reported
- ■ **Contraindications**
  - ▲ Patients with impaired bowel function (e.g., ileus) or perforation
  - ▲ Patients susceptible to aspiration if vomiting occurs

Whole bowel irrigation has been shown to **decrease the bioavailability** of certain toxicants. Although there are no consensus statements regarding specific indications for whole bowel irrigation, this approach may be best suited for intoxications for which the other methods of GI decontamination may not be appropriate. More specifically, whole bowel irrigation may be particularly useful in cases where there has been a **long time lag** between ingestion and treatment and in cases in which **toxicants are released slowly. Current recommendations** suggest that whole bowel irrigation should be used in the following situations:

- ▲ For poisonings with controlled-release substances
- ▲ When there is an extended time between ingestion and treatment (2 hours or more)
- ▲ For toxicants that are not well adsorbed by activated charcoal (e.g., iron tablets)
- ▲ For ingestion of transdermal patches or illicit drug packets

Manipulation of Distribution

After absorption, most toxicants must be distributed to the target tissues to exert harmful effects. Accordingly, another strategy for managing toxicity is to prevent the distribution of toxic substances. In general this is accomplished by **binding the toxic substance in the blood** and preventing access to its site of action.

- ■ General mechanisms of action
  - ▲ **Antibodies**
    - • Generally highly specific for toxicant
    - • Eliminated by renal excretion
    - • Often used as antigen binding fragments (Fab fragments) resulting from the proteolytic digestion of the whole antibody
    - • Use of Fab fragments tends to reduce the incidence of hypersensitivity reactions
    - • Antibody fragments also penetrate more readily to the interstitial spaces to neutralize toxicants that have already undergone distribution
    - • Major adverse effects are hypersensitivity reactions and delayed serum sickness
    - • Examples include:
      - ○ Antivenin
      - ○ Digoxin binding antibodies
  - ▲ **Chelating agents**
    - • Contain reactive sites such as hydroxyl or sulfhydryl groups that bind target molecules
    - • Heavy metal chelators bind to metal ions to form stable complexes
      - ○ Reduces distribution of metal
      - ○ Shields metal from reacting with functional groups on cellular constituents
      - ○ Allows excretion of metal chelates in urine or feces (biliary excretion)
  - ▲ **Edetate calcium disodium** (calcium disodium salt of ethylenediaminetetraacetic acid; EDTA)
    - • Binds iron, lead, copper, manganese, cobalt, and calcium
    - • Primarily used to treat lead intoxication
    - • Not effective for mercury poisoning
    - • Highly charged, so has poor oral bioavailability; requires parenteral administration (intravenous or intramuscular)
    - • When administered intramuscularly, has the propensity to cause pain at the injection site, so it is combined with local anesthetic agents
    - • Used as the calcium salt to prevent excessive binding of endogenous calcium and hypocalcemic tetany
    - • Short half life (<1 hour) necessitates frequent administration
    - • EDTA-lead chelates are excreted primarily in the urine
    - • Main adverse effect is nephrotoxicity

- ▲ Dimercaprol (British antilewisite)
  - Useful in arsenic, mercury, lead, cadmium intoxication
  - Rapidly oxidized in aqueous solutions so given intramuscularly in peanut oil
  - Chelates primarily excreted in urine
  - Thiol-metal ion bonds are labile in acidic solutions; alkalinization of urine is used to prevent release of metal ions in renal tubule and nephrotoxicity
  - Main adverse effects include:
    - Nausea, vomiting
    - Marked hypertension
    - Burning sensations
- ▲ Penicillamine
  - Metabolite of penicillin
  - Oral bioavailability sufficient to allow oral therapy
  - Useful in intoxication from copper (Wilson's disease), mercury, and lead
  - Chelates excreted in urine
  - Main adverse effects include the following:
    - Dermatologic reactions
    - Renal toxicity
    - Hematologic toxicity (e.g., leukopenia)
  - Patients who become intolerant to penicillamine during long-term therapy for copper intoxication can be switched to another copper chelator, **trientine**.
- ▲ Succimer
  - Mercapto (thiol-containing) analogue of succinic acid
  - Oral bioavailability sufficient to allow oral therapy
  - Currently used as a chelator in lead toxicity, but may bind other heavy metals
  - Water-soluble succimer chelates are excreted in the urine
  - Less toxic than dimercaprol
  - Half-life is approximately 2 days
  - Main adverse effects include the following:
    - GI complaints
    - Rash
    - Flulike symptoms
- ▲ Deferoxamine
  - Poor bioavailability necessitates parental administration via intramuscular, subcutaneous, or intravenous (least preferred) route
  - Extremely high affinity for iron; very effective for iron intoxication
  - Eliminated by renal excretion, with a half-life of approximately 6 hours
  - Adverse effects of note include the following:
    - Allergic reactions
    - Hypotension (especially via intravenous route)
  - Reduced compliance with long-term regimens owing to need for parenteral administration
- ▲ Deferiprone
  - Orally available iron chelator
  - Available in European Union but not in Canada or United States
  - Excreted in urine
  - Half-life is less than 1 hour, necessitating frequent administration
  - Major adverse effects include the following:
    - GI disturbances
    - Neutropenia
    - Agranulocytosis
    - Joint pain
  - Up to 40% of patients on long-term therapy discontinue use.
- ▲ Deferasirox
  - Orally available iron chelator
  - Excreted primarily in the feces by biliary excretion
  - Half life is 8 to 16 hours, allowing once-a-day administration
  - Major adverse effects include the following:
    - GI disturbances
    - Skin rashes
    - Mild decrease in glomerular filtration rate
  - May be preferred over other iron chelators because deferasirox has more convenient administration and a good safety profile

Manipulation of Biotransformation

As discussed in the pharmacokinetics chapter, once a substance has been absorbed into the bloodstream it is subject to biotransformation. Biotransformation in most cases causes inactivation of substances. In theory, then, one strategy for reducing toxicity would be to **accelerate inactivation** of the toxicant. This could be achieved through metabolic enzyme induction. However, in most cases the time course of **enzyme induction is too slow** to be an effective treatment strategy.

In some cases, the primary toxicants are not especially harmful but biotransformation results in the formation of reactive intermediates or molecules that mediate the toxic effects. In these situations, an **effective strategy** for the management of toxicity is to **reduce the formation** of the toxic molecule.
- ■ General mechanisms of action
  - ▲ Inhibition of metabolic enzymes that produce toxic molecule
  - ▲ Saturation of an enzyme with substrate that is converted to nonharmful substance
  - ▲ Scavenging of reactive metabolites
  - ▲ Treatments most effective when applied before formation of the toxic metabolite

Examples of this approach will be provided later in the discussion of treatment approaches for specific toxicants. (See treatment of acetaminophen toxicity, treatment of ethylene glycol toxicity.)

Enhancement of Toxin Excretion

Ultimately, the therapeutic goal in treating toxicity is to **remove the toxicant** from the body completely or at least to the point at which plasma concentrations decline to a nontoxic level. Several strategies have been used to increase removal of toxicant from the plasma or, in other words, to increase clearance. These involve enhancement of endogenous clearance mechanisms such as renal excretion and exogenous mechanisms such as extracorporeal elimination (e.g., hemodialysis, hemofiltration).

Renal Excretion

In principle, renal excretion could be enhanced by **increasing glomerular filtration** and/or **tubular secretion** or by **decreasing tubular reabsorption** of toxicants. The major concepts were discussed in the chapter on pharmacokinetics and are reviewed here only briefly.

Forced Diuresis

- Forced diuresis involves administration of diuretic agents and isotonic saline to increase glomerular filtration rate and urine flow.
- When combined with bicarbonate infusion, it is referred to as **forced alkaline diuresis.**
- Fluid overload, pulmonary edema, and electrolyte disturbances can complicate therapy in compromised patients, especially in the presence of cardiac, renal, or pulmonary dysfunction.
- Although it is important to maintain good urine flow during treatment of toxicities, increasing glomerular filtration through forced diuresis is not encouraged in most intoxications. However, this approach has been used with nephrotoxic drugs because of the dilutional effect on nephrotoxic agents in the renal tubules.

Urine Alkalinization

- As discussed in the pharmacokinetics chapter, many substances are reabsorbed from the renal tubules into the bloodstream, limiting the extent of their urinary excretion.
- Tubular reabsorption is dependent on the substance being in the nonionized form.
- The principles of ion trapping (see pharmacokinetics chapter) can be used to increase urinary excretion.
- Urine is generally acidic, and alkalinizing the urine (generally to above pH 7.5) increases ionization of acidic substances and thereby prevents their tubular reabsorption.
- Because pH is a logarithmic scale, each unit change in pH results in an approximately tenfold change in ionization and presumably excretion.
- Bicarbonate solution is infused intravenously while urine pH is monitored, with a goal of reaching a **urine pH** of 7.5 to 8.
- Urine alkalinization will be most effective for toxicants that are:
  - ▲ Weak acids with a low pK_a value
  - ▲ Cleared primarily by the kidney
- Examples of toxicants whose clearance is increased by urine alkalinization include:
  - ▲ Salicylates
  - ▲ Chlorophenoxy herbicides (e.g., 2,4-D)
  - ▲ Barbiturates
  - ▲ Methotrexate

- Main adverse effect of urine alkalinization is:
  - ▲ Hypokalemia (potassium shifts to intracellular space as a result of alkalemia)

Urine Acidification

- Acidification of urine could *theoretically* assist in renal excretion of toxicants that are weak bases.
- Urine is usually acidic, so it not clear how much additional benefit can be achieved by acidifying urine.
- Acidification of urine also carries the risk of inducing systemic acidosis.
- Acidification of urine is **not encouraged** but can be accomplished with administration of ammonium chloride or ascorbic acid.

Gastrointestinal Excretion

Although the majority of toxins are excreted in the urine, a number may be excreted in the feces. Biliary secretion is an important route of **movement of conjugated toxicants** from the plasma into the lumen of the GI tract. However, in many cases these conjugates are cleaved in the gut and the toxicants can be reabsorbed (enterohepatic cycling). **Interruption of enterohepatic cycling** can increase fecal excretion of toxicants. In addition, **strategies to hold toxicants in the GI tract** until they can be passed in the feces can be an effective means of detoxification.

Interruption of Enterohepatic Cycling

Treatments bind toxicants in the GI tract and prevent their reabsorption after cleavage of toxicant conjugates.

- Activated charcoal, particularly MDAC, may increase toxicant elimination in part by interrupting enterohepatic cycling.
- Special binding substances can be ingested to bind toxicants in the GI tract, interrupt enterohepatic cycling, and increase toxicant elimination in the feces.
  - ▲ Bile acid binding resins increase fecal elimination of digoxin.
  - ▲ Thiol-containing resins can be used to interrupt enterohepatic cycling of mercury.

Enterocapillary Exsorption (Gastrointestinal Dialysis)

Enterocapillary exsorption (GI dialysis) refers to the **removal of toxicants** that have **already been absorbed** into the bloodstream **by increasing their transport into the lumen of the GI tract.**

- Binding of toxicant in gut lumen decreases the free concentration of drug in the gut.
- The very low concentration of free toxicant in the gut lumen means that free toxicant concentrations in the plasma are higher than those in the gut. This blood-to-gut concentration gradient favors diffusion of toxicant from the blood into the gut lumen where the toxicant binds to the charcoal. The charcoal-bound toxicant is eventually excreted in the feces (Figure 7-5). As this cycle repeats itself, the blood is cleared of toxicant.

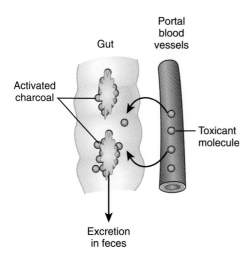

Figure 7-5. Enterocapillary exsorption. Large amounts of activated charcoal in the gut promote drug excretion in the feces.

- Enterocapillary exsorption may contribute to the ability of MDAC to increase the elimination of drugs such as:
  - ▲ Amitriptyline
  - ▲ Carbamazepine
  - ▲ Nadolol
  - ▲ Piroxicam

PHARMACOLOGIC TREATMENT OF SPECIFIC INTOXICATIONS

The types of intoxications that may be encountered in practice are virtually unlimited, making a full discussion of treatment of intoxications beyond the scope of this text. However, it is useful to consider the treatment of some **more common** intoxications to illustrate the general principles discussed previously.

Analgesics

Intoxication with analgesics represents the **most common** form of toxicity requiring hospitalization.

Acetaminophen

- Acetaminophen poisoning causes hepatotoxicity and is one of the more common lethal poisonings in industrialized countries.
- Acetaminophen is present in many combination analgesic preparations. Although intentional overdose is a cause of acetaminophen toxicity, intoxication can also be inadvertent owing to use of multiple acetaminophen-containing analgesics (e.g., combining over-the-counter acetaminophen with prescription opioid-acetaminophen analgesics)
- Acetaminophen is not toxic per se but is metabolized to a **reactive intermediate** that is toxic (Figure 7-6, *A*).
  - ▲ At **therapeutic concentrations**:
    - Phase II conjugation to glucuronate or sulfate accounts for approximately 90% of metabolism.
    - CYP450 metabolism accounts for approximately 5% to 10% of metabolism but results in the production of

an electrophilic molecule, *N*-acetyl-*p*-benzoquinone imine (**NAPQI**).
- NAPQI is **highly reactive** and can form covalent bonds with cellular constituents, leading to cellular death.
- However, under normal conditions the relatively small amount of NAPQI formed is **quickly scavenged** by reaction with intracellular **glutathione**, which prevents NAPQI reaction with cellular constituents.
  - ▲ At **supratherapeutic concentrations**:
    - **Phase II conjugation becomes saturated**, shuttling the bulk acetaminophen metabolism through CYP450 pathways.
    - Increased generation of NAPQI eventually exhausts cellular stores of glutathione, resulting in the **accumulation of free NAPQI** and hepatotoxicity.
- Acetaminophen toxicity may be exacerbated by:
  - ▲ Induction of CYP450 metabolism
    - Chronic alcohol abuse
    - Concurrent anticonvulsant therapy
  - ▲ Depletion of cellular glutathione stores
    - Malnutrition
- **Treatment of acetaminophen poisoning**
  - ▲ **Activated charcoal**
    - Used to decrease absorption of acetaminophen
    - Most effective if given within 2 hours of overdose
  - ▲ ***N*-acetylcysteine (NAC).** A primary treatment strategy for acetaminophen toxicity is replenishment of cellular glutathione via the administration of NAC, a precursor of glutathione (see Figure 7-6, *B*).
    - **Mechanism of action**
      - ○ As a precursor to glutathione, NAC increases production of glutathione.
      - ○ NAC also directly binds to NAPQI.
      - ○ Through these mechanisms, **NAC scavenges NAPQI**, prevents its interaction with cellular constituents, and prevents hepatic cell death.
      - ○ NAC is most effective at preventing acetaminophen toxicity when given within 8 hours of ingestion of the overdose, because it acts by **preventing the accumulation of a toxic metabolite.** However, beneficial effects of NAC can be expected at later times (even >24 hours) if acetaminophen blood concentrations remain above the threshold for saturation of phase II conjugation.
    - **Main adverse effects**
      - ○ Oral formulation is associated with GI symptoms and vomiting.
      - ○ Antiemetics can be used to increase tolerance to oral NAC.
      - ○ Intravenous formulation can trigger anaphylactic reactions (rare).
    - NAC does not react extensively with activated charcoal. The two treatments can be used concurrently.
    - NAC is recognized as the antidote of choice for acetaminophen toxicity.

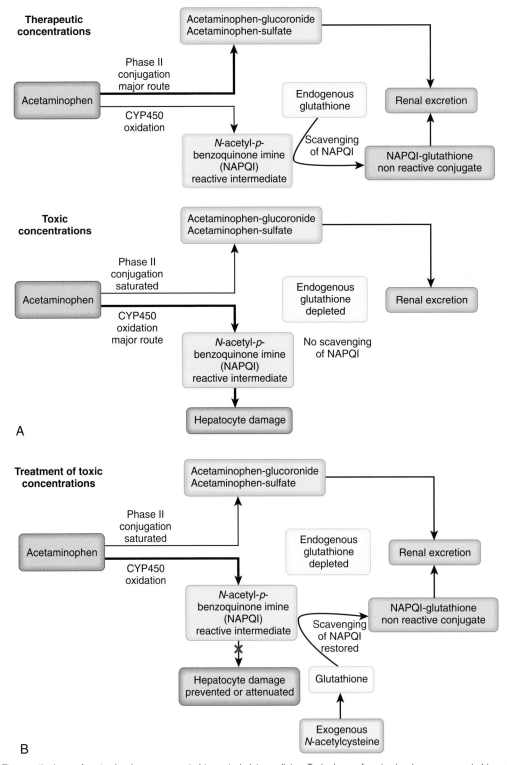

Figure 7-6. A, Therapeutic doses of acetaminophen are converted to nontoxic intermediates. Toxic doses of acetaminophen are converted to reactive intermediates that damage the liver. **B,** Treatment of acetaminophen toxicity involves the use of drugs that scavenge reactive intermediates.

Salicylates

- The salicylates comprise a large group of compounds derived from salicylic acid.
- Acetylsalicylic acid (aspirin) is the most recognizable and one of the oldest and most widely used agents for antiinflammatory, antipyretic, antiplatelet, and analgesic purposes.

- Significant quantities of salicylates are also present in a wide variety of compounds including rubs to treat minor aches and pains (e.g., methyl salicylate rubs) and keratolytics used to treat warts (e.g., salicylic acid) and acne. The antidiarrheal agent Pepto-Bismol contains subsalicylates. Some of these preparations have a **very high salicylate content,** such that even relatively small quantities can produce severe

TABLE 7-1. Salicylate Toxicity			
Toxicodynamics		**Treatment**	
Stage	**Signs and Symptoms**	**Approach**	**Intervention**
Mild	Hyperventilation Respiratory alkalosis Nausea, vomiting Gastrointestinal (GI) pain Tinnitus, hearing loss Dizziness Alkaline urine	Reduce salicylate absorption	**Activated charcoal** Binds salicylate in gut to prevent absorption Multiple-dose activated charcoal (MDAC) useful for intoxication with enteric-coated or slow-release formulations
Moderate	In addition to above: Metabolic acidosis Acidic urine Dehydration Hypotension, tachycardia Slurred speech Fever		**Whole bowel irrigation** Speeds GI transit of drug Useful for intoxications with enteric-coated or slow-release preparations
Severe	In addition to above: Respiratory acidosis Hypoxemia Acidemia Severe dehydration Oliguria Hypotension Myocardial depression Convulsions Coma Cerebral edema Pulmonary edema Cardiopulmonary arrest	Increase salicylate elimination	**MDAC** Useful when salicylate has already been absorbed Decreases free salicylate concentration in gut Promotes diffusion of blood-borne salicylate into the gut for excretion **Urine alkalinization** (bicarbonate diuresis; ion trapping) Intravenous bicarbonate administration Increases urine pH Increases ionization of salicylate Ionization of salicylate prevents reabsorption from renal tubule **Hemodialysis** Directly removes salicylate from blood

toxicity. Oil of wintergreen (methyl salicylate) contains approximately 7000 mg of salicylate per teaspoon, the equivalent of approximately 22 aspirin tablets.

■ **Salicylate toxicity** (Table 7-1)
  ▲ The widespread availability of salicylate preparations has resulted in a relatively high incidence of salicylate poisoning. Acute ingestion of toxic quantities may occur in accidental overdoses or in suicide attempts. Toxicity may also occur chronically because at **high therapeutic doses** (e.g., antiinflammatory doses) **elimination mechanisms** are nearly or completely **saturated** and salicylates exhibit zero-order kinetics. Some of the early-phase signs and symptoms of salicylate poisoning (see later) may be apparent at high therapeutic doses.
  ▲ Salicylic acid is the primary toxicant, and toxicity is related to the amount of free salicylic acid present in the body.
  ▲ Salicylic acid is eliminated primarily by phase II conjugation with subsequent renal excretion of the conjugates. At low concentrations, salicylic acid is cleared by first-order kinetics with a half-life of approximately 2 to 5 hours. However, as mentioned previously, these conjugation mechanisms are near saturation at high therapeutic concentrations. Once the phase II conjugation mechanisms become saturated, elimination follows zero-order kinetics and the half-life may be extended to as much as 18 to 36 hours. In addition, renal excretion of free salicylic acid becomes the primary mechanism for clearance once phase II mechanisms are saturated.

▲ Salicylate toxicity manifests as progressive metabolic, neural, cardiovascular, and renal dysfunction.
▲ Accumulation of free salicylic acid has several toxic effects, which include:
  ● Direct irritation to tissues, especially the GI tract
  ● Stimulation of the chemoreceptor trigger zone to produce nausea and vomiting
  ● Stimulation of the respiratory center in the brain that causes:
    ○ Hyperventilation
    ○ **Respiratory alkalosis**
  ● Uncoupling of oxidative phosphorylation, which:
    ○ Disrupts cellular adenosine triphosphate (ATP) production
    ○ Triggers formation of metabolic acids (e.g., lactic acid)
    ○ Causes **metabolic acidosis**
    ○ Increases heat generation and causes hyperthermia
  ● Neurotoxicity via direct effects and disruption of cellular metabolism and glucose homeostasis, which causes:
    ○ Ringing in the ears, loss of hearing (tinnitus, ototoxicity)
    ○ CNS dysregulation leading to agitation initially with subsequent disorientation, seizures, and coma
  ● Dehydration arising from:
    ○ Diuresis caused by acid-base imbalances
    ○ Insensible water loss caused by hyperventilation and sweating

○ Acidosis-induced increases in capillary permeability
- Cardiovascular collapse from acidosis-induced:
  ○ Cardiac depression
  ○ Vasodilation
  ○ Dehydration

▲ Salicylate poisoning is progressive. The **early (mild) phase** involves:
- Stimulation of respiratory center and secondary compensation
- Direct irritant effects on GI and direct neural effects
- Signs and symptoms of the early phase include:
  ○ Hyperventilation and consequent **respiratory alkalosis** (low P_{CO_2})
  ○ Excretion of **alkaline urine** as the kidney attempts to compensate for respiratory alkalosis
  ○ Nausea, vomiting, abdominal pain
  ○ Hearing loss
  ○ Dizziness
  ○ Mild dehydration
  ○ Fever generally not present

▲ The **moderate phase** of salicylate poisoning involves:
- Progressive disruption of metabolic homeostasis as salicylic acid accumulates in cells and uncouples oxidative phosphorylation
- Activation of compensatory mechanisms to counteract metabolic acidosis
- Appearance of actions on other toxic effect organ systems such as the cardiovascular system
- Signs and symptoms of the moderate phase include:
  ○ Mixed **respiratory alkalosis** (low P_{CO_2}) and **metabolic acidosis** (high lactate, ketones)
  ○ Excretion of **acidic urine** as the kidney excretes metabolic acids
  ○ Worsening of dehydration and neurologic symptoms (e.g., hearing loss, confusion, slurred speech)
  ○ Cardiovascular involvement (tachycardia, hypotension)
  ○ Fever

▲ The **severe (late) phase** of salicylate poisoning involves:
- Worsening of the disruptions of metabolism and organ systems
- Signs and symptoms of the severe phase include:
  ○ Progression of CNS toxicity, wherein hyperventilation may switch to hypoventilation with consequent **respiratory acidosis and hypoxemia**
  ○ Progression of metabolic acidosis to severe levels; **blood pH is lowered** (acidemia)
  ○ Progression of dehydration to severe levels; **urine output is low or absent**
  ○ **Marked CNS dysfunction** including convulsions, coma
  ○ Cardiovascular abnormalities with significant **hypotension, myocardial depression,** and **impaired perfusion** of all organs
  ○ Cerebral and pulmonary edema
  ○ Cardiopulmonary arrest

▲ **Treatment of salicylate poisoning**
- Unfortunately, there are no specific antidotes for salicylate poisoning. Treatments include general measures to support ventilation and renal function and to maintain acid-base balance. **Toxicokinetic treatments** aimed at decreasing the absorption or increasing the elimination of the toxicant, salicylic acid, are also central to the treatment of salicylate poisoning.
- **Reduction of absorption** is attempted.
  ○ Emesis not recommended
  ○ **Activated charcoal** is used to decrease absorption of salicylates. MDAC may increase elimination and shorten the half-life of salicylic acid. MDAC is also useful in poisoning with enteric-coated or slow-release formulations.
- **Whole bowel irrigation** is performed.
  ○ Useful when activated charcoal does not reduce salicylic acid levels or for poisoning with enteric-coated or slow-release preparations.
- Enhancement of elimination is undertaken.
- **Urine alkalinization**
  ○ **Salicylic acid** is a **weak acid** with a pK_a of approximately 3.5 and therefore will be **ionized at alkaline pH.**
  ○ Later stages of toxicity are associated with acidic blood and urine; this acidity promotes the distribution of salicylic acid to the tissues and renal tubular reabsorption, which limits renal excretion.
  ○ Standard of care recommends bicarbonate infusion (usually with potassium supplementation) (sometimes called **bicarbonate diuresis**).
- **Bicarbonate diuresis**
  ○ It maintains normal or slightly alkalemic pH to reduce the distribution of salicylic acid to the intracellular compartment.
  ○ It replenishes bicarbonate lost through renal excretion as the kidney attempts to compensate for respiratory alkalosis caused by hyperventilation.
  ○ Alkalinization of urine converts salicylic acid to its ionized form and prevents its reabsorption from renal tubules (ion trapping).
  ○ Alkalinization of urine from pH 5 to pH 8 may increase renal excretion of salicylic acid by tenfold to twentyfold.
  ○ The main adverse effect is the potential to aggravate pulmonary or cerebral edema.
- Hemodialysis is indicated in cases of severe salicylate poisoning and in patients who exhibit refractory acidosis, refractory hypotension, CNS depression, or evidence of target organ damage (e.g., pulmonary edema, cerebral edema).

Opioid Analgesics

Opioid receptor agonists are used extensively therapeutically for their strong analgesic effect and illicitly for their psychotropic effects.

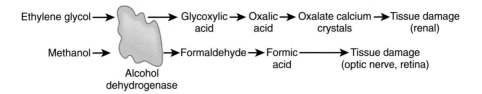

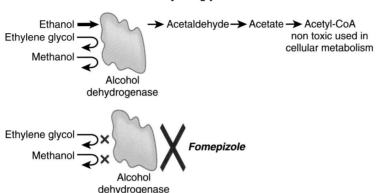

Figure 7-7. Mechanisms and treatment of ethanol or methanol toxicity.

■ **Opioid toxicity**
  ▲ Represents direct extension of the pharmacologic effects of neural depression
  ▲ Characterized by:
    • Miosis (pupillary contraction)
    • Respiratory depression (primary cause of morbidity and mortality)
    • Reduced level of consciousness
    • Hypotension
■ **Treatment of opioid toxicity**
  ▲ **Activated charcoal**
    • Activated charcoal is used to decrease absorption when opioids have been ingested.
    • It is most effective when taken early after ingestion. However, opioids decrease gastric emptying and GI motility. Therefore activated charcoal may still be effective even when there is a substantial lag between ingestion and treatment.
  ▲ **Whole body irrigation**
    • Whole body irrigation is used in cases of toxicity resulting from body packing, in which drug packets are transported by concealing the packets in the GI tract.
  ▲ **Opioid receptor antagonists**
    • Because opioid toxicity is a direct extension of opioid receptor stimulation, opioid receptor antagonists are the most specific and effective treatment (**antidote**) for opioid toxicity.
    • Examples include naloxone (used most frequently), nalmefene, and naltrexone.
    • They may be given orally, intravenously, or intramuscularly.
    • They **compete with opioids for opioid receptor occupancy** and reverse opioid toxicity.

  • Naloxone has a short half-life (1 hour), and opioid toxicity may recur as naloxone concentrations fall.
  • Naloxone may need to be given in multiple doses or intravenously, especially in the case of intoxication with controlled-release preparations or opioids with long half-lives.
  • Because treatment involves competition for opioid receptors, high doses of naloxone may be required for intoxication with opioids that have high receptor affinity (e.g., fentanyl).
  • Main adverse effects:
    ○ Induction of withdrawal symptoms (nausea, vomiting, agitation)
    ○ Aspiration from withdrawal-associated vomiting
  • **Opioid receptor antagonists** are accepted as **specific antidotes** for opioid toxicity.

Ethylene Glycol, Methanol

■ Although relatively infrequent, intoxication with alcohols such as ethylene glycol and methanol can result in a high rate of mortality if not treated appropriately.
■ Ethylene glycol is present in automobile coolants, which may be ingested in suicide attempts or by children because of its sweet taste.
■ Methanol is present in many household products (e.g., paint stripper, windshield washer).
■ Neither **ethylene glycol** nor **methanol** is particularly toxic per se, but these compounds are **biotransformed into toxic metabolites** (Figure 7-7).
■ **Ethylene glycol**
  ▲ Ethylene glycol is converted to glycoxylic acid and then oxalate, which forms crystals with calcium.
  ▲ Oxalate-calcium crystals precipitate in the renal tubules and cause nephrotoxicity.

- **Methanol**
  - ▲ Methanol is converted to formaldehyde and then formic acid.
  - ▲ Formic acid causes metabolic acidosis, which may lead to multiorgan failure and death.
  - ▲ Formic acid causes damage to the retina and optic nerve and blindness.
- **Oxidation** of ethylene glycol and methanol **by alcohol dehydrogenase** is the **initial step** initiating these metabolic cascades.

Treatment of Ethylene Glycol or Methanol Poisoning

The initial step in the production of the toxic metabolites of these alcohols is oxidation via alcohol dehydrogenase. Accordingly, treatment strategies are aimed at reducing the ability of alcohol dehydrogenase to metabolize ethylene glycol or methanol.

- **Inhibition of metabolite formation**
  - ▲ **Ethanol (ethyl alcohol)**
    - Ethanol has a greater affinity than ethylene glycol or methanol for alcohol dehydrogenase.
    - Saturation of alcohol dehydrogenase with ethanol prevents access of ethylene glycol and methanol to alcohol dehydrogenase and their biotransformation to toxic metabolites.
    - The main adverse effect is intoxication with ethanol, which may produce:
      - ○ Altered consciousness
      - ○ CNS depression
      - ○ Hemodynamic compromise
  - ▲ **Fomepizole**
    - Fomepizole is an alcohol dehydrogenase inhibitor that directly inhibits this enzyme and prevents biotransformation of ethylene glycol and methanol to toxic metabolites.
    - Advantages include:
      - ○ Lack of CNS depression
      - ○ High specificity
    - The main adverse effect is burning at the site of infusion.
    - Treatment must be initiated as soon as possible because effectiveness relies on inhibiting the formation of toxic metabolites.
    - **Fomepizole** has replaced ethanol as the treatment of choice and is considered an effective **antidote for** poisoning with **ethylene glycol and methanol.**
  - ▲ **Increasing elimination**
    - In cases of severe poisoning, hemodialysis may be used to increase the clearance of alcohols.

Cardiac Glycosides

- Used clinically in the treatment of heart failure and cardiac arrhythmias.
- Also found in a wide range of plants (e.g., foxglove, milkweed) and herbal remedies (e.g., oleander).
- Have a **low therapeutic index.** Poisonings may result from small changes in absorption or elimination of therapeutic doses or from accidental ingestion of pills or cardiac glycoside–containing plants.
- **Cardiac glycoside toxicity**
  - ▲ Toxicity is a direct extension of the ability of cardiac glycosides to inhibit active transport of sodium and potassium.
  - ▲ The major target organ is the heart, with induction of cardiac arrhythmias.
- **Treatment of cardiac glycoside toxicity**
  - ▲ **Prevention of absorption**
    - Activated charcoal. Cardiac glycosides are well adsorbed by activated charcoal.
    - Gastric lavage has been suggested but has not proven to be of benefit.
    - **Bile acid binding resins** are given orally to sequester cardiac glycosides in the gut lumen.
  - ▲ **Manipulation of distribution or enhancement of elimination**
    - **Immune antibody fragments** (Fab fragments) are derived from proteolytic processing of antibodies against digitalis glycosides, one form of cardiac glycoside. These antibody fragments also bind other cardiac glycosides.
    - Antibody fragments exhibit reduced immunogenicity and are less likely to provoke hypersensitivity reactions.
    - Antibody fragments bind cardiac glycosides in plasma and prevent distribution to site of action.
    - Antibody-bound cardiac glycosides are rapidly cleared by the kidney.
    - **Fab fragments** are considered an effective **antidote** to poisoning with **cardiac glycosides.**

Pesticides

- Many pesticides act as **inhibitors of acetylcholinesterase,** the endogenous enzyme responsible for the degradation of acetylcholine.
- **Organophosphates** (e.g., malathion, parathion) are **time-dependent irreversible inhibitors** of acetylcholinesterase. Organophosphates form a broad group of agents used extensively as insecticides throughout the world and as nerve gas agents.
- **Carbamates** (e.g., carbaryl, carbofuran) are **reversible inhibitors** of acetyl cholinesterase used primarily as insecticides.
- **Toxicity of organophosphate and carbamate pesticides**
  - ▲ The primary mechanism of action of these agents is inhibition of acetylcholinesterase, the enzyme responsible for degrading acetylcholine into choline and acetate, with the resultant accumulation of acetylcholine (ACh) in neuroeffector junctions. Overstimulation of cholinergic receptors is responsible for the signs and symptoms and toxicity of organophosphate and carbamate poisoning (Figure 7-8).

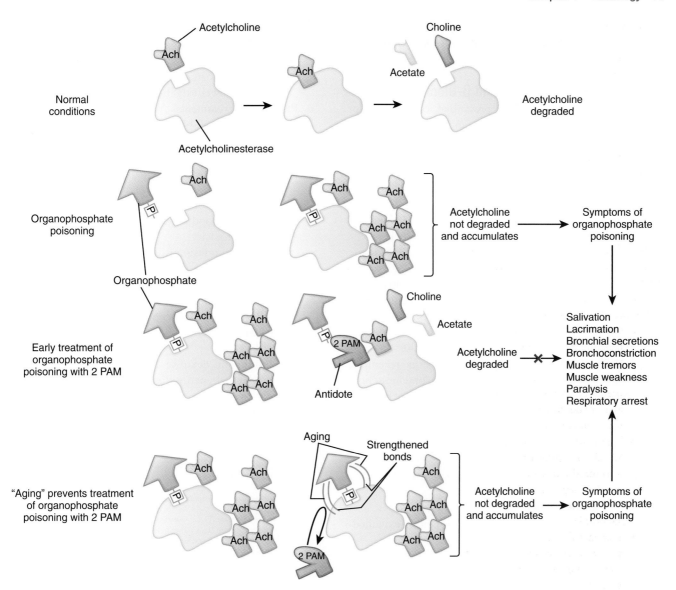

Figure 7-8. Toxicodynamics of organophosphate poisoning.

▲ Excess acetylcholine results in overstimulation of cholinergic **muscarinic and nicotinic** receptors in various tissues.
  - Excess stimulation of **muscarinic** receptors results in:
    ○ Increased salivation and bronchial secretions
    ○ Bronchoconstriction
    ○ Bradycardia
  - Excess stimulation of **nicotinic** receptors results in:
    ○ Muscle tremors
    ○ Muscle weakness and paralysis
  - Respiratory compromise is the major cause of morbidity and mortality.
▲ **Treatment of organophosphate and carbamate pesticide toxicity**
  - **Pharmacological antagonists**
    ○ Atropine, a muscarinic receptor antagonist, is used to reverse the excess muscarinic stimulation resulting from accumulation of acetylcholine.

- **Enzyme activators**—oximes such as pralidoxime [2-PAM]
    ○ 2-PAM disrupts a phophoryl-ester bond (-P- in Figure 7-8) between the organophosphate molecule and acetylcholinesterase to **release the organophosphate from enzyme.**
    ○ **This reactivates acetylcholinesterase** and reverses the effects of cholinesterase inhibitors.
    ○ Organophosphate inhibitors undergo a time-dependent process (called *aging*) that strengthens the bonds between the inhibitor and enzyme. This results in irreversibility of the inhibition. Once aging has occurred, 2-PAM and other oximes are unable to break the bonds between inhibitor and enzyme. Consequently, after aging, oximes are not able to reactivate acetylcholinesterase.
    ○ Oximes must be given before aging has occurred, generally within a few to 24 hours after exposure

depending on the type of organophosphate agent. Thus, early recognition and treatment of organophosphate poisoning are critical.

Calcium Channel Blockers and β-Blockers

■ Calcium channel blockers are prescribed for a number of cardiovascular conditions (e.g., angina, hypertension, tachycardia).

■ β-Blockers are also used extensively for cardiovascular applications (hypertension, heart failure, angina).

■ The widespread use of these drugs has led to an increase in toxicity from overdose, particularly in children, who may become symptomatic with ingestion of a single tablet.

■ **Toxicity of calcium channel blockers and β-blockers**
  ▲ Toxicity is a direct extension of the pharmacologic activity of these agents.
  ▲ Calcium channel blockers decrease calcium entry into:
    • Blood vessels—excessive blockade of calcium entry results in hypotension that may progress to shock
    • Cardiac cells—resulting in decreased force of contraction and conduction of the cardiac impulse
  ▲ β-Blockers reduce stimulation of β-adrenergic receptors, resulting in reduced generation of the second messenger cAMP and reduced function of calcium channels.
  ▲ β-Blocker overdose primarily affects the heart via:
    • Decreased calcium entry
    • Decreased force of contraction
    • Decreased conduction of the cardiac impulse

■ **Treatment of calcium channel blocker and β-blocker toxicity**
  ▲ **Prevention of absorption**
    • These drugs are frequently administered as extended-release preparations.

• Strategies to reduce absorption may have beneficial effects because of continued release of drug in the GI tract.
  ○ Activated charcoal (especially MDAC)
  ○ Whole bowel irrigation

▲ **Physiologic treatments**
  • Calcium channel blocker toxicity
    ○ Supraphysiologic doses of **calcium are infused** to promote the entry of calcium into cells and reverse the effects of calcium channel blockers.
    ○ Direct **vasoconstrictor agents** (e.g., norepinephrine) are used to counteract peripheral vasodilation and raise blood pressure.
  • β-Blocker toxicity
    ○ Glucagon infusion is used to **stimulate cAMP production** via a non–β-adrenergic receptor pathway.
    ○ Increased cAMP generation improves cardiac pumping and cardiac conduction.
  • Insulin-euglycemic clamp has been used to treat both calcium channel blocker and β-adrenergic blocker overdose.
    ○ Insulin and dextrose are infused simultaneously to produce hyperinsulinemia but maintain blood glucose level.
    ○ Precise mechanism is unclear, but it improves cardiac pumping and cardiac conduction.

Websites

American Association of Poison Control Centers: www.aapcc.org
Canadian Association of Poison Control Centres: www.capcc.ca/resources/resources.php
Glossary of toxicologic terms: http://sis.nlm.nih.gov/enviro/iupacglossary/frontmatter.html
National Library of Medicine (U.S.): www.toxnet.nlm.nih.gov
National Toxicology Program (U.S.): http://cerhr.niehs.nih.gov/reports/index.html
World Health Organization: www.who.int/ipcs/poisons/centre/directory/en/index.html

Chapter 8

Herbal Medications

Plants and plant-derived substances have been used as medicines for centuries. Indeed, herbal medications formed the bulk of pharmacopeias until the early twentieth century. Even currently, plants remain an important source of pharmaceuticals. Herbal medications, as defined by the World Health Organization (WHO), include plants, plant components, extracts of plants, and drinks, tablets, and capsules manufactured from plant sources. The WHO has estimated that over 10,000 species of plants have been used for medicinal purposes.

Systematic study of the use of herbals as complementary medicine is relatively sparse. Nevertheless, conservative estimates suggest that approximately 20% to 50% of the general population uses some form of herbal medicine. The prevalence of use is likely underestimated. Some surveys indicate that as many as two thirds of patients are reluctant to divulge use of herbal or complementary medicines to their physicians. Compounding the problems, many physicians fail to ask directly about herbal preparations. In addition, patients fear disapproval of their care providers because most people believe that physicians are dismissive of herbal medications. Moreover, most users of herbal medications believe that the natural sources of these preparations confer a greater degree of safety than conventional pharmaceuticals, and thus these users feel less need to discuss their use.

REGULATORY ISSUES

Initially, in the United States, herbal medications were included with conventional pharmaceuticals for the purposes of regulation. In 1962 a distinction was made between drugs and botanicals, with botanicals assigned to the category of food supplements. As a result, herbal medications have a **lower threshold of burden of evidence.** Subsequently, the Dietary Supplement Health and Education Act (DSHEA; 1994) further delineated regulations pertaining to herbal medications. Herbal medications were defined as compounds containing vitamins, amino acids, herbs, botanical substances, concentrates, or extracts. However, unlike conventional pharmaceuticals, manufacturers are **not required** to provide the Food and Drug Administration (FDA) with data showing

effectiveness and safety—nor are manufacturers required to **report adverse events** to the FDA. Indeed, the regulatory burden is placed on the FDA to show lack of efficacy or safety. Although manufacturers may not claim effectiveness for specific conditions (e.g., angina), they are allowed to make **general claims** of health benefits (e.g., promotes heart health).

The FDA has instituted new regulations that improve labeling and manufacturing specifications. The National Center for Complementary and Alternative Medicine (NCCAM) oversees research activities concerning herbal medications. Lastly, the botanical industry itself has established its own regulatory body, the American Herbal Products Association (AHPA).

Other countries also have various degrees of oversight of the marketing and use of herbal medications. European countries have a much longer history of herbal medication use and regulation. The European Union has a much more stringent oversight system. Similar to conventional drugs, herbal medications are reviewed for safety and efficacy and are licensed by the Committee on Herbal Medicinal Products (HMPC), a branch of the European Medicines Agency. Licensed herbal medications can make specific health claims. The HMPC also publishes monographs describing the applications, efficacy, and side effects for each approved herbal medication. Herbal medications appear on formularies and are prescribed by physicians as well as other healthcare providers.

USE OF HERBAL MEDICINES

Advocates of herbal medicine can find an herbal preparation applicable to virtually any condition. Several factors contribute to the more widespread use of selected herbal medications by a greater segment of the general population. The general public uses herbal medicine as a supplement or substitute for conventional pharmaceuticals most frequently for the treatment of chronic conditions for which conventional pharmaceuticals provide inadequate relief or produce undesirable side effects. The **public often views herbal medication as safer** than traditional pharmaceuticals because herbal medicines are derived from natural sources. Because herbal medications are available without prescription in many cases, convenience and personal control of healthcare decisions also motivate use of herbal medications. Major applications of herbal medicines include the treatment of sleep disorders, cardiovascular disorders, depression, chronic pain, prostatic hypertrophy, obesity, erectile dysfunction, and infection (e.g., the common cold). Given the reluctance of patients to share information concerning the use of herbal medications, physicians should use sound judgment and contextual suspicion to inquire about herbal medication use when treating patients with these conditions.

Practice Points

Despite the scant or contradictory evidence supporting the use of herbal medications for many indications, it is clear that the general public has embraced herbal medications. Accordingly, it is important that physicians be knowledgeable about commonly used herbal medications and ask patients about use of these preparations. Many patients are reluctant to divulge their use of alternative or complementary medicines because they fear the reaction of their physicians. Therefore it is important to inquire about herbal medications in a routine **nonthreatening manner.** If patients acknowledge their use of herbal medications, the physician should determine whether the patient is self-medicating or is receiving guidance from another practitioner (e.g., herbalist, pharmacist). Even if the patient does not acknowledge use of herbal medications, clinicians should **proactively discuss** possible herbal medication candidates. The physician should present a balanced picture regarding herbal medications by indicating that there is evidence both supporting and refuting their use.

- The patient should be informed that just because herbals are natural products, they are **not necessarily any safer** than conventional drugs.
- In addition, it is important to educate patients about the **potential for interaction** between herbal medications and conventional drugs and other interventions (e.g., surgery).
- The physician should refer the patient to reliable sources of patient information on herbals. Most countries maintain a national registry of herbal medications; these registries, which can be found at regulatory agency websites (e.g., NCCAM at the National Institutes of Health [NIH] in the United States and the HMPC monographs in the European Union), serve as valuable sources of information.

RELIABILITY OF HERBAL PRODUCTS

There is a great deal of variability in the safety and efficacy of herbal medications. A number of factors contribute to variability in herbal medications, including the following:

- Constituents
  - ▲ Herbal medications are complex mixtures of substances.
  - ▲ Constituents may interact for beneficial or harmful effects.
  - ▲ Active ingredient(s) providing beneficial effects may not be known.
  - ▲ Constituents vary depending on
    - • Species of plant used (e.g., Echinacea purpurea vs Echinacea angustifolia)

- • Part of plant used—biologically active ingredients may reside in different parts of the plant (e.g., stem vs leaf)
    - • Growing, harvesting, and storage conditions
    - • Processing methods
- Contamination caused by:
  - ▲ Heavy metals, such as lead and mercury
  - ▲ Adulteration with other pharmacologically active substances
- Standardization
  - ▲ Often the active ingredient is not known. Thus standards for ingredients and recommended doses are not established. Similarly, standards for labeling may also not have been established.
  - ▲ Even when the active ingredient is known, herbal medicines have shown considerable variability in consistency. In one analysis of 25 ginseng products, the quantity of active ingredients **varied from 10% to 300%** of the labeled amount. A similar analysis of Echinacea products showed that less than 50% of Echinacea products contained the labeled amount of the herb.
  - ▲ AHPA's *Botanical Safety Handbook* provides relative safety ratings for botanicals.
  - ▲ The FDA has initiated Good Manufacturing Guidelines for herbal medications and dietary supplements that will provide standards for labeling.

EFFICACY OF HERBAL MEDICATIONS

In response to increased demand for herbal products, in 1998 the NIH established NCCAM, which oversees and awards funds for research into complementary and alternative therapies, including herbal medications. In addition, in the European Union, HMPC requires efficacy and safety data before licensing an herbal medication. Nevertheless, compared with mainstream drugs, systematic research into the efficacy of herbal medications is relatively sparse for a number of reasons. The difficulty in obtaining standardized products, lack of knowledge of active principles, and the inability to standardize doses confounds both basic science research and clinical trials. In addition, lack of regulations requiring effectiveness and safety data and lack of patent protection in some countries have limited private investment in herbal research. Moreover, even within existing trials, many conflicting reports exist, perhaps in part because of issues of consistency of products tested (Table 8-1).

SPECIFIC HERBAL MEDICATIONS

Full discussion of the wide array of herbal medications used in various forms is well beyond the scope of this text. However, a relatively short list of the **most commonly used** herbal medications is presented. Table 8-2 presents side effects and drug interactions of some commonly used herbal remedies.

Echinacea

- Derived from *E. purpurea, E. angustifolia,* or *Echinacea pallida*
- Common name: coneflower

TABLE 8-1. Medical Applications of Commonly Used Herbs			
Application	**Herbal Medication**	**Mechanism of Action**	**Efficacy and Evidence***
Relief of benign prostatic hypertrophy	Saw palmetto	Antiandrogen	Unproven
Treatment of erectile dysfunction	Ginseng	Vasodilator	Supportive
Reduction of fatigue	*Ephedra*	CNS stimulation	Proven
	Ginseng	Unknown	Unproven
Reduction of hyperlipidemia	Garlic	HMG-CoA reductase inhibition	Proven
	Soy protein	Unknown	Proven
Reduction in duration of common cold	*Echinacea*	Stimulation of immune cell function and cytokine production	Proven
Treatment of mental disorders Anxiety	Kava	Modulatory effect at GABA receptors	Proven
Depression	St John's wort	Inhibition of norepinephrine, dopamine, and serotonin reuptake	Proven
Enhancement of mental performance	*Ginkgo*	Vasodilator	Unproven
	Ginseng	Unknown	Unproven
Treatment of nausea in motion sickness, pregnancy	Ginger	Serotonin antagonist	Proven
Weight reduction	*Ephedra*	CNS stimulant, catecholaminergic	Proven
	Bitter orange	CNS stimulant, catecholaminergic	Unproven
	Hoodia	Appetite suppressant	Unproven

CNS, Central nervous system; *GABA*, γ-aminobutyric acid.
*Unproven indicates that data are insufficient to support or do not support beneficial effects in this application. Proven indicates that the weight of evidence supports beneficial effect in this application. Supportive evidence indicates that only a few trials are available but data suggest a positive effect.

TABLE 8-2. Side Effects and Drug Interactions of Common Herbal Remedies		
Herbal Medication	**Side Effects**	**Drug Interactions**
Echinacea	Allergic reactions	Potential inhibition of CYP450 isoforms
Ephedra	Excessive adrenergic stimulation Hypertension, myocardial infarction, stroke Excessive CNS stimulation Agitation, sleep disturbances, psychosis	Numerous Synergistic interaction with methylxanthines Synergistic interaction with monoamine oxidase inhibitors Inhibition of antihypertensive effects
Garlic	Odor, diaphoresis, bleeding	Potentiation of anticoagulant and antiplatelet medications Decreased plasma levels of protease inhibitor drug saquinavir
Ginger	No major adverse effects	Potential potentiation of anticoagulant antiplatelet drugs (controversial)
Ginkgo	No major adverse effects	Synergistic interaction with other stimulants (e.g., caffeine)
Ginseng	No major adverse effects	No consistent reports
Kava	Hepatotoxicity	Inhibition of CYP4502E1 Potentiation of other sedatives (benzodiazepines) Inhibition of effects of levodopa in Parkinson's disease patients
St John's wort	Mania in bipolar patients Photosensitivity	Many Serotonin syndrome when combined with selective serotonin reuptake inhibitors or tricyclic antidepressants Reduced plasma concentrations of many drugs such as oral contraceptives, statins, warfarin
Soy	Gastrointestinal disturbance	Inhibition of actions of tamoxifen
Saw palmetto	None	No major interactions reported

CNS, Central nervous system.

- Available as:
  - Capsules
  - Extracts
  - Teas
  - Juice
  - Gels

Suspected Biologically Active Substance(s) and Mechanism(s) of Action

- Echinacosides: cichoric acid, alkylamides, and polysaccharides

- No consensus on primary active ingredient
- Stimulation of immune cell function
- Stimulation of cytokine production

Indications

- Immunostimulant to prevent or treat:
  - Upper respiratory and urinary tract infections
  - Common cold
- Wound healing
- Antibacterial

Evidence-Based Medicine
- Results of clinical trials testing the effectiveness of *Echinacea* in the prevention or treatment of respiratory or urinary tract infections are mixed.
- Recent meta-analysis suggests benefits in reducing duration of the common cold.

Adverse Effects
- Allergic reactions, especially in patients allergic to the daisy family (e.g., ragweed)

Herb-Drug Interactions
- May inhibit CYP450 1A2 and CYP450 3A and interact with drugs eliminated via the cytochrome P-450 enzymes

Ephedra
- Derived from evergreen *Ephedra* shrub (many species—e.g., *Ephedra sinica, Ephedra nevadensis*; different species contain different levels of active alkaloids)
- Common names: ephedra, ma huang, Herbal Fen-Phen, herbal ecstasy
- Available as:
  - ▲ Tablets, capsules
  - ▲ Extracts
  - ▲ Tinctures
  - ▲ Teas
  - ▲ Dried plant parts

Suspected Biologically Active Substance(s) and Mechanism(s) of Action
- Ephedrine is major active constituent
- Direct agonist activity at α- and β-adrenergic receptors
- Indirect adrenergic agonist activities via release of norepinephrine
- Central nervous system (CNS) stimulant, amphetamine-like properties

Indications
- Appetite suppression, weight loss
- Fatigue
- Athletic performance
- Nasal decongestion

Evidence-Based Medicine
- Supports appetite suppressant and weight loss effects

Adverse Effects
- Excessive adrenergic stimulation
- Hypertension, tachycardia
- Myocardial infarction, stroke
- Excessive CNS stimulation
- Anxiety, restlessness
- Sleep disturbances, psychosis

Herb-Drug Interactions
- Methylxanthines, such as caffeine and theophylline, potentiate effects of ephedrine.

- Monoamine oxidase inhibitors potentiate effects of ephedrine.

Note
Despite evidence of effectiveness for weight loss, in the United States the FDA banned the sale of ephedra-containing dietary supplements in 2004 because of the high incidence of cardiovascular-related side effects, some of which were **fatal**. Health Canada has posted several advisories discouraging the use of ephedra and ephedrine-containing products. In the United Kingdom ephedra is a scheduled drug, with specific maximum doses, and is available only under the supervision of a pharmacist.

After the ban on ephedra, nutritional supplement suppliers switched to two other herbal remedies, *Hoodia* and bitter orange. Plants of genus *Hoodia* contain pregane glycosides resembling steroid hormones. *Hoodia* is thought to act as an appetite suppressant. Safety and efficacy data are not established. Bitter orange contains synephrine, which has direct adrenergic pharmacologic activity resembling that of ephedrine, and the adverse effect profile is likely similar, although there has been little systematic investigation of its actions. Bitter orange is frequently found in "ephedra-free" weight loss supplements.

Garlic
- Derived from *Allium sativum* bulb
- Common name: garlic
- Available as:
  - ▲ Tablets
  - ▲ Powders
  - ▲ Whole fresh bulbs
  - ▲ Oils
- Active ingredients are also responsible for the characteristic garlic odor, so *deodorized* preparations lack active ingredients.

Suspected Biologically Active Substance(s) and Mechanism(s) of Action
- Allicin
- Alliin
- Potential inhibition of HMG-CoA reductase
- Vasodilator properties
- Platelet inhibition
- Antioxidant

Indications
- Cholesterol lowering
- Antiatherogenic
- Antibacterial
- Antihypertensive
- Anticancer

Evidence-Based Medicine
- Clinical trials support mild antilipidemic effect.
- Evidence regarding other effects is insufficient.

Adverse Effects

- Diaphoresis
- Dizziness
- Bleeding

Herb-Drug Interactions

- Garlic can cause potentiation of other anticoagulant or antiplatelet therapy or bleeding conditions.
- Discontinue before oral or general surgery.
- Use cautiously in patients with bleeding disorders.
- Garlic causes marked reduction in plasma levels of the anti-AIDS/HIV medication saquinavir.

Ginger

- Derived from *Zingiber officinale* root
- Common name: ginger
- Available as:
  - ▲ Tablets or capsules
  - ▲ Powders
  - ▲ Fresh root
  - ▲ Extracts, tinctures

Suspected Biologically Active Substance(s) and Mechanism(s) of Action

- Shogaol
- Gingerol
- May act as a serotonin antagonist

Indications

- Antiemetic
- Used to control nausea and vomiting related to pregnancy, chemotherapy, or motion or after surgery

Evidence-Based Medicine

- Evidence supports the use of ginger in pregnancy-related nausea and motion sickness.
- Data regarding use in other applications are mixed or insufficient.

Adverse Effects

- No major adverse effects reported

Herb-Drug Interactions

- Antiplatelet activity may potentiate other anticoagulants and antiplatelet drugs.

Ginkgo

- Derived from *Ginkgo biloba* leaves
- Common name: ginkgo
- Available as:
  - ▲ Tablets or capsules
  - ▲ Powders
  - ▲ Extracts, tinctures

Suspected Biologically Active Substance(s) and Mechanism(s) of Action

- *Ginkgo* flavonoids
- Vasodilator properties
- Free radical scavenger
- Inhibition of platelet activating factor

Indications

- Memory, cognitive impairment, dementia, Alzheimer's disease
- Cerebrovascular and peripheral vascular disease
- Sexual dysfunction
- Tinnitus

Evidence-Based Medicine

- Data for effectiveness in cognitive impairment and Alzheimer's disease is mixed.
- Positive effects on intermittent claudication have been reported.
- No evidence of effectiveness for other conditions has been found.

Adverse Effects

- No major adverse effects reported

Herb-Drug Interactions

- May potentiate the activity of anticoagulants and antiplatelet drugs

Ginseng

- Derived from *Panax quinquefolius* roots
- Common names: American, Asian, Korean, or Japanese ginseng; panax; ninjin
- Available as:
  - ▲ Tablets or capsules
  - ▲ Teas
  - ▲ Extracts
  - ▲ Oils
  - ▲ Powders

Suspected Biologically Active Substance(s) and Mechanism(s) of Action

- Ginsenosides (also called *panaxosides*), which are saponins; approximately 40 forms are present in ginseng root.
- Ginsenosides are structurally similar to steroid hormones and may have activity at these receptors.
- Different isoforms of ginsenosides exert different, sometimes opposing, physiologic effects.
- Individual ginsenosides have a multitude of effects. The mechanism(s) of action of the herbal ginseng preparations is not clear and is very dependent on ginsenoside isoform composition.
- Products are often standardized to total ginsenoside content, not to individual ginsenoside isoforms.

Indications

- Increase stamina, energy, and resistance to stress
- Improve mental and physical performance

- Immune system support
- Control of blood glucose
- Control of blood pressure
- Treatment of menopausal symptoms
- Control of blood lipids
- Treatment of erectile dysfunction

Evidence-Based Medicine

- Few well-controlled trials are available, and there are insufficient data to support most health benefits.
- Meta-analyses suggest a positive effect in erectile dysfunction and a blood glucose–lowering effect.

Adverse Effects

- No major adverse effects reported
- May disrupt blood glucose control in diabetics
- May have anticoagulant properties

Herb-Drug Interactions

- May interact synergistically with other stimulants (e.g., caffeine)

Kava

- Derived from root of a pepperlike plant, *Piper methysticum*
- Common names: kava, kawa, tonga, intoxicating pepper
- Available as:
  - Tablets or capsules
  - Drinks
  - Extracts
  - Topical solutions

Suspected Biologically Active Substance(s) and Mechanism(s) of Action

- Kava pyrones found in the root; substances from other parts of the plant may be responsible for liver toxicity
- Acts as a modulator of γ-aminobutyric acid (GABA) receptor function
- Local anesthetic properties
- Muscle relaxant effect

Indications

- Anxiety
- Sleep disturbances
- Depression

Evidence-Based Medicine

- Evidence supports the anxiolytic effect of kava. Current data suggest that effects are comparable to those of conventional anxiolytics such as buspirone.

Adverse Effects

- Serious hepatotoxicity has prompted many countries (United States, Canada, United Kingdom, France) to post health advisories discouraging the use of kava.
- Hepatotoxicity may be caused by the use of plant components other than the root.

Herb-Drug Interactions

- Kava inhibits several isoforms of the hepatic cytochrome P-450 enzymes.
- Kava causes potentiation of other drugs with sedative properties (e.g., alcohol, benzodiazepines).
- Kava may attenuate the effects of dopamine and thereby potentiate the effects of dopamine receptor antagonists used in the treatment of schizophrenia. The same mechanism may interfere with dopamine treatment of Parkinson's disease.

St John's Wort

- Derived from the flowering parts of *Hypericum perforatum*
- Common names: St John's wort, hypericum, goat weed, witches' herb, God's wonder plant
- Available as:
  - Tablets or capsules
  - Tinctures
  - Extracts
  - Teas

Suspected Biologically Active Substance(s) and Mechanism(s) of Action

- Hypericin
- Hyperforin
- Inhibition of norepinephrine, dopamine, and serotonin reuptake
- Suppression of adrenocorticotropic hormone (ACTH) and cortisol secretion

Indications

- Depression
- Anxiety
- Sleep disturbances

Evidence-Based Medicine

- Findings of a large NIH-sponsored trial of efficacy in depression were negative. However, other trials (European) and meta-analyses suggest beneficial effects comparable to those of some conventional antidepressants. The weight of evidence suggests that St John's wort is effective in mild to moderate depression.
- Effectiveness for other indications is not proven.

Adverse Effects

- Relatively rare but include photosensitivity, gastrointestinal disturbances
- May exacerbate mania in bipolar disorder

Herb-Drug Interactions

- Common with St John's wort as it induces several isoforms of the hepatic cytochrome P-450 enzymes and increases P-glycoprotein expression.
- There are numerous reports of decreased plasma concentration of other drugs such as:
  - Oral contraceptives
  - Statins
  - Warfarin

- Excessively elevated levels of serotonin and potential for serotonin syndrome (hypertension, tachycardia, sweating, headache, agitation, confusion, muscle twitches or contraction) are present when St John's wort is combined with selective serotonin reuptake inhibitors (SSRIs) or tricyclic antidepressants.

Saw Palmetto

- Derived from the berries of the American dwarf palm, *Serenoa repens*
- Common names: saw palmetto, palmetto berry, dwarf palm, cabbage palm
- Available as:
  - Fresh or dried berries
  - Tablets or capsules
  - Extracts
  - Tea

Suspected Biologically Active Substance(s) and Mechanism(s) of Action

- Active principles not clearly identified
- May interact with dihydrotestosterone to:
  - Inhibit production
  - Inhibit binding
  - Increase clearance
- May reduce α-adrenergic receptor expression in prostate

Indications

- Benign prostatic hypertrophy
- Prostate cancer

Evidence-Based Medicine

- Evidence is contradictory. A recent meta-analysis suggests that saw palmetto does not have beneficial effects in benign prostatic hypertrophy.

Adverse Effects

- Rare

Herb-Drug Interactions

- None reported

Soy

- Derived from the soy bean produced by the soy bean plant, *Glycine max*
- Common names: soy, soya; dietary products—tofu, tempeh, soy milk
- Available as:
  - Foods
  - Tablets or capsules
  - Protein concentrates

Suspected Biologically Active Substance(s) and Mechanism(s) of Action

- Soy protein
- Isoflavones: genistein, daidzein, and equol (daidzein metabolite)
- Isoflavones act as selective estrogen receptor modulators

Indications

- Hypercholesterolemia
- Hypertension
- Menopausal symptoms
- Osteoporosis
- Cancer of the prostate or breast

Evidence-Based Medicine

- Evidence conflicting for most indications
- Mild lowering of blood lipids
- May improve bone health
- Synthetic isoflavone ipriflavone has beneficial effects on osteoporosis
- Epidemiologic study suggests potential reduction in breast cancer risk
- Insufficient data to support use for other indications

Adverse Effects

- Allergic reactions to soy protein
- Gastrointestinal disturbances
- Caution advised in patients with estrogen-dependent tumors

Herb-Drug Interactions

- May inhibit action of other estrogen receptor modulators, such as tamoxifen

Websites

National Center for Complementary and Alternative Medicine: http://nccam.nih.gov/health

European Medicines Agency: www.emea.europa.eu/htms/human/hmpc/hmpcmonographs.htm

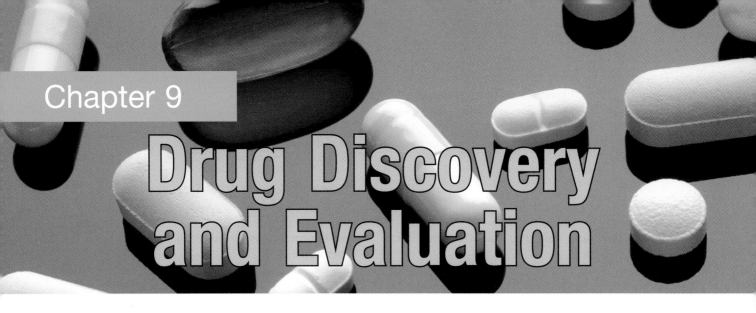

Drug Discovery and Evaluation

The drug discovery and evaluation process can be divided into **preclinical** and **clinical processes.** Preclinical studies are performed before studies in humans. Preclinical studies are typically carried out on animals, although there is increasing interest in using computer modeling to carry out these experiments. Once the safety profile of a drug has been established in the preclinical stage, the developers of the drug can apply to move into the human stages of testing.

PRECLINICAL PROCESS

The preclinical process begins with the discovery of a promising chemical compound. Fundamentally, drug discovery occurs in two ways: through either a **compound-centered** approach or a **target-centered** approach.

Drug Discovery

Compound-Centered Drug Discovery

Compound-centered discovery was the predominant source of new drugs until the late twentieth century. This approach relied very heavily on *serendipity and chemistry*. Receptors were not being characterized until the 1970s, so before the late twentieth century, drug discovery centered on synthesizing compounds that were then tested on biologic targets, typically receptors. The investigators were essentially blind to their biologic targets, and their inspiration for testing a compound in the first place often came from existing substances that either were found in nature or were endogenous to the body.

Natural Products

Naturally derived products were the first *blockbuster* drugs and paved the way for further drug discovery through compound-centered research. Once the efficacy and safety (and potential profitability) of compounds such as penicillin had been established, pharmaceutical chemists set about refining the structures of these agents to achieve specific pharmacologic effects. Table 9-1 lists some common drugs derived from natural sources.

Penicillin Penicillin was discovered in 1928 by Alexander Fleming while he was studying *Staphylococcus* variants. A mold

TABLE 9-1. Common Drugs Derived from Natural Sources

Compound	Source
Penicillin	Penicillium mold
Morphine	Opium poppy
Cyclosporine	Fungus

growing on his culture was causing his bacteria to lyse. The broth in which this fungus was grown proved to be inhibitory for a number of bacteria. The mold belonged to the genus *Penicillium*, leading Fleming to name it penicillin.

It was not until 1941 that the therapeutic potential of penicillin was realized in a small clinical trial. Production methods improved during the 1940s until penicillin could be manufactured in mass quantities by 1950.

Once the chemical structure of penicillin was established, chemists began work on synthesizing new versions, each with its own distinct properties (Figure 9-1). Penicillin-resistant bacteria produce β-lactamase enzymes that attack the penicillin structure. A simple modification of the structure of penicillin created a bulky chemical chain that blocks β-lactamases from the β-lactam site, resulting in the β-lactamase–resistant drug cloxacillin.

Endogenous Ligands

Endogenous agonists such as epinephrine, acetylcholine, and dopamine have a variety of pharmacologic effects. Once the chemical structures of these agonists became known, pharmaceutical chemists began designing drugs that closely resembled these structures, with key modifications to improve their potency and bioavailability or minimize their toxicity. Examples include succinylcholine.

Succinylcholine Recall from the chapter on autonomic pharmacology the mechanism of action of succinylcholine. Succinylcholine is two acetylcholine molecules joined together. This simple modification accounts for the prolonged action of succinylcholine when compared with acetylcholine (Figure 9-2).

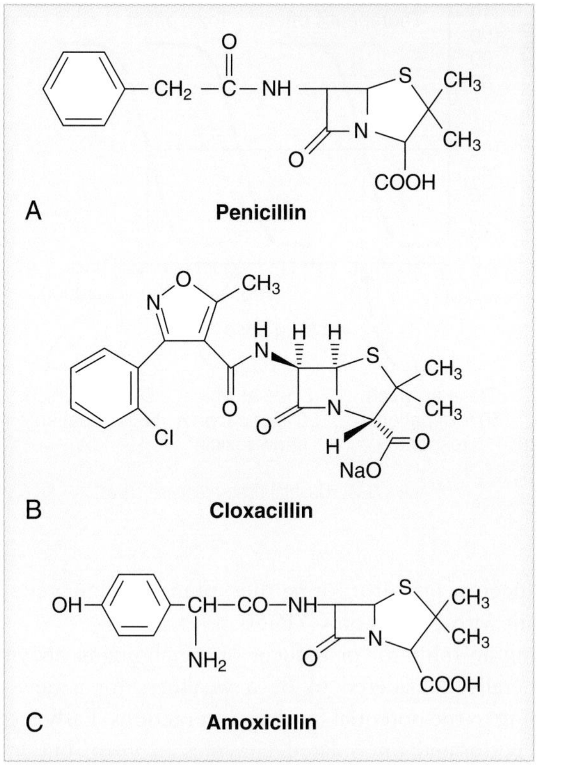

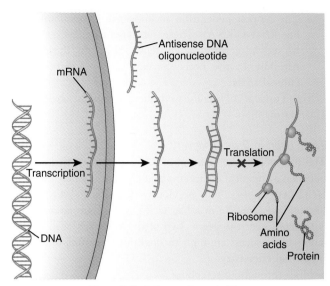

Figure 9-3. Antisense oligonucleotides.

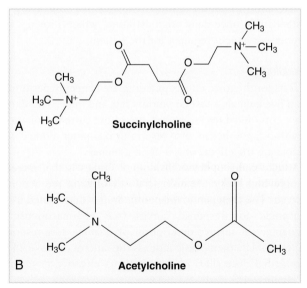

Figure 9-1. A, Penicillin. **B,** Cloxacillin. **C,** Amoxicillin.

Figure 9-2. A, Succinylcholine. **B,** Acetylcholine.

Target-Centered Drug Discovery

Modern analytical techniques such as protein crystallography allow researchers to map the structure of a receptor, so now instead of being *blind* to their biologic targets, investigators can **identify a target first** and then design a drug **to hit that target**. This allows for a significant improvement in receptor **specificity** and accordingly a reduction in side effects. This target-centered approach has been particularly useful in

indications such as cancer, allowing researchers to minimize toxicity of *targeted* therapies.

An understanding of the genetic basis for disease also provides new targets and will lead to gene-based therapies. The ultimate goal will be to selectively target genes that cause or contribute to disease, and prevent their expression. One of the most promising examples of this target-centered approach is antisense (Figure 9-3).

▲ Antisense oligonucleotides are **directed at** specific nucleotide sequences in messenger RNA (**mRNA**).

▲ The sequences in mRNA are known as the "sense" strand, and when these sequences are known, a **complementary** "antisense" strand is designed to bind this sense strand in a sequence-specific manner. Once bound, the antisense strand prevents the mRNA from being translated into a protein.

  • One antisense agent, fomivirsen, has already been approved for use in treatment of cytomegalovirus (CMV) retinitis.

▲ Second-generation antisense agents are designed to signal for destruction of the sense strand, once they have bound to it. The sense strand is destroyed by enzymes (RNAses), allowing the antisense strand to be used again.

  • **Cancer** is an example of a series of diseases that are perfectly suited for antisense therapy. An example is targeting of the **bcl-2** protein, an **antiapoptotic** protein that is **overexpressed** in many cancers.

  • **Apoptosis, or *programmed cell death*,** is an orderly process by which damaged cells quietly facilitate their own death. Prevention of apoptosis through proteins such as bcl-2 is one of the key reasons that cancer cells are so difficult to kill.

  • By targeting its mRNA and selectively **inhibiting the expression** of the bcl-2 protein, antisense agents can remove this survival instinct from a cancer cell, making it much easier to kill with cytotoxic therapies.

▲ The newest generation of antisense is small interfering RNA (siRNA). These substances behave similarly to second-generation antisense, although they occur naturally in the body. Several siRNA agents are in clinical trials.

The concept of gene-based therapeutics is covered in Chapter 6.

Tools Used in Drug Discovery

The first step in the creation of a new drug is to find a *match* between a chemical compound and a promising new molecular target (*receptor*). This previously daunting process, much like finding a needle in a haystack, has become increasingly automated over the years. Two of the key tools used in this automated process are **high throughput screening** and **combinatorial chemistry.**

■ High throughput screening
  ▲ This is an automated system that allows for the rapid screening of thousands of compounds.
  ▲ It allows one to assay for receptor binding and to identify biochemical and cellular targets.
■ Combinatorial chemistry
  ▲ This is an automated method allows for the generation of a large number of compounds from a small number of precursors. This technology allows pharmaceutical companies to create very large libraries of compounds that systematically cover most or all of the possible variations in structure that may occur around a common precursor.

Once a match, also commonly referred to as a *hit*, has been found, this becomes a **lead compound.** This lead compound is typically assigned to a research group, which will then try to make minor adjustments to the compound to maximize its affinity for its receptor, as well as attempt to improve its pharmacokinetic characteristics. This stage, in which scientists try to improve this lead compound, is referred to as **lead optimization.**

Preclinical Testing

After a compound has been synthesized, and appears to have efficacy, fine tuning is then done, focusing on the following issues.

Pharmacodynamics

Tests are performed in vitro to determine receptor binding affinity. Investigators at this point are interested in how specific the drug is for its receptor target, as this will provide an indication of the potential for the drug to cause side effects. Generally speaking, the less specific a drug is for its receptor, the greater the incidence of side effects.

Pharmacokinetics

■ A key step in the development process is to determine the route of metabolism for the drug. If metabolized by CYP450 enzymes, the isoenzymes involved will be identified. Tests will also be performed to determine whether the drug is an

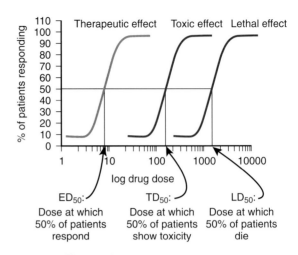

Figure 9-4. Quantal dose-response curve.

inducer or inhibitor (or neither) of metabolizing enzymes, again with a focus on CYP450.

■ Being an inhibitor or inducer of metabolizing enzymes is generally considered to be a weakness for a new drug, owing to the potential for **drug interactions.** Early tests can be performed on isolated enzymes in vitro, but in vivo testing will inevitably be performed to determine the effects of a drug in a whole animal.
■ Pharmacokinetic studies will also provide the **elimination half-life** of a drug, and this information will be used to determine the administration frequency of a drug. The gold standard is once-daily administration, which provides the most convenient regimen for the patient.

Toxicology

■ Tests for the toxic effects of a drug are generally performed on live animals, most commonly rats and mice. These tests are considered necessary because of the current limitations with using either in vitro testing or computer modeling to simulate the effects of a drug in a human.
■ A key feature of these toxicology studies is that **increasingly high,** supraphysiologic doses of drug are administered. The therapeutic index of a drug is determined using quantal dose-response curves (see pharmacodynamics chapter for further description of quantal dose-response curves). The therapeutic index is the ratio of the toxic (TD) or lethal dose (LD) of a drug to its effective dose (ED) (Figure 9-4).
■ One of the limitations of these data is that the doses used are so high that they often have minimal clinical relevance, except in overdose situations. It is not uncommon for widely used drugs to have significant toxicities that emerged in animal studies but have not been evident in humans.

Chemical and Pharmaceutical Development

■ Once the manufacturer has fully characterized the pharmacokinetics, pharmacodynamics, and toxicology of the new chemical, the manufacturer must also consider practical issues, such as how the drug will be produced and what form it will take. The chapter on pharmacokinetics provides a complete description of various dosage forms. Typically, the oral route is the preferred route.

■ At this stage, the manufacturer will also get an idea of the **cost** of producing the new drug. Small molecules, which are simple chemical structures, are typically very inexpensive to produce, often pennies per tablet. At the other end of the spectrum are biologics, which require a much more sophisticated and expensive production procedure. Although not proportional, this increased cost of production is one of the reasons cited for the high price of biologic agents.

Once all preclinical tests have been performed, the company may apply to the appropriate regulatory agency to undergo clinical testing. In the United States, the agent at this stage is referred to as an **investigational new drug** (IND). The regulatory agency that is responsible for approving new drugs in the United States is the Food and Drug Administration, whereas the corresponding agency in Europe is the European Medicines Agency (EMA).

CLINICAL PROCESS
Stages in the Drug Approval Process

Once a new drug application has been filed, manufacturers may begin the process of clinical trials, with the overall goal of proving that the drug is both efficacious and safe. The process is traditionally carried out in phases, with increasingly large numbers of patients in each phase. The manufacturer is responsible for the conduct of these trials, although regulatory agencies may conduct site inspections to confirm that studies are being conducted properly. Table 9-2 lists the key characteristics of each phase of the clinical trial process.

Phase 1

■ Purpose: establish the **pharmacokinetic profile** of the drug. This includes the area under the curve (AUC) and the half-life ($t_{1/2}$), as well as the metabolic routes of the drug.

■ Until recently, this stage was primarily carried out in healthy (usually) male volunteers, because of (among other considerations) concerns over running experiments on sick individuals who might benefit from proven therapies. Males were preferred owing to liability issues from teratogens. Lately, especially in the case of serious diseases such as cancer, phase I trials have included patients as well, providing these individuals with an earlier (faster) exposure to promising new agents.

Phase 2

■ In phase 2 we begin to see the **drug compared with results in a control group**, usually a placebo control. These trials include patients and are of moderate size, usually 100 subjects per group or less. By this time, a range of doses should be established, such that the main purpose is to determine efficacy and safety.

Phase 3

■ Phase 3 represents the **final stage before drug approval** and establishes the **efficacy** of the doses that will be used in the clinic. By this time, obvious safety issues should have been seen, so phase 3 trials are open to a much larger group of patients. However, owing to the size of these trials, less-obvious safety issues may arise, sometimes either preventing the approval of the drug or warranting a strong warning on the labeling.

■ Once a drug has successfully completed phase 3, the manufacturer can apply for a **Notice of Compliance** (**NOC**) from the FDA or equivalent regulatory agency. The FDA will review the efficacy and safety data then make a decision as to whether the drug should be approved for widespread use. Typically around 30 drugs receive an NOC each year in the United States.

Phase IV

■ Phase 4 is also referred to as **postmarketing surveillance**. Regulatory agencies may require double-blind controlled trials in this phase, depending on how many unresolved issues remain from phase 3. Phase 4 has not been a regulatory requirement, although recent events with drugs such as rofecoxib have illustrated the importance of postmarketing surveillance.

	Phase 1	**Phase 2**	**Phase 3**	**Phase 4**
Subjects	Healthy volunteers Patients	Patients	Patients	Patients
Design	No control Open label	Open label Single blind Double blind	Double blind	Surveillance Double blind
Size	Small (<100 subjects)	Medium (>500 subjects)	Large (500 to >1000)	Very large (market)
Duration	Short Single dose to a few weeks	Medium Weeks to months	Long(er) Months but usually <2 years	Very long Years
Primary purpose	Pharmacokinetics Dosage Safety	Efficacy Safety Pharmacokinetics	Efficacy Safety	Safety Effectiveness

TABLE 9-2. Key Characteristics of Phase 1 to Phase 4 Clinical Trials

Limitations of the Drug Approval Process

There are some important limitations to the clinical trial process, which highlight the need for postmarketing surveillance.

- Clinical trials are typically not large enough to reveal **rare but serious** adverse events that may become obvious once the drug is available to the general population.
- Clinical trials are typically of **too short a duration** to reveal serious adverse effects that may take years of continual use to develop.

Note that the commonality between these two limitations is **time**. Large trials take longer to produce results (owing to logistics), and of course longer trials take more time. Time is an important issue for indications such as cancer and human immunodeficiency virus (HIV) infection, and the **fast-tracking** of drugs has become routine in these diseases.

The **International Conference on Harmonisation of Technical Requirements for Registration of Pharmaceuticals for Human Use (ICH)** is an agreement among Europe, the United States, and Japan to improve consistency in the way products are registered.

- ▲ Studies that follow ICH guidelines provide assurance to countries that are using data from these studies that they follow a set of standards.
- ▲ The purpose of ICH is to **reduce duplication** of studies among countries, thus speeding up the approval process and reducing costs.
- ▲ ICH does not, however, guarantee that all of these studies have been performed in a manner that would minimize the potential for bias. Therefore it is important to understand the key features of a good clinical trial, and this will be reviewed in the following section.

Clinical Trial Design

The gold standard in clinical trial design is the **double-blind randomized controlled trial (DBRCT)**. However, simply having a DBRCT design does not guarantee that the study is of sufficient quality to provide reliable results. The key issues are **bias** and avoiding any confounding factors that might influence results either in favor of or against the intervention under review. In a DBRCT the goal is to minimize bias and confounding and thus be as confident as possible that the results are solely a function of the interventions under review.

- **Randomization** is a process by which study participants are randomly assigned to one of the interventions in the trial.
  - ▲ One of the goals of randomization is to stratify groups in the trial so that the composition of each intervention group is identical to that of the other. Demographic and relevant baseline characteristics of the participant's medical condition should be balanced to ensure that comparison groups all begin from the same starting point.
  - ▲ It is also essential that randomization be carried out in a way that ensures that the identity of treatment allocation is not revealed to the investigators (physicians, nurses), the patients, or anyone directly involved in the trial.
  - ▲ Ideally, to maintain allocation concealment, randomization should be carried out by a third party; an automated interactive voice response system (IVRS) is typically used for this purpose. With an IVRS, the patient interacts with a computer (typically over the phone), and the computer randomizes the patient to a treatment group, assigning the patient a number.
- **Blinding** ensures that patients and providers are not influenced by knowledge of their assigned intervention.
  - ▲ This is particularly important for subjective outcomes, such as quality-of-life scales, that rely on a patient's own assessment of well-being. Patients who know they have been assigned to the placebo group, for example, may be less likely to believe they are benefiting from therapy.
  - ▲ Blinding should again be carried out in a way that ensures allocation concealment. The most important step in ensuring allocation concealment is to make sure all interventions are identical in appearance. Therefore the authors of a study should explicitly state that interventions were identical in appearance.

The next considerations are statistical. One of the most common problems with clinical trials is that they are too small to properly answer the questions under review. A study should identify a primary outcome or outcomes; these are endpoints that are considered to be of most importance to the designers of the trial. The plan for statistical analysis, including sample size, is typically based on this primary outcome. Calculation of sample size is also known as **statistical power**. The larger a study is, the more *power* it has to reveal statistical differences between interventions, if they exist. In small or *underpowered* studies, it is difficult to know whether a finding of *no difference* was the result of small sample size or the fact that there were no differences in efficacy between interventions.

Another consideration when calculating sample size is the type of statistical comparison being performed. There are three types of comparisons: **superiority, noninferiority,** and **equivalence**.

- ▲ The simplest design is a **superiority** design, in which one intervention is determined simply to be statistically *superior* to another. Superiority designs typically involve a comparison with placebo.
- ▲ In a **noninferiority** design, the goal is to confirm that a given intervention is **not inferior** to a comparator. Noninferiority trials are typically conducted between two active comparators.
  - A margin for noninferiority is defined before the start of the trial.
  - For example, in a hypertension trial the margin for noninferiority for an intervention is a reduction in diastolic blood pressure of 10 mm Hg.
  - This means that the intervention can reduce diastolic pressure less than its comparator, as long as the difference between the two groups does not exceed 10 mm Hg.
  - If the difference does exceed 10 mm Hg, the intervention is deemed to be *inferior* to its comparator; otherwise it is considered to be *noninferior*.

▲ **Equivalence** trials are rare, and the purpose of an equivalence trial is to determine whether one intervention is statistically *no different* in efficacy than another.
  • The challenge with such a design is that not only is it necessary to prove that the intervention is **not inferior** to its comparator, but the study also must prove simultaneously that the intervention is **not superior.**

Analyzing Data from Clinical Trials
Efficacy Data
In general, data from clinical trials are expressed in two ways: as either **dichotomous** or **continuous** data. Continuous data (e.g., change in blood pressure) are often expressed as a mean difference. Dichotomous data (*all* or *none*) are often expressed as a relative risk (RR) or an absolute risk reduction (ARR).

Relative risk is a ratio of probabilities. For example, the probability of getting heart disease is 10% in smokers, and 5% in smokers who take statin therapy; therefore in smokers the relative risk of heart disease with statin therapy is 0.5 (0.05/0.10). In this case, it can be said that statins reduce the relative risk of developing heart disease by 50% (1 − 0.5).

The **absolute risk** of an event occurring is simply the proportion of patients in whom an event occurs. Continuing with the smoking example, 10% of smokers develop heart disease. The ARR would be the amount by which risk is reduced by an intervention (statins). The risk of heart disease in patients prescribed statin therapy is 5%; therefore statins reduce the absolute risk of heart disease by 5%.

▲ Subsequently, the ARR is expressed as a reciprocal, the number needed to treat (NNT). The NNT is the number of patients who must be treated with a given intervention to prevent an event in one patient.
  • In the example, ARR in heart disease with statin therapy is 5%, and the NNT is 20 (1/0.05). Quite literally, the NNT in this case indicates that 20 patients must be treated with statins to prevent one patient from developing heart disease.
  • The NNT is a popular tool used by clinicians to quickly provide perspective on the efficacy of a drug.

Note that there can be a huge difference in absolute and relative risk, yet the two terms sound similar, and they are often used interchangeably even though they mean two different things. Statin therapy reduced the absolute risk of heart disease by 5% and the relative risk by 50%. The latter sounds more impressive than the former—and that is why improvements in relative risk are often reported in the literature and (especially) by the media, rather than absolute risk.

Another commonly used calculation is the **odds ratio (OR)**. The OR compares the odds of two events occurring.

▲ In the example, out of every 100 smokers who do not take statins, 10 will develop heart disease and 90 will not. Therefore the odds of developing heart disease in these patients are 10/90, or 0.11.
▲ Of every 100 smokers on statin therapy, 5 will develop heart disease and 95 will not. Therefore the odds of developing heart disease in these patients are 5/95, or 0.053.
▲ The OR is the ratio of these two odds: 0.053/0.11 = 0.47.

Note that the OR and RR often yield similar numbers, and OR will also be reported instead of absolute risk. These two ratios are a preferred means for reporting data in the literature, despite the fact that reductions in absolute risk are far more intuitive and easy to grasp for patients and providers.

Safety Data
The version of the NNT used to compare the rate of adverse effects in a study is the number needed to harm (NNH). The NNH is the number of patients who must be treated with an intervention before one patient is harmed.

In a clinical trial, an **adverse event** is any harmful event that occurs to a patient during a trial. An adverse event does **not have to be related to the drug** and therefore is not the same as a side effect. An example of an adverse event is a patient being hit by lightning during the course of the study. Clinical trials also report **serious adverse events,** typically defined as any events that result in death, disability, or prolonged hospitalization. Adverse events and serious adverse events are sometimes collectively referred to as *harms.*

Pooling Data from Studies: the Meta-Analysis
Unless single studies have very large sample sizes, data from these studies are not typically considered to be as reliable as data from multiple studies when one is trying to assess the efficacy or safety of a drug. A **systematic review** is a way of gathering data from separate trials of the same drugs in a scientific manner that promotes reliability and reproducibility.

Authors of a systematic review will design a protocol that defines the *p*opulations, *i*nterventions, *c*omparisons, and *o*utcomes that are of interest in the review, also known by the acronym *PICO*. The protocol is analogous to a protocol in scientific experiments, in that if another investigator were to apply the same protocol to the literature at the same time, he or she should find the same results.

A meta-analysis is a pooled analysis of the papers included in a systematic review. By pooling data from several studies, a meta-analysis is a way of overcoming the limitations associated with single, small studies.

The data from a meta-analysis are often presented as a forest plot (Figure 9-5). The plot provides a quick graphical representation of the data, as well as numeric summaries to the left of the plot.

▲ The plot gives a quick summary of the **direction** of the data. In this case, four of five studies favor the experimental drug over placebo, the only exception being the OUTLIER study.
▲ The plot also provides an indication of the relative **size** of studies. The PANIC study has the largest point estimate (*blue square*) and is the largest study. The OUTLIER study is the smallest study.
▲ The horizontal line running through the point estimate gives an indication of the confidence interval, or the degree of **variation** within the study. Note that larger studies have less variation.

Forest plot comparing number of students who failed an exam taking an experimental memory enhancer (calmmedown) versus placebo

Study or subgroup	Calmmedown Events	Total	Placebo Events	Total	Weight	Risk ratio M–H, Fixed, 95% CI
ANXIOUS study	7	101	20	105	5.6%	0.36 [0.16, 0.82]
HOPE study	67	705	103	697	29.4%	0.64 [0.48. 0.86]
OUTLIER study	25	102	15	97	4.4%	1.58 [0.89, 2.82]
PANIC study	105	653	185	707	50.5%	0.61 [0.50, 0.76]
THINK study	20	458	35	440	10.1%	0.55 [0.32, 0.94]
Total (95% CI)		**2019**		**2046**	**100%**	**0.64 [0.55, 0.75]**
Total events	224		358			

Heterogeneity: $Chi^2 = 11.78$, df = 4 (P = 0.02); $I^2 = 66\%$
Test for overall effect: Z = 5.60 (P < 0.00001)

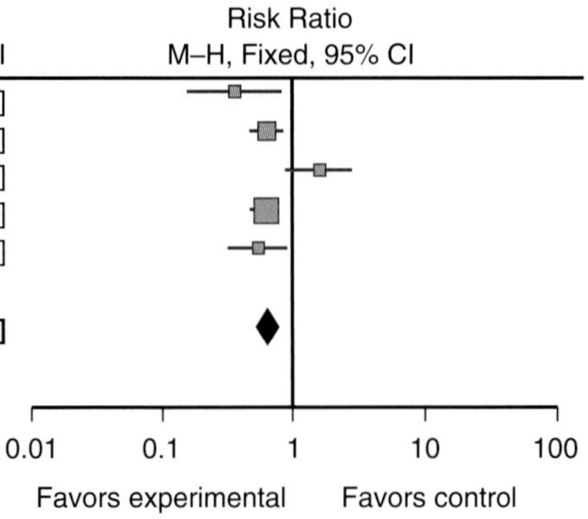

Figure 9-5. Forest plot.

▲ Studies whose point estimate or confidence interval crosses unity (1 on the graph) show no statistical **difference** between comparison groups. In this case, all comparisons are statistically significant except OUTLIER.

▲ The plot also provides a **summary** point estimate, the final black diamond at the bottom. Again, if the black diamond does not cross unity, the results of the meta-analysis are statistically significant, in this case favoring the study drug.

The final key piece of information that a forest plot provides is an indication of the heterogeneity between studies. In Figure 9-5, the results of four studies are fairly consistent, with the exception of the OUTLIER study. An important consideration when assessing the reliability of these data is heterogeneity of the included studies.

▲ The meta-analysis in Figure 9-5 also provides a measure of heterogeneity, expressed as either a P value or an I^2 value. When the test for heterogeneity yields $P < .05$, significant heterogeneity is considered to exist within the meta-analysis. The higher the I^2 value, the greater the heterogeneity. In this case, another analysis should be performed to account for this heterogeneity.

▲ In an **ideal** meta-analysis the design of **included studies,** including baseline characteristics of included populations, would be **identical.** In reality this rarely happens; it is this heterogeneity that weakens the conclusions drawn from a meta-analysis.

▲ Therefore a meta-analysis should comment on the **heterogeneity** of included studies. The more heterogeneous the studies, the less appropriate it would be to rely on the findings of the analysis.

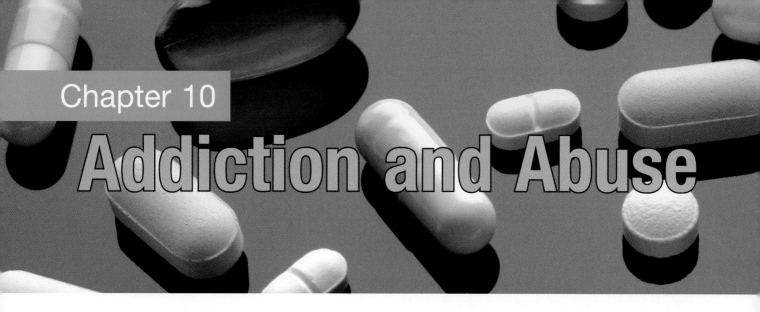

Chapter 10
Addiction and Abuse

There are many variations of the definition of *addiction*. In medical terms, addiction can be characterized as **recurrent** or **relapsing behavior** that results in a **rewarding** experience but also results in **harm**. Other features of addiction include a very **strong motivation** to participate in a given behavior (such as taking a drug), **loss of control** in regulating this behavior, and the presence of an **unpleasant** experience when the behavior is **not performed**. Addictions are chronic problems that are very difficult to treat and overcome.

Addiction can be described as occurring in cycles. The three general cycles include the following:

1. **Behavior** related to the reward (e.g., taking a drug or gambling)
2. **Withdrawal** or negative effect after the behavior is performed (feeling depressed)
3. **Craving** and preoccupation related to future addictive behavior

This chapter focuses on addictions related to substance abuse, but it is important to recognize that addictions can be unrelated to substance abuse and still possess many common neurologic mechanisms; a common example of addiction that is not related to substance abuse is gambling.

SCOPE OF THE SUBSTANCE ABUSE PROBLEM

The statistics in Table 10-1 are from a 2007 survey in the United States by the Substance Abuse and Mental Health Services Administration and provide some information regarding the incidence of substance abuse.

Many different terms are used to describe different components that are related to addiction, and it is important to highlight these terms and provide clear definitions.

- **Dependence**: **Physiologic** condition whereby the absence of a drug results in withdrawal signs and symptoms. It is very closely related to the psychologic processes that occur with addiction, because the body and the mind are not completely separate entities (when you are physically unwell, you do not feel good), but strictly speaking, *dependence* refers to only the physical component of addiction.

TABLE 10-1. Survey by the U.S. Substance Abuse and Mental Health Services Administration (2007)		
Incidence of Substance Use	**Number**	**Proportion of U.S. Population**
Adults who will have engaged in nonmedical or illicit drug use at some time during their lifetime	29 million	15.6%
Adults who will develop substance dependence on illicit drugs during their lifetime	5.4 million	2.9%
People over the age of 12 who are current users of alcohol	120 million	51%
People over the age of 12 who met the criteria for alcohol dependence	18 million	7.7%
People aged 12 or older who were current (past month) users of a tobacco product	70.9 million	28.6%
People aged 12 or older who were current cigarette smokers	60.1 million	24.2%

- **Withdrawal**: **Physical and/or emotional** reaction that occurs when a drug is **not administered** to an individual who is addicted. These experiences are dysphoric (unpleasant) and will be described in more detail.
- **Tolerance**: Phenomenon whereby performing a behavior results in a **smaller reward** than previous, similar behaviors. As a result, the behavior is often *adjusted upward* to reproduce the same magnitude of reward that was previously experienced. **Increasing** the **dose** of a drug would be an example of an upwardly adjusted behavior, as would gambling with a larger amount of money.
- **Obsession**: Recurring **thought**. For example, thinking nonstop about taking a drug would constitute an obsession.
- **Compulsion**: Recurring **behavior**. For example, actually taking a drug over and over would be a compulsion.
- **Impulsiveness**: Tendency toward unplanned behavior without regard for consequences.

▲ **Automaticity:** Behaviors that occur without conscious thought.

▲ **Craving:** Psychologic process similar to craving. It is also characterized by **anticipation and strong desire.**

▲ **Substance abuse:** Pattern of **inappropriate** or **illicit use** of substances for physiologic or psychologic reward.

▲ **Positive reinforcement:** When **exposure** to a stimulus results in a reward and increases the probability of repeating the behavior in future (e.g., getting paid for a job well done).

▲ **Negative reinforcement:** When **removal** of a stimulus avoids or reduces bad feelings (e.g., taking your hand out of boiling water).

A *motivational framework* can be used to help describe the difference between positive and negative reinforcement. In persons who are driven more by **impulse**, there is a state of arousal and tension before the addictive behavior is performed, and the behavior results in pleasant feelings. This would be an example of **positive reinforcement.** In contrast, compulsive behavior is characterized by stress and anxiety before the addictive behavior is performed, and the behavior results in relief from those feeling. This would be an example of **negative reinforcement.**

Throughout the time course of addiction development, the initial behaviors are primarily driven by impulse, whereas the latter stages of addiction are driven by a combination of both impulse and compulsion, and there is a shift from positive reinforcement to negative reinforcement.

NEUROPHYSIOLOGY OF ADDICTION

Studies to determine the neural pathways involved in addiction have involved both human and animal populations and focus on attempts to precisely stimulate or inhibit different regions of the brain and measure outcomes related to these interventions. The pathways are complex and beyond the scope of this text; however, a simplified description of the more important components will be presented.

There are some important details related to neuroanatomy that are relevant to understanding the pathways of addiction; some of them include the following (Figure 10-1):

▲ **Mesolimbic system:** Pathway in the brain that projects from the **ventral tegmental area (VTA)** to the nucleus accumbens, amygdala, limbic system, and other areas of the brain. It is strongly implicated in addiction and dopamine processing.

▲ **VTA:** *Tegment* is Latin for *covering* (*integument* means skin). The VTA is located on the floor of the midbrain and is responsible for reward signaling, motivation, and some psychiatric disorders. It is strongly implicated in dopamine processing.

▲ **Nucleus accumbens:** Pleasure center of the brain.

▲ **Limbic system:** Area of the brain associated with emotions.

▲ **Amygdala:** Latin for *almond*. The amygdala is an almond-shaped group of nuclei deep in the brain near the medial temporal lobes. It is primarily responsible for processing of **emotion**, especially fear and anxiety.

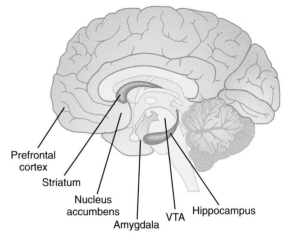

Figure 10-1. Regions of the brain involved in addiction.

Dopamine-Release Theory

All behaviors of addiction activate and increase dopamine signaling in the **mesolimbic** system. However, there is also evidence to suggest that dopamine-**independent** processing occurs in the **nucleus accumbens.**

Associated with the dopamine release theory is the concept of **predicted and actual** reward. This hypothesis suggests that dopamine release in the mesolimbic system represents a learning signal that reinforces constructive behaviors.

▲ An example would be a mouse that learns to pull a lever to obtain food. The pulling of the lever leads to dopamine release, as the animal is predicting a reward, whereas the actual reward (food) does not elicit a response.

▲ Drugs that release dopamine into this pathway generate an "inappropriate" learning signal, one that suggests that the behavior (e.g., taking of the drug) should be repeated.

The degree of importance given to dopamine in addiction remains controversial; however, one thing is clear—several addictive drugs target the dopamine pathway.

A number of classes of compounds are associated with addiction. Some of these, such as the opioids, sedative-hypnotics, cannabinoids, and central nervous system (CNS) stimulants are also covered elsewhere in this textbook. The following summaries focus on the aspects of these compounds that are related to addiction. There are two key common features to note as you progress through the following summaries:

▲ **Speed of onset is vital.** A key distinguishing feature of an addictive substance is a rapid onset of action. This is why most of the substances listed in the following pages are delivered by routes that facilitate quick onset (i.e., intravenous, intranasal, inhalation). This also explains why heroin, which has a rapid onset of action, is considered to be one of the most addictive of opioids.

▲ **Withdrawal is the opposite of the reward.** This is a key reason why substance addictions are so difficult to overcome. If a drug causes euphoria, withdrawal will cause dysphoria; if a drug is a depressant, then withdrawal will cause excitation (anxiety, seizures). Therefore when trying to maintain abstinence, not only must a patient cope with the loss of reward, they must also withstand symptoms that are the opposite of reward.

OPIOIDS

All of the opioids have abuse potential, although their primary use is in analgesia. Heroin is primarily used as a substance of abuse; therefore it is the focus of the following discussion.

Mechanism

Opioids act as agonists at opioid receptors throughout the body; however the μ receptor mediates their euphoric effects.

Actions

- Euphoria
- Sedation

Heroin is much more lipophilic than other opioids and therefore crosses into the brain much more readily, leading to a rapid and dramatic onset of action. It can be injected, smoked or introduced via the intranasal route.

Toxicity

- The main toxicity of concern with use of any opioid is **respiratory depression**, as the patient can eventually stop breathing at high enough doses. Other signs of toxicity include obtundation and miosis (constricted pupils).
- Acute overdose of heroin and other opiates can be treated with intravenous naloxone, an opioid antagonist. The effects of naloxone can be quite dramatic, rapidly reversing the effects of opioid toxicity. However, it must be noted that naloxone also has a relatively short duration of action, and if the elimination half-life of the opioid exceeds that of naloxone, the antagonist may wear off before the opioid has reached safe plasma levels, and respiratory depression can recur. Therefore overdose patients treated with naloxone should be monitored carefully.
- Naloxone can precipitate severe withdrawal symptoms in patients who are physically dependent on opioids.

Important Notes

- Tolerance to opioids does not typically begin until after a few weeks of use. Most of the effects of opioids are prone to tolerance, with the exception of constipation and convulsions. The extent of tolerance can be significant.
- Signs and symptoms of opioid withdrawal include sweating, runny nose, tearing, and yawning initially, followed by:
  - Insomnia
  - Chills
  - Weakness
  - Nausea, vomiting
  - Muscle aches
  - Elevated blood pressure
- Various pharmacologic strategies have been employed to reduce the effects of opioid withdrawal. Opioid antagonists such as naltrexone have been used, but patient adherence is poor.

- Another approach to withdrawal from heroin has been to substitute the longer-acting oral agent methadone. Methadone is eliminated much more slowly than heroin, allowing for a much more gradual withdrawal. It is also an *N*-methyl-D-aspartate (NMDA) antagonist, and this is believed to play a role in preventing tolerance to methadone.
- Opioids such as heroin are often combined with other drugs, one of the more common combinations being heroin and cocaine, known as a *speedball*.

ETHANOL

Ethanol is one of the oldest and definitely the most widely accepted drug of abuse. It is available legally and quite readily in most jurisdictions.

Mechanism

- Ethanol is a **CNS depressant**. It has multiple effects in the CNS, some established and others still in question. The following discussion will focus on established mechanisms.
- Ethanol **potentiates γ-aminobutyric acid (GABA)**, the major inhibitory neurotransmitter in the CNS, as well as **inhibiting glutamate**, the major excitatory neurotransmitter. The effect of both is to promote inhibition.
- The effects on GABA and glutamate neurotransmission are important not only for the effects of ethanol consumption, but also for the withdrawal after chronic use. Removal of the inhibitory effects of ethanol can lead to excess excitation, manifested as seizures.
- Ethanol also releases **endorphins**, which may play a role in the *reward* one gets with consuming alcohol. Secretion of antidiuretic hormone is inhibited, leading to diuresis.
- There are several other effects of ethanol that are less well understood. For example, ethanol alters levels of second messengers; however, the direction of effect seems to vary among tissues, even within different regions of the brain.

Actions

The actions of ethanol are dose dependent and are listed here in order of increasing dose:
- Low doses:
  - Flushing caused by cutaneous vasodilation
  - Sedation or loss of inhibition
- Moderate doses:
  - Slowed reaction time
  - Impaired concentration
- High doses:
  - Impaired judgment
  - Confusion
  - Irrational thinking
  - Impaired memory
- **Death** occurs at or above levels of 5000 mg/L (108 mmol/L) or a **0.5% blood alcohol** concentration.
- Ethanol is metabolized in the liver, oxidized to acetaldehyde primarily by alcohol dehydrogenase with a minor secondary CYP450 pathway, and then oxidized further to acetic acid by aldehyde dehydrogenase. The acetic acid is

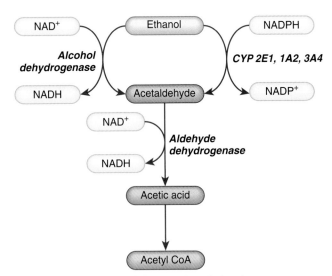

Figure 10-2. Metabolism of ethanol.

broken down to acetyl coenzyme A (CoA) as well as CO_2 and water (Figure 10-2).

- Two steps in this metabolic process require nicotinamide adenine dinucleotide $(NAD)^+$; therefore NAD^+ quickly becomes depleted when ethanol is being metabolized. This limits the amount of ethanol that can be metabolized to a constant amount (*zero-order* kinetics) per unit of time (about 120 mg/kg/hr).
- Depletion of NAD^+, a cofactor in a number of metabolic processes, also leads to the accumulation of lactate and lactic acidosis.
- There are genetic variations in the way ethanol is metabolized, and these polymorphisms may predict propensity for alcohol dependence.

Toxicity

Ethanol has both acute and chronic toxic effects. The acute effects are summarized in the previous section and are dose dependent, up to and including death. Chronic effects of alcohol abuse are listed here.

- **Liver:** The metabolites of ethanol, specifically acetaldehydes, bind proteins, and these adducts can then stimulate an immune reaction, which damages tissue. Eventually this can lead to cirrhosis and liver failure.
- **Brain:** Ethanol inflicts both reversible and irreversible damage to the brain. Chronic abuse leads to cognitive impairment, although it is not clear whether moderate drinking has any effects on the brain.
  - ▲ There are several mechanisms for the brain damage, including up-regulation of glutamate receptors, which leads to excitotoxicity. Chronic ethanol exposure may also deplete neurotrophins, factors that promote neuronal survival. Adduct formation, as noted previously for the liver, is also responsible for some of the damage.
- **Cardiovascular system:** Chronic alcohol abuse has been associated with hypertension, arrhythmias, cardiomyopathy, and stroke. Chronic ethanol abuse leads to oxidative stress and disruption of ion channels and may inhibit

protein synthesis, all of which can lead to cardiovascular complications.

- **Nutritional deficiencies:** Chronic ethanol use is associated with poor diet, as ethanol becomes the dominant source of caloric intake for an alcoholic. The lack of nutrients obtained from diet can lead to a variety of vitamin B deficiencies including Wernicke-Korsakoff syndrome and pellagra.
- **Fetal alcohol syndrome (FAS):** The effects of ethanol use in pregnancy are well documented. FAS is characterized by mental retardation and distinct physical features, including a wide separation between the eyes, a broad upper lip with no philtrum, a small head, and a short nose.

Important Notes

- Acute management of ethanol intoxication involves **maintaining respiration** and providing intravenous support with fluid and electrolytes until the body is able to metabolize the excess down to a safer blood alcohol concentration. In some jurisdictions, metadoxine is used to facilitate the elimination of ethanol.
- **Signs and symptoms** of ethanol **withdrawal** after chronic use include tremor, tachycardia, sweating, anxiety, hallucinations, insomnia, and elevated blood pressure. These signs and symptoms typically begin within 12 hours of the last drink and begin to decline after 4 to 5 days. As noted previously, seizures can also occur.
- **Withdrawal** is often treated with **benzodiazepines**. There is some concern about the use of these agents to treat dependence, given their own tendency to elicit physical dependence. Alternatives that have been tried with some success include nitrous oxide and antiseizure medications.
- **Disulfuram,** a drug that inhibits aldehyde dehydrogenase, has also been used to assist alcoholics in **maintaining abstinence.** Inhibition of this enzyme leads to a **buildup** of **acetaldehyde,** a substance responsible for many of the unpleasant side effects of ethanol: nausea, vomiting, flushing, and headache.
- **Tolerance** to the effects of ethanol can develop. This occurs in part because of induction of ethanol metabolism. As an adjustment to chronic use, the liver will **induce** **CYP450 enzymes** involved in ethanol metabolism. This enzyme induction can also affect the metabolism of other drugs that use those isozymes for their elimination.

CENTRAL NERVOUS SYSTEM STIMULANTS

Cocaine is the most well-known CNS stimulant of abuse. Amphetamines are another class of CNS stimulants that are used as drugs of abuse, and they are discussed in the chapter on CNS stimulants.

Mechanism

- Cocaine is a **sympathomimetic.** It acts as a **reuptake inhibitor,** nonspecifically inhibiting reuptake of several catecholamines, including **dopamine,** which is the neurotransmitter most likely responsible for its reinforcing effects. Inhibition of neurotransmitter reuptake increases the concentration and prolongs the actions of these transmitters in the synapse, enhancing their effects.

- Other neurotransmitters affected by this reuptake inhibition include norepinephrine and serotonin. It is not clear what role enhancing these neurotransmitters plays acutely, but chronic use of cocaine does appear to alter these neurotransmitters and may play a role in withdrawal.

Actions

- Cocaine produces **arousal** and increased **alertness** and enhances **self-confidence** and sense of **well-being. Euphoria** is experienced at higher doses.
- The elimination half-life of cocaine is short, <1 hour, and the onset of action varies between the smoked (rapid vaporization) route and the intranasal route. The drug can also be administered intravenously.
- Cocaine is eliminated primarily by hydrolysis, and its major urinary metabolite, benzoylecgonine, has a much longer half-life than the parent drug and is used to detect cocaine use.

Toxicity

- **Cardiovascular**: cardiac arrhythmias, vasoconstriction (coronary and cerebral vessels), hypertension, congestive heart failure and myocardial infarction
- Neurologic: seizures
- **Psychiatric**: anxiety, psychosis (hallucinations and paranoia), depression

Important Notes

- Signs and symptoms of cocaine **withdrawal** are typically the opposite of the effects seen with the drug: **fatigue, dysphoria, depression,** and **bradycardia.**
- Symptoms of withdrawal from cocaine are usually relatively mild and do not typically need to be managed by other drug therapy. Behavioral interventions are the primary strategy employed to promote and sustain abstinence.
- When drug therapy is attempted, agents that enhance GABA are often used, including benzodiazepines and baclofen (GABA_B agonist). The inhibitory effects of GABA are thought to ease withdrawal from the stimulatory effects of cocaine. Clonidine is also used to treat withdrawal.
- Perhaps because of the milder withdrawal symptoms, cocaine tends to be used less regularly than other addictive substances such as nicotine and opioids.
- *Crack* cocaine is a form of cocaine that is smoked rather than snorted. It is essentially cocaine mixed with sodium bicarbonate *(baking soda)*. Smoking achieves faster onset of action; therefore crack cocaine is considered to be more addictive.
- *Freebase* cocaine is an oily, water-insoluble form of cocaine. Cocaine is typically available as a salt. Freebase cocaine is also smoked.

CANNABIS

The use of cannabis and related compounds in therapeutics is covered in Chapter 15. In this section, the focus will be on the use of cannabis as a substance of abuse.

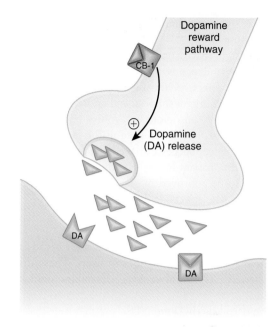

Figure 10-3. Cannabinoids.

Mechanism

Cannabinoid (CB1) receptors in the reward pathways of the brain are stimulated by cannabinoids such as cannabis, leading to the euphoric effects associated with this drug (Figure 10-3).

Actions

- Sedation
- Euphoria

Cannabis is highly lipid soluble and when smoked has a rapid onset of action. The onset is much slower when the drug is swallowed.

Toxicity

- Cannabis is considered to be a relatively safe drug in acute use. Acutely, psychiatric disturbances, including **psychotic episodes,** have been reported.
- Chronically, side effects are controversial, but some data suggest **cognitive effects** such as mental *slowing* and memory loss.
- There are also some studies, typically conducted in animals, suggesting that chronic cannabis use may adversely affect **fertility.**

Important Notes

- Cannabis is not a drug commonly associated with overdose situations, and there are therefore no drugs that are typically used to manage overdose with cannabis.
- For a number of years, the conventional wisdom was that cannabis was not *addictive*. However, with the current understanding of the mechanism of cannabis—namely that it activates the same dopamine reward pathways as many other addictive substances—it is believed that it is possible to develop a physical dependence on cannabis.

This has significant implications for treatment of chronic cannabis use.

- Another sign that cannabis may be capable of eliciting physical dependence is that it has been associated with a withdrawal effect. Cannabis withdrawal may include anxiety, irritability, dysphoria, and anorexia.
- Both naltrexone, an opioid antagonist, and rimonabant, a CB1 antagonist, have been used in the facilitation of cannabis abstinence. Successes have been reported with each, although rimonabant has been withdrawn from the market or failed to be approved in many jurisdictions because of psychiatric side effects, including suicide.

HALLUCINOGENS

The term *hallucinogen* is often used to describe a broad category of drugs that cause hallucinations in users. These drugs are also referred to as *psychedelics*. Examples include the following:

- Lysergic acid diethylamide (LSD)
  - ▲ Others: Mescaline, psilocybin
- Phencyclidine (*angel dust* or PCP)
  - ▲ Other: Ketamine

Mechanism

- LSD interacts with multiple serotonin receptors in the brain; however, its primary actions are believed to be mediated by agonist activity at serotonin 5-HT$_{2A}$ receptors in the prefrontal cortex.
- PCP is primarily an antagonist of the glutamate NMDA receptor. It has several other actions on other neurotransmitters and ion channels, but these are less well understood and are not thought to play as important a role in its effects.

Actions
LSD

- LSD has perceptual, psychologic, and somatic effects.
- **Disorders of perception** include altered shapes and colors, sharpened sense of hearing, and difficulty focusing on objects.
- **Somatic changes** include weakness, tremor, nausea, dizziness, and paresthesias.
- **Psychologic effects** include changes in mood, lapses in judgment, impaired ability to express thoughts, and hallucinations.
- **Physiologic signs** are primarily a result of activation of the sympathetic nervous system:
  - ▲ Mydriasis
  - ▲ Tachycardia
  - ▲ Alertness
  - ▲ Tremor
  - ▲ Increased blood pressure (slight)

PCP

- PCP induces **dissociation** and **distorted body image**. Its use, both clinically and in animal models, has been associated with onset of psychosis.

Toxicity
LSD

- Acutely, LSD and LSD-related hallucinogens do not appear to have any direct serious effects on the body in overdose situations.
- However, the altered perception and hallucinations can have indirect effects, leading to serious accidents involving users who believe they possess superhuman qualities, such as the ability to fly.
- In everyday use, the main toxicities are psychiatric, including the potential for inducing psychosis. Although this is a rare complication (<0.1% of users) it is well documented.

PCP

- **Aggressive behavior:** Users may become physically violent if they believe their hallucinations are becoming a threat to them. This can create problems for medical personnel trying to treat them, as they become part of the hallucination and may be perceived as a threat.
- At higher doses, PCP may induce stupor, muscle rigidity and rhabdomyolysis, as well as coma.

Important Notes

- LSD users can experience a *bad trip*, essentially a negative hallucinatory experience, which can be quite stressful and lead to agitation. Patients are usually treated supportively, with reassurance, although an anxiolytic such as diazepam may also be indicated.
- With the exception of LSD itself, the LSD-related hallucinogens do not act through the dopamine reward pathway. It is therefore believed they might have less propensity for dependence.
- LSD does stimulate the dopamine reward pathway, and there are some indications that dependence is more likely with this agent.
- No agents are available that can reverse the pharmacologic effects of PCP; therefore management of overdose is largely supportive. In cases of PCP overdose, acidification of the urine may help to facilitate excretion.
- In contrast to LSD and related agents, PCP can be fatal in overdose.

INHALANTS

Inhalants—agents that are abused via the inhalational route— range from the anesthetic gases such as nitrous oxide, described elsewhere in this textbook, to industrial solvents such as gasoline, to organic nitrates. Industrial solvents and organic nitrates are considered here.

Agents

- **Industrial solvents:** toluene (sources: paints, adhesives, cleaning solvents, paint thinner)
- **Nitrates:** amyl nitrate (*poppers*), butyl nitrate, nitrous oxide

Mechanism

■ Solvents have a variety of effects in the CNS. They appear to potentiate $GABA_A$ and glycine, enhance $5HT_3$ receptor function, and inhibit NMDA receptors.

Actions

■ **Acute effects** include euphoria, ataxia, and headache.

Toxicity

■ Industrial solvents can cause **damage to numerous organs**, including the liver, kidneys, and brain.
■ **Deaths** from cardiac arrhythmia have been reported at higher doses. This effect may be mediated by the effects these agents have on sodium channels.

■ **Neurotoxic** effects include impaired cognition, ataxia, optic neuropathy, and hearing loss.
■ Chronic low level exposure has also resulted in what has been described as the *painter's syndrome* fatigue, impairments in memory and concentration, as well as changes in personality.

Important Note

■ Nitrous oxide can be obtained from the propellant used in industrial spray canisters.

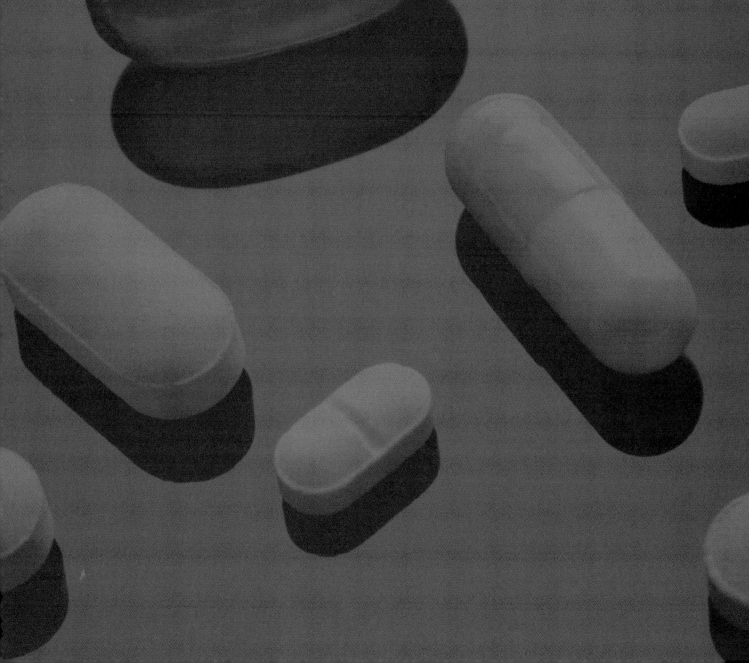

Section II
DRUG CLASSES

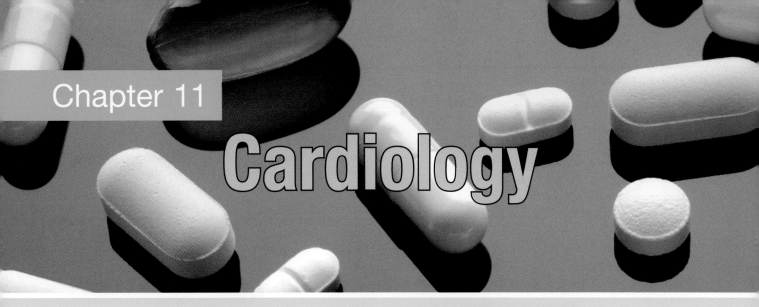

Chapter 11

Cardiology

Angiotensin-Converting Enzyme Inhibitors (ACEIs)

DESCRIPTION
Inhibitors of the angiotensin-converting enzyme (ACE)

PROTOTYPE AND COMMON DRUGS
- Prototype: capto**pril**
- Others: rami**pril**, enala**pril**, fosino**pril**, lisino**pril**, perindo**pril**, quina**pril**, benaze**pril**, cilaza**pril**

MOA (MECHANISM OF ACTION)
- ACE performs two functions:
  - ▲ Catalyzing the conversion of angiotensin I to angiotensin II
  - ▲ Breaking down bradykinin
- Through inhibition of ACE with an ACEI, the following effects occur:
  1. Lower levels of angiotensin II are produced.
     - Angiotensin II is a direct vasoconstrictor.
     - Angiotensin II results in aldosterone secretion, which causes Na and water reabsorption in the kidney.
  2. Higher levels of bradykinin are produced.
     - Bradykinin is a vasodilator.
- **Net result**: Because angiotensin II levels are lower and bradykinin levels are higher, there is more vasodilation; **SVR** (systemic vascular resistance) and **afterload** are lowered. Because aldosterone levels are lower, less Na and water are reabsorbed in the kidney; therefore **preload** is reduced (Figure 11-1).

PHARMACOKINETICS
- Most ACEIs are cleared predominantly by the kidneys. Dose adjustment should be considered in renal impairment.
- With the exception of captopril, all ACEIs have intermediate (12 to 24 hours) durations of action and thus have the advantage of once-daily administration. The duration of

action of captopril is shorter (6 to 12 hours); therefore it is given two or three times daily.

INDICATIONS
- Hypertension (HTN)
- Chronic congestive heart failure (CHF)
- After myocardial infarction (MI)

CONTRAINDICATIONS
- **Pregnancy**: During the second and third trimesters, the teratogenic effects are thought to be caused in part by fetal hypotension.
- **Renal dysfunction**: See side effects.

SIDE EFFECTS
- **Dry cough**: Attributed to increased bradykinin levels. Can be persistent enough to affect compliance and may lead to discontinuation.
- **Hyperkalemia**: Particularly in combination with K^+-*sparing diuretics*. Hyperkalemia occurs via the reduction in aldosterone but is usually clinically significant only with the addition of oral K^+ or in patients with renal dysfunction.
- **Hypotension**: Caused by vasodilation from lower levels of angiotensin II. Patients with ventricular dysfunction (low ejection fraction) are at greater risk.
- **Renal dysfunction**: Angiotensin II plays an important role in maintaining glomerular filtration rate (GFR) by constricting the efferent (outgoing) arteriole of the glomerulus. This is particularly important when the blood flow to the kidneys has been compromised. ACEIs cause vasodilation of the efferent arteriole. This decreases the glomerular pressure and reduces GFR. Volume depletion amplifies this effect.
- **Angioedema**: A rare but serious adverse effect, often attributed to the increased bradykinin levels, although a definitive mechanism has not been established. Angioedema is edema caused by pathologically leaky blood vessels. It can

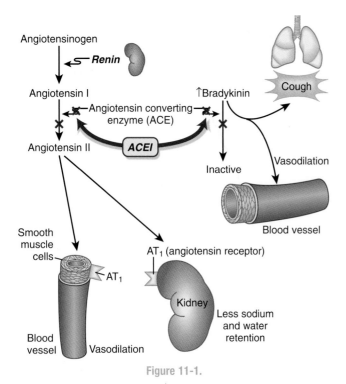

Figure 11-1.

cause swollen lips or tongue, and death can also result from airway obstruction.

IMPORTANT NOTES

- The renin-angiotensin system (RAS) plays an important role in the body's compensation for a failing heart. Activation of the sympathetic nervous system (SNS) leads to the release of renin, which in turn increases vascular tone and sodium and water retention.
- ACEIs might be of particular use in the management of HTN in the diabetic patient, as they may delay the development of diabetic nephropathy. This is primarily because of a reduction in intraglomerular pressure, through relaxation of the efferent arteriole and the overall reduction in systemic blood pressure (BP).

Advanced

- In addition to the beneficial effects of RAS inhibitors in diabetic nephropathy, there is emerging evidence that RAS

inhibitors may reduce the incidence of new-onset diabetes. Potential mechanisms for this effect include improvements in blood flow that improve the delivery of insulin and glucose to skeletal muscle, as well as effects on glucose transport and insulin signaling. **If this preventative effect of RAS inhibition in diabetes becomes established, it could change the way these agents are used.**

- ONTARGET (Ongoing Telmisartan Alone and in Combination with Ramipril Global Endpoint Trial) was a large (approximately 8500 patients per arm), long-term (median follow-up of 56 months) study comparing an angiotensin-receptor blocker (ARB), an ACEI, and a combination of the two in patients with vascular disease or high-risk diabetes. The study found that the combination of ARB and ACEI failed to demonstrate benefit versus either agent alone, with an increased incidence of adverse events in this population.

EVIDENCE
Hypertension

- A 2009 Cochrane review (24 trials, N = 58,040 participants) compared benefits and harms of first-line antihypertensives with those of placebo or no treatment over a minimum of 1 year in patients with hypertension. ACEIs (three trials) reduced mortality (relative risk [RR] 0.83), stroke (RR 0.65), coronary heart disease (RR 0.81), and cardiovascular events (RR 0.76).

FYI NOTES

- It has yet to be shown that any one ACEI is significantly superior to another.
- *Brady* means slow (e.g., bradycardia). *Bradykinin* is so named because it causes slow contractions of the gastrointestinal (GI) tract.
- Bradykinin is also implicated in the edema that accompanies sepsis, allergic reactions, and carcinoid syndrome. Angioedema is associated with a deficiency of C1 esterase, an enzyme that cleaves bradykinin.
- Several ACEIs are available in fixed-dose combinations with hydrochlorothiazide.

Angiotensin Receptor Blockers (ARBs)

DESCRIPTION
ARBs antagonize the angiotensin receptor.

PROTOTYPE AND COMMON DRUGS
- Prototype: losartan
- Others: candesartan, irbesartan, valsartan, eprosartan, telmisartan

MOA (MECHANISM OF ACTION)

- ARBs are antagonists of the angiotensin-1 (AT1) receptor. Therefore they block the actions of angiotensin II.
- Angiotensin II is a vasoactive hormone that induces vasoconstriction and stimulates the secretion of aldosterone by the adrenal cortex, which results in sodium and water retention.

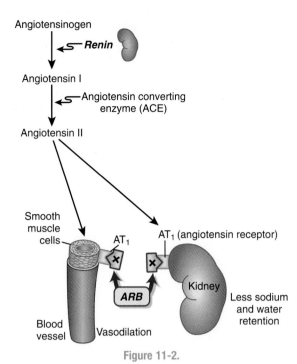

Figure 11-2.

- Blocking AT1 results in **vasodilation, natriuresis** (renal loss of sodium), and **diuresis** (renal loss of water).
- Effects of ARBs are *downstream* of ACE.
- ACEIs block the degradation of bradykinins. ARBs have no effect on bradykinin levels. Because bradykinins are vasodilators, ARBs might not produce as much vasodilation as ACEIs.
- Conversely, ACE is **not** the only enzyme that forms angiotensin II. Thus ARBs might provide more complete inhibition of the vasopressor activity of angiotensin II compared with ACEIs (Figure 11-2).

PHARMACOKINETICS
- All ARBs have intermediate (12 to 24 hour) half-lives and thus provide the advantage of once-daily dosing.
- Losartan has an active metabolite (EXP 3174) that is a more potent inhibitor of the AT1 receptor than the parent drug.

INDICATIONS
- Hypertension (HTN)
- Chronic congestive heart failure (CHF)
- For patients who require an ACEI but cannot tolerate it because of cough

CONTRAINDICATION
- **Pregnancy,** because of teratogenicity

SIDE EFFECTS
- ARBs are well tolerated.
- The most *common* side effects are **dizziness** and **hypotension.**
- **Hyperkalemia** (high potassium) can occur when combined with K^+ supplements or K^+-sparing diuretics.

- **Renal failure** can occur in patients whose renal function is marginal or highly dependent on the RAS, because of the same mechanism seen with ACEIs.
- Angioedema occurs less often than with the ACEIs.

IMPORTANT NOTES
- Perhaps because of the lack of increased bradykinin levels, ARBs are not typically associated with the side effect of cough, which can be a significant limitation to the use of ACEIs.
- The mechanism behind the cough has not been established.

Advanced
- In addition to the beneficial effects of RAS inhibitors in diabetic nephropathy, there is emerging evidence that RAS inhibitors may reduce the incidence of new-onset diabetes. Potential mechanisms for this effect include improvements in blood flow that improve the delivery of insulin and glucose to skeletal muscle, as well as effects on glucose transport and insulin signaling. **If this preventative effect of RAS inhibition in diabetes becomes established, it could change the way these agents are used.**
- ACEIs reduce the effect of both AT1 and AT2 receptors by lowering levels of angiotensin II; only AT1 receptors are inhibited by ARBs. Chronic stimulation of the AT2 receptor may be beneficial in providing neuroprotection in older patients with HTN and thus could mean that ARBs have a potential advantage in this patient subset.
- ONTARGET (Ongoing Telmisartan Alone and in Combination with Ramipril Global Endpoint Trial) was a large (approximately 8500 patients per arm), long-term (median follow-up of 56 months) study comparing an ARB, an ACEI, and a combination of the two in patients with *vascular disease* or *high-risk diabetes*. The study found that the combination of ARB and ACEI failed to demonstrate benefit versus either agent alone, with an increased incidence of adverse events in this population.

Pharmacogenetics
- People of African descent have a smaller average BP response to ARBs.

EVIDENCE
Hypertension
- A 2009 Cochrane review (24 trials, N = 58,040 participants) compared benefits and harms of first-line antihypertensives with those of placebo or no treatment over a minimum of 1 year. No studies were found that included ARBs.

FYI NOTES
- All ARBs except eprosartan (the newest ARB) are also available in combination (i.e., same pill, two drugs) with hydrochlorothiazide.
- Candesartan is actually candesartan cilexetil, a prodrug that is hydrolyzed to the active form, candesartan, during absorption from the GI tract.

Direct Renin Inhibitors

DESCRIPTION
Agents that directly inhibit renin, an enzyme in the RAS

PROTOTYPE AND COMMON DRUGS
- Prototype: aliskiren

MOA (MECHANISM OF ACTION)
- Renin is an enzyme released from the kidneys that converts angiotensinogen to angiotensin I. It is considered to be the rate-limiting step in the eventual formation of angiotensin II.
- Renin and its inactive precursor, prorenin, are stored in the juxtaglomerular cells of the kidney. Renin is released in response to three different stimuli:
  - Change in Na and Cl reabsorption at the macula densa
  - Change in BP (via the baroreceptor pathway)
  - β_1-receptor stimulation
- Angiotensin II performs two main functions via the AT1 receptor:
  - Direct vasoconstriction
  - Stimulation of aldosterone secretion which leads to Na^+ and H_2O reabsorption
- Other agents that target the RAS, such as the ACEIs and ARBs, elicit a *compensatory increase* in plasma renin activity, resulting in increased binding of angiotensin II to AT1 receptors and other AT receptors.
- It is not yet clear what the implications are of activating these other AT receptors.
- Therefore, one *potential* advantage of renin antagonists over ACEIs and ARBs is avoiding the compensatory increase in the RAS. It is yet to be established whether these theoretical advantages translate into clinically meaningful advantages (Figure 11-3).

PHARMACOKINETICS
- The elimination half-life of aliskiren is approximately 40 hours, meaning that it is administered once daily.

INDICATIONS
- HTN
- Chronic congestive heart failure (currently being investigated)

CONTRAINDICATION
- **Pregnancy:** As with other agents that act in the RAS, renin antagonists are contraindicated in pregnancy.

SIDE EFFECTS
- Generally well tolerated.
- **Diarrhea:** mechanism not established.
- **Angioedema (rare):** swelling of face and neck. This side effect also rarely occurs with ACEIs.

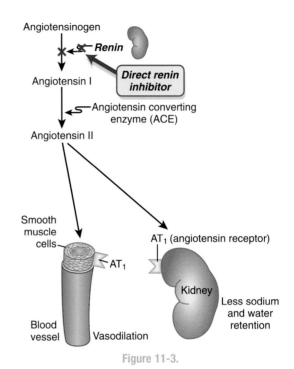

Figure 11-3.

IMPORTANT NOTES
- Angiotensin II binding at the AT1 is also believed to have several other less well-defined effects:
  - Possible contribution to the generation of reactive oxygen species
  - Endothelial dysfunction
  - Mitogenic effects that may further contribute to endothelial disease (and thus vascular disease)

EVIDENCE
Blood-Pressure Lowering Efficacy versus Placebo
- A 2008 Cochrane review (six trials, 3694 participants) compared the blood-pressure–lowering efficacy of renin inhibitors versus placebo in primary HTN. The authors found that aliskiren elicits a dose-dependent reduction in both systolic and diastolic pressure similar to that seen with ACEIs or ARBs. In the included trials, aliskiren did not increase withdrawals due to adverse events versus placebo.

FYI NOTES
- Renin was first identified in 1898, when it was extracted from kidneys and discovered to have pressor properties. It would be another 40 years before it was determined that renin was an enzyme that catalyzed the formation of a pressor substance (angiotensin II), rather than being the pressor itself.

■ Although renin inhibitors were considered to be the most obvious target for inhibition of the RAS, it took several decades to develop the first direct renin inhibitor. Two main hurdles were finding an agent with sufficient bioavailability and an agent with high affinity for the active site of the renin enzyme.

■ Early renin inhibitors were all peptides and therefore were unsuitable for oral administration. Given that all commonly used antihypertensives are delivered via the oral route, renin inhibitors were not considered feasible until a nonpeptide, oral version could be developed.

Sodium Channel Blockers (Class I Antiarrhythmics)

DESCRIPTION
Na channel blockers are Vaughan Williams class I antiarrhythmics. There are three subclasses: Ia, Ib, and Ic. The use of Na channel blockers as local anesthetics is discussed in the discussion of local anesthetics in Chapter 21.

PROTOTYPES
■ Class Ia: procainamide, disopyramide, and quinidine
■ Class Ib: lidocaine
■ Class Ic: propafenone and flecainide

MOA (MECHANISM OF ACTION)
■ Na channels are blocked, so Na ion movement during **phase 0** of the action potential is inhibited. The result is a "slow" phase 0, which results in a wider (and slower) QRS wave on the electrocardiogram (ECG). The net result is **slower conduction** (Figure 11-4).
■ Phase 3 can be longer or shorter, depending on the subclass (a, b, or c). This is omitted in the diagram for simplicity.
■ Changing the **duration of the action potential** (not shown in diagram) influences the QT interval (distance from the QRS to the T wave). This distance can be thought of as the *refractory period* of the ECG. Therefore changing the action potential durations will change the **refractory times** of atrial, Purkinje or ventricular tissues.

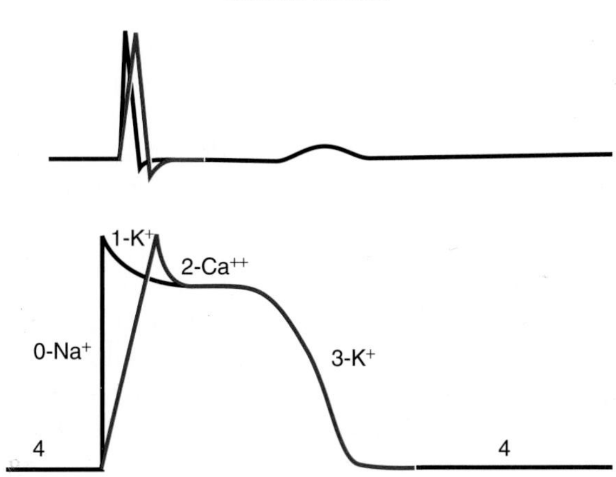

■ Because abnormal electrical circuits require a delicate balance between conduction speed and refractory times, changing these parameters will sometimes terminate dysrhythmias *or create new ones.*

Specific Differences Among the Subclasses (Table 11-1)
Class Ia
■ Moderate slowing of phase 0 (medium Na blockade)
■ Action potential duration is longer, therefore longer QT interval on the ECG

Class Ib
■ Minimal slowing of phase 0 (least Na blockade)
■ Action potential duration is shorter, therefore shorter QT interval
■ Because of the weak Na blockade:
  ▲ The agents basically act only on diseased or ischemic tissue
  ▲ They have basically no effect on atrial tissue

Class Ic
■ Maximal slowing of phase 0 (greatest Na blockade)
■ Action potential duration essentially unchanged
■ Most pronounced slowing of phase 0 in all cardiac tissues; therefore:
  ▲ Can inhibit the *slow* Na channels of the atrioventricular (AV) node and therefore can prolong the AV node refractory period and thus prolong the PR interval

Sodium blocker

Figure 11-4.

	Na Blockade	Action Potential Duration	Indications	Contraindications
Ia	Medium	Longer	Atrial and ventricular	
Ib	Minimum	Shorter	Ventricular only	
Ic	Maximum	No change	Atrial fibrillation	↑ Mortality with myocardial infarction

TABLE 11-1. Sodium Channel Blocker Summary Chart

PHARMACOKINETICS

- **Quinidine interacts with digoxin (CP450).** This can result in increased levels of digoxin, a toxic drug with a narrow therapeutic index. Both drugs are antiarrhythmic drugs and have the potential to be coadministered.
- **Lidocaine** has a very short half-life (about 20 minutes) and is administered intravenously, because of a large first-pass metabolism effect.

CONTRAINDICATIONS

- Class Ic antiarrhythmics *increase* mortality in infarct- and ischemia-related dysrhythmias; therefore they are not used in these settings. They also increase mortality in patients with poor left ventricular function (decreased ejection fraction).

SIDE EFFECTS

- **Proarrhythmic:** As with all antiarrhythmics, changing the delicate balance of conduction speed and refractory times might provoke another area of the conducting system into developing a dysrhythmia.
- **Nervous system dysfunction:** Na channels are required for nerve function. Numbness and tingling of the lips and tongue, ringing in the ear, inappropriate behavior, decreased consciousness, and seizures can all occur.
- Nausea and vomiting may occur.

IMPORTANT NOTES

- Procainamide and lidocaine are used on *crash carts* for cardiac arrest resuscitation. They are used for ventricular fibrillation and ventricular tachycardia but have been mostly replaced by amiodarone as the first-line drug used for ventricular fibrillation and ventricular tachycardia.

EVIDENCE

- **Atrial fibrillation and prevention of recurrence:** A Cochrane review in 2007 (45 studies, 12,559 patients) evaluated the efficacy and safety of multiple different antiarrhythmics in patients who had previously experienced atrial fibrillation (a very common arrhythmia). Class Ia antiarrhythmics were associated with **increased mortality** compared with controls (odds ratio [OR] 2.39; number needed to harm [NNH] 109). Class Ia and Ic were associated with reduced occurrences of atrial fibrillation (OR 0.19 to 0.6). There were many withdrawals from treatment because of side effects for all antiarrhythmics (NNH 17 to 36).

FYI NOTES

- Lidocaine is most commonly used as a local anesthetic.
- Class Ia drugs work fast and can be remembered by the acronym PDQ (pretty darn quick) for procainamide, disopyramide, and quinidine.

β Antagonists (β-Blockers)

DESCRIPTION

β-Blockers antagonize β receptors of the SNS.

PROTOTYPE AND COMMON DRUGS

- Propran**olol**
- β-Blockers are a heterogeneous family and can be subclassified according to the receptors they antagonize (it is important to know which are β_1 selective):
  - ▲ Cardioselective (β_1): aten**olol**, metopr**olol**, nebiv**olol**, esm**olol**
  - ▲ Noncardioselective (β_1, β_2): propran**olol**, nad**olol**, tim**olol**
  - ▲ Mixed α and β: labet**olol**, carved**olol**
  - ▲ **Partial agonists** (stimulate mildly when receptor is inactive, inhibit when active): pind**olol**, acebut**olol**
- **Selectivity is relative.** This means that β_1-selective blockers will block β_2 receptors, but to a much lower degree than nonselective β-blockers.

MOA (MECHANISM OF ACTION)

To understand β-blockers, you must understand the effects of the adrenergic system and which effects are mediated via β receptors. β-Blockers competitively antagonize the action of catecholamines at β receptors. There are many cardiac and noncardiac consequences of β-blockade. More details on the autonomic nervous system are described in Chapter 3.

Hypertension

- Antagonism of β_1 receptors results in reductions in heart rate (HR) and stroke volume (SV). Recall:

$$CO = HR \times SV$$

- Cardiac output (CO) is therefore reduced, which leads to a reduction in BP. Recall:

$$BP = CO \times SVR$$

where SVR = systemic vascular resistance.

- In addition, β_1 antagonism leads to a reduction in renin secretion, which in turn reduces production of angiotensin II, a hormone that induces vasoconstriction and, via aldosterone, sodium retention.
- The utility of β-blockers in myocardial ischemia and infarction results from their ability to reduce HR and contractility and therefore lower O_2 demand. They have also proven useful after a MI for the same reason, reducing the workload of the heart.
- β-Blockers also have direct inhibitory effects on the SNS.

■ Mixed α and β antagonists will additionally cause vasodilation via α-blockade.

Tachycardia and Arrhythmia

The properties of β-blockers that make them antitachycardics include the following:

1. **Depression of the sinoatrial (SA) node (slows automaticity)**
   ▲ Catecholamine β_1 *stimulation* results in an increase in the slow Na$^+$ current (I_f) of the action potential phase 4 in the SA node. This results in a faster rising (and shorter) phase 4, a shorter time to the next heartbeat, and thus a faster HR. β-Blockers will oppose this action, slowing the SA pacemaker rate.
   ▲ This mechanism is useful in sinus tachycardia only.
2. **Depression of the AV node (prolongs the refractory period)**
   ▲ Same mechanism as SA node: a decrease in the slow Na$^+$ current (I_f) leaves the AV node in a refractory state longer.
   ▲ This mechanism is useful in making the AV node a *protector* of the ventricles. In situations (atrial fibrillation and atrial flutter) in which the AV node is bombarded by electrical signals from the atria, the depressed AV node can permit only a fraction of these signals to enter into the ventricular conducting system, controlling the ventricular rate.
   ▲ This mechanism may also be able to terminate a **reentry circuit** that involves the AV node.
   ▲ This mechanism can result in a long PR interval and first-degree AV block.
3. **Prevention of after-depolarizations**
   ▲ After-depolarizations can produce premature ventricular contractions (PVCs), which can deteriorate into ventricular tachycardia or ventricular fibrillation.
4. **Membrane stabilization**
   ▲ This is probably not a significant mechanism; however, it is frequently described.
   ▲ Some of the β-blockers are designated as having membrane-stabilizing properties.
   ▲ Membrane stabilization is mediated through Na$^+$ channel blockade (class I antiarrhythmic effect).
5. **Special antiarrhythmic β-blockers include the following:**
   ▲ Sotalol:
     • Also has class III properties (and often is listed as a class III drug)
     • Prolongs the action potential and thus atrial and ventricular refractoriness
     • Used for ventricular tachycardia (other β-blockers are not) because it can influence ventricular refractoriness
   ▲ Acebutolol:
     • Also has class I properties
     • Used for PVC suppression

Myocardial Ischemia and Infarction

■ One of the main cornerstones of treating myocardial ischemia and infarction is to **increase oxygen supply** to and **decrease oxygen demand** of the myocardium. β-Blockers result in the following:
   ▲ Slower HR = less work = lower oxygen demand
   ▲ Slower HR = longer diastolic time = more time for myocardial perfusion (which occurs only during diastole)
   ▲ Lower contractility = less work = lower oxygen demand
   ▲ Lower BP = less work = lower oxygen demand

Chronic Congestive Heart Failure

■ Patients with a dysfunctional cardiovascular system have an inefficient system and thus require extra support; this support is in the form of increased levels of SNS activation, renin-angiotensin activity, endothelin activity, and many other compensatory mechanisms.
■ Sustained activation of the SNS results in fibrosis and apoptosis of myocytes. Through low level blockade of the SNS, the fibrosis and apoptosis (and other damaging mechanisms) are slowed or inhibited.
■ Unfortunately, the long-term (years) gain of using β-blockers in heart failure is often counterbalanced by the short-term (months) worsening of symptoms, and therefore β-blocker titration in chronic heart failure must be made carefully and judiciously.

PHARMACOKINETICS

■ **Shorter half-lives (3 to 4 hours):** propranolol, metoprolol (sustained-release forms with longer half-lives are available)
■ **Long(er) half-lives (10 to 20 hours):** nadolol (longest), atenolol
■ Distribution to the central nervous system (CNS) has been implicated as a source of drug-induced confusion with some β-blockers. Specifically, metoprolol is lipid soluble and therefore crosses the blood-brain barrier, whereas atenolol, another selective β_1 blocker does not.
■ Esmolol is designed to be broken down by esterases and therefore has a very short half-life of 9 minutes. It is given only intravenously as a single bolus for short-term HR or BP control or as an infusion.

INDICATIONS

■ HTN
■ Chronic congestive heart failure
   ▲ After MI (a damaged heart is a risk for CHF)
■ Tachyarrhythmias
   ▲ Sinus tachycardia
     • Hyperthyroidism
     • Cocaine abuse
     • Pheochromocytoma (adrenaline secreting tumor—very rare)
   ▲ Atrial fibrillation and atrial flutter
   ▲ Prevention of ventricular tachycardia and ventricular fibrillation
■ Angina and MI
■ Noncardiac indications
   ▲ Migraine prevention, public speaking, anxiety, glaucoma (eye drops), tremor

CONTRAINDICATIONS

- **Asthmatics** should not use nonselective (β_1, β_2) β-blockers, as blocking β_2 receptors may lead to bronchoconstriction. Stimulation of β_2 receptors in the airways causes smooth muscle relaxation of the bronchioles and is the basis of bronchodilators that are β_2 agonists.
  - ▲ Cardioselective β_1-blockers are **usually** safe in asthmatics, but some patients can have severe bronchoconstriction in response to these drugs.
- **Second-degree heart block**: It can be converted to third-degree heart block, resulting in very low HRs.
- **Bradycardia**: β-Blockers could make the already slow heart so slow that CO and BP fall below levels that are required by the body for adequate perfusion.
- *Acute* **heart failure**: Note that *chronic* heart failure is an indication for β-blockers, and *acute* heart failure is a contraindication. In acute heart failure the patient is decompensated and probably being kept alive by the SNS being ramped up. Blocking the effects of the flight-or-fight response would further decompensate the patient and potentially kill him or her.

SIDE EFFECTS

- **Hypotension**: β-Blockers are negative chronotropes and inotropes.
- **CHF**: β-Blockers are negative inotropes.
- **Asthma and bronchoconstriction**: Nonselective β-blockers block β_2 receptors in the airways.
- **Bradycardia and heart block**: The SA and AV nodes are under adrenergic influence.
- **Raynaud's phenomenon**: Cold extremities (fingers in particular) may result from antagonism of β_2 receptors, leading to vasoconstriction in the periphery.
- **Impotence**: Erectile function is dependent on changes in blood flow and vasodilation in the corpora cavernosa, and these mechanisms can be blocked by β-blockers.
- **Fatigue**: This is likely a result of the reduction in CO.
- **Hypoglycemia**: Nonselective β-blockers may interfere with recovery from hypoglycemia in type 1 (insulin-dependent) diabetes, as they antagonize the ability of catecholamines to promote glycogenolysis and mobilize glucose. Also, in diabetics, the β-blockade prevents symptoms caused by hypoglycemia and so masks early mild hypoglycemia, which can then deteriorate.
- **CNS effects**: Insomnia, nightmares, and depression are side effects. The mechanism is not well understood, but in theory these effects should occur more frequently with lipophilic drugs that cross the blood-brain barrier, such as propranolol and metoprolol.
- **Lipid profiles**: β-Blockers (except partial agonists) increase triglyceride levels and reduce high-density lipoprotein (HDL), without changing total cholesterol. The long-term effects of these changes are not known.

IMPORTANT NOTES

- β-blockers should not be discontinued abruptly, because of a *rebound* effect that might result in tachycardia and exacerbate the symptoms of coronary artery disease or might induce a hypertensive effect. The rebound appears to be an overactivity of the SNS, caused perhaps by receptor up-regulation.
- The use of β-blockers for HTN is generally avoided in elderly patients, whereas younger hypertensive patients tend to respond well to these agents.
- Not only might β-blockers impair the response to hypoglycemia in type 1 diabetes, but the negative chronotropic effects of these agents may mask the tachycardia that normally provides an *important indicator of hypoglycemia* to the diabetic. Despite these concerns, β-blockers have proven effective in the treatment of people with type 1 diabetes who have experienced an MI, and thus the decision whether to use them is one of risk versus benefit in this population.
- β-blockers were once contraindicated in chronic heart failure, but current evidence is very strong that they reduce mortality. It is very important to note that β-blockers are contraindicated in patients with acute decompensated heart failure.

Advanced

- Intrinsic sympathomimetic activity (ISA) is described for some β-blockers. ISA refers to a partial agonist effect in which the drug mostly blocks β receptors but does have a very small amount of agonist activity (however, far less than if compared with no drug at all).

EVIDENCE
Chronic Heart Failure

- A meta analysis in 2009 (23 studies, N = 19,209 patients) shows a reduction in mortality with β-blockers for patients with chronic heart failure (RR 0.76) when compared with placebo. Decreases in HR were statistically associated with lower mortality.

After Myocardial Infarction

- Evidence for the role of β-blockers in **secondary prevention** after an MI comes from several trials and was summarized in a 1999 systematic review (82 trials, N = 54,234 patients). There was a 23% reduction in the odds of death in long-term trials but only a 4% reduction in short-term trials. The review found that the number needed to treat (NNT) to avoid a fatality over the course of 2 years is 42. The greatest amount of evidence available was for propranolol, timolol, and metoprolol.

Hypertension and Associated Stroke and Coronary Artery Disease

- A Cochrane review in 2007 (13 studies, N = 91,561 patients) compared β-blockers with other agents for HTN. Atenolol was the β-blocker most frequently used. The authors found that β-blockers had only weak effects in reducing stroke and no effect on coronary heart disease versus placebo.

There was also a trend toward worse outcomes when compared with calcium channel blockers (CCBs), RAS inhibitors, and thiazides, prompting the authors to suggest that β-blockers should not be considered as *first-line agents* for HTN.

Obstructive Airway Disease (Asthma and Chronic Obstructive Pulmonary Disease)

- A Cochrane review in 2002 (29 studies, N = 381 patients) examined the impact of single-dose or short-term *selective* β₁-blockers in patients with mild to moderate obstructive airway disease. There were no differences in pulmonary flow measurements compared with placebo except for a small decrease in FEV_1 after the first treatment—an effect that disappeared with subsequent doses.

FYI NOTES

- Nervous about public speaking? β-blockers have been used to reduce HR, palpitations, and sweating just before public speaking engagements.
- Metoprolol (selective β₁) is currently one of the most commonly used β-blockers for cardiac indications.

Potassium Channel Blockers (Class III Antiarrhythmics)

DESCRIPTION

K channel blockers are Vaughan Williams class III antiarrhythmics. Amiodarone is currently one of the most commonly used K channel blocker antiarrhythmics, and therefore this section will focus on amiodarone.

PROTOTYPES AND OTHER DRUGS

- Prototype: bretylium (now discontinued)
- Other drugs in this class:
  - ▲ Amio**darone**, drone**darone**
  - ▲ Ibut**ilide**, dofet**ilide**, azim**ilide**
  - ▲ Sotalol (also a β-blocker)

MOA (MECHANISM OF ACTION)

- Blocking K channels in phase 3 of the action potential slows the efflux of K back out of the myocyte, which slows the rate at which the cell repolarizes and therefore lengthens the plateau phase of the action potential. This increases the **refractory period** of atrial, ventricular, and Purkinje cells. This also increases the QT interval on the ECG (Figure 11-5).
- Amiodarone contains multiple antiarrhythmic properties and is an Na blocker, a K blocker, a Ca blocker, and β-blocker, all rolled into one chemical. However, it is primarily referred to as a class III drug.

PHARMACOKINETICS

- Amiodarone has a half-life of 25 to 60 days (extremely long).
- Drug interactions:
  - ▲ Amiodarone and dronedarone are metabolized by and are inhibitors of CYP3A4; this is important because other drugs used in the control of dysrhythmias, including verapamil and diltiazem, are also metabolized by CYP3A4, and drug levels can be increased when drugs are coadministered.

Potassium blocker

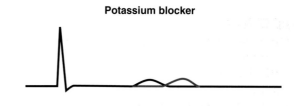

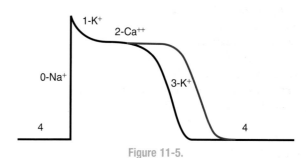

Figure 11-5.

- ▲ There is an interaction with digoxin, another drug used for treatment of arrhythmias: levels of digoxin can be increased up to 2.5 times as a result of P-glycoprotein interactions at the kidney.
- ▲ Dronedarone is also a CYP2D6 inhibitor and can increase levels of metoprolol in some patients.
- It is administered orally and intravenously.

INDICATIONS

- Acute treatment and prevention of atrial fibrillation and flutter
- Acute treatment and prevention of ventricular fibrillation and ventricular tachycardia

CONTRAINDICATIONS

- Caution must be exercised when giving amiodarone to patients with hypotension.

- Second- or third-degree heart block: conduction blocks can become worse (e.g., second-degree can progress to third-degree block) and escape rhythms (ventricular rhythm in 3rd degree block) can be suppressed, leading to no ventricular contractions and cardiac standstill.

SIDE EFFECTS

- Side effects of amiodarone are rare but serious. They can be categorized as cardiac (usually not too serious) and non-cardiac (more serious).
  - ▲ Cardiac:
    - Bradycardia and heart block
    - Hypotension
  - ▲ Noncardiac:
    - Pulmonary fibrosis (interstitial lung disease)
    - Thyroid dysfunction (hyperfunction or hypofunction)
    - Blue skin
    - Nausea, constipation, anorexia (loss of appetite)
    - Liver damage (shown as an increase in *liver enzymes* in the blood)
- Dronedarone appears to have fewer side effects related to the thyroid, lung fibrosis, skin discoloration, and liver enzymes; however, it is associated with more GI side effects.

IMPORTANT NOTES

- Dronedarone is a newer class III drug. Indications for its use, compared with amiodarone, are still being evaluated in clinical trials.

EVIDENCE

- **Atrial fibrillation (AF) and multiple outcomes:** A Cochrane review in 2007 (45 studies, 12,559 patients) evaluated the efficacy and safety of multiple different antiarrhythmics in patients who had previously experienced atrial fibrillation (the most common arrhythmia).
  - ▲ **Mortality:** When compared with controls, amiodarone showed no significant difference in mortality. Compared with class I drugs, amiodarone showed a significant reduction in mortality (OR 0.39, NNT 17).
  - ▲ **AF recurrence:** Amiodarone appeared to be the most effective of the antiarrhythmics at preventing AF recurrence; the NNT was 3 to prevent 1 recurrence of AF in 1 year.
  - ▲ **Adverse effects:** Amiodarone did not appear to show any increased proarrhythmic effects, but there were more withdrawals caused by other side effects than there were with placebo.

FYI NOTES

- There is similarity between the molecular structure of thyroid hormone and that of both amiodarone and dronedarone; it is likely that the structural similarity is the basis for the thyroid-related side effects seen with amiodarone.

Calcium Channel Blockers

DESCRIPTION

CCBs are agents that act by blocking calcium channels, either in the heart or on blood vessels. There are two major classes within CCBs: dihydropyridine (DHP) and non-DHP.

PROTOTYPE AND COMMON DRUGS
Dihydropyridines

- Prototype: nife**dipine**
- Others: amlo**dipine**, felo**dipine**, nicar**dipine**, nimo**dipine**, clevi**dipine**

Nondihydropyridines

- Prototypes: diltiazem, verapamil

MOA (MECHANISM OF ACTION)
Hypertension

- Calcium channels are designated as L-, T-, P/Q-, N-, and R-type, depending on kinetics and receptor specificity. *L* means long duration, and *T* means transient.

- L-type calcium channels are located on the heart, skeletal muscle, neurons, vascular smooth muscle, and uterus.
- All CCBs are antagonists of **L-type** calcium channels. By blocking the influx of calcium through L-type channels, these agents inhibit contraction of smooth muscle (Figure 11-6).
- The **dihydropyridine (DHP)** CCBs have greater selectivity for the vasculature than either diltiazem or verapamil, the non-DHP CCBs.
- DHPs have little effect on the *recovery* of the calcium channel and thus **minimal effects on cardiac** Ca channels involved with automaticity (HR), conduction speed, and refractory periods (important with regard to the AV node).
- As a result, the DHPs have a greater vasodilatory effect than the non-DHPs and essentially no direct clinical effect on the heart. In other words, DHPs are vasodilators, and non-DHPs are cardiac depressants with some vasodilator activity.

Calcium channel blocker

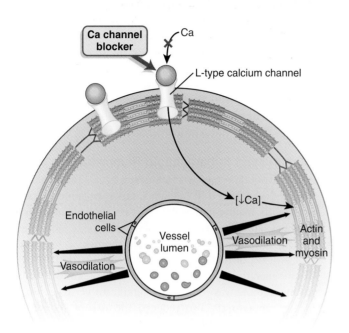

Figure 11-6.

Calcium channel blockers

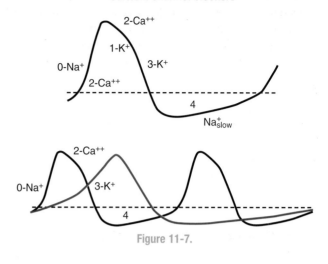

Figure 11-7.

Tachycardia and Arrhythmia

The **non-DHPs** (but not the DPHs) are also **class IV antiarrhythmics**.

Blocking Ca^{+2} channels in phase 0 of the action potential lengthens the depolarizing current in SA and AV nodal cells. This results in more time before the next action potential. In the SA node, the result is a slower pacemaker. In the AV node, the result is a longer refractory period (Figure 11-7).

PHARMACOKINETICS

- Amlodipine has a **slow onset** and much **longer half-life** (40 hours) than nifedipine (4 hours). This slow onset helps to mitigate the reflex tachycardia commonly seen with these agents, particularly nifedipine.
- Clevidipine is a newer DHP that is metabolized by esterases and therefore has a short half-life of 10 minutes. It is given only by intravenous infusion because of its short half-life.
- Oral verapamil undergoes extensive hepatic metabolism. Therefore the oral dose is much greater than the intravenous dose (80 to 160 mg orally [PO] versus 2.5 to 5 mg intravenously [IV]).

INDICATIONS
Nondihydropyridines

- Stable angina
- Sinus tachycardia
- Atrial tachycardia
- Reentry tachycardias
- HTN (diltiazem)

Dihydropyridines

- HTN
- To prevent or treat coronary spasm in variant angina (Prinzmetal's angina)
- To prevent or treat cerebral artery spasm after brain hemorrhage
- Preterm labor

CONTRAINDICATIONS
Nondihydropyridines

- **Wolff-Parkinson-White (WPW) syndrome:** In WPW the accessory pathway (bundle of Kent) is not blocked by Ca^{+2} channel blockers, but the AV node is. Therefore the use of Ca^{+2} channel blockers will promote conduction through the accessory pathway. Because the accessory pathway does not have a conduction delay as the AV node does, conduction through the accessory pathway can result in *very* high ventricular rates in the presence of atrial fibrillation or atrial flutter.
- **Hypotension:** Ca^{+2} channel blockers lower BP and should not be used in patients who already have low BP.
- **Acute CHF:** Non-DHPs have a depressant effect on the heart and **must** be avoided in acute CHF.
- **AV blocks:** Ca^{+2} channel blockers can make an AV block more severe.

Dihydropyridines

- **Pregnancy**—teratogenic effects seen in animals
- Conditions in which **tachycardia** is harmful:
  - ▲ **Coronary artery disease**
  - ▲ **Aortic stenosis**
  - ▲ **Mitral stenosis**

SIDE EFFECTS
Nondihydropyridines
- **Bradycardia**: caused by SA node or AV node suppression
- **Heart failure and hypotension**: secondary to reduced contractility

Dihydropyridines
- **Vasodilation-related symptoms**:
  - ▲ **Flushing**: Caused by cutaneous vasodilation
  - ▲ **Dizziness**: Caused by decreased cerebral perfusion from low BP
  - ▲ **Headache**: Caused by cerebral vasodilation
  - ▲ **Tachycardia**: A baroreceptor reflex response to decreased BP

IMPORTANT NOTES
- Vasodilation results in lower BP, and low BP often induces a baroreceptor-mediated reflex tachycardia. An important clinical consequence of DHPs is that they can indirectly induce tachycardia, which can be very dangerous in conditions in which tachycardia is contraindicated (e.g., coronary artery disease).

Advanced
- The DHPs are predominantly metabolized by the **CYP3A4** enzyme system and thus have numerous interactions with either inducers or inhibitors of this enzyme.
- **Grapefruit juice**: The bioflavonoids in grapefruit juices inhibit the metabolism of most DHPs, especially felodipine. Evidence suggests that amlodipine is not affected by this interaction.

EVIDENCE
As First-Line Agents in Hypertension
- A 2009 Cochrane review (24 trials, N = 58,040 participants) compared benefits and harms of first-line antihypertensives with those of placebo or no treatment over a minimum of 1 year. Only one randomized controlled trial (RCT) was found that included a CCB, and in this trial it reduced stroke (RR 0.58) but not coronary heart disease or mortality. Thiazides (19 trials) reduced mortality (RR 0.89), stroke (RR 0.63), and coronary heart disease (RR 0.84).

For Aneurysmal Subarachnoid Hemorrhage
- A 2007 Cochrane review (16 studies, N = 3361 patients) examined whether DHP calcium antagonists alone or combined with magnesium sulfate (three studies) improved outcomes in patients with subarachnoid hemorrhage. Overall, calcium antagonists reduced the risk of poor outcomes (death or disability), with an NNT of 19 (1 to 51). When separated by individual calcium antagonists, only oral nimodipine was statistically significant versus control. Calcium antagonists also reduced the risk of secondary ischemia.

FYI NOTES
- Patients have been known to take advantage of the interaction between felodipine and grapefruit juice to save themselves a few dollars on the drug cost. They will reduce their dose of felodipine by consuming grapefruit juice on a consistent basis. The bioflavonoids are found in the peel, however, so patients who grind their own juice may find they are not getting adequate drug levels if they do not include the peel.
- Remember, when trying to distinguish between DHP and non-DHP CCBs: dihydropyridines dilate.

Anticholinergics

DESCRIPTION
Antagonists of cholinergic (muscarinic) receptors relevant to the cardiovascular system are discussed here. Because of the diverse range of effects, anticholinergics as a class are also discussed elsewhere.

PROTOTYPE AND COMMON DRUGS
- Prototype is **atropine**
- Others:
  - ▲ Glycopyrrolate
  - ▲ Scopolamine
  - ▲ Benz**tropine**
  - ▲ See other chapters for more examples of non-cardiac anticholinergics
    - Autonomics (Chapter 3)
    - Anticholinergics for airways section (Chapter 24)
    - Anticholinergics for overactive bladder (Chapter 25)

MOA (MECHANISM OF ACTION)
- Anticholinergics block the activity of acetylcholine (ACh) of the parasympathetic system at muscarinic receptors (M).
- With respect to the cardiovascular system, this effect is most pronounced on the SA node and AV node, resulting in increased pacemaker rates of the SA node and *sometimes* increased conduction through the AV node. The primary result is a faster HR. The effect of AV node conduction is not clinically important unless a conduction block such as first-, second-, or third-degree AV block is present.
- Another (less clinically important) cardiovascular effect is reversal of vasodilation of some vascular beds, such as the mesentery (intestinal) vessels. ACh liberates NO from the endothelium, and atropine counteracts this.
- Atropine does not preferentially act on cardiovascular tissues; muscarinic receptors are present throughout the

TABLE 11-2. Effects of Anticholinergic Drugs	
Heart	Increased heart rate
Airways	Bronchodilation
Secretions	Reduced
Pupils	Dilated
Urinary function	Decreased
Gastrointestinal motility	Decreased
Central nervous system	Increased temperature, confusion

body, and therefore the actions of atropine and other anticholinergics are determined by the effects of the parasympathetic nervous system on each organ (Table 11-2).

INDICATIONS

Cardiovascular

- Sinus bradycardia with hypotension
- May be useful in second-degree heart block causing bradycardia
- Usually not effective in third-degree heart block, but can be tried
- Treatment of anticholinesterase side effects (common) or poisoning (rare)

Noncardiovascular

- To dry oral and bronchial secretions (for bronchoscopy)
- To relax the bladder (see also section on anticholinergics and overactive bladder)

CONTRAINDICATIONS

- Caution must be exercised in situations in which tachycardia is dangerous. This includes patients with coronary artery disease, aortic (valve) stenosis, and mitral (valve) stenosis.

SIDE EFFECTS

These side effects can be predicted by understanding the effects (and consequences of blockade) of the parasympathetic nervous system on the different organs and tissues in the body.
- Cardiac
  - ▲ Tachycardia
- Noncardiac
  - ▲ Dry mouth
  - ▲ Flushing
  - ▲ Urinary retention (inability to empty bladder)

- CNS: These effects are not strictly considered part of the autonomic nervous system:
  - ▲ Hyperthermia
  - ▲ Delirium

IMPORTANT NOTES

- Red, hot, dry, and confused is a tetrad of **atropine overdose**.
- Glycopyrrolate has a weaker tachycardia profile and is therefore good for drying secretions for airway procedures such as bronchoscopy because it does not cause excessive increases in HR.
- Many antiarrhythmic drugs (classified I to IV) also possess some degree of muscarinic blockade, but to a lesser degree than their primary mechanism of action.

FYI NOTES

- One chemical used in a form of chemical warfare is an anticholinesterase. An anticholinesterase blocks cholinesterase, which is an enzyme that degrades ACh. The result is too much ACh, which mimics an overactive parasympathetic system and can even cause paralysis from overstimulation of the nicotinic receptor in the neuromuscular junction. Atropine is the antidote.
- One class of anesthetic drug is a neuromuscular blocking *reversal* drug. It is an anticholinesterase and is used to increase the concentration of ACh in the neuromuscular junction. However, in addition to increased ACh in the neuromuscular junction, increased ACh at all other muscarinic receptors also occurs, leading to muscarinic side effects. Usual side effects of a normal dose include bradycardia and bronchorrhea (bronchial secretions). Antimuscarinic drugs including atropine and glycopyrrolate are used to minimize the side effects of these medications.
- A massive outpouring of parasympathetic activity (via the vagus nerve) caused by stress or fear is called a vasovagal attack. It results in bradycardia and hypotension and sometimes loss of consciousness.
- A scopolamine patch is used as an antinauseant.
- Benztropine is used to help motor control in the management of Parkinson's disease. This is an effect in the brain and not related to the autonomic nervous system.
- Ipratropium can be used as an alternative to β_2-agonists for bronchodilation in the management of asthma, particularly in the elderly. This drug is covered in Chapter 24 on inhaled anticholinergics.

Adenosine

DESCRIPTION

Adenosine is an antiarrhythmic that does not fall into the Vaughan Williams classification (class I to IV) scheme.

MOA (MECHANISM OF ACTION)

- Adenosine stimulates adenosine A_1 receptors in the AV node, which results in:
  - Increased outward K^+ currents
  - Decreased inward Ca^{+2} currents
  - Decreased inward Na^+ currents (I_f)
- These ionic actions **hyperpolarize** the cell (i.e., make the inside of the cell more negative because there are fewer positive ions inside the cell) and render it refractory for a prolonged period (a few seconds or more).
- Essentially, the AV node is completely **turned off** for a brief period of time, creating a third-degree heart block for a few seconds. Through this action, tachycardias that originate in the atria can be diagnosed more easily because all the QRSs are absent from the ECG for a few seconds.
- Because the AV node is turned off, any **reentry circuit** that was **originating inside or travelling through** the AV node will be terminated. Through this action, reentry circuits can be treated and normal sinus rhythm resumes (Figure 11-8).

PHARMACOKINETICS

- Adenosine has a half-life of about 10 seconds. It must be given as an intravenous *push* (quickly) with a saline flush (otherwise it will be metabolized in the arm veins before it gets to the heart, where it exerts its effects).
- Caffeine acts on the same adenosine A_1 receptor and can block the action of adenosine.

INDICATIONS

- Adenosine is used for the diagnosis and treatment of supraventricular tachycardias (SVTs).

Adenosine reentry

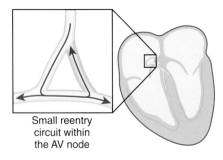
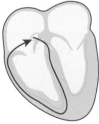

Small reentry circuit within the AV node

Large reentry circuit involving atrium, ventricle, AV node, and accessory pathway

Figure 11-8.

CONTRAINDICATION

- None of major significance.

SIDE EFFECTS

- Because the half-life of adenosine is very short, side effects usually last for only a few minutes.
- **Dyspnea (shortness of breath)** is caused by adenosine agonism in the bronchioles.
- **Angina** and feelings of **extreme discomfort** and unpleasantness may occur. Adenosine is liberated when there is a deficiency of ATP, which occurs when there is a deficiency of oxygen; adenosine is one of the mediators of symptoms when myocardial ischemia occurs.
- **Nausea** may occur.
- **Transient complete heart block** is common (and in fact is the method by which adenosine is diagnostic for SVTs). Therefore ECG monitoring is required during adenosine administration.

IMPORTANT NOTES

- *Diagnostic* for SVT: If the HR is so fast that you cannot determine what the underlying rhythm is, then adenosine will temporarily shut down the AV node, which will block conduction that leads to ventricular activity. This gives the observer an opportunity to assess the underlying atrial activity.
- *Treatment* for reentry tachycardias: When adenosine is given, the AV node is turned off for a few seconds. This is usually sufficient to completely abolish a reentry tachycardia (which almost always uses the AV node as part of its pathway).
- If a patient's heart converts to sinus rhythm after the administration of adenosine, then a diagnosis of reentry tachycardia is confirmed.
- If a patient's heart resumes the SVT after an ECG pause, then the rhythm is probably atrial fibrillation, flutter, or tachycardia or sinus tachycardia and should be diagnosable while the ventricles are temporarily stopped.
- Patients sometimes refuse the drug if they have had it before because of the severity of the unpleasant sensation.

EVIDENCE
Adenosine versus Verapamil for Supraventricular Tachycardia

- A Cochrane review in 2006 (eight trials, N = 577 patients) found that both drugs were 90% effective in treating SVTs and that there were no differences in efficacy; however, adenosine converted heart rhythm to sinus rhythm a little bit faster than verapamil did. Adenosine caused unpleasant side effects in about 10% of patients, and verapamil caused hypotension in 2% of patients.

FYI NOTES

■ Adenosine is an endogenous nucleotide (i.e., occurs naturally) that is part of the well known ATP molecule. In the body, adenosine is liberated during ischemia and in fact is a mediator of the symptoms of cardiac ischemia.

■ Warn the patient how terrible he or she will feel for about 3 minutes.

■ Sometimes adenosine has absolutely no effect (caffeine blocks its effect).

Digoxin

DESCRIPTION

Digoxin is classified as a cardiac glycoside. It is an inotrope that does not have its effects mediated through β receptors.
Digoxin is also loosely classified as an antidysrhythmic.

PROTOTYPE AND COMMON DRUGS

■ Protoype: **digoxin**
■ Others include **dig**itoxin and **dig**italis (much less commonly used)

MOA (MECHANISM OF ACTION)

Digoxin has two mechanisms of action:

1. Inotropic action:
   ▲ Through the action of Na/K/ATP ion pump blockade (Figure 11-9), the following sequence of ionic events occurs:
      • ↓ Na exits the cell
      • ↑ Intracellular Na
      • ↓ Na electrochemical gradient for Na-Ca exchanger
      • ↓ Ca exits the cell
      • ↑ **Intracellular Ca**
   ▲ The increase in intracellular calcium results in **increased contractility, SV, and CO.**
   ▲ In heart failure, sympathetic tone is increased as a compensatory mechanism to increase CO. Digoxin increases

contractility and hence SV and CO, therefore reducing the need for sympathetic compensation; thus digoxin reduces the sympathetic tone in heart failure.

2. Increased parasympathetic nervous system activity:
   ▲ In addition to the indirect reduction of the SNS as outlined previously, there is a **direct increase in the parasympathetic system.**
   ▲ Digoxin sensitizes arterial baroreceptors in the carotid sinus and activates the vagal nuclei (in the brainstem). These baroreceptors induce a response via the vagus nerve that **decreases HR** and causes vasodilation when the receptors are stretched (which occurs with high BP). HR decreases owing to increased parasympathetic tone of the SA and AV nodes. By this mechanism on the **AV node,** digoxin is useful in patients with atrial fibrillation.

PHARMACOKINETICS

■ **The therapeutic index is very low.** The therapeutic range for digoxin is 0.5 to 2.5 nmol/L (in the blood). The probability of toxicity is significant when the level is > 2.6, and toxicity is virtually guaranteed when the level is >3. Contrast this to acetaminophen (Tylenol), in which the toxic oral dose is *10 times* the normal dose.

■ Children experience less toxicity than adults and have a higher therapeutic range (2.5 to 3.5).

■ **It is estimated that 20% of patients taking digoxin will experience toxicity.**

■ **Signs or symptoms of toxicity may not correlate well with digoxin levels.** A *normal* level of digoxin does not rule out toxicity.

■ The half-life is 30 hours in normal adults.

■ Clearance is via the kidneys. **Renal dysfunction** increases the elimination half-time, which increases digoxin levels and increases the risk of toxicity. The dose must be reduced accordingly.

■ **Certain drug interactions increase digoxin levels.**
   ▲ **Diuretics:** spironolactone, amiloride, triamterene
   ▲ **Antiarrhythmics:** quinidine (most commonly cited in books), amiodarone
   ▲ **Calcium antagonists:** verapamil only
   ▲ **HMG-CoA reductase inhibitors:** atorvastatin at high doses (80 mg daily)

■ Factors that increase digoxin sensitivity (and thus increase toxicity risk):
   ▲ **Hypokalemia** (most common cause)
   ▲ Hypercalcemia (less common)

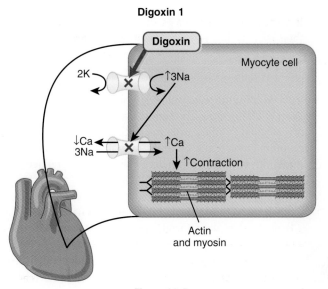

Digoxin 1

Digoxin

Myocyte cell

2K ✕ ↑3Na

↓Ca
3Na ✕ ↑Ca

↑Contraction

Actin
and myosin

Figure 11-9.

- ▲ Hypomagnesemia (less common)
- ▲ Hypothyroidism
- ▲ Hypoxia, acidosis

INDICATIONS
- ■ CHF (third-line drug in adults, first-line drug in children)
  - ▲ Digoxin increases contractility.
- ■ Atrial fibrillation
  - ▲ Digoxin decreases AV node conduction and slows the ventricular rate.

CONTRAINDICATION
- ■ Care must be exercised when prescribing to patients at risk for toxicity (see later).

SIDE EFFECTS (TOXICITY)
Signs and Symptoms
- ■ GI: Nausea, vomiting, diarrhea, abdominal pain and anorexia (loss of appetite)
- ■ CNS: Confusion, dizziness, and agitation
- ■ Cardiovascular: Arrhythmias and heart block
- ■ Visual: Orange tinted vision, visual disturbances

Electrocardiographic Changes
- ■ Increased automaticity occurs. Atrial or ventricular dysrhythmias such as premature atrial contractions (PAC's), premature ventricular contractions (PVC's), atrial or ventricular tachycardia can occur. The mechanisms include the following:
  - ▲ After depolarizations
  - ▲ Decreased slope of phase 0
  - ▲ Increased slope of phase 4
- ■ Long PR interval or AV block (caused by slow AV suppression) may be present.
- ■ Ventricular fibrillation can occur and may result in sudden death.
- ■ *Scooping* of ST segment can occur (Figure 11-10).

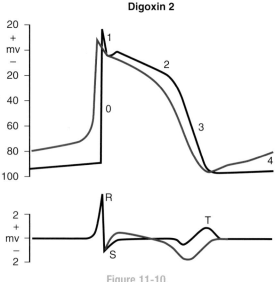

Digoxin 2

Figure 11-10.

IMPORTANT NOTES
- ■ The toxicity of digoxin is very important to understand because toxicity is so common. Treatment is to stop giving the drug for a short period, or, if there are severe cardiac arrhythmias, an antibody called Digibind can be given; Digibind binds digoxin and increases the rate of clearance.

FYI NOTES
- ■ Digoxin is the most commonly used cardiac glycoside, but its use in adults has decreased over the last two decades.
- ■ Differences between digoxin and digitalis are that digitalis has better oral absorption, a longer elimination half-life (5 to 7 days), and hepatic clearance.
- ■ Digitalis is derived from the foxglove plant (*Digitalis purpurea*). This purple flower looks like fingers of a glove, and the name **digitalis** means *relating to fingers*. What color do you think purpuric rashes are?

Inhibitors of Cholesterol Synthesis: Statins

DESCRIPTION
Statins are designed to reduce low-density–lipoprotein (LDL) cholesterol and raise HDL cholesterol.

PROTOTYPE AND COMMON DRUGS
- ■ Prototype: ator**vastatin**
- ■ Others: sim**vastatin**, prava**statin**, lova**statin**, flu**vastatin**, rosu**vastatin**, pita**vastatin**

MOA (MECHANISM OF ACTION)
- ■ These drugs are HMG-CoA reductase inhibitors. HMG-CoA reductase mediates the first step in the biosynthesis of cholesterol.

- ■ Reduced biosynthesis of cholesterol causes *an increase in the number of LDL receptors*, through the actions of sterol regulatory element binding proteins (SREBPs). Additional LDL receptors increase the catabolic rate of LDL, and the liver's extraction of LDL precursors. These actions reduce the plasma pool of LDL (Figure 11-11).
- ■ Other effects of statins include the following:
  - ▲ Small increase in plasma HDL (approximately 5%)
  - ▲ Reduction in plasma triglycerides by 10% to 25%
- ■ Statins are also increasingly being recognized for a large number of effects that are independent of cholesterol-lowering. See advanced notes, later, for further details.

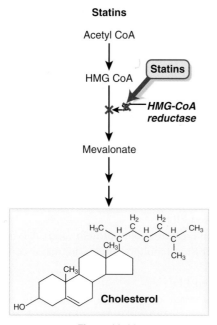

Statins

Acetyl CoA

HMG CoA ← **Statins**

HMG-CoA reductase

Mevalonate

Cholesterol

Figure 11-11.

PHARMACOKINETICS

- **Atorvastatin, simvastatin,** and **lovastatin** are metabolized by CYP3A4; thus drug interactions are of concern with these agents.
  - ▲ **Pravastatin** is the only statin that is not metabolized by the CYP450 enzyme pathways.

INDICATIONS

- Used as first-line agents in the management of hyperlipidemia

CONTRAINDICATIONS

- **Pregnancy:** HMG-CoA reductase inhibitors cause birth defects and should not be used in pregnancy.

SIDE EFFECTS

- Statins are generally well tolerated.
- **Myalgia:** muscle pain and associated weakness. The pathophysiology is not fully understood, and it is probable that this is a very mild form of myositis. This occurs in about 10% of patients.

Rare, Serious Side Effects

- **Myositis and rhabdomyolysis** are rare (1% for myositis) but serious adverse effects of statin therapy, which tend to occur at higher doses or when a drug interaction is present.
  - ▲ **Myositis** is inflammation of muscle cells and is associated with a 10 times increase in CK levels in the blood.
  - ▲ **Rhabdomyolysis** is an extreme form of myositis and results in lysis of skeletal muscle cells and release of **myoglobin** in high quantities, which results in damage to renal glomeruli and renal failure. This condition usually occurs in the presence of other risk factors in addition to statin administration, such as coadministra-

tion with cyclosporine (an immunosuppressant) or gemfibrozil (another lipid-lowering agent).
- **Hepatotoxicity:** Increases in serum aminotransferase have been observed in <1% of patients. As long as the elevations are not too great, patients who have no other risk factors for liver impairment can continue taking the statin without undue risk for liver injury, provided close monitoring is maintained.

IMPORTANT NOTES

- Statins can be used in combination with other agents such as bile acid sequestrants or inhibitors of cholesterol absorption. Fibrates and niacin (other drugs used to achieve a more favorable lipid profile) should be used with caution, as both can interact with statins.
- Ezetimibe is a cholesterol-lowering agent that is used in combination with the statins. Unlike the statins, which lower cholesterol by inhibiting its synthesis, ezetimibe reduces the absorption of cholesterol from the intestine. The fact that these two classes use distinct and complementary strategies to lowering cholesterol has made them a natural fit for combination therapy.

Advanced

- Statins are being studied for their potential role in neuroprotection, with indications such as Alzheimer's disease, Parkinson's disease, stroke, and multiple sclerosis (MS). Statins appear to activate neuroprotective pathways and also may play a role in neurogenesis. The mechanisms of all these effects are still being worked out; however, some researchers believe that the use of statins may become even more widespread than it is today.
- Statins may also improve vascular function. Studies have shown that they can reduce the generation of reactive oxygen species and regulate nitric oxide (NO) production. Other potential applications include sepsis and infection.

EVIDENCE
Patients with Cardiac Risk Factors But Without Cardiac Disease (Primary Prevention)

- A 2009 systematic review (10 studies, N = 70,388 participants) examined the use of statins in people without established cardiovascular disease but with cardiovascular risk factors. The included studies had a mean follow-up of 4.1 years. Statins reduced the risk of all-cause mortality (OR 0.88), major coronary events (OR 0.70), and major cerebrovascular events (OR 0.81).

Prevention of Stroke Recurrence (Secondary Prevention)

- A 2009 Cochrane review (eight studies, N ≅ 10,000 participants) examined the effect of altering serum lipids for prevention of subsequent cardiovascular disease and stroke in patients with a history of stroke. Statins marginally reduced subsequent cerebrovascular events (OR 0.88) but not all-cause mortality or sudden deaths. Three trials showed a subsequent reduction in serious vascular events (OR 0.74).

FYI NOTES
- Statins are among the most often-prescribed drugs worldwide. Their use has become so routine and their safety profile is thought to be so innocuous that consideration has been given in the United Kingdom and the United States to making them available without a prescription.
- Cerivastatin was withdrawn from the market earlier this decade owing to concerns over serious drug interactions, which lead to a higher risk of rhabdomyolysis.

Fibrates

DESCRIPTION
Fibrates are lipid-modifying agents used to reduce the risk of cardiovascular disease.

PROTOTYPE AND COMMON DRUGS
- Prototype: clofibrate
- Others: gemfibrozil, fenofibrate

MOA (MECHANISM OF ACTION) (Figure 11-12)
- **Transcription factors** are proteins that bind DNA and increase or decrease transcription (production of RNA and thus proteins) of selected genes.
- Fibrates activate transcription factors called peroxisome proliferator–activated receptors (**PPARs**). These are nuclear hormone receptors that respond to lipid based ligands, including hormones, vitamins, and fatty acids.
- Very-low–density–lipid (VLDL) particles are converted into fibrate agonism, resulting in:

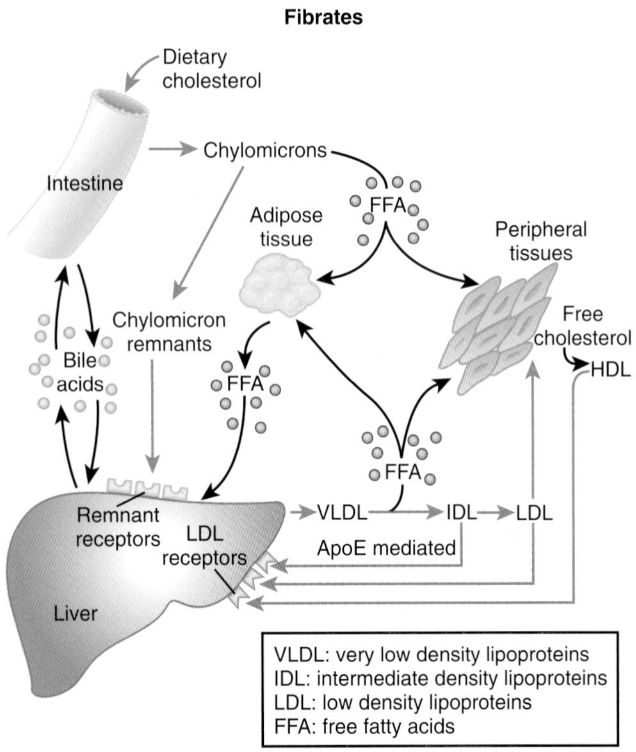

  - ▲ **Increased HDL**
    - Via increased apolipoprotein (apo) A-I and apo A-II expression (apolipoproteins are major constituents of HDL)
  - ▲ **Reduced LDL**
    - As a result of increased hepatic fatty acid uptake, conversion and catabolism of free fatty acids
    - Reduced production of VLDL particles
    - Increased catabolism via lipoprotein lipase, an enzyme that breaks down VLDL particles

PHARMACOKINETICS
- No significant issues; fibrates are well absorbed orally
- Eliminated renally and hepatically

Drug Interactions
- Gemfibrozil competes for the same glucuronosyltransferases that metabolize **statins**. This is important because statins are used for the same indication (high cholesterol) as fibrates are, and both drugs can cause muscle breakdown and muscle pain (rhabdomyositis). Coadministration can result in increased levels of both drugs and an increase in the risk for this side effect.
- Fibrates can potentiate **warfarin**, an anticoagulant. Anticoagulation levels (measured by the international normalized ratio [INR]) should be measured more closely if fibrates are initiated in a patient already taking warfarin.

INDICATIONS
- To reduce the risk of cardiovascular complications in patients with:
  - ▲ Elevated LDL or triglycerides
  - ▲ Reduced HDL

CONTRAINDICATIONS
- Renal or hepatic failure (because of excretion issues)

SIDE EFFECTS
- **Rash**
- **GI symptoms**, specifically **cholelithiasis** (gallstones)
  - ▲ Clofibrate is the fibrate most likely to result in gallstones.
- **Hepatic**: Small elevations in **liver enzymes**

Fibrates

Dietary cholesterol
Chylomicrons
Intestine
Adipose tissue
FFA
Peripheral tissues
Chylomicron remnants
Bile acids
FFA
Free cholesterol
HDL
FFA
Remnant receptors
LDL receptors
VLDL → IDL → LDL
ApoE mediated
Liver

VLDL: very low density lipoproteins
IDL: intermediate density lipoproteins
LDL: low density lipoproteins
FFA: free fatty acids

Figure 11-12.

Rare Side Effects

- **Pancreatitis**
- Reversible **decreased renal function** (indicated by an increased serum creatinine)
- Myositis, myopathy, or **rhabdomyositis**: all terms generally refer to the same process of skeletal muscle lysis resulting in pain and release of the enzyme creatinine kinase (CK) into the blood, causing CK levels to become elevated.

IMPORTANT NOTES

- Fibrates are usually administered in combination with statins and are not frequently first-line single agents.
- Chylomicron and VLDL particles are triglyceride rich.
- *Good* cholesterols lower atherosclerotic risk and include HDL and apolipoproteins apo A, apo B, and apo E.
- *Bad* cholesterols raise atherosclerotic risk and include chylomicrons, VLDL, LDL, and triglycerides.

Advanced

- Fenofibrate is metabolized by different hepatic enzymes, and these enzymes are not involved in statin glucuronidation. Thus, fenofibrate-statin combinations are less likely to cause myopathy than are other fibrate-statin combinations.

EVIDENCE
Fibrates and Cholesterol and Cardiovascular Endpoints

- A 2007 meta-analysis (10 RCTs, N = 36,489 patients) demonstrated the following:

  ▲ Fibrates did **not** significantly reduce the odds of:
  - Cardiovascular mortality
  - Fatal MI
  - Stroke

  ▲ But fibrates **did** significantly:
  - Reduce total cholesterol by 8% (versus placebo)
  - Reduce triglycerides by 30% (versus placebo)
  - Increase HDL by 9% (versus placebo)
  - Reduce the odds of nonfatal MI by about 22% ($P < .00001$)

  ▲ The odds of developing cancer were not significantly higher with the use of fibrates.

FYI NOTES

- Although the word *fibrate* is suggestive of *fiber*, the fibrates do not act as GI lipid-absorbing fiber resins. This mechanism of action belongs to a class of drug called *bile acid sequestrants.*
- Clofibrate was approved for use in 1967 in the United States. An initial study (1978) that was not properly analyzed led to the belief that clofibrate increased mortality, but these results were not supported by subsequent data and analyses.
- There have been concerns that fibrates could increase the incidence of cancer based on data from studies published in the mid 1990s. The evidence is not strong, and the association was not supported in the previously quoted meta-analysis.

Bile Acid Sequestrants

DESCRIPTION

Bile acid sequestrants comprise a family of drugs that share the physicochemical property of binding to negatively charged ions in the gut.

PROTOTYPE AND COMMON DRUGS

- Prototype: cholestyramine
- Others: colestipol, colesevelam

MOA (MECHANISM OF ACTION)

- Bile acids facilitate the digestion and absorption of dietary fats. The bile acids are normally enterohepatically recycled, which means they are secreted into the GI tract through the bile duct and then reabsorbed and transported back to the liver for the cycle to repeat (Figure 11-13).
- Bile acid binding resins carry a large **positive charge** and are therefore attracted to and **bind negatively charged bile acids** in the gut. The resins are large and therefore **not absorbed**, so the bound bile acids are excreted with the resins in the feces.
- The binding of bile acids by the resins therefore interrupts the process of enterohepatic recycling, depleting the pool of bile acids. With a deficiency of recycled bile acids the liver must synthesize more.
- Cholesterol is a precursor of bile acids, so to create more bile acids the liver must obtain more cholesterol. It does this by increasing the number of LDL receptors, which in turn leads to a **lowering of plasma LDL and total cholesterol.**
- The bile acid binding resins are not designed to increase HDL levels, and they have a **minimal impact on HDL.**

PHARMACOKINETICS

- Cholestyramine and colestipol are available in powdered dosage forms, which are administered by suspending in water and drinking.
- The bile acid binding resins are not absorbed, and they exert their actions only within the GI tract.
- Binding to negatively charged molecules can interfere with the absorption of a number of different negatively charged

Bile acid sequestrants

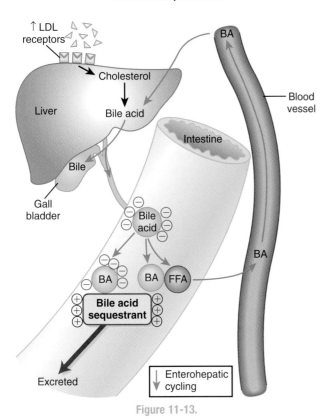

Figure 11-13.

drugs. Some of the more notable examples include thiazide diuretics, furosemide, propranolol, digoxin, and warfarin. Because of the large number of drugs that may be affected by this interaction, it is typically recommended that the administration of bile acid resins be separated from administration of other drugs by at least 1 hour if taken before the resin, or by 3 hours if taken after the resin.

■ Bile acids also facilitate the absorption of fat-soluble vitamins. Because these drugs sequester bile acids, the absorption of vitamins A, D, E, and K may be reduced in the presence of bile acid binding resins.

INDICATIONS
■ Hypercholesterolemia
■ Pruritus associated with partial biliary obstruction
■ Diarrhea associated with excess fecal bile acids in short bowel syndrome

CONTRAINDICATIONS
■ Hypertriglyceridemia

SIDE EFFECTS
■ **GI**: constipation is the most common side effect. Others can include bloating, gas, nausea, and upper abdominal pain.

Serious Side Effects
■ **Hyperchloremic acidosis (rare):** The bile acid binding resins are chloride salts and in susceptible individuals (typically **children**) may increase chloride levels enough to induce acidosis. Chloride and bicarbonate are the primary anions in the blood, and if one goes up, the other usually goes down to maintain electrical neutrality. Dropping bicarbonate results in metabolic acidosis.

IMPORTANT NOTES
■ To compensate for the actions of the bile acid binding resins, **upregulation** occurs in the activity of the HMG-CoA reductase enzyme, which is the rate-limiting enzyme in the production of cholesterol. This is the rationale for using the *statins*, which are HMG-CoA reductase inhibitors, in combination with the bile acid binding resins.

■ Interruption of enterohepatic recycling by the bile acid binding resins leads to an **increase in plasma triglyceride levels**. This is because the activity of the enzyme phosphatidic acid phosphatase, which is involved in triglyceride formation, is suppressed when the enterohepatic recycling system is functioning normally. When enterohepatic recycling is interrupted, it can lead to problematic increases in triglyceride levels, and patients who have preexisting problems with hypertriglyceridemia should avoid taking these agents.

■ The GI side effects of the powdered formulations may be reduced by allowing the suspension to sit, refrigerated, for several hours before consumption.

■ Some patients with chronic diarrhea caused by malabsorption of bile acids respond favorably to the bile acid binding resins.

■ There is some indication that bile acid sequestrants may lower blood glucose levels in patients with hyperglycemia. The mechanism behind this effect has not been identified.

FYI NOTE
■ Cholestyramine powder is also available in *light* formulations that are sugar-free.

Inotropes and Pressors

DESCRIPTION
An inotrope is a drug that results in an increase in inotropy (contractility). Pressors are drugs that primarily cause vasoconstriction. Both drugs are given to increase BP in an attempt to maintain adequate organ perfusion. This section focuses only on drugs that are administered intravenously.

COMMON DRUGS
- Dopamine
- Dobutamine
- Norepinephrine
- Epinephrine
- Phenylephrine

METABOLISM
- The synthesis of natural catecholamines is as follows:

$$tyrosine \rightarrow dopamine\,(+OH) \rightarrow$$
$$norepinephrine\,(+CH_3) \rightarrow epinephrine$$

- Hydroxylation (addition of OH) of dopamine yields norepinephrine. Methylation (addition of CH_3) of norepinephrine yields epinephrine.
- Dobutamine and phenylephrine are synthetic compounds.

MOA (MECHANISM OF ACTION)
- These drugs all exert their actions via the autonomic nervous system α and β receptors. In addition to these receptors, dopamine (and only dopamine) also acts via dopaminergic (DA) receptors.
- Drugs that are β_1 agonists are inotropes; drugs that are α_1 agonists are pressors. Activation of DA receptors results in mesenteric and renal vasodilation. Note: β_2 agonists are *vasodilators (on skeletal muscle)*.
- Most drugs are agonists to both the α *and* β receptors. However, each drug has different potencies for the receptors. Thus at low doses some drugs are primarily agonists for one receptor. At higher doses, both receptors will be stimulated, but one receptor will be more stimulated. The exception to this rule is phenylephrine. It is a pure α_1 agonist.
- Stimulation of a β receptor activates the class of proteins called *G proteins*. This results in increased cyclic adenosine monophosphate (cAMP) levels, which then stimulate protein kinases, which result in increased intracellular calcium. Calcium enhances the actin-myosin interaction and results in increased myocardial contractile force.
- Stimulation of an α_1 receptor results in increased inositol triphosphate (IP$_3$), which results in increased smooth muscle intracellular calcium, resulting in increased contractile force and increased vascular tone (vasoconstriction).
- In simple summary, dobutamine is an inotrope but not a pressor (in fact, it is a dilator). Norepinephrine and phen-

ylephrine are primarily pressors. Epinephrine and dopamine are both pressors and inotropes (Table 11-3).

PHARMACOKINETICS
- These drugs are all administered intravenously. They have short half-lives (minutes) and therefore mostly are given as infusions.
- Phenylephrine is commonly used in anesthesia and is given in small intravenous boluses.
- An exception to infusions is the administration of bolus epinephrine in cardiac arrest resuscitations (code blue) or for the treatment of anaphylaxis using syringes preloaded with epinephrine.

INDICATIONS
1. Hypotension
2. Circulatory shock (severe form of hypotension)
   - Cardiogenic shock (shock caused by a weakly contracting heart)
   - Septic shock (shock caused by vasodilation resulting from sepsis)
   - Anaphylactic shock (extreme vasodilation caused by massive histamine release)
   - Neurogenic shock (loss of sympathetic nervous system activity from spinal cord injury, causing vasodilation)
3. Acute CHF (but not chronic CHF)
   - Dobutamine and dopamine are the most commonly used for CHF

CONTRAINDICATIONS
- Usually the need for hemodynamic support outweighs most other factors. Therefore when inotropes or pressors are indicated, there is little to prevent their use. Side effects of the drugs (tachycardia, extreme vasoconstriction, increased myocardial work) can limit their maximum dose.

SIDE EFFECTS
- **Increased myocardial work**: secondary to $\uparrow$ contractility, $\uparrow$ afterload, and $\uparrow$ HR
- **Tachycardia**: β_1 agonists are also positive chronotropes.

TABLE 11-3. Properties of Inotropes and Pressors

	Receptors				Main Effects			
	α_1	β_1	β_2	DA	HR	CO	SVR	BP
Dobutamine	0	++	+	0	++	++	−	0
Dopamine	++	++	+	++	++	++	++	++
Epinephrine	+	++	++	0	++	++	++	++
Norepinephrine	+++	+	0	0	0	0	+++	+++
Phenylephrine	+++	0	0	0	0	0	+++	+++

0, No effect; *BP*, blood pressure; *CO*, cardiac output; *DA*, dopaminergic; *HR*, heart rate; *SVR*, systemic vascular resistance; +, weak positive effect; ++ moderate positive effect; +++ strong positive effect; − weak negative effect.

- **Decreased organ and tissue perfusion**: extreme vasoconstriction will increase BP but decrease flow to tissues or organs.

IMPORTANT NOTES

- A thorough assessment to determine the specific cause(s) of hypotension or shock must always be performed, and the primary cause of the problem must be corrected. For example, a patient who is bleeding and has hypotension has a *preload* (volume) problem, and therefore the preload should be corrected before the contractility or afterload is manipulated.
- Phosphodiesterase-3 (PDE3) inhibitors are also inotropes, but they are strong vasodilators and are covered separately; however, phosphodiesterase inhibitors are frequently used together with other inotropes and pressors.

FYI NOTES

- A mnemonic for the *nor* of norepinephrine is "**no radical.**" Remember that a radical is a CH group. Therefore, adding a CH_3 group to *norepi* produces *epi*.
- *Epi* starts with a vowel but stimulates the nonvowel (β) receptor more.
- *Norepi* starts with a nonvowel but stimulates the vowel (α) receptor more.
- Oxymetazoline and xylometazoline are both α_1-agonist decongestants but are not used systemically; they are prepared as nasal sprays and function to decrease nasal stuffiness and congestion by vasoconstricting vessels in the nasal mucosa. However, frequent use of these medications results in a rebound congestion when they are stopped, and therefore they must be used sparingly. They are more commonly recognized by their brand names, which in North America include Otrivin and Dristan.

Phosphodiesterase-3 Inhibitors

DESCRIPTION

PDE3 inhibitors are inodilators used in heart failure. They increase contractility and dilate vessels.

PROTOTYPE AND COMMON DRUGS

- Prototype: am**rinone**
- Others: mil**rinone**

MOA (MECHANISM OF ACTION) (Figure 11-14)

- PDE breaks down intracellular cAMP and cyclic guanosine monophosphate (cGMP).
- PDE inhibitors therefore result in **increased intracellular cAMP and cGMP**, which cause increased intracellular calcium. Which cell or tissue type is affected will dictate the effect of the PDE inhibitor.
- PDE3 is distributed in the body primarily in cardiac tissue, vascular smooth muscle, and platelets; thus its effects primarily involve these cell and tissue types.
- Increased cAMP results in increased intracellular calcium, which causes increased inotropy (contraction).
- PDE3 inhibitors also have intracellular actions that *should theoretically* improve diastolic function:
  - Stimulation of intracellular calcium uptake into the sarcoplasmic reticulum (SR) during diastole; the net effects are a lower calcium concentration during diastole and improved relaxation of actin and myosin coupling.
  - Increased cAMP results in increased protein kinase A (PKA) activity, which increases the phosphorylation of a protein called *titin*; this results in a more compliant form of titin, and this helps the cell elongate (relax) during diastole.
- PDE3 inhibitors result in the following physiologic changes:
  - Increased CO
  - Decreased end diastolic pressures
  - Mild increases in HR (because of vasodilation and baroreceptor reflex)
  - No change in myocardial work

PHARMACOKINETICS

- The half-life is about 6 hours. This is important because it is administered as an intravenous infusion. Most cardiovascular drugs (e.g., dopamine, nitroglycerin [NTG]) that are administered as intravenous infusions (to optimize BP and CO) have half-lives of 3 to 5 minutes. Therefore, milrinone is less titratable than these other drugs, and the drug levels can become unexpectedly high.
- Because PDE3 inhibitors are renally cleared, they can accumulate and result in overdose when given to patients with renal dysfunction. This manifests as excessive vasodilation and hypotension.

INDICATION

- Acute heart failure

CONTRAINDICATIONS

- Renal failure is a relative contraindication because the steady state plasma levels with an infusion can become dangerously elevated.

SIDE EFFECTS

- **Hypotension** secondary to vasodilation: This is a very important side effect. Because of the relatively long half-life of milrinone and the fact that it is administered as an infusion, the potential for **steadily increasing serum levels** of drug over a period of many hours after the start of the infusion, especially in patients with renal dysfunction, results in hypotension being a frequent side effect. Hypotension induced by PDE3 infusions is treated with

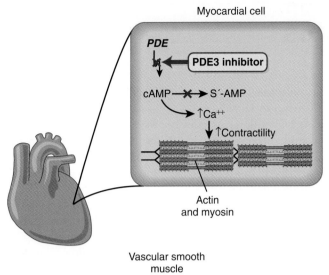

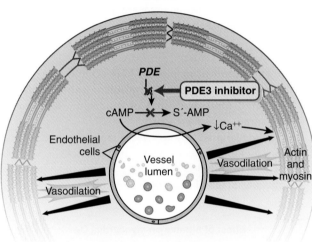

Figure 11-14.

vasoconstrictors (usually norepinephrine) and by decreasing the infusion rate. With the longer half-life, hypotension usually persists for many hours even after the infusion is decreased.

- **Thrombocytopenia:** Amrinone causes a decrease in platelet count in about 30% of patients. Milrinone causes decreased platelet counts in far fewer patients.

IMPORTANT NOTES

- Milrinone is not used for *chronic* heart failure. It is used only in select patients with severe *acute* heart failure.
- PDE3 inhibitors have a physiologic effect similar to that of β agonists because β agonists also result in increased cAMP, leading to:
  - ▲ Increased contractility
  - ▲ Increased vasodilation (with β agonism it is the result of β₂ receptors)

- However, there are important clinical differences between the two PDE3 inhibitors and β agonists:
  - ▲ PDE3 inhibitors are not direct positive chronotropes (increased HR), whereas β agonists are. Lack of a chronotropic effect can be a benefit when the patient is already tachycardic or has disease in which tachycardia would be undesirable (e.g., coronary artery disease).
  - ▲ PDE3 inhibitors do not use β receptors, which are frequently **down-regulated** or often already maximally stimulated by endogenous catecholamines, rendering them virtually unresponsive to additional exogenous β stimulation. Thus PDE3 inhibitors usually are clinically much *stronger* drugs in the setting of acute decompensated heart failure.
- PDE3 inhibitors are frequently used with a pulmonary artery catheter in a critical care setting, and the cardiac index (which is CO divided by body mass index) is used for titrating the dose and for determining when the patient can be weaned off the drug.
- PDE3 inhibitors *increase* myocardial work via increased contractility but *decrease* myocardial work via afterload reduction through vasodilation. The net effect on total myocardial work is difficult to predict but is usually about neutral.

Advanced

- PDE3 breaks down both cAMP and cGMP. The subtype of PDE determines the ratio of activity against cAMP versus cGMP. PDE3 preferentially acts on cAMP 10 times more than it does cGMP. The changes in cAMP and cGMP in different cells dictate the clinical effects seen in either the heart or the vasculature.
- PDEs are a superfamily. There are 11 subtypes. Currently, the other PDE inhibitor in clinical use is PDE5, used for treatment of erectile dysfunction.

EVIDENCE

- In an RCT of 1,088 patients in 1991, long-term treatment of *chronic* congestive heart failure with oral milrinone was associated with a 28% increased risk of mortality, primarily attributed to increased arrhythmias. PDE3 inhibitors are not used at all in chronic heart failure.

FYI NOTES

- cAMP was first identified in 1958 by Earl Sutherland, for which he received the 1971 Nobel Prize in Physiology or Medicine "for his discoveries concerning the mechanisms of the action of hormones."
- Caffeine is a weak, nonspecific PDE inhibitor. This results in increased HR and paradoxically (compared with PDE5 inhibitors) vasoconstriction.
- Theophylline, used in treatment of airway disease, is also a PDE (see also methylxanthines).
- Amrinone is also called inamrinone, a rare example of a drug having two generic names.

Nitrates

DESCRIPTION
Nitrates are agents that release nitric oxide (NO).

PROTOTYPE AND COMMON DRUGS
- Prototype: nitroglycerin (NTG)
- Others: isosorbide dinitrate (ISDN), isosorbide-5-mono-nitrate

MOA (MECHANISM OF ACTION)
- These agents all release NO, through a variety of incompletely understood biochemical mechanisms.
- NO, also known as *endothelium-derived relaxing factor (EDRF)*, induces vasodilation primarily on the venous side of the circulation (**venodilation**). It does this by activating guanylyl cyclase, an enzyme that produces **cGMP**, which decreases Ca^+ entry into cells and causes relaxation of vascular smooth muscle (Figure 11-15).
- This venodilatory effect produces a pooling of blood in the venous capacitance vessels, resulting in a reduction in venous return, preload, and end diastolic pressure, which:
  - Lowers ventricular wall tension and reduces oxygen demand
  - Improves the coronary pressure gradient, which is calculated as:

Pressure gradient = Coronary pressure − End diastolic pressure

  - These two mechanisms improve the supply-demand balance of the myocardium and are the primary mechanisms by which NTG relieves angina (Figure 11-16).
- At higher doses, nitrates can have a vasodilatory (arterial) effect; however, this is not the major mechanism in the management of stable angina. The vasodilation reduces afterload, again reducing ventricular wall tension and oxygen demand.
- To a minor extent, these agents also dilate coronary arteries, although this is again of secondary importance in their antianginal effects. It is important to realize that atherosclerotic plaques do not dilate in response to drugs, but that collateral coronary vessels *might* provide an increase in blood flow to an ischemic myocardium that is downstream from such a blockage.

PHARMACOKINETICS
- The elimination half-time of NTG is 1.5 minutes.
- NTG has very low oral bioavailability and therefore is administered topically (patch or ointment), sublingually (pill or spray), or intravenously.
- The sublingual preparations have a rapid onset and therefore are useful in relieving acute angina attacks.
- ISDN and isosorbide mononitrate have longer half-lives and the advantage of oral administration.

Effect of nitrates on vessels

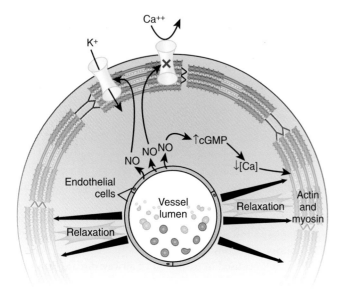

Figure 11-15.

Effect of nitrates on myocardial O₂

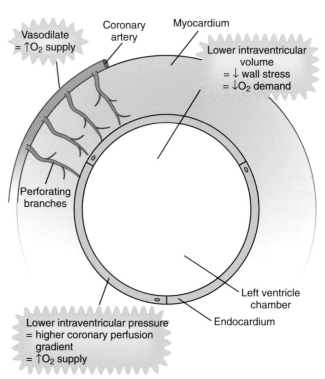

Figure 11-16.

■ Tolerance can develop to nitrates (the mechanism of tolerance is unclear). This is particularly true of long-acting agents. Patches are therefore usually worn 12 hours on and then 12 hours off.

INDICATIONS
■ Stable angina: treatment and prevention
■ Acute coronary syndromes (ACSs):
  ▲ Unstable angina
  ▲ Acute MI
■ CHF
■ Hypertensive emergency
■ To decrease uterine muscle tone (a less common use):
  ▲ To treat premature labor
  ▲ To treat fetal distress caused by high uterine contraction

CONTRAINDICATIONS
■ **Hypotension**
■ Coadministration of **PDE5 inhibitors**
■ **Elevated intracranial pressure (ICP)**—Vasodilation of cerebral arteries increases cerebral blood volume, which further increases ICP.

SIDE EFFECTS
■ **Headache:** A direct result of the cerebral dilation
■ **Flushing:** Caused by cutaneous vasodilation
■ **Orthostatic hypotension:** Low BP upon standing
■ **Presyncope or syncope:** Caused by the hypotensive effect

IMPORTANT NOTES
■ The drug interaction with PDE5 inhibitors (vasodilators used for treatment of erectile dysfunction) is significant. Many men with erectile dysfunction are older and have heart problems, such as angina. Both classes of drugs increase intracellular cGMP, and the hypotension that develops from the profound vasodilation can be severe and refractory to treatment. Hence there is great potential for this interaction to occur and for potentially serious consequences if it does occur.
■ NTG can relax any and all smooth muscle. **Esophageal spasm** can mimic angina. NTG will relax the esophagus and trick the healthcare provider into thinking that the patient does indeed have cardiac ischemia when the "angina equivalent" is relieved.

Advanced
■ Nitrates have some antiplatelet and antithrombotic properties; however, the clinical importance of these effects is unclear.
■ Formation of NO from nitrates requires the enzyme mitochondrial aldehyde dehydrogenase (ALDH2). The gene for this enzyme is often homozygous and sometimes missing in Chinese people, and they demonstrate reduced response to NTG.

EVIDENCE
■ Nitrates have not been as well studied as β-blockers and CCBs in the prevention of stable angina. A meta-analysis measuring a variety of outcomes, including mortality, found that the efficacy of long-acting nitrates did not differ significantly from that of β-blockers or CCBs.
■ There is no evidence that nitrates reduce mortality or cardiovascular complications associated with coronary artery disease. However, nitrates are effective at relieving symptoms associated with coronary artery disease.

FYI NOTES
■ NTG was the first medication used for angina pectoris, in 1879 by William Murrell.
■ The tolerance that has become a characteristic feature of nitrate therapy was discovered accidentally. *TNT* stands for *trinitrotoluene* and has three nitrate groups. Munitions workers exposed to high levels of nitrates found that the headaches they experienced diminished as the work week progressed, only to reappear with intensity after the start of each new week. These "Monday morning headaches" were originally attributed to heavy drinking over the weekend. It was later determined that the workers were actually experiencing side effects of nitrates at the start of the week and then developed tolerance during the course of the week. The tolerance wore off during the weekend, when no exposure occurred.
■ cAMP and cGMP sometimes have opposing effects on Ca^+ levels in cells.
■ NTG and ISDN have very different chemical structures.

Vasodilators

DESCRIPTION

Vasodilators cause dilation of arterioles and, to a lesser extent, veins. Not included in this section are vasodilators that act via α_1-blockade.

PROTOTYPE AND COMMON DRUGS

- Prototype: Hydralazine
- Others: Sodium nitroprusside (SNP)

MOA (MECHANISM OF ACTION)

- The underlying mechanism of **vasodilation** of arteriolar smooth muscle by the direct vasodilators is still not confirmed, but theories include interference with the release of Ca^{+2} from the SR and activation of potassium channels.

Hydralazine

- Hydralazine is **not** a coronary artery dilator.
- It does **not** relax venous smooth muscle (i.e., is not a venodilator). Hence, it will have no effect on preload. For this reason it is not a very useful drug for treatment of chronic heart failure.

Sodium Nitroprusside

- SNP is a prodrug that breaks apart to liberate NO, a mediator of dilation.
- It dilates arterioles and, to a lesser extent, veins.

PHARMACOKINETICS

Hydralazine

- Metabolized in the bowel and/or liver by acetylation. The rate of acetylation varies among individuals, with "fast acetylators" requiring higher doses of the drug.
- If given by intravenous bolus, hydralazine has a peak action 20 minutes after administration. It is also available in an oral form, although the oral form is rarely used.

Sodium Nitroprusside

- Has a virtually immediate onset of action and very short duration (minutes) and is administered only by intravenous infusion.
- SNP breaks down in red blood cells, using hemoglobin as a carrier for cyanide, the primary breakdown product.

INDICATIONS

- HTN

CONTRAINDICATIONS

- Vasodilators drop SVR. The cardiovascular system compensates for low BP from SVR by increasing CO, primarily by increasing HR and contractility via sympathetic nervous stimulation. Therefore situations in which **tachycardia** is harmful would be contraindications:
  - ▲ Coronary artery disease
  - ▲ Aortic stenosis
  - ▲ Mitral stenosis

Hydralazine

- **Systemic lupus erythematosus (SLE)** can provoke an SLE-like effect, including glomerulonephritis, in some patients. The mechanism of these immunologic reactions is not known.

SIDE EFFECTS

- **Tachycardia:** Caused by SNS compensation
- **Palpitations:** Caused by tachycardia
- **Flushing:** When the vessels in the skin dilate, the skin turns more pink.
- **Hypotension**

Hydralazine

- **Immunologic effects** (see list of contraindications). The mechanism is unknown.

Sodium Nitroprusside

- **Cyanide poisoning:** The human body can detoxify a certain amount of cyanide. When this amount is exceeded, then cyanide toxicity ensues.
- **Methemoglobinemia:** See FYI notes.

IMPORTANT NOTES

- The role of hydralazine in treating chronic HTN has severely diminished over time, and its use is now limited largely to hypertensive emergencies. Because of their toxicities, both SNP and hydralazine are considered second-line agents for hypertensive emergencies in many jurisdictions.

FYI NOTES

- These agents are rarely ever prescribed anymore because significant compensatory responses and numerous side effects limit their usefulness in the management of HTN.
- The iron (Fe) molecule in hemoglobin is normally in the Fe^{2+} state and can bind O_2 appropriately. If the iron is oxidized to Fe^{3+}, then the hemoglobin is called methemoglobin. Methemoglobin is *unable to bind oxygen*. In normal humans, about 0.5% of hemoglobin is in the form of methemoglobin. Methemoglobinemia reduces the oxygen carrying capacity of blood.
- SNP is 33% cyanide by weight.

Natriuretic Peptides

DESCRIPTION

Also called *natriuretic factors*, natriuretic peptides are endogenous hormones that are used to treat heart failure. The drug is recombinant human brain natriuretic peptide (BNP). Despite the name, the main source of BNP is the ventricle.

PROTOTYPE

- Prototype: Nesiritide

MOA (MECHANISM OF ACTION)

- A number of hormonal and neurologic mechanisms are activated in heart failure, of which natriuretic factors (peptides) are one.
- Endogenous natriuretic factors are increased during heart failure in response to atrial stretch and ventricular stretch, when the chambers are volume overloaded because of heart failure.
- BNP binds to BNP receptors on blood vessels and kidneys, which activates the cGMP system, resulting in the following effects:
  - ▲ Blood vessels: vasodilation
  - ▲ Kidneys: natriuresis and diuresis
  - ▲ Kidneys: inhibition of renin and aldosterone
- Through these effects, the abnormally high preload (filling volume) of the heart is reduced and abnormally high afterload (vasoconstriction) is also reduced. Both reduction of preload and reduction of afterload are important components of treating patients with heart failure (Figure 11-17).

PHARMACOKINETICS

- Natriuretic factor is a peptide. Taken orally, it would be digested down to amino acids and would therefore be completely ineffective.
- BNP has a half-life of 21 minutes. Therefore it is given as an intravenous infusion, because intermittent administration is not convenient, nor does it result in stable serum levels of drugs with such short half-lives.

INDICATION

- Advanced decompensated acute heart failure

CONTRAINDICATION

- Hypotension: Vasodilators will exacerbate low BP.

SIDE EFFECTS

- Hypotension: caused by vasodilation
- *Possible* worsening renal dysfunction (current evidence not conclusive)

IMPORTANT NOTES

- Endogenous BNP is elevated in patients with heart failure. Most systems that are activated in heart failure (such as the

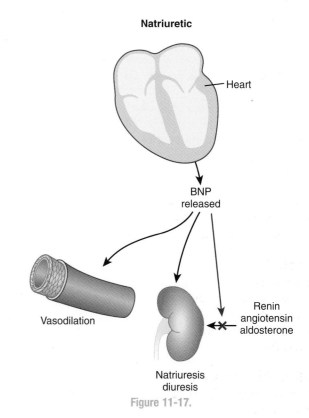

Natriuretic

Heart

BNP released

Vasodilation

Renin angiotensin aldosterone

Natriuresis diuresis

Figure 11-17.

renin-angiotensin-aldosterone system and the SNS) result in vasoconstriction and water retention, which is the opposite effect of BNP. Therefore BNP acts as a counterbalancing hormone system in heart failure.

Advanced

- The body produces proBNP (inactive), which is subsequently cleaved into BNP (active) and NT-proBNP (inactive).
- *NT* refers to the N terminal end of the original (proBNP) protein.
- Both BNP and NT-proBNP can be measured in patients with heart failure.
- Heart failure is not the only pathologic condition in which BNP is elevated. Other conditions, including shock, hypoxia, renal failure, and pulmonary HTN, can also increase circulating levels of BNP and NT-proBNP.

EVIDENCE

- A meta-analysis in 2005 (three trials, N = 862 patients) showed a possibility of *increased* death and renal dysfunction in patients with acute decompensated heart failure treated with nesiritide. All studies were double blinded. However, another meta-analysis in 2006 (seven trials, N = 1717 patients) **did not** show increased mortality or renal failure in patients with acute heart failure treated with nesiritide. Two of the trials were not blinded.

- A third meta-analysis in 2009 (14 trials, N = 934 patients) evaluating the effect of nesiritide on renal function in patients *immediately after cardiac surgery* demonstrated reduced need for dialysis in patients treated with nesiritide (OR = 0.32). However, all studies included were small and underpowered to provide statistical significance on their own.

- More evidence is required to clearly understand the effects of exogenous administration of BNP on mortality and renal function when administered to patients with acute heart failure.

FYI NOTES

- The body produces several different forms of natriuretic factor:
  - ▲ Atrial (type A or ANP)
  - ▲ Ventricular, also called *brain* (type B or BNP)
  - ▲ Vascular (type C)
- Natriuretic factor was identified first in pig brain in 1988, which is why it is called *brain natriuretic peptide* and not *ventricular natriuretic peptide.*
- *Natrium* is the Latin word for *sodium,* and *uresis* refers to *in the urine.*
- *Natriuresis* means losing sodium in the urine.
- *Diuresis* means losing water in the urine.
- *Enuresis* means involuntary passing of urine.

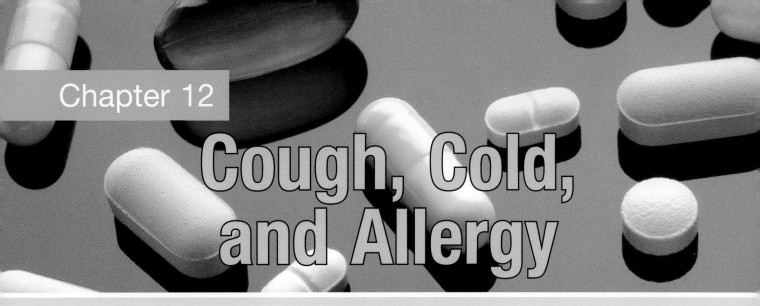

Chapter 12

Cough, Cold, and Allergy

Antitussives

DESCRIPTION

Antitussives constitute a heterogeneous class of compounds that inhibit cough through either a central or a peripheral mechanism, or a mixture of the two.

PROTOTYPE AND COMMON DRUGS
Centrally Acting
- Prototype: dextromethorphan
- Others: codeine, hydrocodone

Peripherally Acting
- Prototype: camphor and menthol
- Others: eucalyptus oil, benzonatate, levodropropizine

MOA (MECHANISM OF ACTION)
- Antitussives are cough suppressants. There are two ways to inhibit coughing: centrally and peripherally.
- Cough is normally produced through the stimulation of sensory receptors of the glossopharyngeal and vagus nerves, innervating the mucous membranes of the lower pharynx, larynx, trachea, and smaller airways of the respiratory system. The receptors then transmit the signal to the cough center in the brain, which then triggers a reflex motor response that results in contraction of the muscles to close the glottis (vocal cords) and contraction of the muscles of expiration. The result is a sudden increase in intrathoracic pressure, followed by relaxation of the vocal cords, resulting in rapid expulsion of air (Figure 12-1).
- Centrally acting agents such as dextromethorphan work by inhibiting the cough center in the brain, elevating the threshold for coughing. The exact mechanism by which they do this is still poorly understood. Dextromethorphan, for example, is an N-methyl-D-aspartate (NMDA) antagonist, although it is not known what contribution this has to its antitussive effects.

- Opiates such as codeine and hydrocodone also work through a central mechanism.
- Peripheral-acting agents work either by anesthetizing the local nerve endings or acting as demulcents. Demulcents have a soothing effect on the throat.

PHARMACOKINETICS
- Dextromethorphan has an onset of action of 15 to 30 minutes and a duration of 3 to 6 hours.
- Camphor and menthol are used topically or are inhaled through a vaporizer. When the medication is applied topically, the vapors are inhaled.

INDICATION
- Cough

CONTRAINDICATIONS
- None of major significance

SIDE EFFECTS
Dextromethorphan
- Drowsiness
- Nausea
- Dizziness

Opiates
Main side effects are **sedation** and **constipation** at the lower doses used to suppress cough. Several other side effects, many seen at higher doses or with chronic use, are reviewed in Chapter 21.

IMPORTANT NOTES
- **Dextromethorphan** was developed in an attempt to create a cough suppressant with the efficacy of codeine but with none of the central nervous system (CNS) side effects such

Antitussives and expectorants

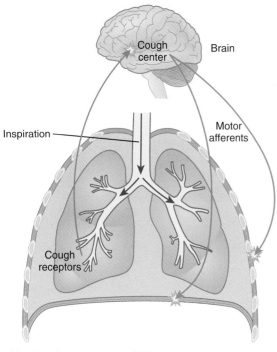

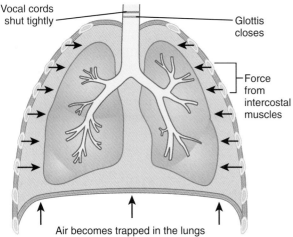

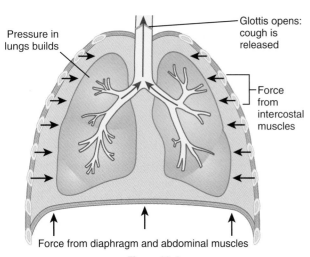

Figure 12-1.

as euphoria. Dextromethorphan therefore has **little or no** ability to induce **euphoria** and therefore is available without a prescription and without pharmacist consultation in most jurisdictions.

■ However, **very high** doses of dextromethorphan can cause **dissociative** effects similar to those seen with phencyclidine (**PCP**). PCP and dextromethorphan are both **NMDA antagonists**, and this is believed to be why they share similar effects. The doses needed to achieve this effect with dextromethorphan are high enough to cause **toxicities** resulting in hypertension, tachycardia, and respiratory depression.

■ **Codeine** can be an effective antitussive at **lower doses** than required for analgesia. Therefore some of the more important side effects of codeine, such as respiratory depression, can generally be avoided at the antitussive dose. The exception appears to be young children (≤5 years of age) who may be more sensitive to the respiratory depression. Codeine is therefore **not recommended** for children **under the age of 2** and should be used with caution in children 2 to 5 years old.

■ The use of **cough and cold preparations** in **children**, particularly combination products, has come under close scrutiny owing to concerns over deaths attributed to overdose. The use of multiple combination products facilitates overdose, as parents can be easily confused by the duplication of ingredients among products. In addition, the lack of clear evidence of efficacy of these products in young children has prompted many to question why they are used at all.

■ The three most common **causes** of **chronic cough** include:
▲ Asthma
▲ Postnasal drip
▲ Gastroesophageal reflux

■ Treatment of chronic cough must include investigations into the possible cause of the cough in addition to symptomatic treatment.

EVIDENCE
Over-the-Counter Preparations for Acute Cough

■ A 2008 Cochrane review (25 trials, N = 3492 participants) assessed the effects of over-the-counter (OTC) cough preparations for acute cough. Six trials in adults had **variable results** for antitussives **versus placebo.** Of the two trials involving expectorants, one showed benefit versus placebo whereas the other did not. In children, antitussives (two trials), antihistamines (two trials), antihistamine-decongestant combinations (two trials), and antitussive-bronchodilator combinations were no more effective than placebo. No trials were found of expectorants, but one trial showed benefit of a mucolytic versus placebo.

FYI NOTES

■ Paradoxically, when **high-potency opioids** are administered intravenously (so that they have a rapid increase in levels in the blood and brain), they can **induce cough**. This is common with the opioid called *fentanyl*, which is commonly used in conjunction with general anesthetics.

■ **Older**-generation **antihistamines** (dexbrompheniramine, diphenhydramine) have also been used as **antitussives** with some success. The mechanism behind their use is not well understood. Other agents that have been used as cough suppressants include amitriptyline and baclofen.

Expectorants

DESCRIPTION

Expectorants comprise a heterogeneous collection of compounds that facilitate the removal of mucous from the respiratory tract.

PROTOTYPE AND COMMON DRUGS

■ Prototype: guaifenesin
■ Others: ammonium chloride, terpin hydrate, potassium iodide, iodinated glycerol

MOA (MECHANISM OF ACTION)

■ Mucus serves as an airway lubricant and functions as a first level of immune defense. When mucus becomes thickened and/or dried out by infections, the functions of the mucus, including the clearing of infections, becomes impaired.
■ Expectorants typically work by increasing the amount of fluid in the respiratory tract, which increases flow and clearance of local irritants as well as reducing the viscosity of mucus.
■ It is not clear exactly how guaifenesin increases respiratory fluid, but it may be through a local irritant effect.

PHARMACOKINETICS

■ Guaifenesin is most commonly available as an oral syrup.

INDICATION

■ Loosening of mucus in upper respiratory tract infections

CONTRAINDICATIONS

■ **Guaifenesin:** none of major significance

SIDE EFFECTS

■ **Guaifenesin:** Generally well tolerated; side effects occur infrequently.
  ▲ **Nausea:** mechanism unknown
  ▲ **Drowsiness:** mechanism unknown
  ▲ **Vomiting:** typically only seen at high doses

IMPORTANT NOTES

■ There has been a longstanding controversy over the use of expectorants. This is partly because of the limited data demonstrating their efficacy.
■ The use of cough and cold preparations in children, particularly combination products, has come under close scrutiny because of concerns over deaths attributed to overdose. The use of multiple combination products facilitates overdose, as parents can be easily confused by the duplication of ingredients among products. In addition, the lack of clear evidence of efficacy of these products in young children has prompted many to question why they are used at all.
■ Guaifenesin is the most widely used expectorant. Other agents that have been used as expectorants include ammonium chloride, which can cause acidosis in patients with renal failure; terpin hydrate, which can cause nausea and vomiting; potassium iodide, which has several side effects; and iodinated glycerol.

EVIDENCE
Over-the-Counter Preparations for Acute Cough

■ A 2008 Cochrane review (25 trials, N = 3492 participants) assessed the effects of OTC cough preparations for acute cough. Of the two trials involving expectorants, one showed benefit versus placebo whereas the other did not. In children, no trials were found of expectorants, but one trial showed benefit of a mucolytic versus placebo.

FYI NOTES

■ Guaifenesin is a derivative of guiacol, which is a constituent of guaiac resin from the wood of *Guajacum officinale*. Guiacol has been used in cough extracts in the past but has been largely supplanted by guaifenesin.

Decongestants

DESCRIPTION

Decongestants are a heterogeneous class of compounds that are related by therapeutic use. These agents are typically available without a prescription.

PROTOTYPE AND COMMON DRUGS

Direct α₁ Agonists

- Prototype: phenylephrine
- Others: oxymetazoline, xylometazoline, naphazoline

Indirect α₁ Agonists

- Prototype: pseudoephedrine
- Others: ephedrine, phenylpropanolamine

MOA (MECHANISM OF ACTION) (Figure 12-2)

- **Nasal congestion** occurs when the nasal passages become **edematous,** usually a result of an inflammatory response to an upper respiratory tract infection, an allergic response, or a response to chemical irritant
- All decongestants are **vasoconstrictors.**
- The main mechanism by which they reduce nasal congestion is by constricting precapillary blood vessels, which **reduces** capillary **hydrostatic pressure,** blood flow, and volume. Hydrostatic pressure is one of the forces that pushes plasma out of a blood vessel into the tissues, causing edema. Capillary permeability and oncotic pressure are the two other factors that influence the formation of tissue edema.
- By **reducing hydrostatic pressure,** the outward force that pushes fluid out of the vessel becomes an **inward force** that drives fluid into the vessel. The net effect is to reduce leakage in blood vessels, therefore reducing congestion.

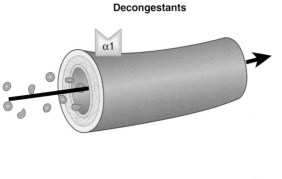

Decongestants

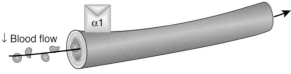

↓ Blood flow

Figure 12-2.

- Through reduction of blood flow and volume, a **smaller amount of fluid** is made available to the leaky capillaries, and thus edema formation decreases as well.
- The **vasoconstriction** is mediated by stimulation of **α₁** receptors. These receptors are stimulated either by direct agonists or indirectly. **Direct agonists** tend to be analogs of norepinephrine, although with greater selectivity for the **α₁** receptor.
- **Indirect agonists** work by increasing levels of endogenous norepinephrine.

PHARMACOKINETICS

- Decongestants come in either **oral** (pseudoephedrine) or **topical** (xylometazoline and oxymetazoline) formulations, or both (phenylephrine). The topical agents have a faster onset of action than the oral agents and have fewer systemic effects.
- Pseudoephedrine has an onset of action of 30 minutes and a duration of 4 to 6 hours.

INDICATION

- Nasal congestion

CONTRAINDICATIONS

- **Concomitant use with monoamine oxidase inhibitors (MAOIs):** Monoamine oxidase **breaks down** amines such as **norepinephrine.** Concomitant use of MAOIs with indirect-acting decongestants such as pseudoephedrine that increase norepinephrine can lead to excess norepinephrine and hypertensive crisis. MOAIs are used to treat depression and are not commonly used because newer agents have replaced them.
- **Severe hypertension and coronary disease:** Decongestants all cause vasoconstriction, which may cause a dangerous **rise in blood pressure** in those with hypertension or may reduce coronary blood flow in patients with heart disease.

SIDE EFFECTS

- **CNS stimulation:** The phenylamines (phenylephrine, ephedrine, pseudoephedrine) share common structural features with amphetamine, and therefore they also stimulate the CNS. This manifests as:
  - ▲ Agitation
  - ▲ Anxiety
  - ▲ Insomnia
- **Rhinitis medicamentosa: Rebound congestion** is typically only seen with topical agents. This is a pharmacologic phenomenon that occurs with chronic use, secondary to changes in receptor density. Patients will find that their decongestant does not work as well, that their congestion is much worse when they miss a dose of the drug, or both.

The net effect is that the patient finds that he or she is unable to discontinue the decongestant.

■ **Increased blood pressure:** Constriction caused by peripheral α_1 receptors leads to **increased resistance** and therefore increased blood pressure. This problem is more likely to be seen with oral agents and is usually a problem only in patients who have hypertension.

■ **Urinary retention:** Stimulation of α_1 receptors in the bladder leads to **constriction** of the **urinary sphincter,** restricting the flow of urine. This is typically a problem only in patients with preexisting urinary retention or in conditions such as enlarged prostate, in which patients are more prone to urinary retention.

■ **Other side effects associated with adrenergic stimulation:** Other effects include dry mouth and sweating.

■ **Local (topical agents only):** Local effects include stinging, burning, and dryness of the nasal mucosa.

IMPORTANT NOTES

■ **Rhinitis medicamentosa** is an uncomfortable complication of topical decongestant use. However, because it is a simple pharmacodynamic phenomenon, patients should **inevitably improve** once receptor densities have returned to their predrug state. This typically **takes 1 to 2 weeks,** and in the intervening period the patient may benefit from oral decongestants to get through the periods of severe congestion.

■ Vasoconstrictors have the greatest efficacy among decongestants; however, there are **other agents** that are used to relieve nasal congestion. **Camphor, menthol,** and **eucalyptus oil** are all considered to be relatively innocuous, although their efficacy in treating nasal congestion and the mechanism by which they exert their effects are not well studied.

■ The use of **cough and cold** preparations in **children,** particularly combination products, has come under close scrutiny because of **concerns** over deaths attributed to overdose. The use of multiple combination products facilitates overdose, as parents can be easily confused by the duplication of ingredients among products. In addition, the lack of clear evidence of efficacy of these products in young children has prompted many to question why they are used at all.

EVIDENCE
Nasal Congestion in the Common Cold

■ A 2009 Cochrane review (seven trials, all in adults) assessed the efficacy of nasal decongestants in reducing symptoms of nasal congestion in adults and children with the common cold. There was a **6% decrease in subjective symptoms** after a single oral dose of decongestant versus placebo. From a clinical standpoint, this is a **small difference.** With repeated use over 3 to 5 days, the benefit decreased to 4%. Only two trials reported safety measures, but in these two trials there was a small increased risk of insomnia versus placebo.

FYI NOTES

■ Ephedrine is structurally related to the amphetamines. The main difference from a pharmacologic perspective is that ephedrine and pseudoephedrine have less effect on the CNS. Ephedrine is also used to raise heart rate and blood pressure, most commonly in anesthetized patients. It is given intravenously for this indication.

■ Although phenylpropanolamine is also supposed to have fewer CNS effects than amphetamine, its use in children has come under scrutiny because of CNS adverse effects such as agitation, irritability, and insomnia. Most jurisdictions have removed phenylpropanolamine from the market or severely restricted access to it.

■ Decongestants are available without a prescription in most jurisdictions. However, their use is often still monitored closely, as they have become drugs of abuse for their stimulant properties. Ephedrine and pseudoephedrine can also readily be converted into amphetamine derivatives such as methamphetamine (also known as *crystal meth*).

■ Pseudoephedrine is available in several different combination products with antitussives (dextromethorphan), expectorants (guaifenesin), and analgesics (acetaminophen).

H$_1$ Antagonists

DESCRIPTION

H$_1$ antagonists are agents that antagonize the allergic responses and other effects mediated by histamine. These are also known as *antihistamines.*

PROTOTYPE AND COMMON DRUGS
First Generation

■ Prototype: diphenhydramine
■ Others: dimenhydrinate, chlorpheniramine, brompheniramine, hydroxyzine, cyclizine, meclizine, promethazine, cyproheptadine, carbinoxamine, clemastine, pyrilamine, tripelennamine, phenindamine

Second Generation

■ Prototype: loratadine
■ Others: cetirizine, desloratadine, fexofenadine, levocetirizine, olopatadine, acrivastine, azelastine, levocabastine, ebastine, mizolastine

MOA (MECHANISM OF ACTION)

■ Histamine is mainly **synthesized** in **mast cells** and basophils of the immune system, enterochromaffin-like cells in gastric mucosa, and certain neurons that release it as a neurotransmitter.

Antihistamines

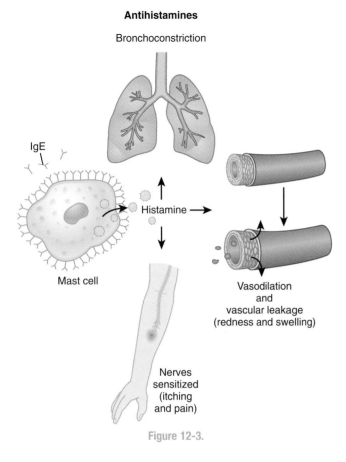

Figure 12-3.

- Histamine plays a key role in **allergic reactions,** also known as *immunoglobulin E (IgE)–mediated hypersensitivity reactions.* The role of histamine in the immune response is largely mediated by H_1 **receptors.** Classic hallmarks of an immune response that is mediated by H_1 include the following (Figure 12-3):
  - ▲ **Lungs:** bronchoconstriction
    - Chest tightness, asthmalike symptoms
  - ▲ **Vascular smooth muscle:** vasodilation
    - Redness from shunting of blood flow to skin
    - Physiologic purpose is to enhance blood flow and thus transport of nutrients to injured or infected areas
  - ▲ **Vascular endothelial cells:** contraction, separation
    - Leakiness of blood vessels leading to edema
  - ▲ **Nerves:** sensitization of afferent nerve terminals
    - Itching, pain
- H_1-receptor antagonists competitively antagonize histamine at these receptors, mitigating the immune response to an allergen.
- Many of the **first-generation** antihistamines also possess **anticholinergic** activity. This might contribute to some of the side effects associated with these agents, but it also might contribute to their efficacy in the treatment of **nausea.**

PHARMACOKINETICS

- Antihistamines vary in their ability to cross the blood-brain barrier. **Second-generation** agents **penetrate** much more slowly and in **lower quantities** compared with first-generation agents. This is one reason why second-generation agents are much **less sedating** than first-generation agents.
- **Fexofenadine** is an **active metabolite** of terfenadine. Terfenadine was a very popular antihistamine before being withdrawn from the market over safety concerns (fatal arrhythmias). Fexofenadine is not metabolized further before being excreted unchanged.
- Several of the first-generation antihistamines are also available in injectable forms.

INDICATIONS

- Allergic rhinitis
- Urticaria (swelling and itching) caused by allergy-related dermatologic disorders
- Nasal symptoms associated with common cold
- Nausea (first-generation agents)

CONTRAINDICATIONS

- None of major significance
- For use in pregnancy, see Advanced section

SIDE EFFECTS

- **Sedation:** H_1 receptors in the CNS mediate wakefulness, so antagonism of these receptors leads to drowsiness. Some antihistamines also antagonize serotonin receptors, and this might also contribute to sedation.
- **Anticholinergic side effects (first-generation agents):** dry mouth, urinary retention

IMPORTANT NOTES

- **Two factors** appear to play a role in distinguishing **sedating** from nonsedating antihistamines. Aside from the pharmacokinetic property of being able to cross into the CNS, some antihistamines also **antagonize serotonin** (5-HT_2) receptors. For the agents that cross into the CNS, this contributes further to their sedating properties.
- **Antihistamines** are **not** typically useful for life-threatening **anaphylactic** reactions, which are managed acutely with an injection of epinephrine. Antihistamines typically do not work quickly enough to be useful in these situations, but they also fail to address many of the most important characteristics of anaphylaxis, such as hypotension and bronchoconstriction. Although histamine elicits these life-threatening responses, it is believed that this is possibly mediated by another histamine receptor and therefore is not addressed through H_1 blockade.
- The use of **cough and cold preparations** in **children,** particularly combination products, has come under close scrutiny because of concerns over **deaths** attributed to overdose. The use of multiple combination products facilitates overdose, as parents can be easily confused by the duplication of ingredients among products. In addition, the lack of clear evidence of efficacy of these products in young children has prompted many to question why they are used at all.

Advanced

- There are also **H₃ receptors**, associated with the nervous system, and **H₄ receptors**, associated with leukocytes, that are current targets of drug development for unrelated indications.
- The **antiinflammatory** effects of antihistamines are currently being studied for their potential role in treating **asthma**. Studies to date have shown mixed success with antihistamines in asthma.

Pregnancy

- The **safety** of antihistamines for the fetus varies **greatly**. Fexofenadine and hydroxyzine are considered to have teratogenic effects in animals, whereas cetirizine, loratadine, chlorpheniramine, and diphenhydramine have not demonstrated these effects.

Lactation

- **First-generation** antihistamines are more likely to **cross** into breast milk, and this may lead to excess sedation in the nursing infant.

EVIDENCE
For the Common Cold

- A 2003 Cochrane review (32 trials, N = 8930 participants) assessed the effects of antihistamines in reducing nasal symptoms in patients with **common cold**. First-generation antihistamines were found to have a small effect on rhinorrhea and sneezing, but this was not considered to be clinically significant. First-generation agents also were associated with the side effect of sedation. Combinations of antihistamines and decongestants were not found to be effective in young children.

FYI NOTES

- Many of the first-generation antihistamines, particularly dimenhydrinate, are used off-label as sleep aids owing to their propensity for inducing sedation.
- The efficacy and safety of second-generation antihistamines has been more thoroughly studied compared with first-generation agents.
- Doxepin, which is classed as a tricyclic antidepressant, also possesses significant antihistamine activity. It is actually much more potent than most marketed antihistamines.
- Sensitization of afferent nerve terminals is the reason why a mosquito bite stings and itches.
- Name alert: **Diphenhydramine** and **dimenhydrinate** are also known in North America by their proprietary names Benadryl and Gravol, respectively.
- Desloratadine is the active metabolite of loratadine.

Mast Cell Stabilizers

DESCRIPTION

Mast cell stabilizers inhibit allergic responses by preventing degranulation of mast cells. They are often referred to as *chromones*.

PROTOTYPE AND COMMON DRUGS

- Prototype: cromolyn sodium
- Others: nedocromil, lodoxamide

MOA (MECHANISM OF ACTION)

- The **degranulation of mast cells** and eosinophils is an important step in the response to an allergen. Degranulation leads to release of a variety of proinflammatory factors, including histamine, leukotrienes, and various cytokines. These factors then act on tissues to elicit the classic signs of an allergic reaction.
- **Mast cell stabilizers** work by preventing this degranulation from occurring. The mechanism by which they accomplish this is still not confirmed.
- Mast cell stabilizers have a variety of other actions that may contribute to their efficacy. They suppress the actions of chemotactic factors on eosinophils, neutrophils, and monocytes, and they may reduce movement of leukocytes in asthmatic airways (Figure 12-4).

PHARMACOKINETICS

- The chromones are generally delivered topically, either by the inhalational route or as drops for ophthalmic use. They have a very low oral bioavailability (1%); therefore any topical drug that happens to be swallowed will have minimal systemic effects.

INDICATIONS

- Conditions with an allergic component:
  - ▲ Asthma (mild to moderate)
  - ▲ Rhinitis
  - ▲ Conjunctivitis
- Systemic mastocytosis (excessive proliferation of mast cells in tissues—this is an extremely rare disorder)

CONTRAINDICATIONS

- None of major significance

SIDE EFFECTS

- **Generally well tolerated**
- Side effects generally related to topical application
- **Cough** from irritation of the throat
- **Nasal irritation**—local irritation from sprays

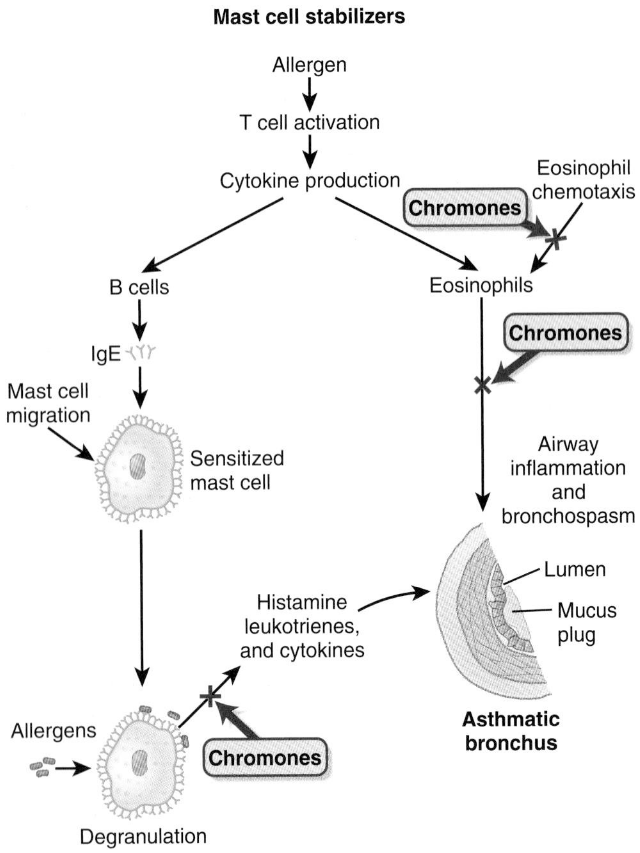

Mast cell stabilizers

Figure 12-4.

IMPORTANT NOTE

■ Cromolyn and related compounds do not posses bronchodilator activity and are therefore not useful in acute asthma attacks.

EVIDENCE

Sodium Cromoglycate versus Placebo in Pediatric Asthma

■ A 2008 Cochrane review (23 trials, N = 1026 participants) examined the efficacy of sodium cromoglycate versus placebo in prophylactic treatment of pediatric asthma. Most of the studies had small sample sizes, and most were crossover studies, thus limiting confidence in the results. The authors concluded that there is insufficient evidence to be certain about the beneficial effects of sodium cromoglycate for this indication and in this population.

Sodium Cromoglycate versus Inhaled Corticosteroids in Chronic Asthma

■ A 2006 Cochrane review (17 trials, N = 1279 children; eight trials, N = 321 adults) compared inhaled corticosteroids with sodium cromoglycate in adults and children with chronic asthma. In children and adults, sodium cromoglycate was inferior to inhaled corticosteroids with respect to use of rescue bronchodilators and improved performance on pulmonary function tests. Sodium cromoglycate was also inferior with respect to improvement of symptoms, although in adults these improvements were significant only in crossover trials and not in those of parallel design. There were no differences in adverse effects between inhaled corticosteroids and sodium cromoglycate in either children or adults.

FYI NOTES

■ The chromones are derived from the *Ammi visnaga* plant and have been used as spasmolytics for many centuries, dating back to ancient Egypt.

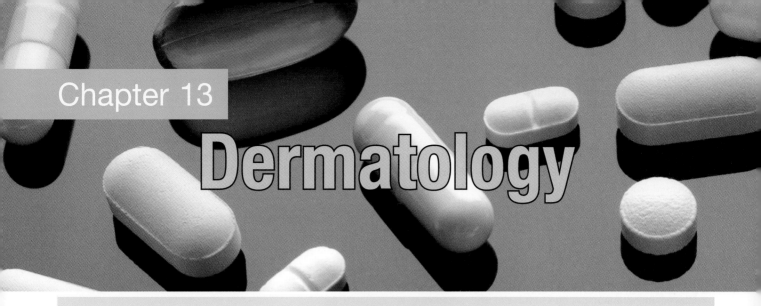

Chapter 13

Dermatology

Retinoids

DESCRIPTION
Retinoids activate retinoic acid receptors (RARs).

PROTOTYPE AND COMMON DRUGS
Topical
- Adapalene, tazarotene

Oral
- First-generation agents: tretinoin (also called *all-trans retinoic acid* [ATRA]), isotretinoin
- Second-generation agent: acitretin
- Third-generation agent: bexarotene

MOA (MECHANISM OF ACTION)
- A retinoid is a molecule (or a metabolite of a molecule) that binds to and activates RARs. There are also retinoid X receptors (RXRs), which also play a role in transducing retinoid signaling (Figure 13-1).
- Retinoid receptors are intranuclear and act as **transcription factors**; they bind to regulatory regions in DNA called *hormone response elements* and activate gene transcription.
- Increased **growth factors** are then released, which results in **epidermal hyperplasia** and thickened skin, caused by the increased proliferation of basal keratinocytes.
- As a consequence of the hyperplasia, subsequent desquamation and peeling of the skin occur.

Acne
- Isotretinoin decreases sebum secretion and sebaceous gland size, the main contributors to the oily characteristic of the skin of patients with severe acne.
- Isotretinoin reduces the abnormal follicular epithelial differentiation and desquamation that play an important role in the pathogenesis of acne.
- Isotretinoin reduces comedogenesis (a comedone is a *blackhead* that occurs when excess oils accumulate in sebaceous glands).

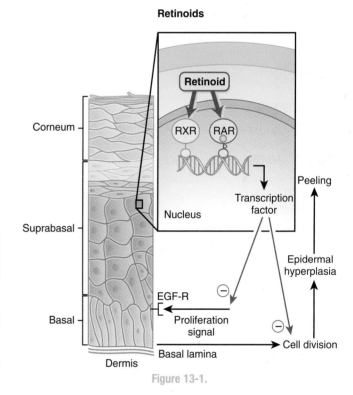

Retinoids

Figure 13-1.

- Isotretinoin reduces colonization with *Propionibacterium acnes*, a bacterium implicated in acne.

Photoaged Skin
- Partial restoration of markedly reduced levels of collagen in sun-exposed skin is one of the mechanisms of benefit for patients with photoaged skin.

Cutaneous T-Cell Lymphoma
- Bexarotene is 100 times more potent for RXR than for the RAR. This results in the following:

▲ Blocking of cell cycle progression
▲ Induction of apoptosis and differentiation
▲ Prevention of multidrug resistance
▲ Inhibition of angiogenesis and metastasis

PHARMACOKINETICS

- Oral retinoids are lipophilic, and their absorption is increased when they are taken with fatty foods.
- Adapalene and tazarotene are not taken orally; they are topically applied.
- Topically applied retinoids do not demonstrate appreciable systemic absorption; however, because the skin lesions treated with retinoids are not life-threatening, it is strongly recommended that topical retinoid application be delayed in pregnant patients until *after* the pregnancy is complete.
- All retinoids are metabolized by the liver.
- Acitretin has a half-life of 2 days, but etretinate, a related drug, has a half-life of 120 days because of storage in adipose tissue (as it is highly lipophilic). If **taken with alcohol**, acitretin is converted to etretinate. Therefore pregnancy must be avoided for 2 years (3 years in the United States) after acitretin is discontinued, according to a manufacturer's warning.

INDICATIONS
Isotretinoin, Adapalene, Tazarotene

- Acne
- Photoaged (sun damaged) skin

Acitretin

- Psoriasis
- Other keratinizing disorders

Bexarotene

- Cutaneous T-cell lymphoma, but not as first-line treatment

CONTRAINDICATIONS

- **Pregnancy:** Retinoids are teratogens. Acne treatment commonly occurs in patients during teenage years. Special attention to pregnancy avoidance must be discussed with **patients at higher risk for unplanned pregnancy.**
- **Tetracycline coadministration:** there is a risk of increased intracranial hypertension. Note that tetracycline also is often used to treat acne.

SIDE EFFECTS
Common

- **Mucocutaneous** side effects:
  ▲ Cheilitis: dry, cracked, chapped lips
  ▲ Xeroderma: dry skin; also called *xerosis*
  ▲ Skin peeling
  ▲ Sicca (dry eyes) resulting in conjunctivitis
  ▲ Epistaxis (nose bleeds) from dry mucosa in the nasal passages

- **Myalgias** (back pain and joint pain)
  ▲ Occur in up to 50% of patients; usually not severe but are worse with exercise
- **Hyperostosis** (excessive bone growth)
  ▲ After 5 years of treatment, hyperostosis occurs in most patients but is usually asymptomatic. Younger patients who are still growing have a *very* small risk of premature growth plate closure (leading to short stature).

Less Common

- Reversible increase in **liver enzyme** test values
- **Hypothyroidism** (bexarotene only)
- **Elevated cholesterol**
- **Loss of color or night vision**

Uncommon

- **Pseudotumor cerebri** (benign intracranial hypertension): Diagnosed as new onset of headache and visual changes. This is more common when retinoids are coadministered with tetracycline (an antibiotic also used to treat acne); therefore they should not be coadministered with tetracycline.
- **Depression and psychosis:** There is an increased risk of psychiatric disturbances.
- **Inflammatory bowel disease:** Retinoids *might* be associated with an increased risk of inflammatory bowel disease.

IMPORTANT NOTES

- Liver enzyme measurements need to be performed at baseline, before the patient starts taking isotretinoin, and again 1 to 2 months after the patient has started to take the medication, to look for an elevation in enzymes.
- Photoaged skin demonstrates increased wrinkles and pigmentation. Treatment for several weeks with isotretinoin or tazarotene has demonstrated improvement.
- **Cheilitis** occurs in virtually all patients taking isotretinoin, and if it does not occur, it should be considered an indication of treatment failure or noncompliance.

Advanced

- Ultraviolet irradiation results in functional impairment of receptor-dependent retinoid responsiveness in human skin. Thus stimulation of these receptors is the basis from which to counter the aging process that occurs from sun damage.

EVIDENCE
Photoaged Skin

- A Cochrane review in 2005 (eight studies, N = 460) showed that topical tretinoin cream in concentrations of 0.02% or higher was superior to placebo for participants with mild to severe photodamage on the face and forearms. The relative risk of improvement for 0.05% tretinoin cream compared with placebo (three studies) at 24 weeks was 1.73. This effect was not seen for 0.001% (one study) or 0.01% (three studies) topical tretinoin. A dose-response relationship was evident for both effectiveness and skin irritation.

Acne

- A systematic review of topical retinoids found evidence to support the following:
  - ▲ Retinoids are superior to placebo.
  - ▲ **0.1% tazarotene was more effective** than 0.025% tretinoin, 0.1% tretinoin microsphere gel, and 0.1% adapalene.
  - ▲ **0.1% adapalene showed fewer side effects** than 0.025 to 0.05% tretinoin creams or gels.

FYI
Nomenclature

- *Xero-* is from the Greek, meaning dry. *Xerostomia* means dry mouth. *Xerophagia* means eating dry foods, something that might be difficult if you already had xerostomia.

- The company Xerox got its name from *xerography*, which means dry writing.
- Sjögren's syndrome is an autoimmune condition that results in a dry mouth and dry eyes.
- Retinoids have biologic activity that is similar to that of vitamin A. Tretinoin is in fact the acid form of vitamin A. Remember that vitamin A is important for vision, so visual problems are a rare risk of retinoids.
- Alitretinoin is a retinoid that has not yet received U.S. Food and Drug Administration (FDA) approval but has been studied as a treatment for chronic refractory eczema and Kaposi's sarcoma. Kaposi's sarcoma is a cancer that is seen most commonly in patients with acquired immunodeficiency syndrome (AIDS).
- RARs have a lot of similarity to hormone and steroid receptors.

Steroids, Topical

DESCRIPTION
Topical steroids are corticosteroids that are used on the skin.

COMMON DRUGS
Organized by nomenclature for easier recall:

- Hydrocort**isone**, betameth**asone**, dexameth**asone**, flutic**asone**, flumeth**asone**, momet**asone**, diflor**asone**, desoximet**asone**
- Triamcin**olone**, prednis**olone**, methylprednis**olone**
- Des**onide**, bud**esonide**, halcin**onide**, fluocin**onide**, amcin**onide**, flurandren**olide**
- Halo**betasol**, clo**betasol**

MOA (MECHANISM OF ACTION)

- As topical agents, steroids are used for their **antiinflammatory** properties, which are exerted through the following mechanisms:
  - ▲ Inhibition of the release of phospholipase A_2, which is the principle enzyme for the formation of arachidonic acid–based inflammatory mediators prostaglandins and leukotrienes.
  - ▲ Inhibition of transcription factors that are involved in the activation of proinflammatory genes. Transcription factors increase or decrease gene expression; two examples are activator protein 1 and nuclear factor kappa B (NF-κB).
    - • Another example: lipocortin I is up-regulated by steroids. It inhibits phospholipase A_2.
  - ▲ Decrease in the release of interleukin-1 (IL-1) (a proinflammatory cytokine) from keratinocytes.

  - ▲ Inhibition of phagocytosis and stabilization of lysosomal membranes of phagocytizing cells.
  - ▲ This property benefits *inflammatory* skin lesions.
- The second benefit topical steroids provide to skin is **immunosuppression**, which is mediated through the following:
  - ▲ Suppressing the production and effects of mediators involved in the inflammatory response, including tumor necrosis factor (TNF), granulocyte-macrophage colony-stimulating factor, IL-1, and IL-8.
  - ▲ Inhibiting leukocyte migration and chemotaxis to sites of inflammation.
  - ▲ Interfering with the function of endothelial cells, granulocytes, mast cells, and fibroblasts.
  - ▲ Depleting mast cells in the skin.
  - ▲ This property also benefits *inflammatory* skin lesions.
- The third benefit of topical steroids is **antimitotic**, or **antiproliferative**, mediated through the following:
  - ▲ Inhibition of DNA synthesis and mitosis.
  - ▲ Inhibition of fibroblast activity and collagen formation.
  - ▲ This property benefits conditions that demonstrate abnormally *high proliferation*, such as scaling lesions, but is also the mechanism responsible for the side effect of thin skin.
- The fourth benefit of topical steroids is as a **vasoconstrictor:**
  - ▲ The mechanism is unclear, but inhibition of vasodilating inflammatory mediators could be responsible for part of this effect.

▲ The **potency** of topical steroids is quantified by the degree of vasoconstriction caused in a vasoconstriction bioassay.

▲ Vasoconstriction could be of benefit in that it results in less redness of the skin (cosmetic effect only) and reduces blood flood, resulting in less swelling.

PHARMACOKINETICS
Absorption

■ Corticosteroids are only minimally absorbed after application to normal skin—for example, approximately 1% of a dose of hydrocortisone solution is absorbed.

■ Occlusion of drug with an impermeable film such as plastic wrap increases absorption by a factor of 10.

■ Absorption depends on the body part to which the medication is applied. Relative to the arm, absorption ratios are as follows: plantar foot, 0.14; palm, 0.83; scalp, 3.5; forehead, 6; vulva, 9; scrotum, 42. Also:

▲ Inflamed skin results in increased absorption.

▲ Exfoliative skin results in decreased absorption.

Potency

■ Topical steroids are graded on a scale from 1 to 7 for potency, with class 1 being the most potent.

■ The **delivery vehicle** can exert a large influence on the potency of a topical steroid. Combinations of powders, oils, and water-based liquids comprise the vehicles. Combinations of ingredients in these three forms in varying proportions make up the most commonly used and are vehicles:

▲ **Ointments** are water suspended in oil and are the **most potent** because of their occlusive effect, but are greasy and not useful on hairy areas. Ointments should be applied two or three times per day, particularly after the skin has been moistened. They are useful for **dry lesions** because they form a water barrier.

▲ **Creams** are semisolid emulsions of oil in 20% to 50% water and are not greasy. Creams are less potent than ointments.

▲ **Lotions** are powder in water formulations and are the **least potent**. They are useful for hairy areas and when large areas have to be treated. Lotions evaporate, providing a cooling and drying effect, making them useful for treating **moist lesions**.

▲ **Gels** are an oil-in-water emulsion with alcohol in the base but are not greasy. They liquefy on contact with skin and are useful for hair-covered areas.

▲ **Foams** are pressurized collections of gaseous bubbles in a liquid film. Foam preparations spread readily and are easier to apply.

■ The **salt (ester derivative)** to which the steroid is bound also influences potency. Topical steroids are named according to the ester to which they are bound. For example, betamethasone exists as betamethasone valerate, betamethasone dipropionate, and betamethasone benzoate, each with a different potency. Furthermore, each chemical can be delivered in a different vehicle (cream versus ointment and therefore a range of potencies can be produced using the same original steroid chemical).

▲ Common examples of ester derivatives include acetate, aceponate, acetonide, benzoate, butyrate, diacetate, dipropionate, furoate, probutate, propionate, and valerate.

■ **Concentration** of the topical steroid (expressed as a percentage) also influences potency. Higher concentrations are more potent.

■ One of the highest-potency agents (clobetasol propionate ointment) is approximately 1000 times more potent than one of the lowest potency agents (1% hydrocortisone).

List of Topical Steroid Potencies
Class 1—Superpotent

■ Betamethasone dipropionate 0.05% optimized vehicle
■ Clobetasol propionate 0.05%
■ Diflorasone diacetate 0.05%
■ Fluocinonide 0.1% optimized vehicle
■ Flurandrenolide, 4 mg/cm^2
■ Halobetasol propionate 0.05%

Class 2—Potent

■ Amcinonide 0.1%
■ Betamethasone dipropionate 0.05%
■ Desoximetasone 0.25% to 0.5%
■ Diflorasone diacetate 0.05%
■ Fluocinonide 0.05%
■ Halcinonide 0.1%
■ Mometasone furoate 0.1%

Class 3—Potent, Upper Midstrength

■ Amcinonide 0.1%
■ Betamethasone valerate 0.1%
■ Diflorasone diacetate 0.05%
■ Fluocinonide 0.05%
■ Fluticasone propionate 0.005%

Class 4—Midstrength

■ Betamethasone valerate 0.12%
■ Desoximetasone 0.05%
■ Fluocinolone acetonide 0.025%
■ Flurandrenolide 0.05%
■ Hydrocortisone probutate 0.1%
■ Hydrocortisone valerate 0.2%
■ Mometasone furoate 0.1%
■ Triamcinolone acetonide 0.1%

Class 5—Lower Midstrength

■ Betamethasone dipropionate 0.05%
■ Betamethasone valerate 0.1%
■ Fluocinolone acetonide 0.025%
■ Flurandrenolide 0.05%
■ Fluticasone propionate 0.05%
■ Hydrocortisone butyrate 0.1%
■ Triamcinolone acetonide 0.1%

Class 6—Mild Strength

■ Desonide 0.05%
■ Fluocinolone acetonide 0.01%

Class 7—Least Potent
- Dexamethasone 0.1%
- Flumethasone
- Hydrocortisone 0.1% to 2.0%
- The **insoluble** corticosteroids are sometimes injected. When injected, the drug is slowly released for 3 to 4 weeks. This method of administration is often reserved for refractory lesions. Drugs that are injected include triamcinolone and betamethasone.

INDICATIONS
- The list of skin conditions that are treatable with topical steroids is long. This incomplete list represents only the most *common and responsive* conditions:
  - ▲ Psoriasis
  - ▲ Atopic dermatitis
  - ▲ Eczema
  - ▲ Seborrheic dermatitis
  - ▲ Contact or irritant dermatitis

CONTRAINDICATION
- Active infection in skin: Because of the immunosuppressive property of topical steroids, application to known active infections should be avoided.

SIDE EFFECTS
- All side effects are more common with higher-potency steroids, larger surface areas treated, and longer durations of treatment.
- **Skin atrophy:** Skin atrophy is demonstrated by thin shiny-appearing skin, telangiectasia (small readily visible blood vessels), ecchymoses (bruises), striae (stretch marks), hypertrichosis (increased hair), redness, and pigmentation changes.
  - ▲ Hydrocortisone aceponate, prednicarbate, fluticasone propionate, and methylprednisolone aceponate have the lowest capacity to induce skin atrophy.
    - • Therefore they can be used to treat the face, scrotum, and large body surface areas in children, with minimal adverse effects.
  - ▲ Higher-potency steroids can induce changes in as little as 2 weeks.
- **Systemic absorption,** leading to systemic side effects. Systemic side effects can occur but are not common. Systemic side effects include the following:
  - ▲ Adrenal suppression
  - ▲ Cushing's syndrome, notably hyperglycemia (glucocorticoid effect)
  - ▲ Sodium retention (mineralocorticoid effect)
  - ▲ Hypertension (mineralocorticoid effect)
  - ▲ Mood changes

- Other
  - ▲ **Glaucoma:** Glaucoma occurs when the drug is administered periorbitally (around the eyes). This side effect is rare.

IMPORTANT NOTES
- There are many different topical steroids. Through modification of the original steroid (hydrocortisone), the antiinflammatory potency, mineralocorticoid versus glucocorticoid ratio, and side effects are changed.
- Many topical steroids are **combined with antibacterial or antifungal** medications. These combination drugs simultaneously treat two problems (inflammation and infection), and if the diagnosis of the lesion is unclear or it appears to be a mixed problem, then these drugs can be useful. Of course, if the lesion worsens, then the medication should be stopped, and further investigations are required.
  - ▲ Combination drugs are more expensive than monotherapy.
  - ▲ A KOH (potassium hydroxide) scraping is a quick diagnostic test for fungal elements in a skin lesion.
- Lower-potency steroids should be used on sensitive areas (face, genitals) and on children.
- Short duration (<3 weeks) should be the goal of steroid treatment if possible; longer duration increases the probability of side effects.

Advanced
- A **fluorine molecule** at specific sites in the corticosteroid molecules results in enhanced corticosteroid selectivity and potency.
- Changing **hydroxyl groups** increases the molecule's lipophilicity, increasing the rate of percutaneous absorption as well as the corticosteroid receptor binding activity.

EVIDENCE
Steroids and Psoriasis
- A 2009 Cochrane review (16 studies, N = 1916 patients) found that use of potent and very potent steroids over a 2- to 3-week period by patients with psoriasis resulted in statistically significant improvement, as measured by an "investigator assessment of overall global improvement." Note that duration of effect investigated is short and that psoriasis is a chronic disease.

FYI
- Steroids are discussed further in Chapters 17 (systemic steroids) and 24 (inhaled steroids).

Keratolytics

DESCRIPTION
Keratolytics break down keratin in the skin.

PROTOTYPE AND COMMON DRUGS
α-Hydroxy Acids
- Prototype: salicylic acid
- Others: lactic acid, glycolic acid

Urea

MOA (MECHANISM OF ACTION)
- **Keratin** is a fibrous insoluble protein found in the skin, hair, and nails. In some dermatologic conditions the amount of keratin is increased, resulting in a thicker epidermis termed **hyperkeratosis**. One of the most commonly recognized causes of hyperkeratosis is **warts**. **Psoriasis** and **eczema** are two other common hyperkeratotic conditions.
- The **stratum corneum** is the outermost layer of the **epidermis** where the keratin is present; it is composed of the dead squamous cells that are produced in the stratum germinativum. The primary roles of the stratum corneum are to prevent water evaporation and to impart physical strength to the skin (Figure 13-2).

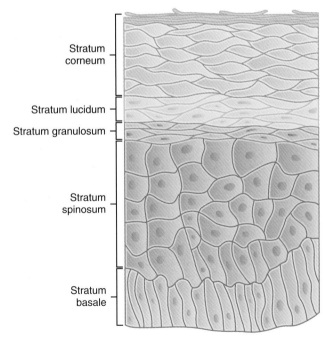

Keratolytics

Stratum corneum

Stratum lucidum

Stratum granulosum

Stratum spinosum

Stratum basale

Figure 13-2.

- **Desmosomes** are structures that contain both intracellular and extracellular components; they are important because they are attached to keratin and function to impart cell-to-cell adhesion and create resistance to physical stresses on the epithelium.
- Keratolytics reduce the thickness of the stratum corneum by incompletely understood mechanisms, but probably via a combination of the following:
  - Acids directly solubilize the protein components of desmosomes.
  - Acids activate endogenous hydrolytic enzymes by changing the pH of the stratum corneum.
  - Acids diffuse into the stratum corneum and bind water; the acids act as **humectants** (they increase the water content) of the stratum corneum. Increasing the water content softens the tissues, making them easier to physically debride.

PHARMACOKINETICS
- Salicylic acid is available in concentrations ranging from 0.5% to 60%. In concentrations over 6%, salicylic acid is destructive to tissue.
- Systemic absorption does occur with salicylic acid and can cause salicylate overdose. Increased concentrations increase this complication.
- Keratolytics are applied topically in various bases: cream, ointment, and plasters. Plasters are applied for a few days (4 to 5) and then removed, and an occlusive dressing is commonly applied over the topical agent to prevent it from being washed away and to prevent application to normal skin.

INDICATIONS
- Hyperkeratotic lesions: warts and many other less common dermatologic conditions
- Cosmetic: *chemical peels*

CONTRAINDICATION
- Open wounds should not be treated with keratolytics.

SIDE EFFECTS
- **Local skin irritation**
  - Redness, itching, and tenderness may occur.
- **Salicylic acid toxicity**
  - Absorption of salicylic acid occurs, and at higher concentrations of salicylic acid, children are at increased risk for systemic toxicity.

IMPORTANT NOTES
- Salicylic acid is the most commonly used keratolytic for warts. Treatment duration depends on the size and depth of the warts. Treatment can persist for many weeks before all tissue containing the human papillomavirus (HPV) is destroyed and debrided.
- **Anhydrous** (without water) preparations are less irritating, allowing higher concentrations of acid to be tolerated.

■ Higher concentrations of keratolytic increase the probability of increased irritation in the skin.

■ Molluscum contagiosum is a skin condition caused by the pox virus that results in very small papules and has been treated with keratolytics.

EVIDENCE
Warts

■ **Salicylic acid versus placebo**: A Cochrane review in 2006 (five studies, N = 322) demonstrated increased efficacy of salicylic acid (73%) over placebo (48%), a relative risk (RR) of 1.6 for cure.

Molluscum Contagiosum

■ A Cochrane review in 2009 (nine studies, N = 495) did not find strong evidence to support the use of salicylic acid in patients with molluscum contagiosum.

Imiquimod

DESCRIPTION
Imiquimod modifies the immune response in skin.

PROTOTYPE
■ Imiquimod

MOA (MECHANISM OF ACTION)

■ Imiquimod enhances both the innate and the acquired immune systems and thereby stimulates a response against abnormal skin cells, which are then eliminated through the body's own mechanisms.

■ Imiquimod exerts its actions through the following sequence of events:
  ▲ Binding to **Toll-like receptors** on B cells
  ▲ Increased release of inflammatory mediators, including **interferon, TNF,** and many interleukins: IL-1, IL-6, IL-8, and IL-10
  ▲ Increased immune cell activity:
    • Activating macrophages and Langerhans cells
    • Inducing proliferation and maturation of B lymphocytes
    • Increasing natural killer T cell activity

■ Imiquimod also has direct apoptosis activity with tumor cells.

■ The net effect of applying topical imiquimod to the skin is an **increased inflammatory reaction** in the dermis, and through this reaction, abnormal cells are destroyed in the heightened inflammatory environment.

PHARMACOKINETICS

■ Imiquimod is supplied as a 5% cream. It has a half-life of 2 to 4 hours and needs to remain on the skin (without being washed) for 10 hours after application.

■ A typical course of therapy consists of application three to seven times a week for 6 to 16 weeks, depending on the lesion that is being treated.

INDICATIONS

■ Genital and perianal warts *resistant* to conventional therapy
■ Actinic keratoses
■ Basal cell carcinoma

CONTRAINDICATIONS
■ None

SIDE EFFECTS

■ **Local** skin reactions:
  ▲ **Mild** burning, stinging, itching, redness, or swelling, mostly related to the inflammatory response produced by the drug

■ **Long-term** skin reactions:
  ▲ Pigmentation changes, including hypopigmentation and hyperpigmentation. The mechanism for development of hypopigmented lesions is not fully understood but could involve antimelanocyte autoantibodies and/or other inflammatory processes that selectively destroy melanocytes.

■ Skin reactions **of concern** that require assessment by a physician:
  ▲ Blistering, flaking, crusting, open sores, or any type of severe form of reactions listed previously

■ **Systemic** reactions (related to a mild widespread inflammatory response):
  ▲ Fatigue, diarrhea, flulike symptoms, headache

IMPORTANT NOTES

■ Lesions suspected to be cancerous (basal cell carcinoma) should be **biopsy proven** before therapy is started. Treatment success rates are about 80% with imiquimod alone.

■ Actinic keratosis lesions that do not respond to treatment should undergo biopsy to ensure that there is no carcinoma within the lesion.

■ Typical therapy for genital warts is through physical destruction (ablation), such as cryoablation (freezing to a temperature that destroys the cells) using liquid nitrogen (temperature of −196° C). Liquid nitrogen is applied to a small applicator (e.g., a cotton-tipped swab) and applied to the wart for 10 to 20 seconds.
  ▲ Imiquimod is **not** first-line treatment for warts because cheaper effective treatments exist that require less treatment time. Resistance to first-line treatment is more common in patients who are immunocompromised—for example, patients with AIDS.

■ Imiquimod is much more expensive than other therapies for warts.

Advanced

■ Differentiating squamous cell carcinoma from (benign) actinic keratoses can be difficult but is important because **squamous cell carcinomas should generally not be treated with imiquimod**. The following five characteristics increase the probability that the lesion is carcinoma and not keratosis:
  ▲ **Hyperkeratosis:** How raised is the lesion above normal skin?
  ▲ **Full thickness:** Does the lesion feel superficial, or does it extend deep into the skin?
  ▲ **Surrounding induration:** thickness or indrawing in the tissue adjacent to the lesion
  ▲ **Surrounding erythema**
  ▲ **Tenderness**
■ Toll-like receptors are important in mediating the innate immune response. At least 15 different receptors have been identified.

EVIDENCE
Imiquimod versus Vehicle (Placebo) for Basal Cell Carcinoma

■ A Cochrane review in 2007 (five studies N = 1145 patients) found a short-term success rate (defined histologically with biopsy) of 87% to 88% at 6 weeks and 76% at 12 weeks. This was a not a comparison with other therapy, but a trial comparing surgery with imiquimod is underway. Furthermore, 12 weeks is a very short period of time to declare success in cancer treatment. More studies are required to define the usefulness of imiquimod in treatment of basal cell carcinoma.

Imiquimod for Anogenital Warts

■ A review of four studies (1641 patients) found complete clearance rates of 37% to 52% in patients treated with imiquimod and partial clearance in 50% to 90% of patients. Recurrence rates were as high as 19% at 3 months.

FYI

■ Warts are caused by HPV. There are different subtypes of this virus; some subtypes cause warts, and some subtypes cause cancer of the cervix (and precancer of the cervix called *cervical dysplasia*). There now exists a vaccine against some of the subtypes that cause cervical cancer.
■ Resiquimod is a more potent Toll-like receptor agonist in development.

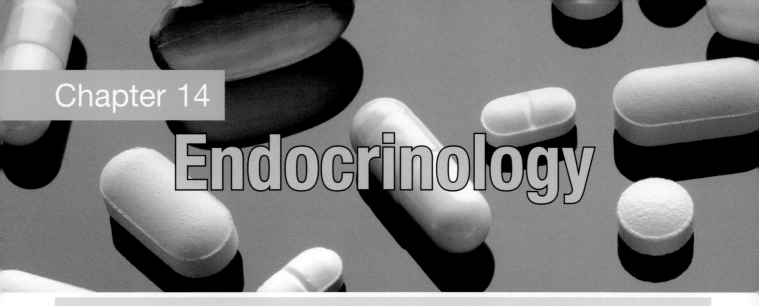

Chapter 14
Endocrinology

α-Glucosidase Inhibitors (AGIs)

DESCRIPTION

α-Glucosidase inhibitors (AGIs) are agents that reduce blood glucose by inhibiting the breakdown of carbohydrates to glucose in the gut.

PROTOTYPE AND COMMON DRUGS

- Prototype: acarbose
- Others: miglitol, voglibose

MOA (MECHANISM OF ACTION)

- Glucosidases (GSs) such as maltase, dextranase, sucrase, and glucoamylase aid in carbohydrate absorption by cleaving complex carbohydrates to yield glucose. Only monosaccharides such as glucose or fructose can be absorbed into the bloodstream (Figure 14-1).
- The AGIs are carbohydrate analogues that bind reversibly and with much greater affinity than carbohydrates to these GS enzymes.
- The competitive inhibition of these GSs delays the absorption of carbohydrates along the gastrointestinal (GI) tract. These agents are therefore useful in reducing the spike in blood sugar that occurs after a meal.
- The different AGIs differ slightly in the target enzymes they inhibit. Acarbose also has a small effect on α-amylase, whereas miglitol inhibits isomaltase and β-glucosidases. The β-glucosidases cleave β-linked sugars such as lactose.

PHARMACOKINETICS

- Acarbose is meant to act locally in the GI tract and therefore has minimal systemic bioavailability (approximately 2%).
- Metabolism occurs within the GI tract, by the action of intestinal bacteria and digestive enzymes.

INDICATIONS

- Diabetes mellitus (type 2), for:
  - ▲ Predominantly postprandial hyperglycemia
  - ▲ New-onset diabetes with mild hyperglycemia

Alpha glucosidase inhibitors

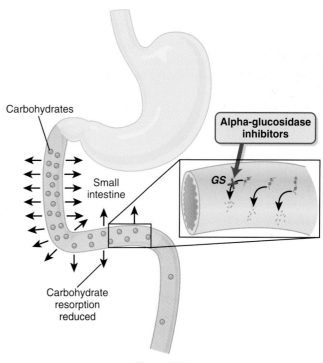

Figure 14-1.

CONTRAINDICATIONS

- **Irritable bowel syndrome (IBS), inflammatory bowel disease:** The GI side effects associated with the use of AGIs (see later) may exacerbate the symptoms of IBS.

SIDE EFFECTS

- **GI (flatulence, bloating, abdominal discomfort, diarrhea):** GI side effects are all caused by the actions of bacteria on undigested carbohydrates that reach the large intestine. The carbohydrate load that reaches the large intestine is a substrate for bacteria, which generate gas when they consume the carbohydrate. This side effect seems to be reduced with time, possibly because of an up-regulation of α-glucosidase enzymes in the distal small intestine.

- **Hypoglycemia**: Hypoglycemia is typically seen only with concomitant administration of sulfonylureas. The hypoglycemia should be managed with glucose and not sucrose, as the breakdown of sucrose might be inhibited by the actions of the α-glucosidase inhibition.

Rare

- **Increased serum aminotransferases**: Reversible elevations in aminotransferase levels (one of the liver enzymes) have been seen with these agents, although this is considered to be a rare phenomenon.

IMPORTANT NOTES

- The effects of AGIs are generally considered *additive* to those of other antidiabetics.
- Acarbose has been shown in some studies to have potential beneficial cardiovascular effects beyond that of simply lowering blood glucose.
- Because of their mechanism of action, namely reducing postprandial glucose levels, there has been considerable interest in the potential for AGIs to *prevent* onset of type 2 diabetes mellitus. Postprandial hyperglycemia is considered to be an early warning sign for development of type 2 diabetes. The STOP-NIDDM trial was a large (N = 1429 participants) double-blind randomized controlled trial that found that the number needed to treat (NNT) for preventing one new case of diabetes over 3 years was 11 for acarbose. Given that these results are from only one study, they should be interpreted with caution; however these findings do suggest further investigation is warranted.

EVIDENCE
α-Glucosidase Inhibitors versus Placebo or Other Antidiabetics in Type 2 Diabetes Mellitus

- A 2005 Cochrane review (41 trials, N = 8130 patients) included studies largely 24 to 52 weeks in duration, with all the various AGIs. Few data on mortality, morbidity, or quality of life were available. The AGIs improved surrogate markers such as HbA_{1c} (−0.8%), fasting blood glucose (−1.1 mmol/L), and postload blood glucose (−2.3 mmol/L) versus placebo.

FYI

- Lactase is a β-glucosidase that breaks down lactose, a disaccharide composed of glucose and galactose. Because acarbose is specific for α-glucosidases, the metabolism of lactose is unaffected.

Biguanides

DESCRIPTION
Biguanides reduce blood glucose without stimulating insulin secretion.

PROTOTYPE
- Metformin

MOA (MECHANISM OF ACTION)
- There are several proposed mechanisms behind the glucose-reducing effects of biguanides (Figure 14-2):
  - ▲ **Reduced gluconeogenesis**
    - Gluconeogenesis is the formation of glucose from noncarbohydrate precursors.
    - Adenosine monophosphate (AMP) kinase is believed to mediate some of this effect by inhibiting enzymes involved in gluconeogenesis.
    - AMP kinase plays a role in energy homeostasis and has become a focal point for research into new therapies for diabetes mellitus and other metabolic conditions.
  - ▲ **Increased action of insulin** in muscle and fat
    - This is also believed to occur through stimulation of the actions of AMP kinase.
  - ▲ **Delayed glucose absorption** from GI tract
  - ▲ **Direct stimulation of glycolysis** in tissue with increased glucose removal from blood

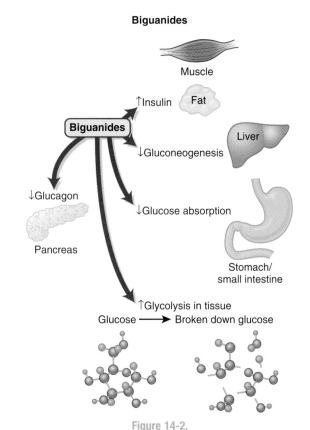

Figure 14-2.

- Glycolysis is the breakdown of glucose.
  ▲ **Reduced plasma glucagon**
    - Glucagon is a hormone that increases glucose levels by breaking down glycogen.

PHARMACOKINETICS

- Metformin is not metabolized and is excreted in urine unchanged. Renal clearance occurs mainly through tubular secretion.

INDICATION

- Type 2 diabetes mellitus

CONTRAINDICATION

- **Metabolic acidosis:** See Side Effects.

SIDE EFFECTS

- **GI:** Abdominal pain, nausea, diarrhea. Mechanism unknown.
- **Reduced absorption of vitamin B_{12} and folate:** Mechanism is unknown, but the risk of reduced vitamin B_{12} appears to increase with dose and duration of therapy.
- **Hypoglycemia:** There is a low risk of hypoglycemia.

Serious

- **Lactic acidosis (rare):** Typically not seen at recommended doses. Patients who have renal impairment are at higher risk. Metformin must be discontinued if this occurs.

IMPORTANT NOTES

- Because metformin does not stimulate the release of insulin, it is less likely to cause hypoglycemia than the oral hypoglycemics.
- Metformin is also used in the management of polycystic ovarian syndrome (PCOS). Hyperinsulinemia is believed to contribute to PCOS by stimulating excess testosterone production by the ovaries and decreasing synthesis of sex hormone binding globulin in the liver. Metformin reduces insulin levels, therefore inhibiting this process.

- Lactic acidosis was a major concern with this drug class, as an original member of this class (phenformin) was withdrawn from the market in the 1970s because of this potentially fatal side effect. The incidence of lactic acidosis with metformin is actually very low (less than one case per 1000 patient years). This risk can increase substantially if metformin is given with other agents that cause acidosis or in patients with renal impairment.

Advanced

- There is increasing evidence from animal and now human studies that metformin may have beneficial effects that extend beyond its known effects in reducing blood glucose. In particular, metformin may have beneficial cardiovascular effects, including a reduction in microvascular complications and improved endothelial function.

EVIDENCE
Metformin Monotherapy in Type 2 Diabetes Mellitus

- A 2005 Cochrane review compared metformin with sulfonylureas (13 trials, N = 1167 participants), placebo (12 trials, N = 702), diet (three trials, N = 493), thiazolidinediones (TZDs) (three trials, N = 132), insulin (two trials, N = 439), meglitinides (two trials, N = 208), and glucosidase inhibitors (two trials, N = 111). Obese participants with type 2 diabetes who were treated with intensive metformin therapy had a reduced risk for any clinical endpoint related to type 2 diabetes, including all-cause mortality and stroke compared with intensive therapy with chlorpropamide, glibenclamide, or insulin. The authors described metformin as eliciting a strong benefit for HbA_{1c} compared with placebo or diet.

FYI

- The biguanides originated from the French lilac plant, which had been used for centuries to treat symptoms of diabetes mellitus. Guanidine is believed to be a major active ingredient in the plant, and two molecules were joined together to form the biguanides.

Incretins

DESCRIPTION

Incretins are oral hypoglycemic agents.

PROTOTYPES AND COMMON DRUGS
Dipeptidyl Peptidase (DPP)–4 Inhibitors (Also Known As the "Gliptins")

- Prototype: sita**gliptin**
- Others: saxa**gliptin**, vilda**gliptin**

Incretin Mimetics

- Prototype: exenatide

MOA (MECHANISM OF ACTION)

- Patients with type 2 diabetes mellitus appear to have an impaired insulin response (insulin resistance) and an inappropriate increase in glucagon release compared with normal individuals. Glucagon is a hormone that does the opposite of insulin—it increases blood glucose.
- Incretin hormones such as glucagon-like peptide-1 (GLP-1) and glucose-dependent insulinotropic polypeptide (GIP) **lower blood glucose.** They accomplish this by a number of mechanisms:

▲ GLP-1 and GIP stimulate insulin release from pancreatic beta cells under conditions of normal or elevated blood glucose.

▲ GLP-1 also lowers glucagon secretion from alpha cells, reduces appetite, slows gastric emptying, and regulates beta-cell growth (Figure 14-3).

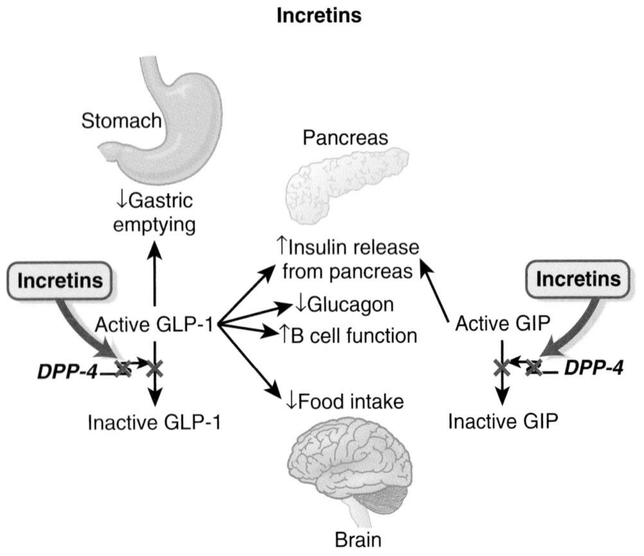

Incretins

Figure 14-3.

■ The DPP-4 enzyme **inactivates incretin hormones**, and therefore agents that overcome the actions of this enzyme enhance the effects of incretins (see Figure 14-3).

■ Two approaches have been taken to enhance incretin hormones. Incretin mimetics are **GLP-1 analogues** that are not degraded by DPP-4 and thus act as GLP-1 agonists. The gliptins work by inhibiting the DPP-4 enzyme, which prevents the breakdown of incretins, thus enhancing their actions.

■ The net effects of incretins are an **increase in insulin** release and a **decrease in glucagon**.

PHARMACOKINETICS
■ Exenatide is administered by subcutaneous injection. It has a circulating half-life of 60 to 90 minutes.
■ Unlike exenatide, the gliptins are administered orally.

INDICATION
■ Diabetes mellitus (type 2)

CONTRAINDICATIONS
■ None of major significance

SIDE EFFECTS
■ The incretins are generally well tolerated.

■ **Hypersensitivity reactions**: DPP-4 contributes to the activation of T cells, so inhibition of the activity of this enzyme might affect immune function.
■ **Increased incidence of infection**: This was observed with sitagliptin in clinical trials, but the mechanism has not been explained. Once again, there might be a connection with immune function.

IMPORTANT NOTES
■ The first indication that incretins exist came from the observation that an oral glucose load is more effective at stimulating insulin secretion than glucose given intravenously. It was subsequently discovered that two hormones (GIP and GLP-1) that are released from the upper and lower bowel enhance glucose-dependent insulin release. This increased effect of oral glucose on insulin secretion is identified as the incretin effect.

Advanced
Pregnancy
■ The safety of sitagliptin in pregnancy has not been established.

EVIDENCE
DPP-4 Inhibitors versus Other Antidiabetics and Placebo in Type 2 Diabetes Mellitus
■ A 2008 Cochrane review included studies of sitagliptin (11 trials, N = 6743 patients) and vildagliptin (14 trials, N = 6121 patients) from 12 to 52 weeks' duration. No data were published for mortality, diabetic complications, or quality of life. Compared with placebo, absolute reductions in HbA_{1c} were sitagliptin 0.7% and vildagliptin 0.6%. Compared with the effects of other agents, no improvements in metabolic control were detected.
■ All-cause infections increased with sitagliptin and with vildagliptin, but the difference was statistically significant only with sitagliptin. Otherwise the agents were well tolerated.

FYI
■ Exenatide is a synthetic analogue of exendin-4, a peptide found in the venom of the Gila monster, a large lizard.
■ Original attempts to use GLP-1 therapeutically were thwarted by its rapid inactivation by DPP-4. The actions on GLP-1 lasted for only a few minutes; therefore it had to be administered by continuous infusion. Exenatide acts as an agonist at GLP-1 receptors but is not broken down to an appreciable extent by DPP-4; thus it represents the first clinically feasible incretin analogue.

Insulins

DESCRIPTION
Insulin is a naturally occurring hormone that reduces blood glucose.

PROTOTYPES AND COMMON DRUGS
Short-Acting Insulin
- Prototype: insulin R (regular)
- Others: insulin aspart, insulin lispro, insulin glulisine

Intermediate-Acting Insulin
- Prototype: Neutral Protamine Hagedorn (NPH) insulin
- Others: insulin Lente

Long-Acting Insulin
- Prototype: insulin ultralente
- Others: insulin protamine zinc, insulin glargine, insulin detemir

MOA (MECHANISM OF ACTION)
- Insulin is a hormone secreted by beta cells of the islets of Langerhans in the pancreas. It has several functions, many of which serve to lower blood glucose (Figure 14-4):
  - ▲ Controls the uptake, use, and storage of cellular nutrients:

- The most widely known function of insulin is to promote the uptake of glucose by cells. Insulin does this by mobilizing glucose transporters (GLUT-4) on the surface of muscle and adipose tissue.
- In the liver and in muscle, insulin leads to increased glycogen deposition by increasing its synthesis and inhibiting its degradation. Glycogen is the primary means for storing glucose in the body.
- In the liver, insulin inhibits the synthesis of glucose (gluconeogenesis).
- In muscle, insulin facilitates uptake of amino acids, promoting protein synthesis.
- In adipose, insulin promotes synthesis of triglycerides and inhibits lipolysis.
- Aside from its multiple metabolic effects, insulin also binds to the insulin-like growth factor receptor (IGF-1) and appears to have growth-promoting effects.

PHARMACOKINETICS
- As is the case with most peptides, insulin cannot be administered orally. It is most frequently delivered parenterally, typically subcutaneously.
- An inhaled formulation of insulin is now available in some jurisdictions.
- A wide variety of insulins is available, characterized by onset and duration of action, summarized in Table 14-1.
- There is considerable interindividual variability in the pharmacokinetics of insulin, thus creating variability and unpredictability in the time to peak hypoglycemic effect.
- The Lente insulins absorb more slowly because of their crystal size.

Insulin

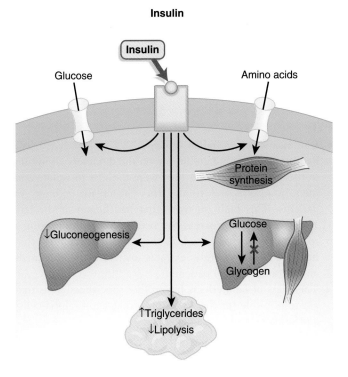

Figure 14-4.

TABLE 14-1. Insulin Formulations			
Type	**Onset (hours)**	**Peak (hours)**	**Duration (hours)**
Rapid Acting			
Glulisine	—	0.5-1.5	1-2.5
Aspart	0.25	0.6-0.8	3-5
Lispro	0.25	0.5-1.5	2-5
Regular	0.5-0.7	1.5-1.4	5-8
Intermediate Acting			
NPH	1-2	6-12	18-24
Lente	1-2	6-12	18-24
Glargine	2-5	5-24	18-24
Slow Acting			
Ultralente	4-6	16-18	20-36
Protamine zinc	4-6	14-20	24-36

INDICATION

- Diabetes mellitus (type 1 and type 2)

CONTRAINDICATIONS

- None of major significance

SIDE EFFECTS

- **Hypoglycemia**: seen with overdose or a missed meal; signs and symptoms include:
  - ▲ Sweating
  - ▲ Tachycardia
  - ▲ Tremor
  - ▲ Weakness
  - ▲ Hunger
  - ▲ Blurred vision
  - ▲ Confusion
  - ▲ Convulsions
  - ▲ Coma
- Most of these signs and symptoms are secondary to the release of counterregulatory hormones such as epinephrine, glucagon, growth hormone (GH), cortisol, and norepinephrine, with epinephrine and glucagon playing the most important roles.
- Mild hypoglycemia is typically managed by patients with intake of sugar, preferably glucose. More severe cases can be managed with intravenous glucose, or with glucagon, a hormone with actions opposite to those of insulin.
- **Lipodystrophy**: Insulin injections can lead to localized atrophy of subcutaneous fat (lipoatrophy) or enlargement of fat deposits (lipohypertrophy). Lipoatrophy may be caused by an immune response, whereas lipohypertrophy may be caused by generation of fat cells.
- **Edema**: Edema is attributed to Na^+ retention.

IMPORTANT NOTES

- Recombinant human insulin was a very early example of the use of biotechnology in drug development. Insulins were originally derived from beef (bovine) or pork (porcine) sources, and these forms of insulin are still used in some areas of the world. As they were not of human origin, bovine and porcine insulins elicited immune responses that either made their administration unpredictable or in some cases led to hypersensitivity reactions. Porcine insulin differs from human by one amino acid, and bovine by three amino acids; therefore bovine insulin is more prone to cause immunogenic reactions.
- The beta cells of the pancreas actually secrete a 110–amino acid polypeptide called preproinsulin, which is cleaved to proinsulin in the endoplasmic reticulum and then to insulin in the Golgi and secretory granules. Insulin is composed of two polypeptide chains: an A chain of 21 amino acids and a B chain of 30 amino acids. Modification of these chains has yielded several different analogues of insulin with different onset times and duration.

Advanced

- The use of units for insulin dosages dates back to the time when insulin had to be standardized because of the use of impure hormone. One unit of insulin was the amount required to lower blood glucose in a fasting rabbit to 2.5 mM (45 mg/dL).
- Homogeneous preparations of human insulin contain 25 to 30 units/mg, and most insulin preparations are supplied in concentrations of 100 units/mL, or about 3.6 mg/mL.

EVIDENCE

Short-Acting Analogues versus Regular Insulin

- A 2006 Cochrane review (49 trials, N = 8274 participants) assessed the effects of short-acting insulin analogues versus regular human insulin. There were minimal differences in efficacy. In patients with type 1 diabetes, the weighted mean difference (WMD) of HbA_{1c} was −0.1% in favor of short-acting insulin analogues versus insulin, and in patients with type 2 diabetes there was no difference. In type 1 diabetes the incidence of **severe hypoglycemia was lower** for insulin analogues versus insulin (median 22 versus 46 episodes per 100 person-years). In type 2 diabetes there were also fewer severe hypoglycemia events with analogues versus insulin (median 0.3 versus 1.4 per 100 person-years).

Gestational Diabetes Mellitus

- A 2009 Cochrane review (eight trials, N = 1418 women) compared the effects of various treatment policies with one another or with routine antenatal care for gestational diabetes mellitus (GDM) on both maternal and infant outcomes. Intensive management (including dietary advice and insulin) reduced the risk of preeclampsia compared with results of routine antenatal care (relative risk [RR] 0.65), based on one trial of 1000 participants. The risk of the composite outcome of perinatal morbidity (death, shoulder dystocia, bone fracture, and nerve palsy) was also reduced for those on intensive therapy for mild GDM versus routine antenatal care (RR 0.32), based on one trial of 1030 infants. Note that gestational diabetes leads to large babies, which can then experience complications in the birthing process because of their size.

FYI

- *Lente* means *slow* in Italian.
- Banting and Best are credited with the discovery of insulin in the 1920s. In essence, they were the first to isolate and identify insulin and to use this "pancreatic extract" in patients. This built on work that had begun in the late 1880s, when the pancreas had been identified as playing a role in diabetes, and work at the turn of the century that had first used pancreatic extracts to treat diabetic animals and (unsuccessfully) patients.
- The islets of Langerhans have other specialized cells that are responsible for the secretion of glucagon (alpha cells) and somatostatin (delta cells).
- NPH insulin is created by treating regular insulin with *protamine* and zinc at a *neutral* pH (7.2). This results in a fine precipitate of protamine zinc insulin that provides for slow and even absorption when administered subcutaneously. Hagedorn (the H in NPH) was the name of the scientist who created the formulation.

- In an attempt to create a long-acting heparin injection, protamine was also originally added to heparin. However, the two chemicals formed a precipitate, and it was this discovery that led to the use of protamine as a reversal agent for heparin.

- Protamine is manufactured from salmon sperm.

Meglitinides

DESCRIPTION

Meglitinides are oral agents that lower blood glucose by increasing insulin secretion.

PROTOTYPE AND COMMON DRUGS

- Prototype: repa**glinide**
- Others: nate**glinide**

MOA (MECHANISM OF ACTION)

- The meglitinides are insulin secretagogues, **stimulating the release of insulin** from pancreatic beta cells in a manner similar to that of the sulfonylureas (Figure 14-5).

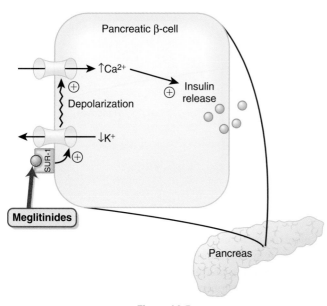

Meglitinides

Figure 14-5.

- They bind to a beta cell sulfonylurea receptor (SUR-1) that is associated with an inward rectifier adenosine triphosphate (ATP)–sensitive potassium channel. Binding leads to depolarization, which then opens a voltage-gated calcium channel, leading to calcium influx and insulin release.

- Meglitinides therefore rely on **functioning beta cells** in order to achieve their pharmacologic effect. They are thus not useful in type 1 diabetes mellitus.

PHARMACOKINETICS

- The meglitinides are rapidly and completely absorbed, achieving peak plasma concentrations in less than 1 hour after oral administration.

- They are metabolized in the liver, and have a short elimination half-life of 1 to 2 hours. Dose adjustments should be considered in patients with impaired liver function.

- Nateglinide acts more quickly than repaglinide and also has a shorter duration of action. Because both of these agents have a rapid onset and offset, they are typically administered just before meals for the management of postprandial hyperglycemia.

- Food increases the absorption of nateglinide but has minimal impact on repaglinide absorption.

INDICATION

- Diabetes mellitus (type 2)

CONTRAINDICATION

- **Concomitant gemfibrozil and repaglinide:** Gemfibrozil (a fibrate) significantly reduces the metabolism of repaglinide, leading to as much as an *eightfold* increase in repaglinide levels. In some cases this has lead to severe episodes of hypoglycemia. Gemfibrozil is used to lower cholesterol; multiple risk-reduction strategies are frequently used in patients with multiple risk factors for atherosclerosis and thus there is a risk that these two drugs can be co-administered.

SIDE EFFECTS

- **Hypoglycemia:** Although less common than with the sulfonylureas, hypoglycemia still occurs in approximately 1% of patients. This side effect is treated in the same manner as hypoglycemia seen with other insulin secretagogues.

IMPORTANT NOTES

- The rapid onset of action of the meglitinides, particularly nateglinide, makes them useful agents in the management of postprandial hyperglycemia. Patients can take these agents just before eating, allowing them flexibility in choosing the timing of their meals. The sulfonylureas do not allow for this much flexibility.

EVIDENCE

Meglitinides versus One Another, Metformin, and Placebo

- A 2007 Cochrane review (15 trials, N = 3781 patients) did not find any studies that reported on morbidity or mortality. Compared with the effects of placebo, HbA_{1c} was reduced by both repaglinide (0.1% to 2.1%) and nateglinide (0.2% to 0.6%). In trials comparing the two agents, repaglinide performed better than nateglinide with respect to reducing HbA$_{1c}$. Repaglinide had similar reductions in HbA$_{1c}$ to metformin (three studies, N = 248 patients), whereas nateglinide had similar or slightly less of an effect on HbA$_{1c}$ compared to metformin (one study, N = 355 patients).

■ Weight gain was generally greater with meglitinides versus metformin; diarrhea occurred less frequently and hypoglycemia more frequently with meglitinides versus metformin.

FYI

■ The meglitinides were approved 40 years after the approval of the first sulfonylurea, tolbutamide.

Sulfonylureas

DESCRIPTION

Sulfonylureas are oral agents that lower blood glucose by increasing insulin secretion.

PROTOTYPES AND COMMON DRUGS
First-Generation Agents

■ Prototype: Tolbut**amide**
■ Others: Chlorprop**amide**, tolaz**amide**, acetohex**amide**

Second-Generation Agents

■ Prototype: Glybur**ide**
■ Others: Glipiz**ide**, gliclaz**ide**, glimepir**ide**

MOA (MECHANISM OF ACTION)

■ Patients with type 2 diabetes mellitus appear to have an impaired insulin response (insulin resistance) and an inappropriate increase in glucagon release compared with normal individuals. Glucagon is a hormone that does the opposite of insulin—it increases blood glucose.

■ The sulfonylureas are insulin secretagogues, meaning that they **stimulate insulin release** from the beta cells of the pancreas.

■ They bind to a **beta-cell sulfonylurea receptor** (SUR-1) that is associated with an inward rectifier ATP-sensitive potassium channel. Binding leads to depolarization, which then opens a voltage-gated calcium channel, leading to calcium influx and insulin release (Figure 14-6).

■ Sulfonylureas also **reduce serum glucagon levels.** Although the mechanism behind this has not been definitively established, sulfonylureas enhance the release of insulin and somatostatin, and it is believed that one or both of these effects may in turn lead to a reduction in glucagon release from pancreatic alpha cells.

PHARMACOKINETICS

■ The elimination half-lives of first-generation agents vary considerably, whereas the half-lives of second-generation agents are typically short (3 to 5 hours). However, the biologic half-lives, the amount of time for which they are effective, is longer than their elimination half-lives would suggest, for reasons that are still unknown.

■ All sulfonylureas are metabolized by the liver and excreted in urine. Because of the risk of hypoglycemia, dose adjust-

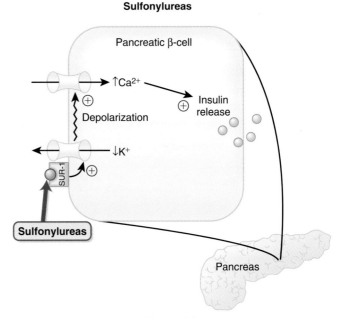

Sulfonylureas

Figure 14-6.

ments must be considered in patients with hepatic impairment. A small proportion is also excreted unchanged in urine, therefore caution should also be exercised in patients with renal impairment.

INDICATION

■ Diabetes mellitus (type 2)

CONTRAINDICATIONS

None of major significance.

SIDE EFFECTS

■ **Hypoglycemia:** Hypoglycemia is caused by oversecretion of insulin and occurs more frequently with glyburide. Glyburide may impair the body's ability to prevent endogenous insulin secretion during hypoglycemia.

■ **Flushing:** Flushing occurs when these drugs are taken with alcohol and is more common with older agents like chlorpropamide.

- **Weight gain:** Weight gain is caused by increased insulin activity in adipose. It occurs less frequently with the second-generation sulfonylureas.

Rare, Serious
- **Hematologic toxicities:** Anemias and thrombocytopenias occur and are mainly seen with chlorpropamide.

IMPORTANT NOTES
- Because of concerns over hypoglycemia, the sulfonylureas, particularly glyburide, should be **initiated at a low dose**, and patients should be observed carefully for changes in blood glucose over the first few weeks of therapy. Patients with irregular diets or who drink ethanol to excess are at increased risk for hypoglycemia.
- The hypoglycemic effects of the sulfonylureas tend to diminish with time. The most likely explanation for this **reduced response** is progressive loss of beta cells from diabetes.
- Patients with type 1 diabetes mellitus are unable to secrete appreciable amounts of insulin; therefore a drug that promotes insulin secretion will not work in these patients.

Advanced
Pregnancy
- Patients with gestational diabetes should not be treated with sulfonylureas, but should instead be treated with insulin.

EVIDENCE
Glyburide for Hypoglycemic Events and Cardiovascular Risk
- A 2007 systematic review (21 trials, N = 7047 patients) compared glyburide with other insulin secretagogues and insulin for hypoglycemic and cardiovascular events. The authors found that glyburide was associated with a greater risk of experiencing a hypoglycemic event compared with other secretagogues (RR 1.52) or other sulfonylureas (1.83). Glyburide was not associated with an increased risk of cardiovascular events, death, or end-of-trial weight gain compared with other secretagogues.

FYI
- The sulfonylureas were the first oral agents for type 2 diabetes and have been in use for over 50 years.
- After a large study conducted in the 1970s found increased cardiovascular mortality with sulfonylureas, for many years there was an association drawn between this class and elevated cardiovascular risk. Subsequent studies have not found this association, although this class is still believed in some circles to carry this risk.

Thiazolidinediones

DESCRIPTION
The thiazolidinediones (TZDs) are oral agents that lower blood glucose by increasing the sensitivity of cells to insulin.

PROTOTYPE AND COMMON DRUGS
- Prototype: rosi**glitazone**
- Others: pio**glitazone**

MOA (MECHANISM OF ACTION)
- The TZDs are peroxisome proliferator–activated receptor–gamma (**PPAR-γ**) agonists.
- The PPAR-γ receptors are a complex family of receptors found in the cell nucleus in muscle, fat, and liver. Among other roles, they regulate expression of genes responsible for lipid and protein metabolism, insulin signal transduction, and adipocyte and other tissue differentiation. It is through a combination of these effects that they are thought to decrease insulin resistance, although the relative importance of each has not been established (Figure 14-7).
- The TZDs are thought to exert their effects at PPAR-γ receptors in adipose tissue by promoting uptake and storage

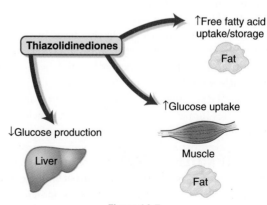

Figure 14-7.

of free fatty acids (FFAs) in adipose tissue. They accomplish this by increasing the number of small adipocytes that store FFAs while decreasing the number of large adipocytes that release FFAs. Through a variety of poorly understood mechanisms, high concentrations of FFAs are thought to promote **insulin resistance.**

- The TZDs also promote the expression and translocation of glucose transporters in muscle and adipose tissue. This increases glucose uptake into muscle and adipose tissue. The TZDs also may reduce hepatic production of glucose, although the mechanism by which this is accomplished is unclear.
- Activation of the PPAR-γ receptor also has several other effects, including inhibition of proinflammatory genes and cytokine production, as well as increased adiponectin production. Adiponectin is thought to play several protective roles in the body, stimulating glucose uptake in muscle, protecting against atherosclerosis and endothelial cell apoptosis, and stabilizing plaques.

PHARMACOKINETICS

- Rosiglitazone peak plasma levels are seen 1 hour after administration, and absorption is not significantly affected by food.
- Pioglitazone reaches its peak in 2 hours. It has two active metabolites (M-III and M-IV).
- Both rosiglitazone and pioglitazone are metabolized by hepatic CYP450 enzymes. They do not appear to induce or inhibit any CYP450 isozymes.

INDICATION

- Diabetes mellitus (type 2)

CONTRAINDICATION

- **Heart failure:** See Side Effects.

SIDE EFFECTS

- **Weight gain:** Weight gain is caused by redistribution of adipocytes from visceral to subcutaneous regions.
- **Edema:** TZDs promote retention of sodium and water by up-regulating tubular transporters for sodium and reducing glomerular filtration rate (GFR).
- **Cardiovascular:** Heart failure is likely caused by the edema described previously, observed with rosiglitazone in a large clinical trial. Myocardial ischemia has also been reported with rosiglitazone.
- **Fractures:** TZDs appear to impair osteoblasts, and higher fracture rates (upper arm, hand, or foot) in female subjects were observed in a large clinical trial.

IMPORTANT NOTES

- The PPAR-γ receptor has an extensive list of biologic actions, making it difficult to sort out the actions of agonists such as the TZDs. The most difficult effects to sort out are the cardiovascular effects. The TZDs initially appeared to have beneficial cardiovascular effects, but recently adverse cardiovascular effects, specifically heart failure, have emerged.

Advanced

- The TZDs appear to have variable effects on triglycerides and LDL, although they consistently raise HDL. Pioglitazone appears to have greater beneficial effects on lipid profiles compared with rosiglitazone.

Pregnancy

- Oral antidiabetics are generally not recommended. Insulin is the recommended treatment for diabetes during pregnancy.

Lactation

- Pioglitazone is secreted in breast milk in rats, and although human studies have not been performed, the TZDs are not recommended for breastfeeding women.

Drug Interactions

- Rosiglitazone is extensively metabolized by CYP2C8, with a minor contribution from CYP2C9.
- Pioglitazone is extensively metabolized by CYP2C8 and CYP3A4.

EVIDENCE
Rosiglitazone versus Oral Antidiabetics or Placebo in Type 2 Diabetes Mellitus

- A 2007 Cochrane review (18 trials, N = 3888 patients) found no improvement in mortality, morbidity, adverse effects, and quality of life in trials with a follow-up of at least 24 weeks. HbA$_{1c}$ was not improved by rosiglitazone compared with other oral antidiabetic agents. Edema occurred significantly more frequently in rosiglitazone-treated patients, and the ADOPT study identified an increased risk of cardiovascular events with rosiglitazone. Data from ADOPT and another trial, PROactive, suggest increased risk of fractures in women treated with rosiglitazone.

Pioglitazone versus Oral Antidiabetics or Placebo in Type 2 Diabetes Mellitus

- A 2006 Cochrane review (22 trials, N = 6200 patients) did not find convincing evidence of improvement in mortality, morbidity, adverse effects, and health-related quality of life. Improvements in HbA$_{1c}$ were similar with pioglitazone compared with other oral antidiabetics. Edema occurred significantly more frequently with pioglitazone.

FYI

- The PPAR-γ receptor is very large and has several different distinct ligands, including warfarin, monounsaturated and polyunsaturated fats, some nonsteroidal antiinflammatory drugs (NSAIDs), and the angiotensin receptor blocker (ARB) telmisartan.
- The first marketed TZD, troglitazone, was removed from the market because of concerns over hepatotoxicity.
- Dual PPAR-α and PPAR-γ agonists are being developed in order to maximize the benefits of PPAR agonism on both lipids and glucose. PPAR-α agonists (fibrates) are used to treat hypercholesterolemia.

Glucagon

DESCRIPTION

Glucagon is an endogenous hormone that generally opposes the actions of insulin.

PROTOTYPE

- Glucagon

MOA (MECHANISM OF ACTION)

- Glucagon is a 29–amino acid protein secreted from the alpha cells in the pancreas and has significant homology with secretin, vasoactive intestinal peptide (VIP), and GI inhibitory polypeptide.
- Glucagon secretion is under the control of the sympathetic system and is regulated by the following:
  - ▲ Dietary amino acids, glucose, and fatty acids (stimulation)
  - ▲ Hypoglycemia
  - ▲ Ketones (inhibition)
- The main effects of glucagon are on the **liver**, mediated by G protein–linked glucagon receptors and increased intracellular cyclic adenosine monophosphate (**cAMP**). The important specific actions include the following (Figure 14-8):
  - ▲ **Increased glycogenolysis** via cAMP-stimulated phosphorylation
  - ▲ **Decreased glycogen synthesis** via phosphorylation of glycogen synthase, which inactivates the enzyme
  - ▲ **Increased glycolysis** via reduction in levels of fructose-2,6-bisphosphate, which is an important regulator in the rate-limiting step for glycolysis
  - ▲ **Increased ketogenesis**
- Because glucagon acts to increase blood sugar, it works against insulin, which acts to lower blood sugar.
- In **cardiac tissue** glucagon binds a glucagon receptor and raises cAMP, resulting in a positive inotropic (contractility) and chronotropic (heart rate) effect on the heart. This is the mechanism by which it is therapeutic in β-blocker and calcium channel blocker overdoses; importantly, its action is *independent* of β receptors or calcium channels.
- Secretion of different pancreatic hormones influences other hormones:
  - ▲ Glucagon stimulates endogenous insulin secretion.
  - ▲ Insulin and somatostatin both inhibit glucagon secretion (see also the section on somatostatin analogs in this chapter).

PHARMACOKINETICS

- As a peptide, glucagon cannot be given orally because it will be digested into amino acids.
- Glucagon has a short half-life of 3 to 6 minutes. It is usually given as an intravenous infusion.

Glucagon

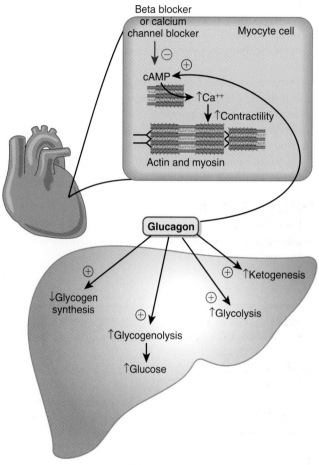

Figure 14-8.

INDICATIONS

- Refractory hypoglycemia (not corrected by glucose administration)
  - ▲ Oral hypoglycemia overdose
  - ▲ Hyperinsulin states
    - • Insulin overdose
    - • Insulinoma (islet cell tumor that secretes insulin)
- Drug overdoses
  - ▲ β-Blockers
  - ▲ Calcium channel blockers
- Intestinal relaxation
  - ▲ To facilitate some radiologic investigations of the GI tract

CONTRAINDICATION

- **Pheochromocytomas:** These are rare catecholamine-secreting tumors and are sensitive to glucagon, which promotes catecholamine secretion from these tumors.

SIDE EFFECTS
- Hyperglycemia
- Hypokalemia
- Nausea and vomiting, caused by delaying gastric emptying and hypotonicity

IMPORTANT NOTES
- Intravenous or oral glucose is the first-line treatment for hypoglycemia. Glucagon is the second-line treatment. Insulin overdoses are usually not treated with glucagon unless hypoglycemia is refractory to glucose administration.
- Glucagon decreases hepatic glycogen but does not decrease skeletal muscle glycogen because there are no glucagon receptors on skeletal muscle.
- Although some drugs that treat acute heart failure result in an increase in cAMP (β agonists and phosphodiesterase inhibitors), glucagon is not used for treating heart failure despite its similar action on cAMP.

Advanced
- Proglucagon is the precursor to glucagon and if cleaved at different locations also gives rise to glucagon-like peptides (GLP-1 and GLP-2), called *incretins*. Incretins are themselves a class of drugs used for diabetes management. GLP-1 and GLP-2 are secreted from intestinal cells and are involved with insulin and glucagon secretion, gastric emptying, intestinal blood flow, and permeability and appetite satiety.

EVIDENCE
- There are no human controlled studies of glucagon use in β-blocker or calcium channel blocker therapy. However, "the available animal data, human clinical experience, and minimal adverse effect profile support the use of glucagon early in the course of both β-blocker and calcium channel blocker toxicity."

FYI
- With the discovery that propranolol did not prevent the positive inotropic action of glucagon in cats and dogs, it was suggested that there was the possibility that glucagon may be useful in the treatment of heart failure induced by β-blockers; subsequently the logic was extended to the treatment of calcium channel blocker overdose.

Estrogens

DESCRIPTION
Estrogen is one of the endogenous female sex hormones. See also the discussions of progestins and hormone contraception.

COMMON DRUGS
- **Bioidentical estrogens**: estrone sulfate (E1), estropipate (E1), 17β-estradiol (E2), estriol (E3)
- **Esterified estrogens**: ethinyl estradiol, mestranol, quinestrol, equilin
- **Conjugated equine estrogens (CEEs)**: dienestrol

MOA (MECHANISM OF ACTION)
- Estrogens are transcription factors; they modify messenger RNA (mRNA) synthesis directly.
- Estrogens enter the cell passively (no receptor required) and bind to estrogen receptors in the nucleus, which then dimerize and bind DNA directly to regions called **estrogen-responsive elements** (EREs) and influence gene transcription.
- Important effects of estrogen include the following (Figure 14-9):
  - Reproductive:
    - Female sexual maturation (neonatal and pubescent)
    - Endometrial growth stimulation
    - Breast tissue stimulation
  - Hematologic:
    - Increased tendency for clotting via increased circulating levels of factors II, VII, IX, and X (vitamin K–dependant factors) and decreased antithrombin III
  - Skin and mucosa:
    - Increased pigmentation (melasma)
    - Increased skin collagen content and skin thickness
    - Maintenance of skin moisture by increasing acid mucopolysaccharides and hyaluronic acid
  - Metabolic:
    - Decreased bone resorption via antagonism of parathyroid hormone and interleukin-6 (IL-6)
    - Increased high-density lipoprotein (HDL); decreased low-density lipoprotein (LDL); increased triglycerides

PHARMACOKINETICS
- Estrogen preparations include oral tablets, creams, and patches.

INDICATIONS
- Prevention of pregnancy (contraception)
- Menopausal hormone replacement therapy (HRT)
- Endometriosis
- Dysfunctional uterine bleeding (DUB)

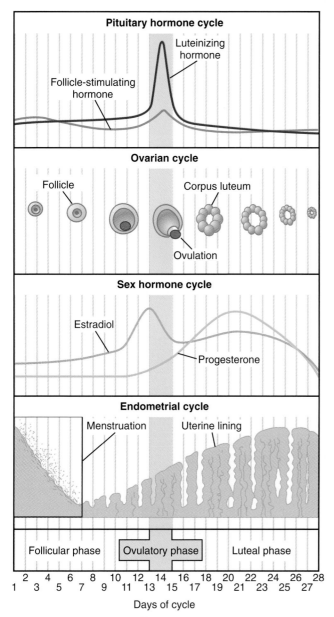

Pituitary hormone cycle

Luteinizing hormone

Follicle-stimulating hormone

Ovarian cycle

Follicle

Corpus luteum

Ovulation

Sex hormone cycle

Estradiol

Progesterone

Endometrial cycle

Menstruation

Uterine lining

Follicular phase

Ovulatory phase

Luteal phase

2 4 6 8 10 12 14 16 18 20 22 24 26 28
1 3 5 7 9 11 13 15 17 19 21 23 25 27

Days of cycle

Figure 14-9.

- Urogenital atrophy: thinning and drying of vaginal mucosa
- Anti-androgen therapy: acne, hirsutism
- Infertility
- Polycystic ovarian syndrome (PCOS)

CONTRAINDICATIONS

- **Hypercoagulable states:** Estrogen is a procoagulant, and estrogen administration is a risk factor for pathologic thromboses (deep vein thrombosis [DVT] and pulmonary embolus [PE]).
- **Cancers** that could demonstrate increased growth in response to estrogen: breast, ovarian, uterine, endometrial.
- **Strong risk factors for atherosclerosis:** hypertension (HTN), diabetes, high cholesterol, family history.

SIDE EFFECTS

- Migraine headaches
- Water retention
  - ▲ Abdominal bloating
  - ▲ Weight gain
- Stimulation of reproductive organ tissues:
  - ▲ Vaginal bleeding or spotting (because of growth of endometrial tissue)
  - ▲ Enlarged fibroids
  - ▲ Breast tenderness
- **Gall bladder** disease (primarily stones)
- **Nausea** (this is particularly common with higher doses used with postintercourse contraception, also called the "morning after" pill)
- **Thrombosis:** (estrogen is a procoagulant)
  - ▲ DVT and PE
  - ▲ Stroke
  - ▲ Coronary heart disease
- Skin rashes
- Increased triglycerides

IMPORTANT NOTES

- Progesterone is often co-administered with estrogen.
- Estrogen stimulates endometrial growth and can also stimulate cancers of reproductive tissues.
- Estrogens do not cause HTN at the doses in which they are currently prescribed but can cause HTN at very high doses.
- Estrogen is prothrombotic. It increases the probability of clot formation. Bleeding is a potential complication of natural childbirth, and the prothrombotic effects of estrogen are therefore beneficial during this time.
- The natural progression of sex hormone synthesis is as follows: progestins → androgens → estrogens (Figure 14-10). The similarity to aldosterone probably accounts for the water retention properties of sex hormones.

Advanced

- The cause of water retention is not fully understood, but it is possibly mediated by the following:
  - ▲ Changes in the thresholds for antidiuretic hormone (ADH) secretion and osmotic thirst, resulting in increased body water
  - ▲ Increases in the renin-angiotensin-aldosterone system by estrogen or progesterone
  - ▲ Nitric oxide–mediated vasodilation (thus increasing total blood volume) because of estrogen
- The mechanism by which estrogens increase the prevalence of migraines is complex, but it probably involves the following:
  - ▲ Vasodilation mediated by nitric oxide
  - ▲ Neuronal excitability mediated by increased calcium and decreased magnesium

EVIDENCE

(Note that many studies also include progesterone.)

- Many studies, often with different methodologies, have resulted in many results; summarizing is difficult because of

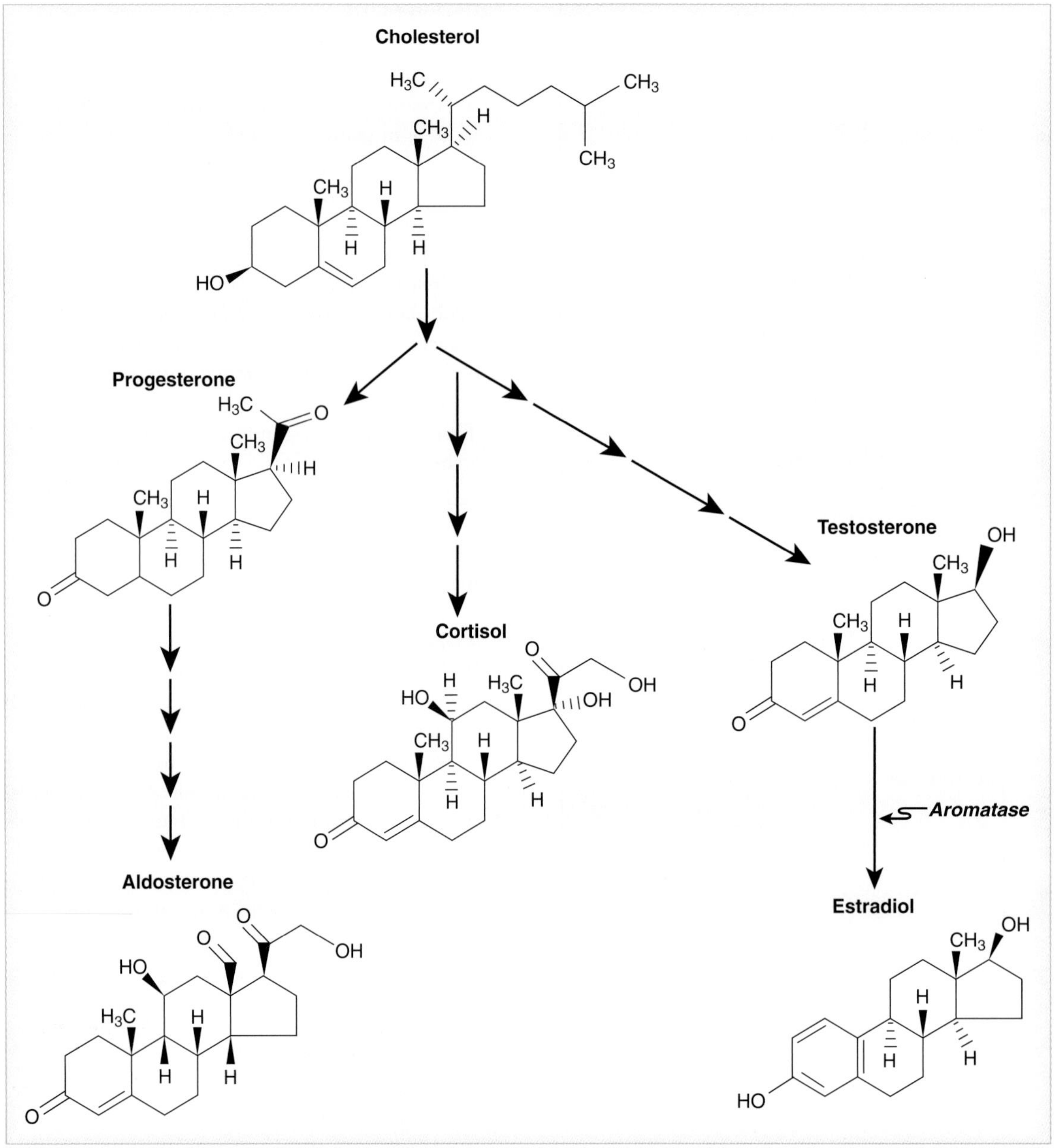

Figure 14-10.

the heterogeneity of studies that exists. Patient differences (age, gravida status, time since menopause) and drug differences (estrogen only versus estrogen with progesterone, dose, duration, estrogen formulation, estrogen delivery method) are some examples of the differences among studies. A very small subset of the evidence is presented here.

▲ **Endometrial cancer risk**: An analysis of 45 RCTs with 38,702 **postmenopausal** women demonstrated that *unopposed* estrogen (without any progesterone coadministered) of any dose for a duration of only 1 year increases risk of endometrial hyperplasia (and by extension, endometrial cancer) in patients being treated for menopausal symptoms. This effect increased with increasing dose of estrogen and increasing duration of administration.

▲ **Cardiovascular risk**: A single large double-blind RCT of 10,739 **postmenopausal** women comparing estrogen with placebo demonstrated no difference in myocardial infarction or cardiac death. However, the hazard ratio for stroke was 1.39, indicating an almost 40% increase in risk for stroke. Average follow-up time was 6.8 years.

▲ **Bone health (bone density, fractures)**:
  • An analysis in 2008 of 13 RCTs (two were placebo controlled), provides evidence that *combined* hormone oral contraceptives does not affect bone health. Depot progesterone alone (depot medroxyprogesterone acetate or DMPA) was associated with decreased bone density. Note that oral contraceptives would be administered to women of **childbearing age**.
  • A single large double blind RCT of 10,739 **postmenopausal women** comparing estrogen with placebo

demonstrated a hazard ratio of 0.61 for hip fractures (reduction of risk by 40%) and 0.70 for all fractures in the estrogen group. Average follow-up time was 6.8 years.

▲ **DVT risk:** In a 2006 RCT, 10,739 women followed for an average of 7.1 years demonstrated a rate of venous thrombosis of 3.0 *per 1000 person-years* in the estrogen group versus 2.2 in the placebo group. This represents a statistically significant *hazard ratio* of 1.47 (47% more likely to get a blood clot if on estrogen). Compared with estrogen plus progesterone, it appears that the risk is greater with combination therapy versus estrogen alone.

▲ **Cognitive function:** A meta-analysis in 2007 of 16 studies with 10,114 women with normal brain function demonstrated no benefit in prevention of cognitive decline over a period of 3 to 5 years compared with placebo. In fact, there was a slight trend toward better function with placebo. It has been previously suggested that estrogen deficiency is associated with decreased cognitive function.

▲ **Weight gain:** An analysis of available literature in 2008 included five RCTs (957 women) comparing hormone with placebo and did not find strong evidence to support an association between weight gain and the use of oral contraceptives; however, most studies were not designed to study this particular outcome.

▲ **Acne:** A meta-analysis in 2009 found 25 trials evaluating combined hormones and acne treatment. Of the 25, seven were placebo controlled, and these studies showed improvement in acne with hormone therapy. The remaining studies compared different hormone combinations and doses. Hormones containing cyproterone acetate *might* be superior in treating acne, but data are somewhat conflicting.

FYI

■ A state of **estr**us in mammals (excluding humans) is the time around ovulation when the female is receptive to sexual activity (being *in heat*); **estr**ogen peaks right before this time in the cycle.

■ Simplified memory tip: Estrogen is like *fertilizer* for the endometrium. Progesterone is like the *lawnmower*.

■ Fibroids are benign tumors of the uterus, composed of myometrium.

■ *Gravida* status refers to the number of previous pregnancies.

■ *Dysfunctional uterine bleeding* is defined as bleeding outside the normal menstrual period.

■ *Menorrhagia* is heavy menstrual bleeding.

■ *Dysmenorrhea* is a condition of having excessively painful menstrual periods.

Estrogen Receptor Antagonists

DESCRIPTION

Estrogen receptor antagonists are drugs that block estrogen receptors. See also the section on aromatase inhibitors (AIs) in this chapter for drugs that inhibit estrogen *synthesis*.

PROTOTYPE AND COMMON DRUGS
Selective Estrogen Receptor Modulators (SERMs)

■ Prototype: tamoxi**fen**
■ Others: toremi**fen**e, raloxi**fen**e

Estrogen Receptor Antagonists

■ Prototype: clomiphene
■ Others: fulvestrant

MOA (MECHANISM OF ACTION)

■ There are several forms of estrogen, but **17β-estradiol** is the predominant form intracellularly. Estrogens have multiple effects in females, from maintaining bone to regulating the menstrual cycle and development. Important effects of estrogen include the following:
  ▲ Reproductive:
    • Female sexual maturation (neonatal and pubescent)
    • Endometrial growth stimulation
    • Breast tissue stimulation
  ▲ Hematologic:
    • Increased tendency for clotting via increased circulating levels of factors II, VII, IX, and X (vitamin K–dependant factors) and decreased antithrombin III
  ▲ Skin and mucosa
    • Increased pigmentation (melasma)
    • Increased skin collagen content and skin thickness
    • Maintenance of skin moisture by increasing acid mucopolysaccharides and hyaluronic acid
  ▲ Metabolic:
    • Decreased bone resorption via antagonism of parathyroid hormone and IL-6
    • Increased HDL; decreased LDL; increased triglycerides

■ Estrogens also mediate cell proliferation, in both normal and malignant cells. There are two estrogen receptors (ERα and ERβ), both of which either increase or decrease transcription of target genes.

■ On binding of estrogen, the receptors dimerize (join together) and then bind to EREs, typically found in the promoter region of target genes. A promoter is a region of a gene that facilitates transcription. Binding of agonist to the estrogen receptor also recruits coactivators, which help to stimulate transcription. The net effect of all of this is to initiate transcription (Figure 14-11).

Estrogen receptor antagonists

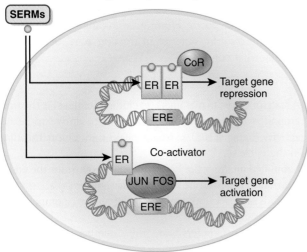

Figure 14-11.

■ Estrogen receptor antagonists inhibit transcription by promoting the binding of co-repressors (CoRs) to the ERE. CoRs inhibit transcription.

■ The SERMs are **partial agonists**, *antagonizing* the effects of estrogen in some tissues (breast) and *stimulating* estrogen receptors in others (bone, brain, liver). This is in contrast to the estrogen antagonists (e.g., clomiphene), which block estrogen receptors in *all tissues*.

■ Some breast cancers express estrogen receptors, and estrogen antagonists are used to treat these tumors.

■ Clomiphene has a unique mechanism in that it **stimulates the release of follicle-stimulating hormone (FSH)**. It does this by antagonizing the negative feedback of estrogen on gonadotropin-releasing hormone (GnRH). Estrogen normally has an inhibitory effect on GnRH, so through blocking of this inhibitory effect, more FSH is released, promoting ovulation in patients with infertility.

PHARMACOKINETICS

■ Tamoxifen's elimination is biphasic, as the parent drug has a much shorter half-life (6 hours) than the active metabolite (5 to 10 days). The major route of elimination for tamoxifen is through metabolism by CYP3A4 and CYP2D6.

■ Toremifene is an active metabolite of tamoxifen.

■ Raloxifene and clomiphene do not undergo extensive CYP metabolism. Clomiphene has a long elimination half-life of 5 to 7 days.

■ Fulvestrant is available in a depot injection, which can be administered on a monthly basis.

INDICATIONS

■ Breast cancer (estrogen-receptor positive)
■ Prevention of breast cancer in high-risk women
■ Osteoporosis
■ Infertility

CONTRAINDICATIONS
Pregnancy

■ Estrogen plays an important role in maintenance of pregnancy.

SIDE EFFECTS

■ **Endometrial:** Some of the partial agonists have estrogen *agonist* effects on the endometrium, leading to abnormal cell growth. This can manifest as increased endometrial thickness, endometrial polyps, leiomyomas, and even endometrial cancer.

■ **Thromboembolism:** Increased risk of thromboembolic events, including pulmonary embolism, have been observed in large studies.

■ **Stroke:** Stroke has been observed in large studies.

■ **Hot flashes:** Hot flashes mimic the physiology of menopause.

■ **Nausea, vomiting**

■ **Menstrual irregularities:** Oligomenorrhea (infrequent periods) and amenorrhea (absent periods) may occur.

■ **Cataracts**

IMPORTANT NOTES

■ Although they are all partial agonists, the SERMs are a heterogeneous drug class because they have different effects (agonist or antagonist) depending on the tissue they target.

■ Raloxifene does not have the endometrial side effects seen with tamoxifen (see Side Effects).

■ Raloxifene began as an investigational drug for treatment of breast cancer but was first approved for its beneficial effects in osteoporosis in postmenopausal women. Since then it has been "rediscovered" as a preventive therapy for postmenopausal women at high risk of invasive breast cancer.

■ Several large trials have reported a benefit of tamoxifen in the prevention of breast cancer, particularly in high-risk groups. The National Surgical Adjuvant Breast and Bowel Project (NSABP) P-1 trial randomized 13,388 high-risk women to either tamoxifen or placebo. The risk of estrogen receptor–positive breast cancer was reduced by 69% at 5 years. The International Breast Cancer Intervention Study (IBIS) randomized 7154 women to tamoxifen or placebo and also found a 32% reduction in the overall risk of breast cancer.

EVIDENCE
Tamoxifen and Breast Cancer Treatment

■ A 1998 meta-analysis (55 trials, N = 37,000) clearly established the role of tamoxifen in the treatment of estrogen receptor–positive breast cancer. The analysis included women with early breast cancer, finding that adjuvant tamoxifen for approximately 5 years reduced breast cancer recurrence by 42% and mortality by 22%.

Aromatase Inhibitors (AIs)

DESCRIPTION
AIs block the synthesis of estrogen.

PROTOTYPE AND COMMON DRUGS
- Prototype: first- and second-generation AIs are discussed in the FYI section.
- Others: third-generation AIs:
  - ▲ Steroid (type I): exemestane
  - ▲ Nonsteroids (type II): ana**strozole**, le**trozole**

MOA (MECHANISM OF ACTION)
- **Aromatization** is the process of converting a nonaromatic ring into an aromatic ring and is catalyzed by **aromatase**, a P450 enzyme. Aromatization converts androgens into estrogens. Estrogens contain an aromatic six-carbon ring. Androgens do not (Figure 14-12).
- *Steroid-type* AIs have an androgen structure and bind the substrate binding site in a noncompetitive, irreversible fashion.
- *Nonsteroid-type* AIs bind the cytochrome P450 moiety of the enzyme and are competitive and reversible.
- Aromatase inhibition results in the following:
  - ▲ Lower levels of estradiol, estrone, and estrone sulfate. This is beneficial for conditions that require lower estrogen levels, including breast cancer and precocious puberty.
  - ▲ Decreased negative feedback on the hypothalamic-pituitary axis by estrogen, leading to increased FSH secretion and resultant ovarian follicle growth, which is the mechanism by which AIs are beneficial for infertility.
  - ▲ Higher androgen levels in the ovary, which might promote follicular growth and also help with infertility.

PHARMACOKINETICS
- AIs and tamoxifen, a SERM, are frequently coadministered for cancer therapy. Tamoxifen induces CYP enzymes and so reduces the levels of AIs.

INDICATIONS
- Hormone-sensitive breast cancers
- Precocious puberty (early puberty in young children)
- Endometriosis
- Infertility due to anovulation (absence of ovulation)

CONTRAINDICATION
- Pregnancy (which is a physiologic state requiring increased estrogen)

SIDE EFFECTS
- Reduced bone density and increased fractures
  - ▲ Bone protection measures should be taken. These include bisphosphonates, vitamin D, calcium, and exercise.
- Hot flushes from estrogen deficiency (which mimics perimenopausal symptoms)
- Nonspecific: nausea, fatigue, increased sweating, peripheral edema, and increased appetite

IMPORTANT NOTES
- Comparisons between AIs and SERMs:
  - ▲ AIs inhibit estrogen synthesis; SERMs do not. Therefore estrogen *metabolites* (which could act on tumors) would also be reduced with AIs but not necessarily blocked with SERMs.
  - ▲ AIs will not block exogenous estrogens (e.g., phytoestrogens); SERMs will.
  - ▲ AIs do not bind to the estrogen receptor; SERMs do. Progesterone receptor *up*-regulation in tumors has been observed with SERMs but not with AIs, and this could be a mechanism of tumor resistance.
- Aromatase is present in many tissues, including the ovaries, brain, placenta, adipose tissue, muscle, liver, breast, and estrogen-dependent breast cancer. Adipose is the primary source of estrogen production in both men and postmenopausal women.

Advanced
- Aromatase converts:
  - ▲ Testosterone into estradiol
  - ▲ Androstenedione into estrone
- Type I (steroid) AIs are actually prodrugs; when they bind aromatase, the enzyme converts them to a structure that permanently binds and destroys the enzyme. They are

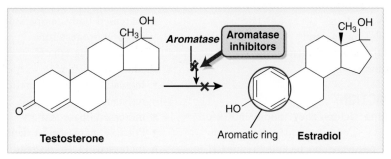

Figure 14-12.

called *suicide* inhibitors because the enzyme is destroyed by the chemical it creates.

EVIDENCE

Advanced Breast Cancer
■ A meta-analysis in 2007 (25 studies, N = 9416 women) showed a pooled hazard ratio for survival of 0.89 (11% benefit) of AIs over other therapy (progesterones or SERMs).

Early Breast Cancer
■ An RCT in 2004 with follow-up in 2007 demonstrated that postmenopausal women *who were cancer free while on tamoxifen* at the 2- to 3-year mark (postsurgery) had increased survival (3.3% absolute increase) at 5 years if they switched to exemestane versus staying on tamoxifen.

Anovulation
■ A 2008 review (9 studies, N = 2573 women) examined the impact of adding letrozole to conventional infertility treatments. There were no statistically significant improvements in ovulatory cycles nor pregnancies per ovulatory cycle. Large RCTs are required to clarify the roles of AIs for anovulation therapy.

Endometriosis
■ Data are currently too limited to recommend AI use with endometriosis, but it is being tried in advanced cases.

FYI
■ The prototype first-generation (aminoglutethimide) and second-generation (fadrozole and formestane) AIs are no longer used because of low potency, lack of specificity, and side effects.
■ The nonsteroidal AIs contain a triazole structure. An azole is a five-membered ring that includes at least one noncarbon atom. Triazoles have three nitrogens. There is also a class of antifungals called "azoles" whose mechanism of action is also inhibition of a P450 enzyme (Figure 14-13).

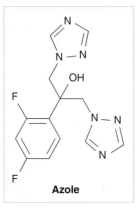

Azole

Figure 14-13.

■ Total body aromatization of plasma androstenedione increased from 0.5% to 10% with a rise in body weight from 100 to 400 pounds in women.
■ An aromatic ring contains an odd number of "lone electrons." It is a very stable structure.
■ Patients with PCOS have reduced aromatase activity within the ovary, which is probably responsible for the production of multiple small follicles, resulting in multiple cysts.

Progestins

DESCRIPTION
Progestins (also called *progestogens*) are one of the endogenous female sex hormones. See the discussions of estrogens and hormone contraception.

COMMON DRUGS
■ **Bioidentical:** progesterone
■ **First-generation** *pregnanes:* megestrol acetate, medroxyprogesterone acetate (MPA)
■ **Second-generation** *estranes:* norethindrone, norethindrone acetate, ethynodiol, lynestrenol
■ **Third-generation** *gonanes:* norgestrel, levonorgestrel, desogestrel, norgestimate, gestodene, dienogest
■ **Nonsteroidal:** drospirenone

MOA (MECHANISM OF ACTION)
■ Progestins are transcription factors; they modify mRNA synthesis directly.
■ Progestins enter the cell passively (no receptor required) and bind to progesterone receptors in the nucleus, which then dimerize and bind DNA directly and influence gene transcription.
■ Important effects of progesterone include the following:
  ▲ Reproductive:
    • Part of feedback loop with luteinizing hormone (LH) and FSH
    • Abrupt decline determines onset of menstruation
    • Changes endocervical glands from watery to viscous; this reduces sperm entry into the uterus
    • Maintenance of pregnancy
    • Increased body temperature because of preovulatory surge in progesterone
    • Mild sedating effects
  ▲ Metabolic:
    • Increased insulin secretion and peripheral insulin resistance
    • Increased lipase activity
    • Possible increased fat deposition
    • Increased LDL; decreased HDL (the opposite of estrogen)

PHARMACOKINETICS

- There are multiple routes of administration: oral, subcutaneous, and depot subcutaneous.
- Additional routes of administration include insertion of foreign bodies that contain and slowly release progesterone. These include implants (which are placed surgically in the arm), intrauterine devices (IUDs), and vaginal rings.

INDICATIONS

- Prevention of pregnancy (contraception)
- Menopausal HRT
- DUB

CONTRAINDICATIONS

- Risks for DVT or PE
- **Severe migraine headache:** There are relationships among estrogen, progesterone, and serotonin levels. Serotonin is implicated in migraine pathophysiology; administration of estrogen or progesterone can potentially exacerbate (or alleviate) migraines.
- **Unexplained vaginal bleeding:** Prolonged progesterone administration can cause vaginal bleeding; it is important to diagnose any pathologic causes of bleeding before starting treatment that could confound other bleeding.
- **Breast cancer:** Female sex hormones can stimulate breast tissue growth.
- **Active liver disease**
- Conditions of concern for hypoestrogenic effects and reduced HDL levels, theoretically increasing cardiovascular risk:
  - ▲ HTN with vascular disease
  - ▲ Current and history of ischemic heart disease
  - ▲ History of stroke
  - ▲ Diabetes for over 20 years or with nephropathy, retinopathy, neuropathy, or vascular disease

SIDE EFFECTS

- **Androgenic activity:** Because of the similarity of progestins to androgens and the conversion of progestins to androgens, androgenic side effects are not uncommon. **Levonorgestrel** is the most androgenic. Third-generation progestins are less androgenic than second-generation progestins.
  - ▲ Acne and hirsutism are the most common signs.
  - ▲ Increased LDL and insulin resistance are also seen.
- **DVT:** Third-generation progestins may be associated with a higher incidence of DVT than second-generation progestins.
- **Vaginal bleeding:** The mechanism is not completely understood.

IMPORTANT NOTES

- Progesterone is secreted by the ovary, mainly by the corpus luteum during the luteal phase (second half) of the menstrual cycle. See Figure 14-9.
- **Bioidentical hormones** are hormones that are chemically identical to what is naturally produced in the human body.

Because minor chemical changes can result in a change in function, some women experience fewer side effects with bioidentical hormones.
- Drospirenone is derived from spironolactone (an aldosterone antagonist) and also has antialdosterone effects.
  - ▲ Reduces estrogen-induced water retention
  - ▲ Also has antiandrogen effects
- Progestins can be administered alone or in combination with estrogens for birth control. Long-term contraception (e.g., depot injections, implants, IUDs) are *progestin only.* Their use is associated with menstrual irregularities, including abnormal bleeding.
- HRT is administered as estrogen only or a combination of estrogen and progesterone, but not progesterone alone.
- Subcutaneous rods can deliver progestins for as long as 5 years.

Advanced
Chemical Structure

- *Pregnanes* have an extra methyl group at C6, which decreases first-pass hepatic metabolism and thus makes these formulations orally available.
- *Estranes* have lost the methyl group at C19, which decreases androgenic activity.
- *Gonanes* have replaced the methyl group at C13 with an ethyl group, which again decreases androgenic activity.

EVIDENCE
Hormone Replacement Therapy and Cardiovascular Outcomes

- A Cochrane review in 2005 (10 studies, N = 24,000 women) compared HRT (estrogen only and estrogen combined with progesterone) with placebo or no treatment and found that there were no protective effects of HRT on all-cause mortality, cardiovascular death, or myocardial infarction. However, there was an *increased* risk of DVT and PE (RR 2.15) and stroke (RR 1.44) in patients treated with HRT.

FYI

- **Gest**ation refers to pregnancy. The man who co-discovered pro**gest**erone in the 1930s, American medical student Willard H. Allen (later to become an obstetrician), described a *pregestational proliferation* of the uterus and coined the names *progestin* and *progesterone.*
- The word root -*sterone* refers to **steroid ketones**, which testosterone is, but estrogen is not. This similarity of progesterone to testosterone is the reason for the androgenic side effect profile of progesterones.
  - ▲ There is no aromatic ring in progesterone (as there is in estrogen). Instead, there is a ketone group (C=O) on the A ring (similar to testosterone).
  - ▲ In addition to the four-ring, 19-carbon steroid structure, there are an extra two carbons at C17 (named 17α), to make the structure a C21 steroid.
  - ▲ See Figure 14-10.

Hormone Contraception

DESCRIPTION

Hormone contraceptives are estrogen and progestin preparations used for the purpose of preventing pregnancy. See also the two sections on estrogens and progestins for further details.

COMMON DRUGS

- Multiple combinations of different estrogens and progestins
  - Estrogens: ethinyl estradiol, mestranol
  - Progestins: many different types

MOA (MECHANISM OF ACTION)
Progestins

- Progestins are primarily responsible for the **contraceptive activity.**
- They prevent the LH surge that is required for release of the ovum; thus the ovum is not released from the ovary.
- They thicken cervical mucus, which impedes sperm entry into uterus.
- They decrease tubal motility, which impedes sperm transit through fallopian tubes.
- They thin the endometrium, which reduces probability of implantation.

Estrogens

- Estrogens are primarily responsible for **cycle control** (bleeding) and to a lesser extent demonstrate some contraceptive activity.
- They stabilize the endometrium, minimizing irregular shedding (bleeding).
- They inhibit release of FSH, preventing the development of the dominant follicle.
- They potentiate the progestin's inhibition of the LH surge.

Combined Hormone versus Progestin-Only Preparations

- Most preparations are a combination of an estrogen plus progestin; however, some preparations contain progestin only. Progestin-only preparations are used in women in whom estrogens are contraindicated or not tolerated.

PHARMACOKINETICS

- Estrogen is metabolized by CYP3A4 liver enzymes, and thus the birth control pill (BCP) can become **less effective if coadministered with** other drugs that are CYP3A4 inducers:
  - Barbiturates (for seizures or, less commonly now, for sedation)
  - Isoniazid (for tuberculosis treatment)
- The BCP is usually administered over a 28-day period:
  - The pill is used for 21 days, followed by 7 days of no pill or placebo.
  - Seven days of no hormone results in withdrawal bleed, creating a menstrual period.
  - Some formulations extend the 21 days of hormone to 24 and shorten the placebo to 4 days.
  - The duration of the hormone administration can be extended even more so that a woman will experience less frequent menstrual bleeding. Administration for 42 or 84 (plus 7 placebo) days of **extended cycle** hormone results in menstrual bleeding once every 2 or 4 months.
- The BCP can be packaged with different administration schedules:
  - **Monophasic:** There is only one dose of hormone throughout the cycle.
  - **Multiphasic** (biphasic or triphasic): There is more than one dose of hormone throughout the cycle.
- Other forms of hormonal contraception administration include the following:
  - **Depot:** slow release injection once every 3 months
  - **Transdermal patch:** changed once a week
  - **Vaginal ring:** changed once a month
  - **IUDs:** can be drug free or hormone eluting
  - **Implants:** progestin-impregnated implants, placed under the skin in the inner arm between the bicep and tricep muscles.

INDICATIONS

- **Planned prevention of conception:** BCP, also called the *oral contraceptive pill* (OCP)
- **Unplanned prevention of conception:** the morning-after pill

CONTRAINDICATIONS

- Smoking is a *relative* contraindication because of the increased risk of thrombus and atherosclerotic disease.
- **Risk for thrombus** should be considered an *absolute* contraindication:
  - Familial **factor V Leiden,** the most common inherited coagulation cascade abnormality that gives rise to pathologic thrombi.
  - **Previous DVT or PE**
- Also see the sections on estrogens and progestins for details.

SIDE EFFECTS

- Side effects are related to the dosages and types of hormone used.
- **Breakthrough bleeding** is common when the BCP is started. Bleeding in cycle 1 (after starting the pill) is often reduced by cycle 4.
- Although doses are not routinely reported in this textbook, doses of hormones in BCPs are important and require mention:
  - Side effects are usually attributed to the estrogen; the higher the dose, the higher the probability of side effects.

▲ Doses of ethinyl estradiol range from 20 mcg to 50 mcg.
  • Doses of **20 to 25 mcg** are considered *ultra-low* doses.
▲ Ethinyl estradiol **50 mcg** has higher incidences of **headache, breast tenderness, DVT, and nausea**. This dose is rarely used anymore.
▲ 35 mcg of ethinyl estradiol is equivalent to 50 mcg of mestranol (both are estrogen compounds).
▲ Patients who develop intolerable estrogen-related side effects might be candidates for progestin-only BCPs.
■ Progestin-related side effects are primarily **androgenic: acne** and **hirsutism**. Levonorgestrel is the *most androgenic* progestin.
■ Different formulations and routes of administration are associated with slightly different side effect profiles:
▲ **Extended cycle:** Side effects include breakthrough bleeding and acne.
▲ **Progestin only:** Side effects include increased breakthrough bleeding and a slightly lower efficacy for preventing pregnancy.
▲ **Depot (progestin only):** Side effects include decreased bone density, which is reversible. Use should be limited to 2 years in adolescents, and all women on the depot injection should take supplemental calcium.
▲ **Morning-after pill:** Because of the high dose of estrogen, nausea is common. Progestin-only formulations are also used which do not carry the same risk of nausea.

IMPORTANT NOTES
■ A few BCPs use iron pills instead of placebo pills during the 7 days of no hormone. This is to help maintain iron levels in women who have low iron stores because of regular menstrual blood loss.
■ Ultra-low–dose estrogen should be **avoided in adolescents** because of the requirement for slightly higher estrogen levels for proper bone development.
■ Side effects are the most common reason for discontinuing BCPs. They include the following:
▲ Dysmenorrhea, anemia, acne, hirsutism, ectopic pregnancy, benign breast disease, endometrial cancer, and ovarian cysts
■ The estrogen-containing morning-after pill has about 3 to 5 times the dose of estrogen compared with the BCP. It is usually prescribed with an antinausea medication.

■ Monophasic and triphasic regimens offer similar rates of abnormal bleeding, discontinuation, and adverse events.
■ Extended cycle formulations are always monophasic.
■ When used correctly, BCPs prevent pregnancy 99% of the time. However, because of incorrect use, the failure rate is about 2% to 3%. Twenty percent to 50% of adolescents do not take the BCP as directed; 20% of users miss one or two pills per cycle.

EVIDENCE
Lactation
■ A meta-analysis in 2008 with five included studies could not find evidence to support or refute an association between hormone contraception and lactation quality or quantity.

Breakthrough Bleeding
■ A systematic review in 2007 did not find a clear association between type or dose of oral BCP and breakthrough bleeding; however, studies were heterogeneous with respect to methodology and reporting of bleeding. Bleeding in cycle 1 (first menstrual cycle after starting the BCP) was higher than in cycle 4.

FYI
■ The BCP was on the front cover of *Time* magazine in 1967.
■ Mestranol was the estrogen used in the first oral contraceptive.
■ Many brands of BCP are named according to the dose of hormone. For example, 1/30 would represent 1000 mcg of a progestin formulation plus 30 mcg of an estrogen formulation.
■ BCPs are also named according to *phases*. For example, if there are three different doses, each for 7 days, then 7/7/7 is used to denote this.
■ Related to reproduction and the coagulation cascade, a hypercoagulable state can give rise to **recurrent spontaneous abortions** (also called *miscarriages*). The mechanism is uteroplacental thrombi resulting in impaired circulation to the placenta. Affected women should be investigated for hypercoagulable states, such as the presence of **factor V Leiden.**
■ Progestins are more closely related to androgens than are estrogens and therefore are the female hormones that give rise to androgenic side effects.

Oxytocin

DESCRIPTION
Oxytocin is a naturally occurring neuropeptide released from the posterior pituitary.

PROTOTYPE AND COMMON DRUGS
■ Prototype: Oxy**tocin**
■ Others: Carbe**tocin**, demoxy**tocin**

MOA (MECHANISM OF ACTION)
■ Oxytocin is produced in the hypothalamus but is secreted by the *posterior* pituitary and acts primarily on smooth muscle of breast and uterine tissue (Figure 14-14):
▲ *Let-down* reflex to release milk from the breast
▲ Myometrial (uterine) contraction during and after delivery

Oxytocin

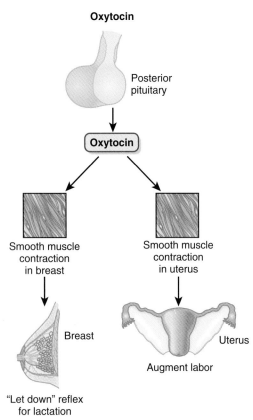

Figure 14-14.

- In the uterus, oxytocin binds oxytocin receptors, which activates G proteins and results in:
  - ▲ Increased intracellular calcium leading directly to increased contraction
  - ▲ Increased levels of prostaglandin (PG) $F_{2\alpha}$, which is a potent vasoconstrictor and oxytocic (uterine constrictor)
- Increased uterine contraction helps to expel the fetus. After delivery, uterine contraction is critical to help stop bleeding; the uterus contracts down on intramyometrial vessels, which clamps them shut.
- Oxytocin is involved in a positive feedback loop: once labor has started, uterine contractions caused by oxytocin induce more oxytocin to be released from the cervix.

PHARMACOKINETICS

- Oxytocin is a peptide, so it cannot be given orally; it is given by intravenous or subcutaneous injection. The half-life of oxytocin is 3 minutes.
- Carbetocin is a synthetic, nonpeptide oxytocin analogue with a duration of action of 1 hour.
- When given to augment labor, oxytocin is given as an intravenous infusion, starting at a low dose and increasing approximately every 30 minutes (to a maximum dose).
- When given to prevent postpartum bleeding, it is given as a subcutaneous injection or intravenous infusion.

INDICATIONS

- Induction of labor
- Augmentation of labor
- Prevention and treatment of postpartum bleeding

CONTRAINDICATION

- Previous uterine rupture

SIDE EFFECTS

- **Hypotension** results when oxytocin is administered rapidly.
- **Abnormally high uterine tone:** Increased contraction can lead to decreased blood flow to the uterus and thus **decreased oxygen delivery to the fetus.** Uterine tone and oxytocin administered must be considered as a cause of **fetal distress.** Reducing the dose or discontinuing the oxytocin is required if oxytocin is thought to be the cause.
- **Uterine rupture:** This is a rare complication (in some reports, about 1 in 6000). Uterine stimulation is one risk factor for this complication. A scarred uterus (from previous caesarian sections) is another risk factor.
- **Antidiuretic effect:** This occurs because of the similarity of oxytocin to vasopressin (ADH).

IMPORTANT NOTES

- The first stage of labor is cervical dilation; the second stage is expulsion of the fetus once the cervix is fully dilated; the third stage is the period after the baby is delivered until the placenta is delivered.
- Uterine atony (loss of tone) is a very common cause of postpartum hemorrhage (PPH) and is treated with drugs that increase uterine tone:
  - ▲ Oxytocin
  - ▲ Prostaglandin ($PGF_{2\alpha}$)
  - ▲ Ergotamine derivatives (ergometrine)
- Postpartum uterine atony can also be caused by prolonged uterine stimulation by exogenous oxytocin.
- Considering that the gravid uterus receives 20% of cardiac output, torrential blood loss can occur in the postpartum period. Blood loss of 500 mL is not unusual for caesarian sections or vaginal deliveries. Blood loss of >1000 mL becomes medically important.

EVIDENCE
Postpartum Bleeding (Including the Third Stage of Labor)

- **Oxytocin versus nothing:** In a meta-analysis in 2004 (seven trials, N = 3000 women), prophylactic oxytocin was found to reduce blood loss with an RR of 0.50 for blood loss greater than 500 mL.
- **Oxytocin versus ergot alkaloids:** A meta-analysis in 2004 (six trials, N = 2800 women) demonstrated little difference. Manual placenta removals were less frequent with oxytocin (RR 0.57).
- **Oxytocin versus oxytocin plus ergot alkaloids:** A meta-analysis in 2007 (six trials, N = 9332 women) demonstrated that if blood loss was defined as >1000 mL, there was *no*

difference, but if blood loss was defined as >500 mL, then there was a *small reduction* in blood loss with the combination therapy. Combination therapy significantly *increased* the following side effects: HTN, vomiting, and nausea.

- **Carbetocin versus oxytocin**: A meta-analysis in 2007 (four studies, N = 1032 women) did not demonstrate a difference in blood loss or risk of PPH. However, with carbetocin there was a reduction (RR 0.44) in the use of uterotonics and a reduction (RR 0.38) in the need for uterine massage (used to stimulate contraction). There was no difference in side effects.

Induction or Augmentation of Labor

- **Oxytocin versus no treatment**: A meta-analysis in 2001 (26 studies, N = 6660 women) showed that oxytocin reduced the rate of unsuccessful vaginal delivery within 24 hours: 8.3% versus 54% (RR 0.16), but the caesarean section rate was increased: 10.4% versus 8.9% (RR 1.17).
- **Oxytocin versus vaginal PGs**: A meta-analysis in 2001 (27 studies, N = 4649 women) showed that oxytocin was associated with increased unsuccessful vaginal deliveries within 24 hours (52% versus 28%, RR 1.85), irrespective of membrane status (ruptured or not ruptured). There was no difference in caesarean section rates.
- **Oxytocin versus intracervical PGs**: A meta-analysis in 2001 (13 studies, N = 1244 women) showed that oxytocin alone was associated with an increase in unsuccessful vaginal delivery within 24 hours (51% versus 35%, RR 1.49).

FYI

- Oxytocin, vasopressin (AVP), and the AVP analogue DDAVP are structurally very similar; they all contain nine amino acids (they are nonapeptides). There is one amino acid difference between AVP and DDAVP, and there are two amino acid differences between AVP and oxytocin.
- Octreotide has eight amino acids (a somatostatin analogue).
- Oxytocin and AVP evolved from a single peptide in non-mammals called *vasotocin.*
- Tocolysis is *termination* of uterine contractions; oxytocics and uterotonics are *stimulants* of uterine contraction.

Reproductive Prostaglandins (PGs)

DESCRIPTION

PGs are involved with many processes in the body; this section discusses reproductive uses of PGs.

PROTOTYPES

- Miso**prost**ol (PGE$_1$)
- Dino**prost**one (PGE$_2$)
- Carbo**prost** (PGF$_{2\alpha}$)

MOA (MECHANISM OF ACTION)

- PGs act on a family of receptors that are coupled to G proteins. Some G proteins are stimulatory and some are inhibitory, depending on the specific receptor type. Therefore the physiologic effect of a given PG depends on the receptor and the tissue type. The actions are ultimately mediated by changes in cAMP and intracellular calcium concentrations.
- PGs bind PG receptors:
  - ▲ PGE binds EP receptors (four subtypes, 1 to 4)
  - ▲ PGF binds FP receptors (two subtypes, A and B)
- Second messengers associated with PG receptors include G proteins, which link to adenylyl cyclase and phospholipase 3.
- The most dominant effects on the **female reproductive** system include the following (Figure 14-15):
  - ▲ Cervical softening (the firm cervix relaxes before dilation, a necessary step in early labor)
  - ▲ Increased uterine contraction

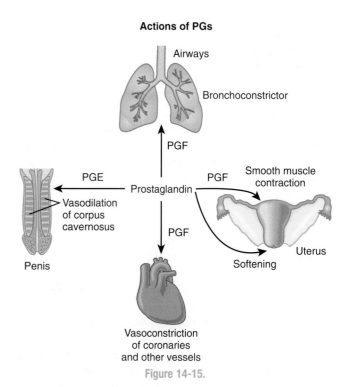

Actions of PGs

Airways

Bronchoconstrictor

PGF

PGE

Prostaglandin

PGF

Vasodilation of corpus cavernosus

Penis

PGF

Smooth muscle contraction

Uterus

Softening

Vasoconstriction of coronaries and other vessels

Figure 14-15.

- The most dominant effects on the **male reproductive** system include the following:
  - ▲ Vasodilation of the vessels in the corpus cavernosum of the penis

PHARMACOKINETICS

- Administration is by different routes:
  - ▲ PGE_1: orally or transurethrally
  - ▲ PGE_2: locally as a gel (vaginally, close to the cervix), suppository
  - ▲ $PGF_{2\alpha}$: intramuscularly or intramyometrially
- Oral administration of $PGF_{2\alpha}$ results in too many GI side effects for the agent to be useful.
- Topically administered PGs (in women, vaginal or intracervical route; in men, intraurethral route) will have minimal absorption.
- PGs have short half-lives; about 95% of the agent is inactivated after one circulation through the pulmonary circulation via enzymes that are specific for PGs.

INDICATIONS (REPRODUCTIVE ONLY)

- PGE_1 and PGE_2
  - ▲ Labor induction and cervical ripening
  - ▲ Missed abortion (miscarriage with products of conception not yet expelled)
  - ▲ Abortion
- PGE_1 only
  - ▲ Erectile dysfunction
- $PGF_{2\alpha}$ only
  - ▲ Treatment of postpartum hemorrhage, but not as first-line treatment
  - ▲ Abortion

CONTRAINDICATIONS

- **Severe asthma**: $PGF_{2\alpha}$ is a potent bronchoconstrictor.
- **Glaucoma**: This is discussed in more detail in the ophthalmology section.
- **Myocardial infarction**: Myocardial infarction occurs because of the risk of vascular constriction to the myocardium.
- Relative contraindications that are **obstetric related** include unexplained vaginal bleeding, chorioamnionitis, ruptured membranes, and previous cesarean section.

SIDE EFFECTS

- **Smooth muscle contraction** of the following:
  - ▲ Airways, leading to an **asthma**-type reaction
  - ▲ Vasculature, leading to **HTN**
  - ▲ GI tract, leading to diarrhea, cramping, and vomiting. PG's also promote movement of water and electrolytes into the intestine; this also increases diarrhea.
- **Fever**: Naturally occurring *E type* PGs are a key element in the fever response (with inflammation); the site of action is in the preoptic area of the hypothalamus. Administration of exogenous PGE_2 therefore causes fever.

IMPORTANT NOTES

- Missed abortions are also commonly treated expectantly (wait for spontaneous passage of products of conception)

or procedurally with dilatation and curettage (D&C), a procedure that involves mechanical dilation of the cervix and then gentle removal of intrauterine contents with a suction catheter or curettage, an instrument that scrapes away the endometrium.

- For erectile dysfunction, the PG must be injected into the penis or inserted into the urethra.
- Both PGE_2 and $PGF_{2\alpha}$ cross the uteroplacental barrier, but fetal toxicity is uncommon.

Advanced

- PG receptors are located in cell membranes and have seven transmembrane segments; they encompass a large family of receptors with four classes and at least 10 different subtypes.
- Dinoprostone comes prepackaged in a viscous gel of colloid with triacetin (antifungal). The syringe is connected to a soft-plastic catheter for intracervical administration.

EVIDENCE
Induction of Labor

- **Intravenous PGs versus oxytocin**: A meta-analysis in 2004 (13 trials, N = 1165 women) showed that *intravenous* PG was associated with higher rates of uterine hyperstimulation, both with changes in the fetal heart rate (RR 6.76) and without (RR 4.25), compared with oxytocin. Use of PG was also associated with significantly more maternal side effects: GI effects, thrombophlebitis, and pyrexia. PG was no more likely to result in vaginal delivery than oxytocin.
- **Vaginal PGs versus oxytocin**: A meta-analysis in 2001 (27 studies, N = 4649 women) showed that *vaginal* PGs were associated with decreased unsuccessful vaginal deliveries within 24 hours (28% versus 52%, RR 0.54), irrespective of membrane status (ruptured or not ruptured). There was no difference in caesarean section rates.
- **Intracervical PGs versus oxytocin**: A meta-analysis in 2001 (13 studies, N = 1244 women) showed that *intracervical* PGs were associated with a decrease in unsuccessful vaginal delivery within 24 hours (35% versus 51%, RR 0.67).

Erectile Dysfunction

- **PGE1 versus placebo or no treatment**: A meta-analysis in 2009 (4 studies, N = 1873 men) demonstrated increased probability (odds ratio [OR] 7.22) of *at least one successful intercourse*. Adverse effects were most frequent in the treated groups and occurred more often and intensely as doses increased. Penile pain and minor urethral trauma were predominant.

FYI

- In 1934, Dr. Ulf von Euler found that extracts of sheep vesicular gland dramatically lowered blood pressure when injected into animals. Human seminal fluid also seemed to possess similar qualities. Von Euler named it prostaglandin, believing that it originated in the prostate gland.

- Nomenclature:
  - ▲ *Eicosa* is Greek for 20. Eicosanoids have 20 carbon atoms. Eicosanoids include PGs, prostacyclins, leukotrienes, and thromboxane. Arachidonic acid is the most abundant precursor.
  - ▲ The letter after *PG* represents a historical designation.
    - Ether and phosphate buffer were first used to separate PGs in Sweden; the PGs that partitioned into ether were called *PGE*, and those in phosphate (spelled *fosfat* in Swedish) were called *PGF*.
    - An additional test, using acid and base, gave rise to *PGA* and *PGB*.
  - ▲ The subscripted number refers to the number of double bonds (C=C).
    - PGE_1 has a double bond at C5; PGE_3 has double bonds at C5, C13, and C17.
  - ▲ The α or β designates the orientation (pointing in front of the molecule or pointing behind) of the second hydroxyl (-OH) group on the ring. Most PGs have only a single hydroxyl group on the ring; PGF has two.
    - $PGF_{2\alpha}$ therefore was fractionated into phosphate, has two double bonds, and has a second hydroxyl group that is oriented behind the ring.

Nonsteroidal Androgen Antagonists (NSAAs)

DESCRIPTION

Nonsteroidal androgen antagonists (NSAAs) are androgen receptor antagonists.

PROTOTYPE AND COMMON DRUGS

- Prototype: **Flutamide**
- Others: **Ni**lutamide, bica**lutamide**

MOA (MECHANISM OF ACTION)

- These are androgen receptor antagonists that act on androgen receptors in the prostate. As their name states, they are not steroids (unlike dihydrotestosterone [DHT], the agonist they block).
- Antagonism of androgen receptors in prostate tissue reduces growth stimulation of prostatic cancer because of their action on modifying transcription factors related to cellular growth.

PHARMACOKINETICS

- NSAAs are hepatically metabolized, so they are contraindicated in patients with severe hepatic dysfunction.
- Bicalutamide can be given orally once a day; its half-life is about 1 week. Flutamide has a shorter half-life and requires 3-times-a-day administration.

INDICATION

- Metastatic prostate cancer

CONTRAINDICATION

- Severe hepatic dysfunction

SIDE EFFECTS

- Direct antiandrogen effects: Breast pain, gynecomastia, and hot flushes may occur.
- Diarrhea, vomiting, and nausea may occur.
- Hematuria (blood in urine): Many patients with prostate cancer already have hematuria; this side effect has been described, but the drug probably does not *cause* the bleeding.
- Asthenia (decreased sensation in skin) and skin rashes may occur.

IMPORTANT NOTES

- Bicalutamide has essentially replaced flutamide because of once-daily dosing (flutamide administration was 3 times a day) and a lower incidence of diarrhea.
- NSAAs are usually used in combination therapy with either chemical or surgical castration in advanced metastatic prostate cancer.
  - ▲ Chemical castration is accomplished with a GnRH agonist, which shuts down testicular function.
- NSAA therapy is **not curative** of prostate cancer. It is palliative. The goal of therapy is to improve both quality and duration of life.
- Estrogen antagonists and other androgens have been used to help reduce the incidence of antiandrogen side effects.

EVIDENCE

A meta-analysis was conducted in 2000 (23 trials, N = 6320 men), looking at treatment of advanced prostate cancer with castration (surgical or chemical) versus castration plus NSAA. The analysis found an absolute 5% reduction with NSAA in mortality at 5 years, thus an NNT was of 20. There were more adverse events in the group receiving NSAAs, and 10% withdrew from treatment because of side effects.

FYI

- Gynecomastia is the feminization of men: breast development, hair pattern changes, and skin changes.

Androgens

DESCRIPTION
Androgens are male sex hormones.

COMMON DRUGS
- Testosterone
- **Testosterone esters**: testosterone undecanoate, testosterone cypionate, testosterone enanthate
- **17α-alkylated androgens**: danazol, methyltestosterone, oxandrolone, stanozolol, fluoxymesterone

MOA (MECHANISM OF ACTION)
- Testosterone can be converted in the body to **DHT** (another physiologically active androgen) and also to estradiol (an estrogen).
- Physiologic androgens will act on androgen receptors to produce the following:
  - ▲ Male sex organ differentiation in utero
  - ▲ Secondary sex characteristics during puberty, including libido (sex drive)
  - ▲ Prostate gland stimulation (growth)
- It is important to note that exogenous androgen administration will result in inhibition of the physiologic sex hormone axis and will significantly inhibit production and secretion of naturally produced sex hormones in both men and women. See Figure 14-10.

PHARMACOKINETICS
- Androgens administered orally undergo extensive first-pass hepatic metabolism. Therefore modifications to the hormone and also alternative methods of delivery have been developed.
- Androgens can be administered via the oral, transdermal, sublingual, or injection route.
- **Testosterone esters** are more lipophilic and therefore well absorbed in fat (subcutaneous injections). A **depot form** of injection (slow release) is the ester testosterone undecanoate.
- **17α-Methylated androgens** (they have a methyl group attached to the 17 carbon) demonstrate reduced hepatic metabolism but also are less androgenic and are hepatotoxic.

INDICATIONS
- Male hypogonadism (reduced testicular secretion of testosterone)
- Low libido states
- Heavy menstrual bleeding

CONTRAINDICATIONS
- Prostate cancer: Androgens stimulate the growth of prostate tissue and thus would stimulate growth of prostate cancer. In fact, creating the opposite (hypoandronergic states) are part of prostate cancer therapy.

SIDE EFFECTS
- Salt and water retention from the mild mineralocorticoid effect (remember that aldosterone is a similar steroid hormone)
- Hepatic toxicity with 17α-methylated androgens only
- Masculinization if used in women: hirsutism, deeper voice, baldness, amenorrhea, breast and uterine atrophy, and infertility
- Consequences of **anabolic steroid abuse** include the following:
  - ▲ Central nervous system (CNS): Aggression and depression are associated but may also have been present before steroid abuse; difficult to differentiate
  - ▲ Cardiovascular system: HTN, accelerated atherosclerosis, sudden death, cardiac hypertrophy, cardiac fibrosis
  - ▲ Male endocrine: testicular atrophy, decreased sperm counts, increased number of abnormal sperm, infertility
  - ▲ Hepatic: increased liver enzymes and gallstones
  - ▲ Musculoskeletal system: premature bone growth plate fusion (shorter stature), tendon ruptures
  - ▲ Skin: increased acne and baldness

EVIDENCE
Female Libido Management
- A Cochrane meta-analysis in 2007 (35 RCTs, N = 4768 women) showed that the addition of testosterone to HRT effectively increased sexual function. Side effects were acne, hair growth, and lower HDL levels.

Heavy Menstrual Bleeding
- A meta-analysis in 2007 (9 RCTs, N = 353 women) showed weak evidence of the superiority of the use of an androgen over NSAIDs or a progesterone IUD for the treatment of heavy bleeding. However, the side effects were greater with the androgen.

FYI
- How to recognize a steroid abuser when you go to the gym:
  - ▲ Back acne
  - ▲ Hypogonadism
  - ▲ Frequently looks at self in mirror
  - ▲ Never shares weights
- Hirsutism is a male pattern of hair distribution on a woman (e.g., facial and chest hair).
- Amenorrhea is cessation of the menstrual cycle.
- Infertility in both men and women can persist for months or years after abuse of anabolic steroids, because of prolonged suppression of gonadal hormone production.
- **Sterone** means a *ketone* derived from a steroid ring. In addition to testosterone, proge**sterone** and aldo**sterone** are also *ketone steroids.*

Somatostatin Analogs

DESCRIPTION
Somatostatin analogs are modifications of somatostatin.

PROTOTYPE AND COMMON DRUGS
- Prototype: Oct**reotide**
- Others: Lan**reotide**, vap**reotide**

MOA (MECHANISM OF ACTION)
- Somatostatin acts on somatostatin receptors; five subtypes have been identified, named SR1 through SR5. Octreotide acts primarily on SR2 and SR5.
- Somatostatin is secreted by the delta cells of the pancreatic islet cells and inhibits the release of the following:
  - ▲ GH, insulin, glucagon, gastrin, VIP
  - ▲ Pancreatic enzymes
- Somatostatin also lowers portal blood pressure, possibly through its inhibitory action of other vasodilating hormones, particularly glucagon. Inhibition of vasodilators results in vasoconstriction that *reduces blood flow into the portal system* and thus reduces the pressure in this system (Figure 14-16).

PHARMACOKINETICS
- Octreotide is an octapeptide (eight amino acids) and therefore must be given parenterally (intravenous or subcutaneous) because it would be digested if taken orally.
- Somatostatin has a half-life of 1 to 2 minutes; octreotide has a half-life of 2 hours.
- There are long-acting formulations of octreotide and lanreotide that require injections only once every 28 days.

INDICATIONS
- Variceal bleeding
- After pancreatic surgery (reduced suppression of pancreatic secretions)
- Suppression of hormones or transmitters:
  - ▲ Acromegaly (GH)
  - ▲ Symptomatic VIP or carcinoid tumors
  - ▲ Functioning islet cell tumors (insulinoma and glucagonomas)
- Severe refractory chemotherapy-induced diarrhea
- Hepatorenal syndrome (renal failure in the setting of advanced liver failure)

CONTRAINDICATION
- Caution with type 1 diabetes: altered glucose metabolism (hypoglycemia) can result.

SIDE EFFECTS
- **Cardiovascular**: sinus bradycardia
- **GI related**: abdominal pain, diarrhea, nausea
- **CNS related**: headache, fatigue

IMPORTANT NOTES
- Variceal bleeding occurs when liver cirrhosis increases resistance to the passage of blood through the liver and hence causes portal HTN, resulting in dilated fragile veins in the esophagus, stomach, and rectum.
- Because of the actions on glucose-mediating hormones (primarily glucagon, insulin, and glucagon-like peptides), administration to patients with type 1 diabetes can result in reduced insulin requirements and thus a risk of hypoglycemia. Paradoxically, administration to patients with type 2 diabetes can result in hyperglycemia.

Advanced
- Somatostatin is also released from other tissues: hypothalamus, stomach, and duodenum.
- Octreotide has been used in patients with advanced cancer. Research is still ongoing.

EVIDENCE
Variceal Bleeding
- A meta-analysis in 2007 (21 studies and 2588 patients) demonstrated no benefit of octreotide versus placebo with

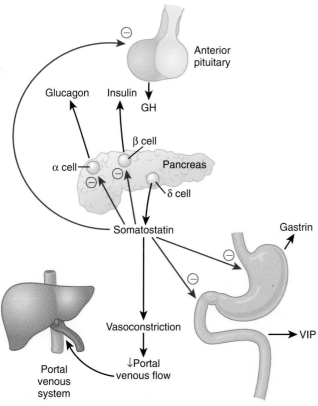

Somatostatin

Figure 14-16.

regard to mortality. Treated patients, on average, required slightly fewer red blood cell transfusions (0.7 units).

Refractory Diarrhea

■ A systematic review in 2001 (30 studies and 712 patients) found that among the eight RCTs included in the review, there was a response (complete or partial resolution of diarrhea) of 64% to therapy compared with 34% in the placebo (control) group.

FYI

■ Somatostatin's inhibition of somatotropin (GH) is the origin of its name. Octreotide's name arises from its **octa**-**pept**ide structure.
■ Islets in the pancreas are multisecretory. In addition, glucagon is secreted from alpha cells and insulin from beta cells in the pancreas.
■ Carcinoid tumors of the gut secrete serotonin, which causes flushing, diarrhea, wheezing, and abdominal pain.

Growth Hormone Antagonists

DESCRIPTION
GH antagonists block the action of GH.

PROTOTYPE
■ Pegvisomant

MOA (MECHANISM OF ACTION)
■ GH antagonists block the action of GH at the GH receptor in the liver.
■ GH is a protein. The substitution of one amino acid converts endogenous GH into an antagonist. Commercial GH antagonists have multiple substitutions to enhance binding affinity.
■ IGF-1 mediates the effects of GH; GH stimulates release of IGF-1 from the liver, and IGF-1 stimulates growth in bone and soft tissues (Figure 14-17).
■ Biologic activities of GH include the following:
   ▲ Skeletal growth
   ▲ Soft tissue growth
   ▲ Insulin antagonism
■ Pathologically high levels of GH result in gigantism (very large stature) and acromegaly, a condition of bone and soft tissue overgrowth that occurs with high GH levels after growth plates have been fused and vertical growth is finished.
■ Because of the insulin antagonism, insulin resistance (diabetes) also occurs with GH overproduction.

PHARMACOKINETICS
■ The addition of polyethylene glycol 500 (PEG-500) to GH (and thus also GH antagonists) increases its half-life from 30 minutes to about 2 days.
■ As a protein, it cannot be taken orally; it is injected subcutaneously.

INDICATION
■ Acromegaly: a rare condition, of which the most common cause is a benign GH (hyper)secreting pituitary adenoma
   ▲ For patients with persistently elevated IGF-1 despite other therapy
   ▲ Possibly as monotherapy (more research required)

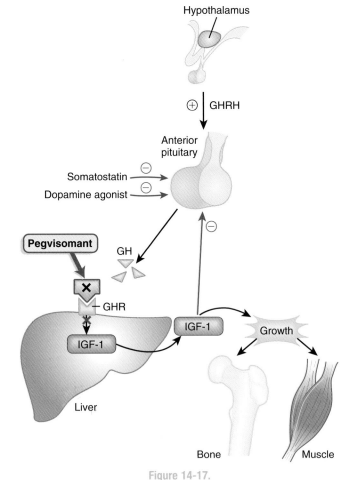

Figure 14-17.

CONTRAINDICATION
■ Severe liver disease (because of risk of liver damage)

SIDE EFFECT
■ Elevated liver enzymes (transaminases) are seen in 25% of patients, indicating liver damage. Liver enzymes must be routinely monitored.

IMPORTANT NOTES

- Surgery, dopamine agonists, and somatostatin are standard first-line treatments for acromegaly. Dopamine agonists and somatostatin are inhibitors of GH *secretion* but are not direct *antagonists* of GH; therefore their mechanism of action is slightly different, and they act at a different location in the biochemical pathway.
- Some signs of acromegaly include coarse facial features (prominent brow, cheekbones, chin), large hands and fingers, large tongue (macroglossia), obstructive sleep apnea (because of the macroglossia), vocal changes, HTN, cardiomegaly, and insulin resistance.
  - ▲ Life expectancy in active acromegaly is 10 years shorter than normal.
- IGF-1 levels are measured to help monitor effectiveness of acromegaly treatment. A drop in levels indicates that GH antagonism has occurred, and drug doses are titrated to IGF-1 levels. It is possible to lower IFG-1 levels to below normal, which is probably undesirable.

Advanced

- Nelson's syndrome is a condition of rapid growth of the pituitary as a result of cortisol absence (lack of negative feedback). Concerns about the development of Nelson's syndrome have been raised with regard to the use of GH antagonists and the resulting loss of negative feedback from IGF-1 on the pituitary. So far, Nelson's syndrome has not been demonstrated.

EVIDENCE
Biochemical Markers

- In an observational study in 2001 (N = 160), it was demonstrated that somatostatin normalizes IGF-1 levels in about 65% of patients. Pegvisomant normalized IGF-1 levels in 97% of patients and reduced insulin and resting glucose levels but not HbA$_{1c}$. However, GH levels almost double. The mechanism of this increase is unknown, but it could be related to loss of negative feedback on the pituitary from IGF-1.

FYI

- Andre the Giant, a professional wrestler in the 1970s who passed away in 1993 from heart failure, had acromegaly.
- *Acro-* means top, height, or summit. The name would suggest that *acromegaly* means large height; however, the term *gigantism* is used instead. *Acromegaly* describes the non–height-related effects of GH excess.
- Somato**trophin** is another name for *endogenously* produced GH; somato**tropin** is the name for *synthetic* GH.
- The name *pegvisomant* reflects the **PEG** and **somato**trophin constituents of the drug.
- Laron dwarfism is caused by a deficiency of IGF-1. Approved in the United States, recombinant IGF-1 is currently being used to treat this condition.

Adrenocorticotropic Hormone (ACTH)

DESCRIPTION

Adrenocorticotropic hormone (ACTH) is secreted by the anterior pituitary and acts on the adrenal glands.

PROTOTYPE

- ACTH (cosyntropin)

MOA (MECHANISM OF ACTION)

- Corticotropin-releasing hormone (CRH) is released from the hypothalamus and stimulates the anterior pituitary.
- ACTH is produced and secreted from the **anterior pituitary**. ACTH binds ACTH receptors on the adrenal cortex. As a result, **cortisol** production and secretion from the **adrenal cortex** are increased (Figure 14-18).
- Activation of the ACTH receptor results in activation of the following signaling process: G proteins → increased cAMP → increased protein kinase A (PKA) → increased intracellular Ca^{2+}, all of which result in:
  - ▲ Increased uptake of lipoprotein and metabolism of cholesterol, for the synthesis of adrenal steroids (cortisol and aldosterone)
  - ▲ Activation of transcription factors for enzymes required for steroid synthesis and release

PHARMACOKINETICS

- The half-life of ACTH is 10 minutes.

INDICATION

- ACTH test: to test adrenal gland function. This test stimulates (or attempts to stimulate) the adrenal gland. The appropriate response is a rise in serum cortisol.

CONTRAINDICATIONS

- None

SIDE EFFECTS

- Minimal when used as a single bolus test

IMPORTANT NOTES

- Cortisol insufficiency is *rarely*, if ever, treated with ACTH. It is usually treated with systemic steroids to replace the cortisol.

Adrenocorticotropic hormone (ACTH)

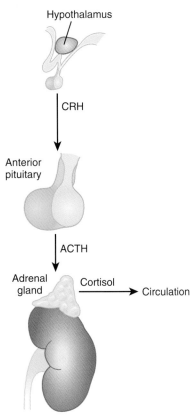

Figure 14-18.

- Cortisol insufficiency can be caused by decreased ACTH secretion or dysfunctional adrenal glands.
- Cortisol insufficiency manifests as:
  - Hypotension (aldosterone raises blood pressure)
  - Hypoglycemia (cortisol raises blood sugar)
  - Hyponatremia *with hyperkalemia* (aldosterone conserves Na^+ and excretes K^+ in the kidney, so deficiency causes Na^+ wasting and K^+ retention)
  - Metabolic acidosis (aldosterone conserves bicarbonate in the kidney; deficiency results in bicarbonate wasting through the kidney, a condition called *renal tubular acidosis* or *type 4 RTA*)
  - Hypercalcemia (probably from decreased renal excretion)
- Measurements of serum cortisol are difficult to interpret in different disease states because 90% of circulating cortisol is *protein bound* to corticosteroid-binding globulin. During severe illness, the corticosteroid-binding globulin drops by as much as 50%. Most assays measure total cortisol and so will not be able to measure free (unbound) cortisol, which is the fraction that is biologically available. This severely limits the ability to interpret the results.

Advanced

- ACTH is also (in smaller quantities) produced by the immune system, including T cells, B cells, and macrophages. Fighting off infection usually results in the body mounting an increased metabolic response, so the interplay between adrenal function and the immune system is logical.
- The ACTH test usually involves administration of 250 mcg of ACTH. This dose has been criticized for being far too large (supraphysiologic) to be sensitive. A more appropriate dose of 1 mcg has been suggested, but data to recommend the use of this dose are lacking.
- In severe illness, such as septic shock or acute respiratory distress syndrome (ARDS), ACTH stimulation tests are not recommended for identifying patients who require steroid therapy. Confounding the interpretation of this test is the fact that cortisol is protein bound and the active component is unbound. Most assays for serum cortisol measure both bound and unbound components, and in critical illness protein binding is abnormal, so it is difficult to know what the unbound (active) levels of cortisol are with these results.

FYI

- The adrenal glands sit on top of the kidneys. Originally named the *suprarenal glands*, they were renamed to the *adrenal glands*. Each is composed of a cortex and a medulla. Thus, *adrenocortico* refers to action primarily on the adrenal cortex.
- The zona glomerulosa, zona fasciculata, and zona reticularis are the three zones of the adrenal cortex.
  - Aldosterone is produced in the zona glomerulosa.
  - Cortisol is produced in zona fasciculata.
  - Androgens are produced in the zona reticularis.
- Cortisol and aldosterone are referred to as glucocorticoids and mineralocorticoids, respectively; the *corticoid* part of the name is in reference to the adrenal cortex.
- The adrenal *medulla* produces epinephrine and norepinephrine.
- Former U.S. president John F. Kennedy had chronic adrenal insufficiency (Addison's disease).

Thyroid Replacements

DESCRIPTION
Thyroid replacements compensate for low levels of endogenous thyroid hormone.

PROTOTYPES
- Levothyroxine (T_4)
- Liothyronine (T_3)

MOA (MECHANISM OF ACTION)

- Exogenously administered thyroxine replaces deficient endogenous thyroid hormone, a condition called **hypothyroidism.**
- Thyroid-releasing hormone (TRH) from the hypothalamus stimulates the pituitary to release thyroid-stimulating hormone (TSH), which stimulates the thyroid gland to synthesize and release thyroid hormone. Thyroid hormone has negative feedback loop activity on both TRH and TSH.
- There are three major forms of thyroid hormone: T_4, T_3, and rT_3 (reverse T_3).
  - T_3 **is far more active** than T_4, but T_4 is more abundant.
  - Peripheral (nonthyroid) tissues convert T_4 to T_3.
  - rT_3 is not active.
  - T_4 is the most common type of thyroid replacement. Exogenously administered T_4 is converted (**deiodinated**) to the more active form of T_3.
  - T_4 contains four iodine molecules. T_3 and rT_3 both contain three, but the orientation of the iodine is different in the T_3 compared to rT_3.
- Thyroid hormones bind intracellular nuclear thyroid hormone receptors (THRs) and influence RNA transcription directly. THRs have 10 times the affinity for T_3 that they have for T_4.
- Thyroid hormone influences many systems and processes in the body, including the following:
  - **Metabolic:** energy levels, body temperature, weight, lipids, appetite
  - **Cardiovascular:** heart rate, heart rhythm (normal sinus versus other), blood pressure, fluid distribution (because of hydrostatic pressures)
  - **Skin and hair:** composition, thickness, texture
  - **GI:** motility
  - **Musculoskeletal:** bone growth, tendon reflexes
  - **Hematologic:** erythropoiesis (red blood cell production)
  - **Reproductive:** ovulation and spermatogenesis

PHARMACOKINETICS

- Thyroxine (T_4) is administered daily and has good oral availability.
- It has a long half-life of 7 days, meaning that achievement of steady state (five half-lives) requires about 35 days; dose adjustments based on TSH levels should not be made before steady state is reached.
- In contrast, liothyronine (T_3) has a half-life of 1 day, mandating more frequent administration.
- Thyroid hormone is deiodinized (iodine molecule removed) to inactive forms by the liver. Doses might require adjustment in liver disease.
- T_4 is almost always administered orally. An indication for intravenous administration of T_4 is severe life-threatening hypothyroidism (**myxedema coma**).
- *Hypo*thyroidism decreases clearance of T_3 and T_4, whereas *hyper*thyroidism increases clearance.

- Thyroid hormone contains iodine. Therefore other iodinated agents such as amiodarone or iodinated contrast media can inhibit the **5'-deiodinase** necessary for the conversion of T_4 to T_3. β-Blockers, corticosteroids, and severe illness or starvation can also produce the same effect. This results in more T_4 being converted to the inactive form of rT_3.
- Drugs that induce CYP enzymes can result in increased T_4 metabolism to inactive forms.
- Thyroid hormone is strongly bound to **thyroxine-binding globulin (TBG)**, which contributes to its long half-life. Only the unbound hormone is active. Therefore changes in the TBG level can strongly influence the overall activity level.

INDICATION

- Hypothyroidism from any cause

CONTRAINDICATIONS

- Caution must be exercised in conditions in which tachycardia is dangerous (coronary artery disease, aortic stenosis, mitral stenosis) because of the risk of tachycardia if the dose of thyroid replacement is too high.

SIDE EFFECTS

- Hyperthyroidism-related signs and symptoms
  - Cardiac toxicity is one of the most important components:
    - Tachycardia
    - Atrial fibrillation: One must consider thyroid function as a cause of atrial fibrillation, including endogenous (not drug-related) hyperthyroidism.

IMPORTANT NOTES

- **TSH** is the most commonly used test to monitor hypothyroid states. In primary (thyroid gland dysfunction) hypothyroidism, TSH levels are *elevated* in an attempt to further stimulate the thyroid gland. Secondary hypothyroidism (pituitary gland dysfunction) would result in a *low* TSH.
- Adrenal and thyroid hypofunctioning can coexist. Thyroid hormone replacement **without additional corticosteroids** may precipitate acute adrenal insufficiency in patients with impaired adrenal function. The outcome can be fatal; however, patients are usually *very* sick if both adrenal function and thyroid function are significantly abnormal. This can occur in myxedema coma.
- T_4 is preferred over T_3 administration because T_4 has a longer half-life, enabling daily administration, and has a lower potential for cardiac toxicity.
- Diseases associated with abnormal levels of thyroid hormones include the following:
  - **Grave's disease:** Grave's disease consists of elevated T_4 resulting from antibodies *stimulating* the TSH receptors on the thyroid.
  - **Hashimoto's thyroiditis:** Antibodies against the TSH receptor *destroy* the thyroid gland, eventually resulting in hypothyroidism. Through the destruction process, there

can be episodes of increased release of thyroid hormone, causing episodic *hyper*thyroidism.

▲ **Myxedema:** Myxedema is a severe form of hypothyroidism that can be life-threatening. Adrenal function *must* also be assessed in this condition. Patients can manifest hypoglycemia, hyponatremia, hypothermia, bradycardia, hypotension, congestive heart failure, and coma.

▲ **Cretinism:** Cretinism is a severe hypothyroidism in children.

▲ **Thyrotoxic storm:** Thyrotoxic storm is severe hyperthyroidism. It is treated with antithyroid therapy.

Advanced

■ **Subclinical hypothyroidism** is a condition of **elevated TSH** but with **normal T_3 and T_4** levels. Patients are usually healthy and without symptoms.

■ **Sick euthyroid syndrome** is a condition of **normal TSH** but with **decreased T_3**. It is a term used in patients who are *critically ill,* but whose disease is not a primary thyroid disorder.

■ T_3 therapy is rarely ever required but has a faster onset of action than T_4 because T_4 first needs to be converted to T_3.

Myxedema coma would be the only indication for T_3 administration, and evidence is lacking to support that T_3 is superior to T_4 in myxedema coma. In fact, cardiovascular toxicity (tachycardia and arrhythmias) can result from too high a dose or too fast an onset of action—a reason to consider avoiding intravenous T_3 in critically ill patients.

EVIDENCE
Subclinical Hypothyroidism

■ A meta-analysis in 2007 (12 trials, 350 patients) compared levothyroxine replacement with placebo or no treatment for patients with *subclinical* hypothyroidism. No significant differences were found with respect to symptoms, survival or cardiac function. There was some evidence that thyroid replacement slightly improved lipid levels.

FYI

■ *Subclinical* generally means asymptomatic or having too small an effect to be detected by tests.

■ Thyroid hormone with all the iodine molecules removed (thus inactive) is called *thyronine.*

Antithyroids

DESCRIPTION
Antithyroids are used to treat hyperthyroidism.

PROTOTYPE AND COMMON DRUGS
Thioamides
■ Prototype: propylthiouracil (PTU)
■ Others: meth**imazole**, carb**imazole**

Ablative Agents
■ Prototype: radioactive iodine (^{131}I)

MOA (MECHANISM OF ACTION)
■ Synthesis of thyroid hormone requires the following steps:
▲ Uptake of iodide into the thyroid
▲ Through the action of **thyroid peroxidase**, the following occurs:
• Conversion of the ion *iodide* (I^-) to an oxidized form *iodine* (I)
• Iodination (addition of iodine) of the tyrosine groups of **thyroglobulin (Tg)**: addition of one iodine makes **monoiodotyrosine (MIT)**; addition of two iodines makes **diiodotyrosine (DIT)**. Coupling two DITs makes T_4 (a total of four iodines). Coupling an MIT with a DIT makes T_3 (a total of three iodines).
▲ Cleavage of T_3 or T_4 from thyroglobulin occurs via proteases in the lysosome.
▲ T_3 or T_4 is then released from the thyroid gland.

▲ Further deiodination (removal of iodine) of T_4 to T_3. This step occurs outside of the thyroid (*peripheral conversion*) and generates 80% of the total T_3.
■ A simplified way to think about synthesis is that thyroid hormone is really like two tyrosine amino acids combined together with either three or four iodine molecules. Thyroglobulin is the tyrosine amino acid supplier (Figure 14-19).
■ **Thioamides** act primarily by blocking the synthesis of thyroid hormone. They do the following:
▲ Inhibit the **thyroid peroxidase** catalyzed reactions
• Block iodine oxidation (I^- to I)
• Block coupling of the iodinated tyrosines
• Inhibit the peripheral deiodination of T_3 and T_4
▲ *Do not* block uptake of iodide by the gland
▲ Require about **3 to 4 weeks** to exert their effects because of the thyroid precursors of thyroid synthesis that are stored inside the thyroid gland
■ **Radioactive iodine** (^{131}I) destroys the thyroid gland via radiation.
▲ ^{131}I has a half-life of 8 days and emits primarily β-radiation, which penetrates to a depth of 2 mm.
▲ ^{131}I preferentially destroys the thyroid gland because of the avid uptake of I by the thyroid.

PHARMACOKINETICS
■ Antithyroids have good oral availability; dose adjustments are not required in renal or liver disease.

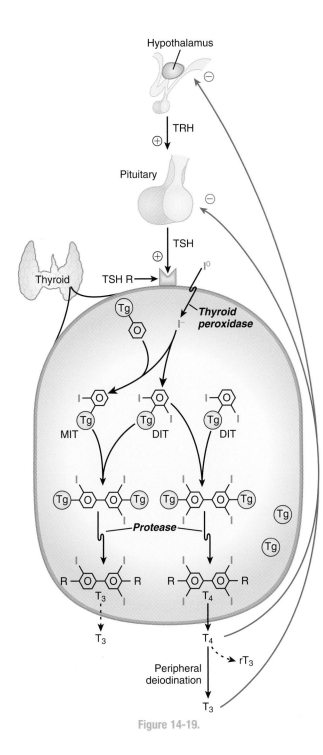

Figure 14-19.

INDICATIONS

- Thioamides:
  - ▲ Hyperthyroidism
- [131]I
  - ▲ Hyperthyroidism
  - ▲ Thyroid cancer

CONTRAINDICATIONS

- Thioamides penetrate the placental barrier and should be used with caution in pregnancy. If required, the lowest dose should be used.

- [131]I is:
  - ▲ *Absolutely* contraindicated in pregnancy because it can ablate the fetal thyroid gland. Furthermore, pregnancy must be avoided for 6 months following administration of [131]I.
  - ▲ Relatively contraindicated in children. There is a small risk of cancer.

SIDE EFFECTS
Thioamides

- The most common side effects (in 6% to 10% of patients) are **skin rash**, fever, and arthralgia (sore joints).

Serious, Rare Side Effects

- **Agranulocytosis:** Patients can develop a serious reduction in the granulocyte count (neutrophil count), which severely impairs the immune system and results in high risk for serious life-threatening infections. Discontinuing the drug results in restoration of the blood count. A blood count should be performed before the drugs are started, and if the patient develops a fever, cough, sore throat, or urinary tract infection or other symptom that might be suggestive of infection, then a blood count must be repeated. The thioamides must be stopped if the granulocyte count is low.
- **Hepatotoxicity:** A small percent (0.2%) of patients develop liver damage, which is an allergic-type response and can result in liver failure, necessity for transplant, or death.
- **Vasculitis:** Vasculitis, an autoimmune process that results in inflammation of blood vessels, is very rare.
- If side effects occur with one thioamide, the probability of side effects occurring with another thioamide is about 50%; so if a severe reaction occurs, then all thioamides are absolutely contraindicated thereafter.

[131]I

- **Hypothyroidism:** Almost all patients require lifelong thyroid replacement after radioactive ablation.
- **Sialadenitis:** Inflammation of the salivary glands occurs because of uptake of [131]I. Salivary damage can result in xerostomia (dry mouth), altered taste, increased dental caries, and pain.
- **Cancer:** Although very small, a risk of cancer arises from the radiation from the [131]I.

IMPORTANT NOTES

- β-Blocker therapy is an important part of hyperthyroidism treatment. However, it treats the *downstream effects* (signs and symptoms) of hyperthyroidism but does not reduce thyroid production or secretion. β-Blocker therapy works within hours of the start of treatment and so is an important component of therapy, because antithyroid medication requires at least 3 to 4 weeks before lowering thyroid hormone levels.
- TSH levels should be tested on a monthly basis and then when symptoms are under control, every 1 to 3 months thereafter.
- Hyperthyroid remission can occur, so treatment with thioamides can be used without thyroid ablation or

thyroidectomy. Choice of therapy is not always straightforward and must balance the risks and benefits of the three different options (surgery, ^{131}I ablation, and suppressive therapy). If a patient could be predicted to go into remission, then suppressive therapy might be the best option; however, predicting remission is difficult.

■ ^{131}I has been suggested to be associated with increased cancer formation (nonthyroid cancers). The evidence is still under debate.

Advanced

■ There are generally two different approaches to administering thioamides:
  ▲ Dose titration: Adjust the dose to effect.
  ▲ Block and replace: Give a high dose, and then give thyroid replacement.
■ Potassium perchlorate is a competitive inhibitor of **iodide transport** and is used only in amiodarone-induced hyperthyroidism.

FYI

■ Nomenclature:
  ▲ Antithyroid (*-imazoles*) should not be confused with *-azoles* (such as fluconazole), which are antifungal agents.
  ▲ Thioamides, as the name suggests, contain a sulfur (thio) and an amide (S = C-NH).
■ Carbimazole is converted to methimazole in the body.
■ Tyrosine is also the precursor for the synthesis of dopamine, norepinephrine, and epinephrine (see discussions of inotropes and pressors in Chapter 11).
■ After ^{131}I treatment, a patient can set off airport radiation alarms for a few months.
■ ^{131}I was released after the Chernobyl accident and is also released after nuclear bomb testing.

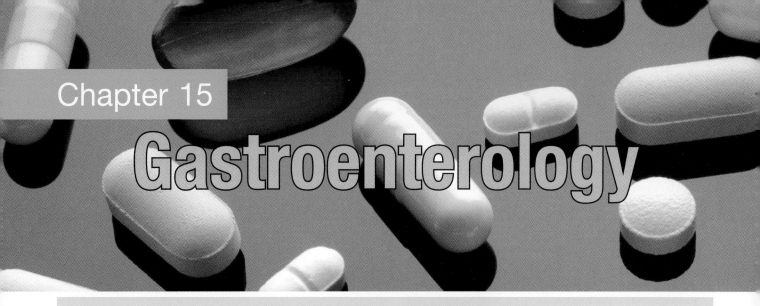

Chapter 15

Gastroenterology

Antacids: Buffers

DESCRIPTION
These are agents that act as buffers in the stomach, neutralizing acid through a simple chemical reaction.

PROTOTYPES
Calcium-Containing Agents
- Prototype: calcium carbonate ($CaCO_3$)

Aluminum-Containing Agents
- Prototype: aluminum hydroxide ($AlOH_3$)

Magnesium-Containing Agents
- Prototype: magnesium hydroxide ($MgOH_2$)

MOA (MECHANISM OF ACTION)
- All buffers act locally in the stomach by reacting with H^+ to increase pH. All buffers are bases; therefore they reduce acidity by reacting with acid in the stomach to form a neutral solution:

$$Acid + Base \rightarrow Neutral$$

PHARMACOKINETICS
- Calcium, magnesium, and aluminum are typically poorly absorbed. However, patients with impaired renal function can have accumulation of these cations.
- Divalent and trivalent cations such as Ca^{2+}, Mg^{2+}, and Al^{3+} may chelate other drugs, interfering with their absorption. Where possible, administration of antacids should be separated from administration of other drugs that require systemic absorption, ideally by 2 hours.
- Antacids administered in suspension may have greater acid-neutralizing efficacy than those administered as tablets or powders.

INDICATIONS
- Hyperacidity, including reflux disease
- Indigestion

CONTRAINDICATIONS
- None of major significance

SIDE EFFECTS
Mg^{2+}-Containing Buffers
- **Diarrhea:** Mg^{2+} salt exerts an osmotic effect on the gut.

Ca^{2+}-Containing Buffers
- **Hypercalcemia (at high doses):** These agents may lead to formation of calculi (milk alkali syndrome). Calculi are solid formations, typically consisting of minerals, which precipitate in organs such as the kidney and obstruct ducts.
- **Bloating, flatulence, belching, nausea:** These effects are caused by the liberation of CO_2 from carbonate-containing antacids.
- **Constipation**

Al^{3+}-Containing Buffers
- **Hypophosphatemia:** Al^{3+} can bind phosphate in the gut, inhibiting its absorption.
- **Constipation**

IMPORTANT NOTES
- Although these agents act locally in the stomach, they are not devoid of systemic adverse effects, particularly at higher doses or with chronic use.
- As with other antacids, buffers may reduce pH enough to interfere with absorption of drugs that require a low pH for absorption.
- Al^{3+} and Mg^{2+} are often combined into one antacid formulation because of their complementary onset of action (Mg^{2+} is rapid, Al^{3+} is slow reacting) and side effects (Mg^{2+} causes diarrhea, Al^{3+} constipation).
- **Simethicone** is a surfactant added to antacids to decrease bloating. A surfactant is a substance that reduces surface tension, in this case reducing large bubbles into smaller

ones. The foaming action of simethicone may also alleviate gastroesophageal reflux.

- Sodium bicarbonate, one of the first antacids, is still used in some regions. This formulation has fallen out of favor because of concerns over systemic alkalosis and the impact of sodium on cardiovascular health.
- **Milk alkali syndrome** is a rare disorder caused by ingestion of large amounts of calcium, resulting in hypercalcemia and alkalosis.

FYI

- Although the agents in this class have traditionally been referred to as *antacids*, the term *antacid* has much wider use and applies to each of the many classes of drugs that reduce acid secretion. The more appropriate term for the agents in this class is *buffer*, as this describes their mechanism and distinguishes them from other classes.

H₂ Antagonists

DESCRIPTION

H₂ antagonists comprise a group of agents that reduce acid secretion in the stomach.

PROTOTYPE AND COMMON DRUGS

- Prototype: rani**tidine**
- Others: cime**tidine**, famo**tidine**, niza**tidine**

MOA (MECHANISM OF ACTION)

- The amount of **gastric acid** is largely determined by the secretion of protons (H⁺) by **parietal cells** in the stomach, as well as volume of stomach contents.
- In the parietal cell, the **proton pump**, H⁺/K⁺ ATPase, creates an ion gradient by pumping H⁺ into the lumen of the stomach. The pump is key to creating the acidic environment of the stomach (pH <1) while maintaining a relatively normal intracellular pH (approximately 7.3).
- The **H₂ receptor** on parietal cells mediates both the **basal and meal-stimulated** release of acid. The binding of histamine to the H₂ receptor stimulates the proton (H⁺/K⁺ ATPase) pump via the second messenger cyclic adenosine monophosphate (cAMP) (Figure 15-1).
- H₂ antagonists competitively block the interaction of histamine with H₂ receptors, thus reducing stimulation of the proton pump through this receptor.
- **Nocturnal** acid secretion depends largely on histamine; thus the H₂ antagonists have a greater impact on nocturnal acid secretion than meal-stimulated acid secretion, which is stimulated by gastrin and acetylcholine (ACh), in addition to histamine.
- An additional mechanism, by which H₂ antagonists are also able to attenuate the **gastrin and ACh-stimulated** release of gastric acid, has been proposed by some sources. ACh, by binding to muscarinic (M3) receptors, and gastrin, by binding to cholecystokinin (CCK2) receptors, also stimulate the proton pump.
- It is not clear how H₂ antagonism attenuates the ability of gastrin and ACh to stimulate activity of the proton pump, but this would most likely be mediated through second messengers.

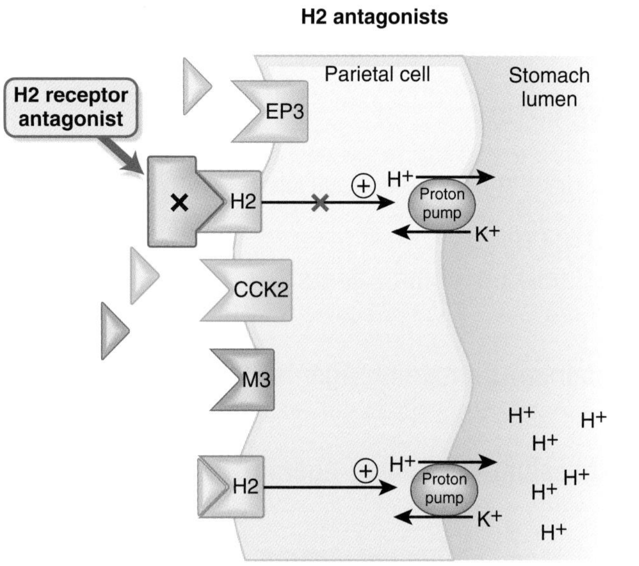

Figure 15-1.

PHARMACOKINETICS

- All the H₂ antagonists are available in oral formulations. Intravenous and intramuscular formulations of cimetidine, ranitidine, and famotidine are also available.
- Oral formulations are all rapidly absorbed, achieving peak plasma concentrations in 1 to 3 hours.
- All of the H₂ antagonists are excreted by the kidneys, both by filtration and by renal tubular secretion; hence it may be necessary to adjust the dose of these agents in patients with impaired renal function.

INDICATIONS

- Gastroesophageal reflux disease (GERD)
- Peptic ulcer disease (with or without bleeding)
- Dyspepsia
- Gastritis
- Gastric protection in patients on life support

CONTRAINDICATIONS

- None of major significance

SIDE EFFECTS
- **Generally well tolerated**
- **Common:** Diarrhea, headache, drowsiness, fatigue, muscle pain, and constipation may occur.
- **Rare central nervous system (CNS) side effects:** Confusion, delirium, hallucinations, slurred speech, and headache can occur and are thought to be caused by antagonism of H_2 receptors in the CNS. These CNS effects are more likely to occur with intravenous administration or in the elderly.
- **Thrombocytopenia (rare):** The mechanism has not been established, but theories include bone marrow suppression due to inhibition of DNA synthesis, and the development of platelet antibodies against H_2 antagonists.

Cimetidine Only
- **Gynecomastia** (breast development in men) and **galactorrhea** (lactation not associated with childbirth): Cimetidine inhibits binding of testosterone to the androgen receptor, and as a CYP450 inhibitor, it inhibits the hydroxylation of estradiol.

IMPORTANT NOTES
- The H_2 antagonists are considered to be less effective than the more expensive proton pump inhibitors (PPIs). However, it is important to note that the H_2 antagonists are able to reduce daily acid secretion by about 60% to 70%.
- Tolerance can develop to the acid-suppressant effects of the H_2 antagonists, occurring as early as 3 days after initiation of therapy. One theory is that secondary hypergastrinemia may stimulate histamine release from enterochromaffin-like cells. Hypergastrinemia is an elevation in gastrin levels in the blood in response to low pH in the stomach. Gastrin stimulates the proton pump to release acid into the stomach.
- Cimetidine may also enhance cell-mediated immunity when administered in high doses. This has lead to its use in treating infections such as candidiasis and herpesvirus in immunocompromised patients, as well as warts.

Advanced
Drug Interactions
- Cimetidine inhibits a variety of CYP450 enzymes; thus drug interactions are common with this agent.

EVIDENCE
Versus Other Agents for Treatment of GERD
- A 2006 Cochrane review (31 studies, N = 9457 patients) found that PPIs were more efficacious for achieving heartburn remission than H_2-receptor antagonists (seven trials, relative risk [RR] 0.66) and prokinetics (two trials, RR 0.53).

Versus Other Agents for *Endoscopy Negative Reflux Disease*
- The same 2006 Cochrane review found that PPIs were more efficacious at achieving heartburn remission compared with H_2 antagonists (three trials, RR 0.78) and compared with prokinetics (one trial, RR 0.72). Endoscopy-negative reflux disease is simply GERD without any evidence of histologic changes on endoscopic examination.

Versus Proton Pump Inhibitors for Acute Bleeding from Peptic Ulcer
- A 2006 Cochrane review (24 studies, N = 4373 patients) found no statistically significant difference between PPIs and H_2 antagonists with regard to the *incidence of surgery* required to treat peptic ulcer bleeding.

Versus Other Agents for Nonulcer Dyspepsia
- A 2006 Cochrane review (73 trials) examined the efficacy of various agents in nonulcer dyspepsia. H_2-receptor antagonists (12 trials, N = 2183 participants) improved dyspepsia in more patients than placebo (54% versus 40%), and PPIs also demonstrated improvement versus placebo (34% versus 25%).

FYI
- Because of their relatively innocuous side effect profile, the H_2 antagonists, particularly ranitidine and famotidine, are available over the counter in most jurisdictions. Because of its propensity for drug interactions, cimetidine is not available over the counter in some jurisdictions.

Proton Pump Inhibitors (PPIs)

DESCRIPTION
PPIs comprise a class of agents that reduce acid secretion by inhibiting the acid (proton)–secreting pump in the stomach. Accordingly, they are also often referred to as antisecretory agents.

PROTOTYPE AND COMMON DRUGS
- Prototype: ome**prazole**
- Others: panto**prazole**, lanso**prazole**, esome**prazole**, rabe**prazole**

MOA (MECHANISM OF ACTION)

■ The amount of **gastric acid** is largely determined by the secretion of protons (H^+) by **parietal cells** in the stomach, as well as the volume of stomach contents.

■ In the parietal cell, the **proton pump**, H^+/K^+ ATPase, creates an ion gradient by pumping H^+ into the lumen of the stomach. The pump is key to creating the acidic environment of the stomach (pH <1) while maintaining a relatively normal intracellular pH (approximately 7.3) (Figure 15-2).

Proton pump inhibitors (PPI)

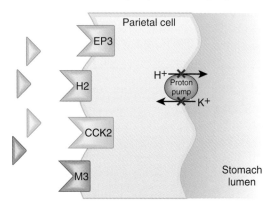

Figure 15-2.

■ PPIs enter the parietal cell and bind to the proton pump, resulting in an irreversible inactivation of the pump. This dramatically reduces the amount of H^+ that is pumped into the lumen of the stomach, and because the binding is irreversible, the effects of PPIs persist until new pumps are synthesized. The reduction in gastric acid secretion can thus persist up to 48 hours after a single dose.

■ The PPIs tend to be particularly adept at reducing acid secretion because the proton pump is the final and key step in secreting acid (H^+) into the lumen of the stomach. All other agents that suppress acid secretion work by reducing gastric H^+ concentration act upstream of the proton pump, rather than directly at the proton pump.

■ The release of gastrin is modulated by intragastric acid levels, such that higher acidity suppresses gastrin release. Gastrin stimulates ECL cell hyperplasia, which may predispose patients to developing malignancies.

PHARMACOKINETICS

■ Although they act on cells in the stomach, PPIs must be absorbed into the systemic circulation from the small intestine. It is from the systemic circulation that they reach the parietal cells of the stomach.

■ This is important because the PPIs (ironically) tend to be unstable in an acidic environment. Hence all PPIs have some form of enteric coating, to protect them until they reach the small intestine and can be absorbed. Disruption of this enteric coating (e.g., by splitting the tablet) will likely reduce the bioavailability of the PPI.

■ All PPIs are prodrugs that are activated in the acidic environment of the parietal cell acid canaliculi. Food intake stimulates acid secretion. Oral PPIs should be taken approximately 30 to 60 minutes before meals. This allows enough time for the PPI to be absorbed into the systemic circulation and to be distributed to the parietal cells. This will also ensure that the PPIs are active at the same time as maximal activation of the proton pumps.

■ All PPIs are cleared primarily by hepatic metabolism.

INDICATIONS

■ Gastric and duodenal ulcers
  ▲ Nonsteroidal antiinflammatory drug (NSAID)-induced ulcers
  ▲ Non–NSAID-induced ulcers
  ▲ *Helicobacter pylori* eradication
■ GERD
■ Upper gastrointestinal (GI) bleeding
■ Pathologic hypersecretory conditions:
  ▲ Zollinger-Ellison syndrome—a rare syndrome characterized by gastric hypersecretion and hyperacidity as well as persistent peptic ulcers

CONTRAINDICATIONS

■ None of major significance

SIDE EFFECTS

■ Generally well tolerated

Common

■ **GI**: nausea, abdominal pain, constipation, diarrhea, flatulence

Less Common

■ **Hypergastrinemia**: Gastrin levels become elevated because of the body's response to chronic gastric acid suppression. This may lead to rebound hypersecretion of gastric acid if the PPI is stopped. There is also concern over the chronic effects of hypergastrinemia, including development of gastric tumors.

IMPORTANT NOTES

■ Of all agents used to treat hyperacidity, PPIs are the most effective at reducing daily acid secretion, capable of reducing acid (basal and stimulated) by 80% to 95%. H_2 antagonists are able to achieve a 60% to 70% reduction in acid.

■ PPIs inhibit only active proton pumps. Not all proton pumps are active at the same time; therefore, although pumps are irreversibly inhibited once bound by the PPI, it takes a few days to achieve the inhibition of proton pumps seen at steady state.

■ PPIs are often prescribed in combination with other GI drugs and antibiotics for eradication of *H. pylori*. By increasing intragastric pH, PPIs appear to enhance the antimicrobial activity of these agents. PPIs may also have a minor antimicrobial effect. Some of the more common combinations are listed in Table 15-1.

TABLE 15-1. Combination Therapy for *H. pylori* Eradication

Proton Pump Inhibitors	Other Agents	
Lansoprazole	Clarithromycin	Amoxicillin
Omeprazole	Clarithromycin	Metronidazole
Pantoprazole		Metronidazole
Rabeprazole	Bismuth subsalicylate	Tetracycline

Advanced
Drug Interactions
■ All PPIs are metabolized by CYP450 enzymes (particularly CYP2C19 and CYP3A4). However, only omeprazole is able to act as both an inhibitor (2C19—phenytoin) and inducer (1A2—antipsychotics) of CYP450 enzymes.

■ Some drugs require an acidic environment for their proper dissolution and absorption. By increasing gastric pH, the PPIs may therefore interfere with the absorption of vitamin B_{12}, ampicillin, and ketoconazole, among others.

Pharmacogenomics
■ Asians are more likely to have the CYP2C19 genotype that correlates with slow metabolism of the PPIs, and this may lead to increased efficacy and/or toxicity in this population.

EVIDENCE
Versus Other Agents for Treatment of Gastroesophageal Reflux Disease
■ A 2006 Cochrane review (31 studies, N = 9457 patients) found that PPIs were more efficacious for achieving heart- burn remission than H_2-receptor antagonists (seven trials, RR 0.66) and prokinetics (two trials, RR 0.53).

Versus Other Agents for Endoscopy Negative Reflux Disease
■ The same 2006 Cochrane review found that PPIs were more efficacious at achieving heartburn remission compared with H_2 antagonists (three trials, RR 0.78) and compared with prokinetics (one trial, RR 0.72). Endoscopy-negative reflux disease is simply GERD without any evidence of histologic changes on endoscopic examination.

Versus H_2 Antagonists for Acute Bleeding from Peptic Ulcer
■ A 2006 Cochrane review (24 studies, N = 4373 patients) found no difference in mortality between PPIs and controls but did find that PPIs reduced rebleeding (incidence of 10.6% for PPI versus 17.3% control) and surgery (6.1% versus 9.3%, respectively) versus control. No benefit was seen for PPIs versus H_2 antagonists with regard to surgery.

FYI
■ Omeprazole is a racemic mixture of *R*- and *S*- isomers, and esomeprazole is the *S*- isomer of omeprazole (*S*-omepra- zole). Because the *S*- isomer is eliminated more slowly than the *R*-isomer, esomeprazole has a longer half-life than omeprazole.

Gastrointestinal Cytoprotectants

DESCRIPTION
Gastrointestinal cytoprotectants are a heterogeneous group of agents that protect cells in the lining of the stomach.

PROTOTYPES AND COMMON DRUGS
■ **Prostaglandin analogue**: misoprostol (prostaglandin E_1 [PGE_1])
■ **Coating agents**: sucralfate, bismuth

MOA (MECHANISM OF ACTION)
Prostaglandin Analogue
■ Protection of the mucosal lining of the stomach can be achieved in two ways: by increasing gastric pH or by enhancing the mucosal barrier that protects the stomach.

■ The prostaglandin E receptor 3 (EP3) receptors are found on parietal cells of the stomach and, when stimulated, have an inhibitory effect on the proton pump. The proton pump stimulates the release of hydrogen ions (acid) into the lumen of the stomach.

■ Endogenous PGE_2 acts as an agonist at EP3 receptors on parietal cells and **reduces** activity of the proton pump, thereby reducing secretion of gastric acid (Figure 15-3).

■ PGE_2 also contributes to maintenance of the mucosal barrier, stimulating secretion of mucin and bicarbonate and enhancing mucosal blood flow. Mucin is a thick substance that has a protective effect on the lining of the stomach. Bicarbonate helps to raise the pH of the stomach, particu- larly in the area close to the mucosal lining.

■ PGE_2 is synthesized through the cyclooxygenase (COX) pathway, largely through the COX-1 enzyme.

■ NSAIDs work by inhibiting COX enzymes, thus reducing the amount of PGE_2 and subsequently reducing the amount of protective mucus in the stomach. Nonselective (i.e., COX-1 and COX-2) inhibitors are thus implicated in damage to the gastric mucosa.

■ Therefore a PGE_1 analogue such as misoprostol is typically given as an adjunct in patients undergoing NSAID therapy,

GI cytoprotectants

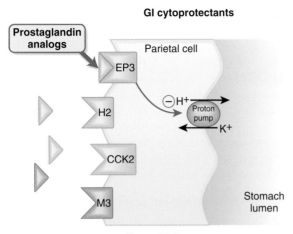

Figure 15-3.

for the purpose of substituting for the PGE lost with NSAID use (Figure 15-4).

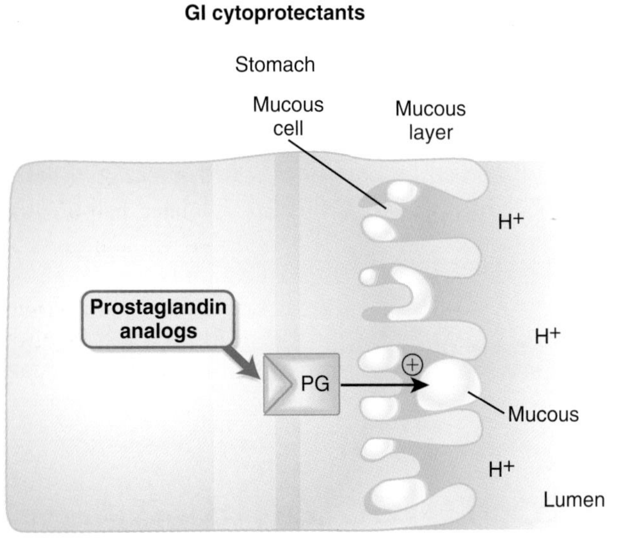

GI cytoprotectants

Figure 15-4.

Sucralfate

- Sucralfate is a complex of sucrose and aluminum hydroxide that forms a viscous paste in aqueous acidic media. This negatively charged paste binds to positively charged proteins in the ulcer, forming a direct protective barrier for up to 6 hours.
- Sucralfate works by multiple mechanisms, both direct and indirect, to enhance the amount of mucus to protect cells lining the stomach.
- Indirectly, sucralfate exerts a mucoprotective effect by stimulating PG synthesis of mucus and secretion of bicarbonate. In addition, sucralfate may stimulate growth factors that promote mucosal repair, although this mechanism has not been confirmed.

Bismuth Salts

- Bismuth salts work by forming a protective barrier on the ulcer and enhancing secretion of PGs, mucus, and bicarbonate.

- They also inhibit the growth of *H. pylori* and prevent adherence of *H. pylori* to gastric mucosa.

PHARMACOKINETICS

- Misoprostol has a short half-life and thus must be administered frequently (3 or 4 times daily).
- Sucralfate primarily acts locally in the GI tract, is only minimally absorbed, and is excreted mainly in the feces. It also must be administered 4 times daily. Sucralfate should be administered 1 hour before meals, as it is activated by acid.
- Every tablet of sucralfate contains aluminum. Although only a very small proportion of aluminum is absorbed, because elimination relies on urinary excretion, caution should be exercised in those with chronic renal failure, as an accumulation of aluminum may occur. This is particularly important if these patients are also receiving aluminum in another form, such as an antacid.

INDICATIONS
Prostaglandins
(See also ophthalmic prostaglandins and vasodilator prostaglandins in Chapters 22 and 24, respectively, for non-GI indications.)

- Prevention of NSAID-induced ulcers

Sucralfate
- Treatment of duodenal and gastric ulcers
- Prevention of ulcer recurrence

Bismuth
- Adjunctive therapy in *H. pylori* eradication
- Acute diarrhea
- Heartburn

CONTRAINDICATIONS
Misoprostol
- **Pregnancy:** Misoprostol stimulates uterine contractions and could induce premature labor.

Bismuth Subsalicylate
- Similar to acetylsalicylic acid (ASA), bismuth subsalicylate may be associated with a higher risk of **Reye's syndrome** in children; therefore it should be avoided in children or teenagers with viral infections such as influenza or chickenpox. Reye's syndrome is an often fatal encephalopathy in children that has been associated with the use of ASA during viral infection.

SIDE EFFECTS
Misoprostol
- **Diarrhea, abdominal cramping:** Diarrhea is the most common side effect and can be very severe. PGs stimulate contractions of smooth muscle in the GI tract. Patients with inflammatory bowel disease may be at increased risk for developing severe diarrhea.
- **Uterine contractions:** PGs stimulate uterine contractions.

Sucralfate

- Sucralfate has minimal systemic effects because it is not absorbed to an appreciable extent.
- **Constipation** occurs rarely, because of the aluminum. It is not clear why aluminum causes constipation.

Bismuth

- **Black tarry stools**: Bismuth causes discoloration of the stool, which may mask the appearance of or be mistaken for blood in stool. Bismuth salts react with hydrogen sulfide to form bismuth sulfide, which turns stool black.
- **Discoloration of tongue**: Bismuth can cause a harmless blackening of tongue.
- **Constipation** may occur.
- **Tinnitus**: Ringing of the ears may occur at high doses because of the salicylate content.

IMPORTANT NOTES

- The acid-suppressant effects of misoprostol are dose related. An oral dose of 100 to 200 mcg inhibits basal acid secretion by up to 95% and meal-stimulated acid secretion by up to 85%.
- Misoprostol is marketed in a fixed-dose combination with diclofenac.
- Because of the high risk of diarrhea, it is recommended that misoprostol be administered with food to mitigate this side effect.
- Bismuth subsalicylate contains **salicylic acid**, with a dose of 30 mL having approximately the same salicylate content as a 325-mg ASA tablet. Thus people who have an allergy or intolerance to ASA must avoid bismuth subsalicylate.

Advanced

- Sucralfate may reduce absorption of other drugs, binding them in the GI tract. Because of these and other unexplained interactions, it is recommended that the administration of sucralfate be separated from that of other orally administered agents.
- Sucralfate requires an acidic environment to be active; therefore agents that reduce gastric acidity will reduce its efficacy. Antacids should not be taken within 30 minutes of sucralfate.

EVIDENCE
Prevention of NSAID-Induced Upper GI Toxicity

- A 2002 Cochrane review (40 studies) compared interventions (PG analogues, H_2-antagonists, PPIs) for prevention of NSAID-induced upper GI toxicity. The review found that although all classes prevented NSAID-related gastric and duodenal ulcers, only misoprostol reduced the risk of ulcer *complications* such as perforation, hemorrhage, and obstruction.
- The authors also concluded that misoprostol is associated with significant adverse effects, particularly at higher doses.

FYI

- Misoprostol is used off-label in many jurisdictions for induction of uterine contractions in abortion and has therefore become a controversial drug.
- Colloidal bismuth subcitrate is a commonly used bismuth compound in the rest of the world, but not in North America.

Prokinetics: Dopamine Antagonists

DESCRIPTION

These are dopamine antagonists that are used to enhance gastric motility.

PROTOTYPE AND COMMON DRUGS

- Prototype: metoclopramide
- Others: domperidone

MOA (MECHANISM OF ACTION)

- Dopamine has an inhibitory effect on GI motility, mediated by the inhibitory effect of D2 receptors on ACh release. These natural inhibitory effects of dopamine include reduction of lower esophageal sphincter tone.
- Therefore D2 antagonists **increase lower esophageal sphincter tone**, and **stimulate contractions** of the stomach and small intestine. The effects of metoclopramide and domperidone are largely confined to the upper GI tract, with minimal effect on the colon (Figure 15-5).

- The increase in lower esophageal sphincter tone is useful in reflux disorders such as GERD because it reduces the volume of gastric acid that enters the esophagus.
- The D2 antagonists also act as **antinauseants** through central inhibition of the vomiting center (chemoreceptor trigger zone).
- Although they share D2 antagonism as a mechanism, the prokinetic actions of metoclopramide are very complex compared with those of domperidone. Metoclopramide also has the following actions:
  - ▲ It acts as an agonist at serotonin-4 (5-HT4) receptors.
  - ▲ It acts as an antagonist at muscarinic receptors and central 5-HT$_3$ receptors.
  - ▲ It may also sensitize muscarinic receptors on smooth muscle.
- It is not clear what the relative contributions of these other receptors are to the actions of metoclopramide.

Prokinetics: Dopamine antagonists

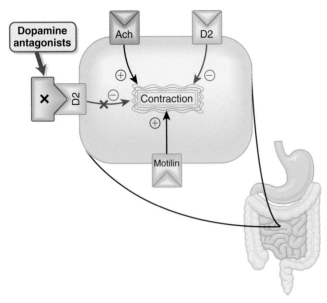

Figure 15-5.

■ Conversely, domperidone is almost exclusively a D2 antagonist.

PHARMACOKINETICS

■ Metoclopramide is rapidly absorbed, undergoes hepatic metabolism, and is excreted mainly in the urine.
■ Domperidone is also rapidly absorbed (peak plasma levels in <30 minutes) but has low oral bioavailability because of an extensive first-pass effect.
■ Although the bioavailability of domperidone is increased with food, food also increases the time to peak plasma concentration. It is recommended that domperidone be taken 15 to 30 minutes before eating.

INDICATIONS

■ Disorders of GI motility:
  ▲ Gastroparesis
  ▲ Nausea, vomiting
■ GERD
■ Diagnostic procedures (adjunct)
■ Facilitation of intubation of the small bowel
■ Contrast radiography of GI Tract
■ Critically ill patients who do not tolerate enteral feeding

CONTRAINDICATIONS

■ Avoid using these prokinetics in situations in which stimulation of GI motility may be harmful, such as in patients with obstruction or perforation.

SIDE EFFECTS
All

■ **Hyperprolactinemia:** DA inhibits prolactin release, so DA antagonism can lead to increased prolactin and the following:
  ▲ **Galactorrhea:** spontaneous flow of milk from the nipple not associated with nursing a baby

▲ **Gynecomastia:** development of breasts in males
▲ **Dysmenorrhea:** painful menstruation

Metoclopramide

■ **Extrapyramidal:** Extrapyramidal effects are analogous to the side effects seen with the antipsychotics that are DA antagonists:
  ▲ **Abnormal muscle tone (acute) and Parkinson-like symptoms (after a few weeks):** Both are reversible and can also be managed with anticholinergics. DA plays an important role in normal movement, so blocking its effects will lead to disordered movement.
  ▲ **Tardive dyskinesia:** These are abnormal, uncontrolled movements, particularly of the face (lips, tongue). They are seen with chronic therapy (months to years) and may not be reversible. Again, these are believed to be caused by inhibiting the effects of DA on normal movement. In this case, blockade of DA receptors may lead to enhanced sensitivity of these receptors, causing uncontrolled movement.
■ **Other CNS effects: Drowsiness, restlessness, insomnia, anxiety, and agitation** may be more common in the elderly. The mechanism has not been established.
■ **Rare:** Methemoglobinemia may occur in premature and full-term neonates. Methemoglobinemia is a condition in which the hemoglobin in blood is not able to carry oxygen.

IMPORTANT NOTES

■ Domperidone does not cross the blood-brain barrier as readily as metoclopramide; therefore it lacks the extrapyramidal side effects associated with metoclopramide. Domperidone still does exert effects on areas that lie outside the blood-brain barrier, including the chemoreceptor trigger zone (nausea, vomiting). Hence domperidone maintains antinauseant effects.
■ The prokinetic activity of domperidone is considered to be relatively weak compared with that of metoclopramide.
■ Children and young adults may be more susceptible to extrapyramidal side effects associated with metoclopramide.

Advanced
Drug Interactions

■ Domperidone is extensively metabolized, primarily by CYP3A4 enzymes.
■ Animal studies suggest that P-glycoprotein transporters may be responsible for the low penetration of domperidone into the CNS.
■ Because of its prokinetic effect and site of action, metoclopramide may decrease the extent of absorption of drugs from the stomach while accelerating absorption from the small intestine. The clinical implications of these interactions are unknown.

Toxicology

■ Metoclopramide is toxic in overdose, oxidizing hemoglobin to methemoglobin. Signs and symptoms of toxicity include cyanosis, nausea, vomiting, vertigo, tachycardia, tachypnea, convulsions, coma, and death. The antidote is methylene blue.

EVIDENCE
Nasoenteral Tube Migration
- A 2002 Cochrane review (four studies, N = 204 patients), updated in 2008, examined the use of intravenous metoclopramide on transpyloric passage of a nasoenteral tube compared with placebo or no intervention. The four included studies were small and did not find a statistically significant improvement in the enhancement of migration of nasoenteral tubes with metoclopramide.

FYI
- Structurally, domperidone is classified as a butyrophenone. This is the same chemical class as haloperidol, a DA antagonist with CNS effects, primarily used in the treatment of schizophrenia.
- Nasoenteral tubes are also known as **small bowel feeding tubes.** Similar tubes that go into the stomach (instead of the small bowel) are commonly referred to as **nasogastric tubes,** or NG tubes. If the same tube is inserted via the mouth, it is called an **orogastric** or OG tube.

Antidiarrheals

DESCRIPTION

Antidiarrheal agents are used to treat diarrhea, either by reducing GI motility or by providing bulk to stool.

PROTOTYPES AND COMMON DRUGS
Opiates
- Prototype: loperamide
- Others: diphenoxylate, difenoxin

Bulk or Hygroscopic ("Water-Attracting") Agents
- Prototype: kaolin/pectin
- Others: attapulgite, bismuth

MOA (MECHANISM OF ACTION)
Opiates
- The bowel contains both μ and δ opioid receptors. The δ receptors mediate intestinal secretion, the μ receptors mediate peristalsis, and both types of receptors play a role in intestinal absorption (Figure 15-6).
- Loperamide and diphenoxylate are piperidines, structurally related to opiates such as meperidine. They are μ agonists, although they have less propensity for eliciting the euphoric effect typically seen with opiate analgesics because of limited CNS penetration.
- μ Agonists reduce or completely abolish peristalsis in the colon, significantly delaying passage of feces through the bowel. The delayed transit through the bowel also increases the opportunity for increased absorption of fluid from the feces, producing a drying effect on the stool that further slows its progress through the bowel.
- In addition, anal sphincter tone is also enhanced, as is the reflex relaxation that normally occurs in response to rectal distension.

Bulk-Forming Agents
- Although bulk-forming agents are used to treat constipation, they have also been successfully used to treat mild

Antidiarrheals

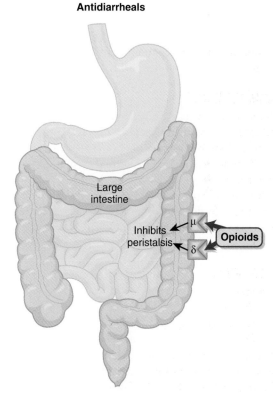

Figure 15-6.

cases of diarrhea. The mechanism is not well understood, but colloids that are insoluble and do not ferment may provide some additional structural integrity to the stool, reducing its viscosity.
- Some of the bulk agents may also work by binding enterotoxins, the bacteria that cause diarrhea in the first place. Kaolin may be one example of a bulk agent that binds enterotoxins.

PHARMACOKINETICS

- Loperamide does not penetrate the blood-brain barrier very readily, in large part because of the actions of the P-glycoprotein (Pgp) transporter. This limits the euphoria experienced with loperamide use. It is not clear whether concomitant administration of Pgp inhibitors is able to increase the euphoria experienced with loperamide.
- Loperamide and diphenoxylate have low solubility; thus they are unlikely to be abused parenterally.
- The bulk-forming or hydroscopic agents are generally clays that are able to absorb a significant amount of water. This absorptive ability is not selective, however, and agents such as kaolin may bind other substances, including drugs and nutrients. It is therefore advised that administration of these agents be separated from the administration of other agents by about 2 to 3 hours.

INDICATION

- Diarrhea

CONTRAINDICATIONS

- The use of opiates in some forms of severe, infectious diarrhea in some cases is contraindicated or warrants extreme caution, as it will interfere with the clearance of these microorganisms from the GI tract and prolong these serious illnesses:
  - ▲ Acute dysentery
  - ▲ Bacterial enterocolitis caused by invasive organisms (*Salmonella, Shigella, Campylobacter*)
  - ▲ Pseudomembranous colitis secondary to broad-spectrum antibiotics
- Severe inflammatory bowel disease in which a reduction in GI motility could lead to serious sequelae such as ileus, megacolon, and toxic megacolon

SIDE EFFECTS
All

- Constipation

Opiates

- **CNS effects, abuse potential:** These effects are possible with higher doses of diphenoxylate or difenoxin. They are likely to occur with only very high (toxic) doses of loperamide.

IMPORTANT NOTES

- Diarrhea is generally considered to be a self-limiting condition that is best treated with oral rehydration and maintenance of electrolytes. In many cases, particularly with infectious diarrhea, treatment with constipating agents may actually prolong the disease, unless accompanied by antibiotic therapy (see evidence section).
- Diphenoxylate and difenoxin are marketed as combination products with atropine. Atropine is an anticholinergic and

will therefore also reduce GI motility. This reduces the need for higher doses of these agents, which in turn reduces the potential for abuse.

- Although studies have shown that loperamide elicits very little euphoria, even at high doses, diphenoxylate does induce an opiate-like euphoric effect at higher doses (40 to 60 mg). Hence diphenoxylate remains a controlled drug, while loperamide is readily available without a prescription.
- Difenoxin is a metabolite of diphenoxylate and has actions similar to those of the parent drug.
- Bismuth compounds are also widely used in the treatment of diarrhea (see the discussion of GI cytoprotectants in this chapter for other actions and details about bismuth compounds). Their mechanism in the treatment of diarrhea is not well defined, although they do contain clays and this might contribute as a bulk-forming agent, as described earlier. The bismuth compounds may also have antisecretory and antimicrobial effects.
- Somatostatin analogues (octreotide, somatostatin) are also used to treat certain forms of diarrhea. See the discussion of somatostatin analogues in Chapter 14.

Advanced

- Racecadotril is a novel antidiarrheal that targets δ opiate receptors indirectly, by inhibiting an enzyme (enkephalinase) that breaks down endogenous enkephalins, hence enhancing their stimulation of this opiate receptor. Thus this agent specifically targets the secretory component of diarrhea. It has been investigated in types of diarrhea characterized by large secretion of fluid.

EVIDENCE
Antimotility Agents in Combination with Antibiotics for Traveler's Diarrhea

- A 2008 systematic review (nine trials, N = 1435 participants) examined the effect of using antimotility agents such as loperamide in conjunction with antibiotics for traveler's diarrhea. The authors found that combinations of loperamide and antibiotics were more likely to produce a cure than antibiotics alone, both after 24 hours (odds ratio [OR] 2.6) and after 48 hours (OR 2.2).

Antimotility Agents for Chronic Diarrhea in Patients with HIV/AIDS

- A 2008 Cochrane review (one trial, N = 91 participants) assessed the effectiveness of antimotility agents in treating chronic diarrhea in patients with human immunodeficiency virus (HIV) infection and acquired immunodeficiency syndrome (AIDS). The authors did not find any trials involving antimotility agents. They found no evidence that the adsorbent attapulgite was superior to placebo in controlling diarrhea.

Laxatives

DESCRIPTION
Laxatives are agents that promote defecation.

PROTOTYPES AND COMMON DRUGS
Stimulants
- Prototype: sennosides
- Others: castor oil, bisacodyl

Bulk
- Prototype: psyllium

Osmotics
- **Sugars:** Prototype—lactulose
- **Salts:** Prototype—magnesium sulfate
- **Others:** magnesium hydroxide, magnesium citrate, sodium phosphate
- **Polyethylene glycol**

Softeners
- Prototype: docusate

Peripheral Opioid Antagonists
- Prototype: methylnaltrexone

MOA (MECHANISM OF ACTION)
Stimulant
- Stimulant laxatives are also known as *irritant* laxatives, and, as the name suggests, they work by irritating the intestinal wall, which leads to an accumulation of fluid and electrolytes and increased motility.
- The method by which stimulant laxatives irritate the intestinal wall has not been clearly defined, although likely mediators include the activation of cAMP and cyclic guanosine monophosphate (cGMP) pathways, inhibition of Na/K-ATPase, and increased platelet activating factor production (Figure 15-7).

Bulk
- Water is the largest determinant of stool volume, making up 70% to 85% of stool. A large amount of fluid is also extracted from stool as it makes its way through the intestines. Interruptions in this extraction of water, either excess extraction (constipation) or reduced extraction (diarrhea) can lead to GI problems.
- Fiber is the component of food that cannot be broken down by digestive enzymes.
- Fiber promotes intestinal motility by increasing the bulk of the stool. This is accomplished by increasing the bacterial content of stool by fermentation of fiber (*fermentable* fiber) or simply by drawing water into the stool (*nonfermentable* fiber). Many substances in the diet perform a combination of the two. Fiber, and specifically the short-chain fatty acids

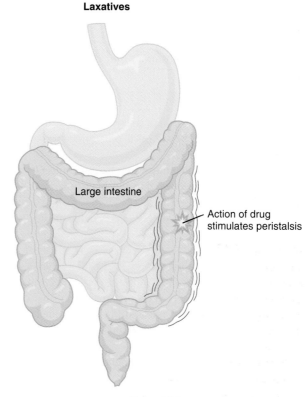

Laxatives

Large intestine

Action of drug stimulates peristalsis

Figure 15-7.

produced by fiber, may also have a direct stimulatory effect on the gut.
- For a list of fermentable versus nonfermentable fibers, see Important Notes, later.

Osmotics
- There are two types of osmotic laxatives: those made of sugars and alcohols and those that are salts of electrolytes.
- A shared mechanism of both types is that they create an osmotic force, pulling water into the stool and creating additional bulk, in a manner analogous to that seen with the bulk agents. The sugars are typically nonabsorbable, such as mannitol, sorbitol, and lactulose.
- Additional mechanisms may contribute to the efficacy of the electrolyte salts, and these agents are generally considered to be more potent than the sugars. For example, magnesium-containing laxatives may stimulate CCK release, which in turn leads to increased fluid and electrolytes within the gut lumen and increased motility.

Softeners

- As the name suggests, softeners are emollients that soften the stool, making defecation easier. They accomplish this in a variety of ways.
- Docusate salts are surfactants that allow mixing of aqueous and fatty substances in the stool. The docusate salts also increase intestinal fluid secretion.
- Mineral oil is not digested to an appreciable extent, so it stays in the gut and is absorbed into the stool, having a direct softening effect.

Opiate Antagonists

- Constipation caused by opiate analgesics such as morphine is a result of agonist effects on μ opiate receptors in the gut.
- Peripheral opiate μ antagonists are charged molecules that have limited ability to cross into the brain; therefore they selectively block the receptors that cause constipation without antagonizing the central analgesic effects of the opiates.

PHARMACOKINETICS

- Laxatives work best when poorly absorbed, as they all act locally within the gut.
- Because they work by a local irritant effect, bisacodyl tablets are designed to be released in the intestine but not before. Crushing or chewing of tablets will lead to irritation of the stomach.
- A number of the osmotic and stimulant laxatives can also be given as enemas or suppositories (bisacodyl).

INDICATIONS

- Constipation
- As cathartics, in preparation for radiologic or surgical procedures

CONTRAINDICATIONS
Fiber

- **Patients with obstructive symptoms or megacolon.** Increasing the bulk of the stool will worsen these conditions.

SIDE EFFECTS

- Laxatives are generally well tolerated when used in moderation, with mild side effects that are typically an extension of their pharmacologic effect
- **Diarrhea:** The osmotic and stimulant agents, in particular, have the potential to cause diarrhea.

Bulk

- **Abdominal distension:** The fermentation process by bacteria contributes to the production of gas, which leads to bloating. This side effect usually improves with time.

Osmotics, Sugars

- **Abdominal distension, flatulence:** These effects are likely caused by increased fermentation of the sugars by bacteria in the large intestine and tend to improve with continued use.

Osmotic Salts

- **Electrolyte abnormalities** are usually seen only at higher doses or in patients with preexisting electrolyte disturbances or renal dysfunction. The osmotic salts should be used with extreme caution (or not at all) in these patients or in patients on diuretic therapy.

Mineral Oil

- **Interferes with vitamin absorption:** Mineral oil interferes with the absorption of fat-soluble substances, including vitamins.
- **Foreign body reactions:** Mineral oil can elicit foreign body reactions in the gut.
- **Lipid pneumonitis** is a rare side effect that occurs when mineral oil has been aspirated.

IMPORTANT NOTES

- Osmotic sugar laxatives are useful in the treatment of constipation caused by opiates, as well as constipation in the elderly.
- Lactulose is used as a treatment for **hepatic encephalopathy** (confusion or decreased level of consciousness caused by liver failure). Patients with severe liver disease have difficulty detoxifying ammonia, which is produced by bacterial metabolism of feces. The actions of lactulose decrease intestinal pH, which traps ammonia within the lumen of the gut, facilitating its exit from the body.
- There are two types of mineral oil, and it is important that their use not be confused. **Light mineral oil** is for topical use as an emollient, whereas **heavy mineral oil** is used as a laxative.
- Composition of various forms of dietary fiber are shown in Table 15-2.

EVIDENCE
Laxatives for Hemorrhoid Symptoms

- A 2005 Cochrane review (seven trials, N = 378 participants) evaluated the ability of laxatives to treat hemorrhoid symptoms. The authors found that the risk of persisting symptoms was significantly reduced with fiber (RR 0.47), as was the risk of bleeding (RR 0.50).

Laxatives for Constipation in Palliative Care Patients

- A 2006 Cochrane review (four trials, N = 280 participants) compared laxatives used for constipation in palliative care patients. All laxatives demonstrated a limited degree of

TABLE 15-2. Dietary Sources of Fiber	
Highly Fermentable	**Poorly Fermentable or Nonfermentable**
Hemicellulose	Lignin
Mucilages and gums	Cellulose
Pectins	

efficacy, although these results were confounded by significant use of rescue laxatives during the studies. The only significantly different treatments were in a comparison of lactulose + senna versus danthron + poloxamer. The authors concluded that there was a paucity of data for this indication in this population.

FYI
- Several of the most commonly used laxatives are plant-derived, including many of the stimulant laxatives such as cascara (bark of the Buckthorn tree), senna (leaflets on pods of *Cassia angustifolia*), and castor oil (bean of the castor plant).
- Castor oil contains ricin, a very toxic protein that has been used in the past as a poison. Although castor oil was one of the original laxatives, the development of safer alternatives has lead to a reduction in its use.
- The stimulant laxatives have a checkered past with respect to safety. Phenolphthalein, the original Ex-Lax and once the most popular stimulant laxative, was withdrawn from the market in the late 1990s because of concerns over potential carcinogenicity.

Cannabinoids

DESCRIPTION
- The cannabinoids are the major active component of *Cannabis sativa*, also known as *marijuana*.

PROTOTYPE AND COMMON DRUGS
Agonists
- Prototype: dro**nabi**nol, also known as Δ^9-tetrahydro-cannabinol (THC)
- Others: **nabi**lone, can**nabi**diol

Antagonists
- Prototype: rimonabant

MOA (MECHANISM OF ACTION)
- The cannabinoid (CB) receptors are G-protein–coupled receptors that are widely distributed throughout the body, most notably in the CNS.
- CB1 receptors are found in the hypothalamus, amygdala, basal ganglia, and cerebellum (Figure 15-8).
- In the periphery, CB1 receptors are found in adipocytes, the adrenal gland, the ovaries, the testes, and the GI tract.
- The location of CB1 receptors in areas of the brain (i.e., the hypothalamus) associated with feeding, coupled with the longstanding observation of the appetite-stimulating effects of cannabis, led to the conclusion that CB1 receptors may play an important role in the treatment of obesity.
- These regions of the brain are also interrelated with the **mesolimbic DA** pathway, also known as the *reward pathway*. This explains another, perhaps more well known effect of cannabis, that of euphoria and reward. The link between the reward pathways in the brain and the hypothalamus might also explain why eating is also associated with reward.
- Evidence of a link between smoking and the endocannabinoid pathway comes from the observation that THC triggers release of DA in the reward pathway via CB1 receptors, in the same way that nicotine stimulates DA release via

Cannabinoids

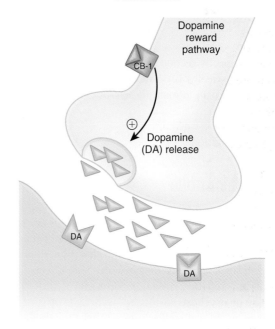

Figure 15-8.

nicotinic receptors. Chronic nicotine administration increases levels of endogenous cannabinoids, which then bind to CB1 receptors and elicit a feeling of reward.
- The potential of CB1 antagonists as antiobesity drugs is supported by the actions of CB1 in adipose tissue. CB1 antagonism may decrease lipogenesis and increase adiponectin levels. Adiponectin is a hormone secreted by adipocytes. It plays a role in lipid and glucose metabolism and also influences response to insulin. Low levels of adiponectin are found in obesity, and high levels are associated with reduced risk of heart attack.

PHARMACOKINETICS
Agonists
- Δ^9-THC is well absorbed but undergoes extensive first-pass metabolism and significant distribution into tissues, thus limiting the amount (10% to 20%) of oral dose that reaches the systemic circulation.
- It has an active metabolite, 11-OH-Δ^9-THC. Both the parent and active metabolite are eliminated by hepatic metabolism.
- The combination of Δ^9-THC and cannabidiol is available as a buccal spray.

Antagonists
- Rimonabant is a lipophilic drug with an exceptionally long elimination half-life ($t_{1/2}$) of 6 to 9 days. This prolonged $t_{1/2}$ is doubled in obese patients (16 days), as drug deposits in fatty tissue.
- Rimonabant undergoes hepatic metabolism, primarily by CYP3A4.

INDICATIONS
Agonists
- Emesis (typically secondary to cancer chemotherapy)
- Anorexia (typically associated with AIDS)
- Neuropathic pain in multiple sclerosis (MS)

Antagonists
- Smoking cessation
- Obesity

CONTRAINDICATIONS
Agonists
- **Serious cardiovascular disease**: Cannabinoids are not recommended for patients with a history of ischemic heart disease, arrhythmia, poorly controlled hypertension, or severe heart failure. See details under Side Effects, later.
- **Significant hepatic or renal impairment**
- **History of psychosis**
- **Pregnancy**: Animal studies suggest that cannabinoids may impair fetal development.

SIDE EFFECTS
Agonists
- **CNS effects consistent with marijuana use**: euphoria, drowsiness, impaired sensory perception
- **Cardiovascular effects**: tachycardia, hypotension

Antagonists
Rimonabant
- **Nausea**: CB agonists have an antinauseant effect, so it is not surprising that antagonizing these receptors will lead to a pronauseant effect.

Serious
- **Depression and suicidality**: The mechanisms is unclear, but at present the simple explanation is that if CB1 agonists can generate euphoria, blocking this receptor may lead to severe dysphoria in some patients.

IMPORTANT NOTES
- The combination of Δ^9-THC and cannabidiol, a nonpsychoactive plant cannabinoid, is being used for neuropathic pain in MS and as an adjunctive analgesic in advanced cancer.
- Concerns over side effects of severe depression and suicidal ideation led to the withdrawal of rimonabant in Europe and lack of approval in the United States. There are other CB1 antagonists in development, and these agents will need to address this safety issue.
- The location of function of CB2 receptors is not as well understood. It is believed that CB2 receptors might mediate antinociception, and thus CB2 agonists may have potential as analgesics.

FYI
- Endocannabinoids such as anandamide are eicosanoids and are therefore derived from arachidonic acid. The name *anandamide* is derived from Sanskrit for *bliss*.
- There are approximately 70 naturally occurring cannabinoids, and THC is the most important psychoactive compound of the group. There are many isomers of THC, but the Δ^9-THC isomer is considered to be the most active.
- The cannabinoids have been investigated in a variety of disorders, including neurologic disorders such as MS and Parkinson's disease. In MS, cannabis is often used to treat spasticity. Cannabis has also been used since the 1970s for glaucoma.
- Legal issues around the use of medicinal marijuana have created problems with the study of cannabinoid agonists. Specific agonists such as dronabinol have been developed to further "medicinalize" the use of THC. However, the problem with using these specific compounds is that they may lose some of the pharmacologic contributions from the variety of other cannabinoids found in marijuana.

Pancreatic Enzymes

DESCRIPTION
Pancreatic enzymes are agents that act as enzyme supplements. They are used in patients with pancreatic enzyme deficiency.

PROTOTYPE AND COMMON DRUGS
- Prototype: **pancre**lipase
- Others: **pancre**atin

MOA (MECHANISM OF ACTION)
- Deficiencies of pancreatic enzymes occur in disorders such as cystic fibrosis and chronic pancreatitis or in people in whom the pancreas has been surgically resected.
- Pancreatic enzyme secretion below 10% of normal interferes with proper digestion of fats and proteins, leading in turn to steatorrhea, azotorrhea, malabsorption of vitamins, and weight loss.
- Pancreatic enzyme supplements contain a mix of amylase, lipase, and proteases.

PHARMACOKINETICS
- As proteins, the pancreatic enzymes are quickly destroyed by gastric acids. For this reason, some formulations are encapsulated with acid-resistant microspheres or microtablets. The non–enteric-coated formulations must be coadministered with acid suppressants such as PPIs or H_2 antagonists.
- Doses are titrated based on patient age and weight, extent of pancreatic insufficiency, and dietary fat intake. Inadequate response to enteric-coated formulations may be caused by insufficient mixing of granules with food and/or slow dissolution and release of enzymes.

INDICATIONS
- Pancreatic enzyme deficiency secondary to the following:
  - ▲ Cystic fibrosis
  - ▲ Chronic pancreatitis
  - ▲ After pancreatectomy
  - ▲ After GI bypass surgery
  - ▲ Duct obstruction from pancreatic tumor

CONTRAINDICATIONS
- None of major significance

SIDE EFFECTS
- **Diarrhea, abdominal pain**: typically only seen with higher doses
- **Hyperuricosuria or renal stones**: caused by the high purine content of the enzyme supplements

IMPORTANT NOTES
- Most cystic fibrosis patients will experience pancreatic insufficiency. Cystic fibrosis is characterized by disruption of chloride transport as well as other transporters for sodium and bicarbonate. Patients have excessive intestinal mucoprotein, increasing the viscosity of the intestinal lumen. The increased viscosity leads to blockade of ducts, which damages acinar cells and causes fibrosis as well as exocrine pancreatic insufficiency.

Serotonin Antagonists

DESCRIPTION
Serotonin antagonists act as antinauseants by blocking serotonin-3 ($5\text{-}HT_3$) receptors.

PROTOTYPE AND COMMON DRUGS
- Prototype: ondan**setron**
- Others: grani**setron**, alo**setron**, tropi**setron**, ramo**setron**, dola**setron**, palono**setron**

MOA (MECHANISM OF ACTION)
- $5\text{-}HT_3$ receptors in the gut mediate contraction of various segments of the GI tract, including the fundus, corpus, and antrum. These receptors also sensitize spinal sensory neurons and participate in vagal signaling of nausea. 5-HT3 receptors in the brain also mediate nausea.
- Chemotherapeutic agents used in cancer stimulate the release of 5-HT from enterochromaffin cells in the GI tract. This 5-HT activates $5\text{-}HT_3$ receptors on vagal sensory afferent neurons, and these neurons project to the emetic center in the brainstem (Figure 15-9).
- $5\text{-}HT_3$ receptor antagonists were thus first developed for, and continue to be first-line agents in the treatment of chemotherapy-induced nausea and vomiting.
- Antagonism of $5\text{-}HT_3$ receptors also appears to slow intestinal transit and secretions of the small bowel and decreases colonic compliance. This accounts for the efficacy of some $5\text{-}HT_3$ antagonists in treating conditions such as irritable bowel syndrome (IBS).
- The first $5\text{-}HT_3$ antagonist to be approved for treatment of IBS (alosetron) is a much more potent antagonist at $5\text{-}HT_3$

Serotonin antagonists

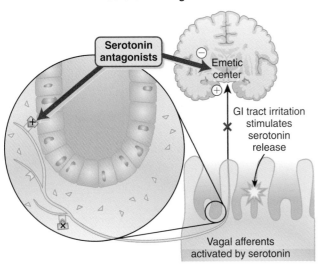

Figure 15-9.

than ondansetron, suggesting that efficacy in IBS may be determined by potency.

PHARMACOKINETICS

- The 5-HT$_3$ antagonists all appear to have a prolonged biologic half-life, with actions persisting well past elimination from the systemic circulation.
- All are well absorbed from the GI tract. All appear to undergo hepatic metabolism, typically via the CYP450 enzymes.
- The 5-HT$_3$ antagonists are also available in parenteral preparations, both intravenous and intramuscular.

INDICATIONS

- Nausea, vomiting
- IBS

CONTRAINDICATIONS

- None of major significance

SIDE EFFECTS

- **Generally well tolerated**
- **Constipation or diarrhea:** Constipation is more common, and likely occurs because of 5-HT$_3$ antagonism in the gut, which slows intestinal transit. The mechanism for the diarrhea is not clear.
- Headache
- Light-headedness

Rare but Serious

- **Ischemic colitis** has been associated with alosetron. This may be related to the ability of alosetron to induce contractions in the GI tract, in this case resulting in severe spasms in certain individuals.
- **Electrocardiographic (ECG) changes:** QT prolongation and other ECG changes have been reported. These changes are typically harmless but rarely may lead to clinically significant arrhythmias. Caution is advised when administering other drugs that may prolong the QT interval or in patients with QT prolongation.

IMPORTANT NOTES

- Alosetron was withdrawn from the U.S. market in 2000 because of concerns over ischemic colitis but was reintroduced in 2002 with a revised indication for women with severe IBS.
- Of all antiemetic agents, the 5-HT$_3$ antagonists are among the most specific, having little if any affinity for any receptors other than serotonin receptors. This specificity may account for their paucity of side effects.
- The 5-HT$_3$ antagonists were considered to be breakthrough drugs in the treatment of chemotherapy-induced nausea and vomiting. However, they do not appear to be efficacious in management of nausea caused by motion sickness.
- Neurokinin (NK1) receptor antagonists are a newer class of antiemetics that are used in combination with 5-HT$_3$ antagonists for chemotherapy-induced nausea and vomiting. These agents work centrally, in the area postrema. The first two NK1 antagonists were aprepitant and fosaprepitant.

EVIDENCE
Prevention of Postoperative Nausea and Vomiting

- A large (>100,000 subjects) 2006 Cochrane review compared a wide variety of agents with placebo and found that ondansetron, granisetron, tropisetron, and dolasetron were among eight drugs that prevented postoperative nausea and vomiting. Others were droperidol, dexamethasone, cyclizine, and metoclopramide.

Relief of Emesis in Pediatric Gastroenteritis

- A 2006 Cochrane review examined the effectiveness of antiemetics in children and adolescents with vomiting induced by gastroenteritis. The conclusions were limited by the small studies (total of 396 subjects over three studies). The results suggested that ondansetron performed better than placebo in reducing the number of vomiting episodes in this population. This was at the expense of an increased incidence of diarrhea, thought to be a result of the retention of toxins that would normally have been eliminated by vomiting.

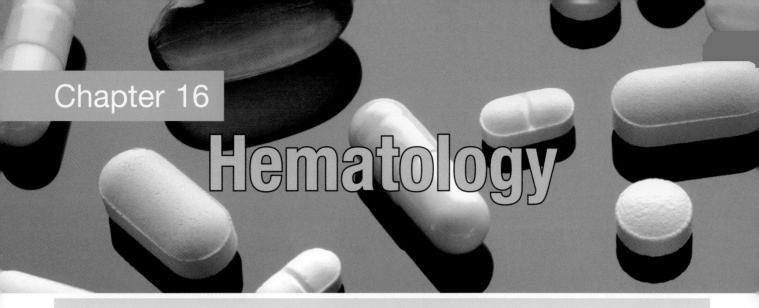

Hematology

Heparins

DESCRIPTION

Heparin belongs to a family of endogenous substances known as glycosaminoglycans (GAGs). Heparin and its synthetic derivatives are anticoagulants.

PROTOTYPE AND COMMON DRUGS

- Prototype: he**parin** (also known as unfractionated heparin [UFH])
- Others: low–molecular-weight heparin (LMWH)
  ▲ Dalte**parin**, enoxa**parin**, nadro**parin**, tinza**parin**

Pentasaccharides

- Prototype: Fonda**parin**ux

Heparinoids

- Prototype: Danaparoid

MOA (MECHANISM OF ACTION)

- The coagulation (clotting) system is composed of many proteins. Most of these proteins are procoagulants, which means they contribute to clotting. Some proteins are anti-coagulants that serve to keep the coagulation system in balance.
- When a protein is *activated*, its name is followed by a small letter *a*. Each activated protein serves as an enzyme for the next protein downstream in the cascade (Figure 16-1).
- Heparins interfere with the coagulation cascade by ampli-fying the anticoagulant effect of **antithrombin III**.
- Antithrombin III, a natural plasma protease inhibitor, is an anticoagulant, and it inhibits **thrombin (IIa) and factor Xa**.
- To inhibit factor Xa, heparins must bind only antithrombin III.
- To inhibit factor IIa, heparins must bind to both antithrombin III and factor IIa (dual binding not shown Figure 16-1).
- LMWHs are typically too small to bind both antithrombin III and factor IIa. Therefore their anticoagulant effects are exerted largely through factor Xa, with minimal effects on factor IIa.

Heparins

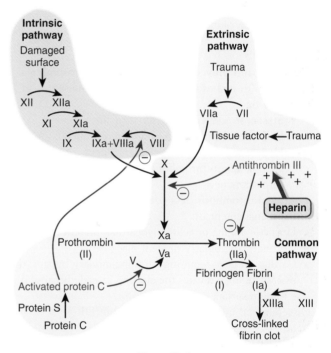

Figure 16-1.

PHARMACOKINETICS
Unfractionated Heparin

- Very complex pharmacokinetics exist because there is a large range in molecular weight of the molecules
- The dose-response curve is difficult to predict, so the dose must be individualized in every patient, with frequent mea-surements (i.e., activated partial thromboplastin time [aPTT]) made to guide titration.
- UFH binds to a variety of plasma proteins, reducing its bioavailability at low concentrations.
  ▲ Levels of these heparin-binding proteins can vary signifi-cantly, requiring the use of very high doses in some patients.

- UFH exhibits saturation kinetics, meaning that the elimination half-life ($t_{1/2}$) increases with increasing dose.
- UFH is administered via the intravenous (IV) or subcutaneous (SC) routes.
  - ▲ UFH acts immediately after IV administration, and effects last a few hours. Infusion is required to maintain continuous anticoagulation.
  - ▲ Onset occurs in 60 minutes when UFH is given subcutaneously.

Low–Molecular-Weight Heparin

- LMWH has a more predictable dose-response curve than UFH because there is a smaller range of molecular weights.
- aPTT is not used to measure LMWH activity, but sometimes factor Xa levels can be measured (not commonly performed).
- LMWH is administered via the subcutaneous route. Compared to UFH, LMWH has:
  - ▲ A longer half-life than heparin
  - ▲ More predictable pharmacokinetic profile
    - Less protein binding
    - First-order kinetics

INDICATIONS

- **Treatment and prevention of inappropriate thrombosis**
  - ▲ Venous thrombosis (and pulmonary embolism [PE]) caused by:
    - **Stasis** (prolonged inactivity: airplane, surgery)
    - **Endothelial damage** (common in orthopedic surgery)
    - **Hypercoagulable states** (the balance of thrombogenesis and thrombolysis inappropriately favors thrombogenesis)
  - ▲ Arterial thrombosis (less common than venous)
- **Initial management of:**
  - ▲ Unstable angina or acute myocardial infarction (MI)
  - ▲ Coronary angioplasty or stent placement
  - ▲ Cardiac surgery requiring cardiopulmonary bypass (the bypass tubing activates the clotting cascade because it is a foreign surface)
- **Disseminated intravascular coagulation (DIC)**

CONTRAINDICATIONS

- **Previous heparin-induced thrombocytopenia syndrome (HITS)** (see Side Effects)
- **Coagulopathies:** hemophilia, thrombocytopenia (low platelet count)
- **Active bleeding:** intracranial hemorrhage, gastrointestinal (GI) ulcers, certain cancers

SIDE EFFECTS

- **HITS**
  - ▲ Antibodies against **platelet factor 4** are produced and bind to platelets.
  - ▲ Platelets get activated and sticky, and this causes:
    - Thromboses (multiple)
    - Platelet consumption resulting in thrombocytopenia
    - Bleeding as a result of thrombocytopenia

- **Hemorrhage** can be reversed with protamine (see later).
- **Osteoporosis** occurs with long-term therapy; the cause is unknown.
- **Hyperkalemia:** Although not a common occurrence, heparin can cause increased serum potassium; it is more likely to occur in patients with diabetes or renal disease. In this regard the action of heparin is similar to that of spironolactone, which is an aldosterone blocker classified as a *K-sparing diuretic*.
- **Fever:** Rarely, heparin can cause a *drug* fever.

IMPORTANT NOTES

- To measure the effect of UFH, the **aPTT** test is used (compare this with prothrombin time [PT] or International Normalized Ratio [INR], which is used with warfarin). It is a measure of time to coagulation (in the laboratory) and is measured in seconds. The higher the number, the more strongly a patient is anticoagulated.
- Unlike UFH, LMWHs do not prolong the aPTT, and they also have a more predictable pharmacokinetic profile. These important differences make LMWH far more convenient for patients to use, with more stable administration and less rigorous monitoring.
- Heparins provide a safe and important alternative to teratogenic warfarin in pregnancy.
- For cases of heparin overdose, protamine sulfate is a strongly basic protein that forms a complex with heparin, acting as a *chemical antagonist*. LMWH does not have an antidote.
- Danaparoid works by the same mechanism as the heparins, but it is **not structurally related** to the heparins; it is therefore considered a *heparinoid*. Therefore it can be used in the management of patients with heparin-induced thrombocytopenia (HIT) too.
- Fondaparinux is synthetic and is based on the structure of the antithrombin binding region of heparin. The binding region of heparin is only 5 saccharide units and is the basis for the pentasaccharide structure of fondaparinux. Fondaparinux could be thought of as *really* low molecular weight heparin.

EVIDENCE

LMWH versus UFH for Treatment of Venous Thromboembolism

- A 2005 Cochrane review (five studies, N = 1508 participants) found that LMWH may be more efficacious than UFH for the initial treatment of venous thromboembolism (VTE). This Cochrane review also found that LMWH was safer than heparin, with significantly fewer hemorrhagic adverse events.

LMWH versus Warfarin for Treatment of Venous Thromboembolism

- A 2001 Cochrane review (seven studies, N = 1137 participants), updated in 2003, compared warfarin with LMWH for long-term treatment of VTE. There was no difference in the risk of recurrent VTE between warfarin and LMWH. There was a lower risk of bleeding with LMWH (odds ratio

[OR] 0.38), and no difference in mortality rates between these two interventions was found.

LMWH and Heparinoids versus UFH for Ischemic Stroke

- A 2008 Cochrane review (nine studies, N = 3137 patients) compared LMWH and heparinoids (danaparoid) with UFH in patients with acute, presumed or confirmed ischemic stroke. The odds of developing a deep vein thrombosis (DVT) were reduced with LMWH compared with UFH (OR 0.55); however, the incidence of key clinical outcomes such as PE, death, and hemorrhage (intracranial or extracranial) was too small to provide a reliable comparison.

FYI

- Heparin was discovered in 1916 by a medical student who was working on a summer research project. He was trying to extract procoagulant substances from various tissues and instead found a potent anticoagulant still used today.
- The name *heparin* reflects the fact that this substance was extracted from the liver (*hepatic*).
- *Thrombo* means blood clot. *Cyto* means cell. Thrombocytes (also known as *platelets*) are cells that contribute to blood clots. *Penia* means decreased. *Thrombocytopenia* means a low platelet count.

Direct Factor Xa Inhibitors

DESCRIPTION

Direct factor Xa inhibitors are agents that inhibit clotting by inhibiting a specific component of the coagulation cascade.

PROTOTYPE

- Prototype: rivaroxaban

MOA (MECHANISM OF ACTION)

- The coagulation system is composed of many proteins: most of these proteins are procoagulants, which means they contribute to clotting. Some proteins are anticoagulants, which serve to keep the coagulation system in balance.
- When a protein is *activated*, its name is given a small letter *a* at the end. Each activated protein serves as an enzyme for the next protein downstream in the cascade (Figure 16-2).
- Factor Xa converts prothrombin to thrombin (factor IIa). **Thrombin** is an enzyme that catalyzes the final step in the coagulation cascade, the conversion of fibrinogen to fibrin.
- Fibrin is a fibrous protein that forms a mesh, providing structural rigidity to a clot. The mesh is created by the cross-linking of fibrin, and this cross-linking step is facilitated by factor XIII.
- In addition to converting fibrinogen to fibrin, thrombin also activates factor XIII; thus thrombin not only catalyzes the creation of the key component of the clot, it also facilitates the provision of structural rigidity to the clot.
- Thrombin also activates factors V, VIII, and XI, therefore amplifying the coagulation cascade. In addition, thrombin activates platelets, leading to their aggregation.
- Direct factor Xa inhibitors directly inhibit the conversion of prothrombin to thrombin without using antithrombin III as an intermediary. The direct inhibition of thrombin **formation** results in an anticoagulant effect.

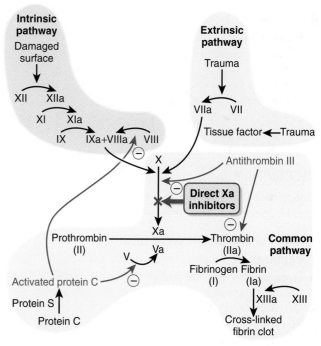

Direct Xa inhibitors

Figure 16-2.

PHARMACOKINETICS

- Rivaroxaban, the first direct factor Xa inhibitor, is administered orally. It is rapidly absorbed, reaching peak plasma concentrations in 2 to 4 hours, and has an elimination half-life of 9 hours.
- One third of rivaroxaban is eliminated unchanged in the kidneys; therefore dose adjustments should be considered in renal impairment, and an alternative drug should be considered in patients with severe renal impairment.

INDICATIONS
- Postsurgical VTE prophylaxis
- As an alternative to heparins in patients with severe HIT

CONTRAINDICATIONS
- Active bleeding
- Pregnancy
- **Patients at increased risk of bleeding**: clotting disorders, history of recent hemorrhagic stroke

SIDE EFFECTS
- **Bleeding**: As with all anticoagulants, bleeding is the major side effect.

IMPORTANT NOTES
- There are no monitoring requirements for rivaroxaban. This and the fact that it is an orally administered agent suggest that drugs in its class, and perhaps the direct thrombin inhibitors, will supplant warfarin as the drugs of choice among oral anticoagulants.

Advanced
Drug Interactions
- CYP450 3A4 enzymes are involved in the metabolism of rivaroxaban; thus the potential exists for pharmacokinetic drug interactions with inhibitors or inducers of this isozyme.

Rivaroxaban is also a P-glycoprotein (Pgp) substrate, and therefore its levels could also be affected by inhibitors or inducers of Pgp.

EVIDENCE
Postsurgical Venous Thromboembolism Prophylaxis
- The RECORD trials were a series of double-blind randomized controlled trials that compared rivaroxaban with enoxaparin for the prophylactic treatment of VTE after total hip replacement (RECORD-1 and RECORD-2) or total knee replacement (RECORD-3 and RECORD-4). The trials were all relatively large, randomizing 2509 to 4541 patients between the two treatment groups. Rivaroxaban-treated patients had fewer events of VTE and all-cause deaths compared with enoxaparin in each of the four studies. The risk of bleeding was slightly higher with rivaroxaban than with enoxaparin.

FYI
- For a quick summary of the difference between two of the newer oral anticoagulants—direct factor Xa and direct thrombin inhibitors. Direct factor Xa inhibitors inhibit the *formation* of thrombin, whereas direct thrombin inhibitors allow thrombin to be formed but interfere with the *actions* of thrombin.

Direct Thrombin Inhibitors

DESCRIPTION
Direct thrombin inhibitors reduce clotting by inhibiting a specific component of the coagulation cascade.

PROTOTYPE AND COMMON DRUGS
Parenteral
- Prototype: hirudin (lepirudin)
- Others: bivalirudin, desirudin

Oral
- Prototype: argatroban
- Others: dabigatran, ximelagatran

MOA (MECHANISM OF ACTION)
- The coagulation (clotting) system is a multistep cascade that eventually leads to the formation of fibrin and development of a clot.
- **Thrombin (factor IIa)** is an enzyme that catalyzes the final step in the coagulation cascade, the conversion of fibrinogen to fibrin (Figure 16-3).
- Fibrin is a fibrous protein that forms a mesh, providing structural rigidity to a clot. The mesh is created by the cross-linking of fibrin, and this cross-linking step is facilitated by factor XIII.

Direct thrombin inhibitors

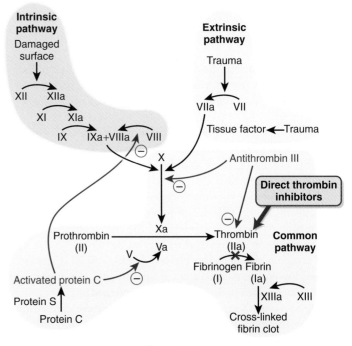

Figure 16-3.

- In addition to converting fibrinogen to fibrin, thrombin also activates factor XIII; thus thrombin not only catalyzes the creation of the key component of the clot, it also facilitates the provision of structural rigidity to the clot.
- Thrombin also activates factors V, VIII, and XI, therefore amplifying the coagulation cascade. Thrombin also has antiplatelet effects.
- Thrombin has an active site as well as two other sites, referred to as exosite 1, which binds fibrin, and exosite 2, which binds heparin.
- Direct thrombin inhibitors all bind to thrombin directly at its active site. The bivalent inhibitors (-irudins) also bind at exosite 1 (hence the term "bivalent", indicating two binding sites), while the univalent inhibitors only bind at the active site.
- The univalent thrombin inhibitors (e.g., argatroban and dabigatran) and bivalirudin all bind reversibly, whereas the other bivalent inhibitors bind thrombin irreversibly.
- The net result of this binding is that the effects of thrombin are inhibited. The inhibition of thrombin results in an anticoagulant effect.

PHARMACOKINETICS

- Argatroban has a short half-life and is typically administered by infusion.
- Hirudin is administered by either IV or SC injection, with elimination half-life of 60 minutes and 120 minutes, respectively. It is cleared by the kidneys.
- Bivalirudin is administered intravenously and has rapid onset and offset, with a half-life of about 25 minutes. It is primarily eliminated by proteolysis, although about 20% of elimination is renal.

INDICATION

- Postsurgical VTE prophylaxis

Bivalirudin

- **Severe heparin-induced thrombocytopenia (HIT)**

CONTRAINDICATIONS

- **Patients who are at high risk of bleeding, such as those with the following conditions:**
  - ▲ Uncontrolled active bleeding
  - ▲ Major bleeding (coagulopathy) disorders
  - ▲ Acute gastric or duodenal ulcer
  - ▲ Recent (<6 months) stroke

SIDE EFFECTS

- **Bleeding:** As with all anticoagulants, bleeding is the major side effect.

IMPORTANT NOTES

- All of the agents in this class are approved for prophylaxis of DVT and VTE after orthopedic surgery. Patients undergoing knee or hip replacement surgeries, in particular, are at high risk for developing a DVT or VTE. The risk is so high that these patients receive prophylactic anticoagulants for several days postsurgery.
- The theoretical advantage of direct over indirect thrombin inhibitors such as LMWHs is that the direct inhibitors inactivate fibrin-bound thrombin, in addition to the thrombin in the fluid phase. This may lead to a greater inhibition of the thrombus. Direct thrombin inhibitors may also provide more predictable anticoagulation, as they are not bound to plasma proteins (unlike heparin) and are not neutralized by platelet factor 4 (a protein secreted by platelets) and other factors generated at the site of vascular injury.
- The anticoagulation of bivalirudin can be monitored using aPTT.
- Warfarin has been the prototypical oral anticoagulant for decades, but with its narrow margin of safety, significant potential for drug-drug and drug-food interactions, and significant variability in response among patients, there is much anticipation that new oral anticoagulants will soon be able to replace it. The direct thrombin inhibitors, which lack any of these limitations associated with warfarin, are one of the classes that might replace warfarin.

FYI

- The -irudins are based on the anticoagulant activity of leeches. Leeches secrete hirudin, and that facilitates their ability to draw blood from their victim. The recombinant form of hirudin, lepirudin, is used clinically.
- Ximelagatran, the first direct thrombin inhibitor, was withdrawn from the market because of concerns over hepatotoxicity.

Vitamin K Antagonists

DESCRIPTION

Vitamin K antagonists are a family of naturally derived anticoagulants, which are also known as coumarins.

PROTOTYPE

- Prototype: warfarin

MOA (MECHANISM OF ACTION)

- Vitamin K is key cofactor in the hepatic activation of four coagulation factors. The four vitamin K-dependent clotting factors are II, VII, IX, and X (Figure 16-4).
- To act as a cofactor, vitamin K must be in its reduced form, vitamin K hydroxyquinone. The enzyme vitamin K

Coumarins

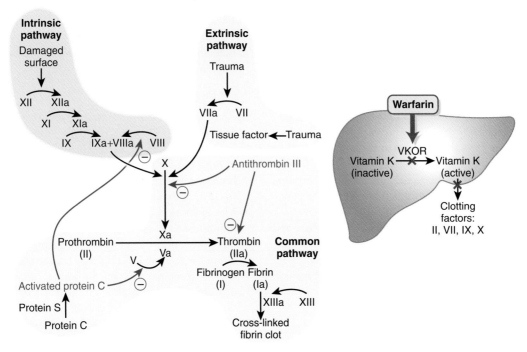

Figure 16-4.

epoxide reductase (VKOR) converts vitamin K to its reduced form.

- Warfarin inhibits the enzyme VKOR. Blocking formation of the reduced form of vitamin K inhibits the activation of these four clotting factors.
- These clotting factors vary in their half-lives (6 to 50 hours), with factor II having the longest half-life and factor VII having the shortest. This delays the onset of action of warfarin, as one must wait until these clotting factors have been mostly depleted before the full anticoagulant effects have been achieved.

PHARMACOKINETICS
- Warfarin is an orally administered anticoagulant.
- Warfarin requires 2 to 3 days of treatment before anticoagulation takes effect. This is because warfarin prevents vitamin K–dependant protein synthesis, and before anticoagulation occurs the plasma proteins must be cleared from the plasma, which takes about 48 hours.
- Drug-drug and drug-food interactions are frequent with this agent.
  - **Pharmacodynamic:** competitive antagonism with vitamin K
    - Foods containing vitamin K will oppose warfarin.
  - **Pharmacokinetic:** enzyme induction or inhibition
    - Warfarin may also inhibit or induce metabolism of *other* drugs.

INDICATIONS
- **Long-term** (home) anticoagulation. Note that heparin would be used first for many of these conditions in the hospital and that warfarin would replace heparin on discharge.

- The most common indications include the following:
  - PE or DVT treatment
  - Atrial fibrillation
  - Prevention of thrombus for mechanical heart valves
  - Chronic hypercoagulable states

CONTRAINDICATIONS
- **Pregnancy:** Warfarin is teratogenic and can also cause fetal bleeding.
- Recent events that predispose to bleeding include the following:
  - Surgery
  - Stroke
- Platelet disorders (If you have dysfunctional clotting *cells* and dysfunctional clotting *proteins*, there really is not much left to form a clot if you should need it.)

SIDE EFFECT
- **Hemorrhage**
  - **Minor:** Small cuts, nosebleeds, easy bruising, hematuria (blood in urine), and bleeding gums may occur.
  - **Major:** Intracranial bleeding is often catastrophic.

IMPORTANT NOTES
- Warfarin therapy is monitored using the International Normalized Ratio (INR), which is a standardized form of the PT test. Because different laboratories use different reagents to test the PT, every laboratory generates a slightly different result, so the INR corrects for this discrepancy among laboratories.
- Patients must undergo regular blood tests to ensure that their INR levels remain "therapeutic," which means being

in the appropriate range for their problem. For example, DVT treatment requires that the INR be 2.0 to 2.5 but for mechanical valves, the INR should be 2.5 to 3.5.

- The anticoagulant effects of warfarin can be reversed by administration of vitamin K. The time required for vitamin K to work is dependent on the time the liver requires to generate more proteins (many hours).
- *Fresh frozen plasma* (plasma from another human) can be transfused to immediately replace clotting factors and is the fastest way to correct an overdose of warfarin.
- When warfarin is being administered, all vitamin K–dependent protein synthesis is inhibited. This includes the *prothrombotic* factors II, VII, IX, and X but also includes the *antithrombotic* factors protein C and protein S. Protein C and S are inhibited very early with warfarin, and thus there can be a short duration of time when *only* the natural anticoagulants are inhibited and a **paradoxical, temporary hypercoagulable** state can be induced with warfarin. Therefore it is important to coadminister heparin with warfarin until the patient's anticoagulation levels (measured by INR) are in the desired range.

Advanced
- Warfarin is actually a racemic mixture of two enantiomers: R (weak) and S (potent). Each is eliminated by different metabolic pathways:
  - S by 2C9
  - R by 1A2 (major) as well as 2C19 and 3A4 (both minor)

Pharmacogenetics
- There is significant genetic variability in responses to warfarin owing to variants in 2C9 that metabolize the drug less efficiently and to variants in VKOR. See Chapter 6 for further details.

EVIDENCE
Warfarin versus LMWH for Treatment of Venous Thromboembolism
- A 2001 Cochrane review (seven studies, N = 1137 participants), updated in 2003, compared warfarin with LMWHs for long-term treatment of VTE. There was no difference in the risk of recurrent VTE between warfarin and LMWH. There was a lower risk of bleeding with LMWH (OR 0.38), and no difference in mortality rates between these two interventions.

Warfarin versus Acetylsalicylic Acid for Atrial Fibrillation
- A 2007 Cochrane review (eight studies, N = 9598 participants) compared warfarin with acetylsalicylic acid (ASA) in atrial fibrillation patients who had not had a prior stroke or transient ischemic attack (TIA). Treatment with warfarin led to a lower risk of stroke (OR 0.68), ischemic stroke (OR 0.53), and systemic emboli (OR 0.48). The risk of intracranial hemorrhage was increased with warfarin (OR 1.98). All-cause mortality and vascular deaths were similar between groups, and disabling or fatal strokes and MI were almost reduced with oral anticoagulants, but this did not reach statistical significance.

FYI
- Coumarins were first isolated from spoiled sweet clover and were discovered when cattle consuming this feed began to develop hemorrhagic disease.
- You may hear warfarin referred to as "rat poison," as it is commonly used as a rodenticide. However, the dose that a rat receives is very high.

Salicylates

DESCRIPTION
Salicylates comprise a heterogeneous group of agents that are related by chemical structure and by their antiinflammatory effects.

PROTOTYPE AND COMMON DRUGS
Salicylates
- Prototype: acetylsalicylic acid
- Others: sodium salicylate, salsalate, sodium thiosalicylate, choline salicylate, magnesium salicylate
- Others (derivative): diflunisal

Aminosalicylates
- Prototype: 5-ASA
- Others: sulfasalazine, olsalazine, balsalazide, mesalamine

MOA (MECHANISM OF ACTION)
Salicylates
- Like nonsteroidal antiinflammatory drugs (NSAIDs), the salicylates work by inhibiting the actions of the cyclooxygenase (COX) enzyme (Figure 16-5).
- ASA works by *irreversibly* inhibiting COX-1, an enzyme that catalyzes the formation of cyclic endoperoxide, which in turn is then converted to the following:
  - **Thromboxane A_2 (TXA_2)** in platelets
    - TXA_2 is a potent inducer of platelet aggregation and release.
    - Inhibition of TXA_2 leads to the antiplatelet effects of ASA (Figure 16-6).
  - **Prostaglandin E_2 (PGE_2)** mediates fever, pain, inflammation, and mucous production.

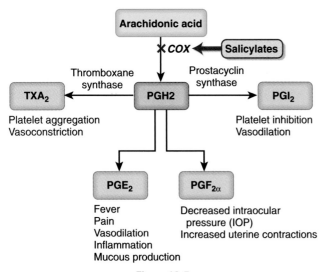

Figure 16-5.

Salicylates

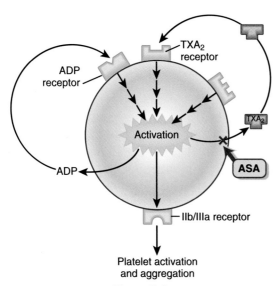

Figure 16-6.

- Inhibition of PGE_2 formation therefore leads to many of the most well known effects of the salicylates, namely their antiinflammatory, analgesic, and antipyretic properties.
  ▲ PGI_2 **(prostacyclin)** in endothelial cells
  - PGI_2 performs essentially the opposite role as TXA_2 (see Figure 16-5).

Aminosalicylates

- Although the **aminosalicylates** are related to salicylates in chemical structure, inhibition of prostaglandin (PG) synthesis is believed to play only a minor role, if any, in their efficacy in inflammatory bowel disease.
- Aminosalicylates appear to inhibit inflammatory cytokines. They appear to do this by inhibiting nuclear factor (NF)–κB, a transcription factor for inflammatory cytokines. Aminosalicylates are also peroxisome proliferator–activated receptor–gamma (PPAR-γ) agonists, and PPAR-γ is believed to play an important role in inflammation in ulcerative colitis.

PHARMACOKINETICS
Salicylates

- Salicylates are also readily absorbed from the skin. They are absorbed to such an extent that systemic poisoning can occur if the agent is applied topically to a large surface area.
- Metabolism of salicylates occurs through glucuronidation and by conjugation to salicyluric acid. A small proportion (approximately 10%) of salicylates is excreted as salicylic acid in the urine, although this proportion can increase with urine that has an alkaline pH and decrease with acidic pH.
- The elimination half-life of ASA is only 20 minutes; however, the salicylate component has a much longer half-life, which is dose dependent (low dose, 2 hours; analgesic dose, 12 hours; high or toxic dose, 15 to 30 hours).

Aminosalicylates

- Aminosalicylates appear to exert their actions directly at the colon and therefore must be delivered directly to the colon.
- These include attaching the drug to a chemical that is then cleaved in the colon, applying an enteric coating that does not dissolve until the drug reaches the distal small intestine, and using microspheres that slowly release drug beginning in the duodenum.
- A newer technology combines a pH-dependent release mechanism initially with a special coating that prolongs release of drug as it passes throughout the colon.

INDICATIONS
Salicylates

- Prevention of MI and ischemic stroke
- As an antiinflammatory, including in rheumatoid arthritis
- Analgesia
- As an antipyretic

Aminosalicylates

- Ulcerative colitis
- Crohn's disease

CONTRAINDICATIONS
Acetylsalicylic Acid

- **Hypersensitivity (allergy) to ASA.** Can be fatal.
- **Not for use in children.** Causes Reye's syndrome, an often fatal encephalopathy in children that has been associated with the use of ASA during viral infection.

SIDE EFFECTS
Salicylates

- **GI:** GI effects are caused by reduced levels of a PG (produced by COX-1) that protects the lining of the stomach. They can range in severity from upset stomach to GI bleeds and ulcers.
- **Bleeding** is caused by the antiplatelet effect.
- **Tinnitus:** Ringing of the ears is typically only seen at higher doses.

Aminosalicylates

- **GI**: nausea, vomiting, dyspepsia
- **Headache**
- **Hypersensitivity reactions**: Many aminosalicylates contain a sulfa moiety, and a number of patients are allergic to sulfur-containing drugs.

IMPORTANT NOTES

- Because the binding of ASA to the platelets is irreversible, the antiplatelet effect of ASA lasts for the lifespan of the platelet, which is about 5 to 7 days. Patients preparing for surgery must stop taking ASA 7 days before surgery.
- As with other NSAIDs, data from long-term epidemiologic studies suggest that ASA might prevent the development of colorectal cancer. The mechanism behind this protective effect has not been clearly established; however, COX is believed to mediate cell growth.
- Salicylates can stimulate respiration. They do this in two ways. Indirectly, they do this by increasing CO_2 production, which in turn leads to an increase in the depth of respiration as the body tries to exhale the excess CO_2. They also directly stimulate the respiratory center in the brain.
- Salicylate poisoning can therefore lead to severe acid-base disturbances. Stimulation of respiration leads to a respiratory alkalosis, which is compensated for by the kidneys (Figure 16-7).

Salicylates

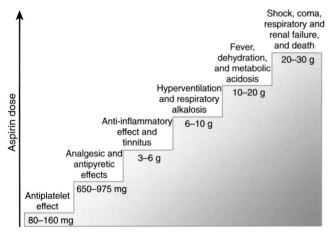

Figure 16-7.

- Diflunisal is a salicylate derivative that is a competitive COX inhibitor and appears to lack antipyretic effects. It appears to be a more potent analgesic and antiinflammatory than ASA.
- Many of the side effects of sulfasalazine have been attributed to the sulfapyridine component. Therefore later compounds were developed without the sulfapyridine group.
- Sulfasalazine may inhibit intestinal absorption of folate, and thus folate supplementation is typically indicated in patients taking sulfasalazine.

Advanced

- Salicylates are rapidly absorbed after oral administration. Despite the fact that salicylates are acids, and are therefore ionized in an alkaline environment, raising the pH of the stomach will enhance dissolution, and the net effect will be to enhance absorption. Therefore buffered preparations confer minimal advantage when it comes to rapid absorption.

EVIDENCE

Aspirin Alone or in Combination with Clopidogrel for Prevention of Cardiovascular Events

- A 2007 Cochrane review (two studies, N = 28,165 patients) compared the combination of clopidogrel and aspirin with aspirin alone for preventing cardiovascular events in patients at high risk for cardiovascular disease and those *with established* cardiovascular disease. The authors included two large trials. CHARISMA patients were at high risk for cardiovascular events, with or without established cardiovascular disease, whereas patients in CURE had had a recent non–ST-segment elevation acute coronary syndrome. In CHARISMA the benefit of combination therapy was minimal: five cardiovascular events avoided and three major bleeds for every 1000 patients over 28 months. In CURE the benefits were more obvious, with 23 events avoided and 10 major bleeds over 9 months.

Single-Dose Aspirin versus Placebo for Acute Pain

- A 1999 Cochrane review (72 trials, N = 3253 participants) compared a single dose of aspirin with placebo for acute pain of moderate to severe intensity. The number needed to treat (NNT) for at least 50% pain relief was 4.4 for 600- to 650-mg doses, 4.0 for a 1000-mg dose, and 2.4 for a 1200-mg dose. A single dose of aspirin produced more drowsiness (number needed to harm [NNH] 28) and gastric irritation (NNH 38) than placebo.

Aspirin for Prevention or Regression of Sporadic Colorectal Adenomas

- A 2004 Cochrane review (nine trials, N = 24,143 participants) examined the use of NSAIDs and aspirin for the prevention or regression of sporadic colorectal adenomas and colorectal cancer. Fewer patients treated with low-dose ASA developed recurrent sporadic colorectal adenomas after 1 to 3 years (NNT 12.5) compared with controls, and these results were driven by one large placebo-controlled study. There was no significant difference in the outcomes for colorectal cancer or for adverse events in any trials.

Aspirin versus Other Antiplatelets for Preventing Serious Vascular Events in High-Risk Patients

- A 2000 Cochrane review (four trials, N = 22,656 patients) compared the thienopyridines ticlopidine and clopidogrel with aspirin for the prevention of serious vascular events in high-risk patients, particularly those who had had previous TIA or ischemic stroke. Thienopyridines reduced the risk of a serious vascular event compared with aspirin, avoiding 11 events per 1000 patients over 2 years (OR 0.91). Thienopyridines also reduced the risk of stroke by seven events per 1000 patients over 2 years. This reduction in risk increased to 16 events per 1000 patients in individuals with a history of TIA or ischemic stroke. The thienopyridines reduced the risk of GI hemorrhage but increased the risk of skin rash and diarrhea versus aspirin. Ticlopidine also significantly increased the risk of neutropenia.

Maintenance of Remission in Ulcerative Colitis

■ A 2006 Cochrane review (16 studies, N = 2479) assessed the newer release formulations of 5-ASA versus placebo or sulfasalazine in the maintenance of remission in ulcerative colitis. Compared with placebo, the NNT for failure to maintain clinical or endoscopic remission was six. However, newer formulations of 5-ASA were less effective than sulfasalazine (OR 1.29). Although the incidence of side effects was similar with 5-ASA and with sulfasalazine, the authors noted that sulfasalazine trials enrolled patients who were already tolerating sulfasalazine, perhaps biasing the comparison of side effects in favor of sulfasalazine.

FYI

■ ASA originated from salicylic acid, derived from the bark of the willow tree. The use of salicylic acid dates back to ancient times, both in North America and in Europe, and its first *official* medical use was ascribed to Hippocrates. Chemists began synthesizing salicylic acid in the later nineteenth century. Salicylic acid had some significant GI side effects, and it was these side effects that led Hoffman, a chemist at Bayer, to acetylate the molecule and create what is still perhaps the most successful nonantibiotic in the history of pharmaceutical development.

■ ASA therapy is very inexpensive when compared with the other antiplatelets. Given that and its long history of use, it is a first-line agent in MI prevention.

■ ASA is more commonly referred to by its original brand name, *Aspirin*. The word *aspirin* has been in use for over a century and was derived from the name for another plant, the meadowsweet (*Spiraea ulmaria*), which has similar properties.

■ The aminosalicylates were originally developed as treatments for rheumatoid arthritis. In clinical trials it was noted that rheumatoid arthritis patients who also had ulcerative colitis appeared to experience greater benefit for their ulcerative colitis than for their rheumatoid arthritis.

Adenosine Diphosphate (ADP) Blockers

DESCRIPTION

Adenosine diphosphate (ADP) blockers inhibit platelet aggregation and/or release and are also known as the *thienopyridines*.

PROTOTYPE AND COMMON DRUGS

■ Prototype: ticlopidine
■ Others: clopidogrel, prasugrel, ticagrelor

MOA (MECHANISM OF ACTION)

■ Platelets are **activated** by adhering to damaged endothelium by linking of glycoprotein Ia (GPIa) receptors with collagen and GPIb receptors with von Willebrand factor (vWF). The activation of platelets leads to aggregation and clot formation.

■ Platelet activation leads to synthesis and release of mediators involved in platelet **aggregation**:
  ▲ TXA$_2$
  ▲ Serotonin (5-HT)
  ▲ **ADP**

■ Mediators such as ADP promote platelet aggregation by increasing GP receptor expression and promoting binding of fibrinogen to GPIIIa/IIb receptors. These actions are mediated by binding of ADP to the P2Y1 and P2Y12 receptors on platelets. Both P2Y1 and P2Y12 are receptors for ADP, and stimulation of both of these receptors is required for platelet activation.

■ **Ticlopidine, prasugrel,** and **clopidogrel** are **irreversible inhibitors of the P2Y12 receptors** and thus inhibit the ADP-dependent pathway of platelet activation and subsequent aggregation (Figure 16-8). Ticagrelor is a reversible inhibitor.

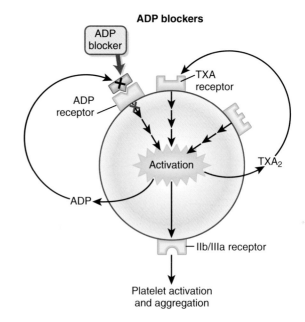

Figure 16-8.

PHARMACOKINETICS

■ Clopidogrel has a relatively slow onset of action, as it requires approximately 5 days to achieve a plateau in platelet inhibition.

■ Because clopidogrel, prasugrel, and ticlopidine are irreversible inhibitors of the ADP receptor, the biologic half-lives of these drugs are longer than their elimination half-lives. The effects of each drug will be notable until the body replenishes its supply of platelets, requiring approximately 5 to 7 days (the life span of a platelet).

INDICATIONS
- Prevention of ischemic stroke in patients intolerant to ASA
- Acute myocardial infarction

CONTRAINDICATIONS
- **Active bleeding**: These agents impair clotting and prolong bleeding.
- **Significant hepatic impairment**: Clopidogrel and ticlopidine agents need a functioning liver in order to be converted to their active metabolites. Hepatic complications have also been reported with both agents but are extremely rare.

Ticlopidine Only
- **Hematopoietic disorders**: See Side Effects.
- **Thrombotic thrombocytopenic purpura (TTP)**: See Side Effects.

SIDE EFFECTS
- Bleeding
- **Rash, diarrhea**: mechanism not known

Serious
- **Severe neutropenia** is a rare side effect associated with ticlopidine but not with clopidogrel. It necessitates discontinuation of the drug.
- **TTP** has been associated with ticlopidine and less commonly with clopidogrel.

IMPORTANT NOTES
- There is a significant range of responses to clopidogrel among patients. The extent of platelet inhibition can range from 5% to 90%, with patients at the lower end of the range (<10%) deemed to be "clopidogrel unresponsive." Genetic polymorphisms are thought to play a role in these variable responses, including alterations in the PGY12 receptor as well as CYP450 mutations.
- Several other ADP-targeting antiplatelet agents are in various stages of clinical development, in an effort to improve on the toxicity issues associated with ticlopidine and the slow onset and prolonged effect of clopidogrel.

Advanced
- TTP is a life-threatening disease caused by abnormal activation and aggregation of platelets because of vWF macromolecules. The platelets aggregate in vessels and form pathologic thrombi, resulting in hemolysis (and anemia), a decreased platelet count (from consumption), central nervous system (CNS) dysfunction or stroke, and renal compromise because of vascular occlusion and fever. These five findings comprise the pentad of TTP.

EVIDENCE
Adenosine Diphosphate Blockers versus Aspirin for Stroke Prevention in High-Risk Patients
- A 2000 Cochrane review (four trials, N = 22,656 patients) compared ADP inhibitors with aspirin for preventing serious vascular events in high-risk patients, including those who had had a prior TIA or ischemic stroke. One large trial (N = 19,185 patients) included clopidogrel, whereas the other three (N = 3471) included ticlopidine. Results suggested that ADP blockers would result in 11 fewer serious vascular events per 1000 patients treated over approximately 2 years. Strokes were also reduced, by seven events per 1000 patients.
- Risk of GI hemorrhage and other GI events was reduced with ADP blockers versus aspirin, but risk of skin rash and diarrhea was increased. The risk of skin rash and diarrhea was greater with ticlopidine than clopidogrel, and ticlopidine was also associated with a higher risk of neutropenia than clopidogrel.

Clopidogrel with or without Aspirin for Preventing Cardiovascular Disease
- A 2007 Cochrane review included two large studies (CHARISMA and CURE, N = 28,165 patients). CHARISMA patients were at high risk for cardiovascular disease but did not necessarily have established cardiovascular disease, whereas patients in CURE had had a recent non–ST-segment elevation acute coronary syndrome. The combination of clopidogrel and aspirin reduced the risk of cardiovascular events by 13 events for every 1000 patients treated; however, six major bleeds would be caused over the same number of patients.
- Results differed between studies, with benefit more evident in CURE (reduction of 23 events and increase of 10 major bleeds over an average of 9 months) than in CHARISMA (reduction of five events and increase of three major bleeds over an average of 28 months).

FYI
- Both ticlopidine and clopidogrel are considerably more expensive than aspirin.

Antiplatelet IIb/IIIa Inhibitors

DESCRIPTION
Antiplatelet IIb/IIIa inhibitors are antiplatelet drugs; they inhibit platelet function.

PROTOTYPE AND COMMON DRUGS
- Abciximab
- Eptifibatide and tirofiban

MOA (MECHANISM OF ACTION)

- IIb/IIIa receptors are located on the outside of platelets, in very high numbers (50,000 to 80,000 per cell); in the resting platelet they are inactive.
- Fibrinogen and vWF bind to IIb/IIIa receptors; once bound, they bind to foreign surfaces and also bridge other platelets to induce platelet **aggregation.**
- These drugs bind to the IIb/IIIa receptor complex on the platelet and prevent binding of endogenous ligands including fibrinogen and vWF, thus inhibiting aggregation of the platelet (Figure 16-9).

Antiplatelets IIb-IIIa

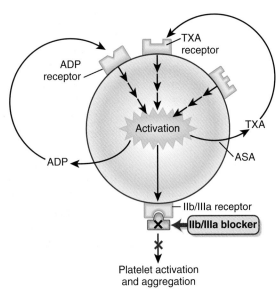

Figure 16-9.

PHARMACOKINETICS

- All drugs are administered intravenously.
- Abciximab has a half-life of 10 minutes, but the effect lasts 24 hours because although the drug is cleared from the blood, it is still bound to platelets.
- Eptifibatide has a half-life of 2 hours; its effects last for the duration of drug levels in the body.
- Tirofiban has a half-life of 2.5 hours; its effects last for the duration of drug levels in body.

INDICATIONS

- Coronary angioplasty
- High-risk patients with acute MI

CONTRAINDICATIONS

- High risk of bleeding, including but not limited to the following:
  - ▲ Recent surgery
  - ▲ Recent stroke
  - ▲ Thrombocytopenia (low platelet count)
  - ▲ Recent GI bleed

SIDE EFFECTS

- **Bleeding**
- **Thrombocytopenia** is the most serious complication. Thrombocytopenia is immune-mediated and occurs in 5% of patients but is severe in 1%.

IMPORTANT NOTES

- The three drugs in this class are all structurally very different:
  - ▲ Abciximab is a monoclonal antibody.
  - ▲ Eptifibatide is a cyclic heptapeptide (seven amino acids).
  - ▲ Tirofiban is a nonpeptide.

Advanced

- Glanzmann's thrombasthenia is a condition of deficient IIb/IIIa receptors and is a bleeding disorder.
- Abciximab is less specific for the receptors it binds; it also binds the vitronectin receptor, which regulates plasminogen activity.

EVIDENCE
Coronary Angioplasty

- A meta-analysis in 2007 (38 trials, N = 58,495 patients) demonstrated that with angioplasty compared with placebo, IIb/IIIa blockers decreased mortality at 30 days (OR 0.74) but not at 6 months. *Death or MI* was decreased both at 30 days (OR 0.67) and at 6 months (OR 0.71), although severe bleeding was increased (OR 1.38; absolute risk increase 8.6 per 1000).

Non–ST-Elevation Myocardial Infarction— No Angioplasty

- A meta-analysis in 2007 (38 trials, N = 58,495 patients) demonstrated that IIb/IIIa blockers did not decrease mortality at 30 days or at 6 months. *Death or MI* was decreased at 30 days (OR 0.92) and at 6 months (OR 0.88). Severe bleeding was increased (OR 1.27; absolute risk increase 1.2 per 1000).

Stroke

- A meta-analysis in 2006 (two studies, N = 414 patients) did not find statistically significant evidence for safety or efficacy of IIb/IIIa inhibitors for the treatment of ischemic stroke.

FYI

- Eptifibatide is based on a rattlesnake venom peptide, which is a toxin that produces coagulopathy.

Fibrinolytics

DESCRIPTION

Fibrinolytics lyse (break up) blood clots. They are also called *clot busters* and *thrombolytics*.

PROTOTYPES AND COMMON DRUGS

- There are two major subclasses.

Fibrin Selective

- Prototype: al**teplase** (also known as recombinant tissue plasminogen activator, or rtPA)
- Others: re**teplase**, tenec**teplase**

Nonselective

- Prototype: strepto**kinase**
- Other: uro**kinase**

MOA (MECHANISM OF ACTION)

- These agents are *plasminogen activators* and cleave **plasminogen** to form **plasmin** (Figure 16-10).
- Plasmin is a protease that digests fibrin (a *fibrinolytic*). Fibrin is a fibrous protein that forms a mesh, providing structural rigidity to a clot. The mesh is created by the cross-linking of fibrin.
- Tissue plasminogen activator is found in the body. It is a serine protease that is released from endothelial cells in response to injury. Its physiologic purpose is to gradually dissolve clots that have formed because of injury. Urokinase is also secreted endogenously and serves the same purpose, although it has some important differences, especially selectivity of action.

- The plasminogen activators can work either in the presence (alteplase, reteplase) or absence (streptokinase, urokinase) of fibrin.
- The physiologic advantage of requiring fibrin for activity is that the fibrinolytic effects will be (mainly) localized to the clot.
- The thrombolytics that do not need fibrin to enhance their activity will activate both bound and circulating plasmin. In addition to fibrin, plasmin also degrades fibrinogen and some clotting factors; thus circulating coagulation factors will be depleted. Therefore these agents are not considered to be "clot specific," and this *in theory* may make them less safe to use than agents that need fibrin to work optimally.

PHARMACOKINETICS

- The agents in this class are all administered intravenously.
- They all have short elimination half-lives, most around 15 to 20 minutes, although the half-life of alteplase is only 5 minutes. Because of its short half-life, alteplase is typically delivered by infusion after an initial IV bolus, whereas the longer-acting agents can be given with repeat bolus injections.

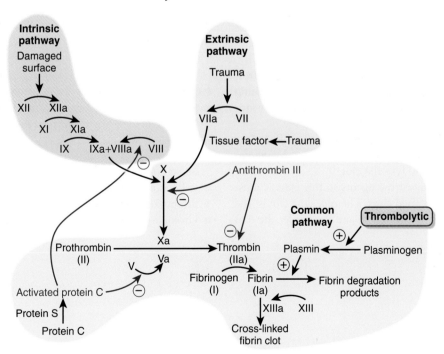

Fibrinolytics

Figure 16-10.

- Tenecteplase demonstrates biphasic clearance, meaning that it is eliminated in two phases. Therefore its total elimination half-life may be as long as 2 hours.
- These drugs are sometimes trickled in through a long catheter right to the site of a pathologic thrombus so that the concentration of drug is high at the site of the thrombus but low(er) in all other areas of the body.

INDICATIONS

- Acute ST elevation myocardial infarction (STEMI)
- Massive pulmonary embolus
- Thrombotic stroke (very specific criteria must be met)

CONTRAINDICATIONS

- Any potential source for major bleeding, including the following:
  - Prior hemorrhagic stroke
  - Active internal bleeding
  - Recent surgery

SIDE EFFECTS

- **Hemorrhage** is such a major concern that these drugs are used only when very strict criteria are met, because the risk of bleeding can outweigh the benefit of thrombolysis.
- **Hypersensitivity: Streptokinase** and **urokinase** are both antigenic.

IMPORTANT NOTES

- There are advantages and disadvantages to using streptokinase versus rt-PA. rt-PA is more *clot selective* than urokinase or streptokinase, as it does a poor job of activating plasminogen in the absence of fibrin. However streptokinase is much cheaper than rt-PA. Streptokinase also elicits an immune response that can harm the patient.
- The use of streptokinase results in the patient developing antibodies to the drug. If a patient receives streptokinase and subsequently requires repeat fibrinolytic therapy (days to months later), then reteplase should be used.
- Tenecteplase is more fibrin specific than alteplase. It is therefore believed to be less likely to elicit serious bleeding than alteplase, which is the major side effect of concern for drugs in this class.
- Reteplase is believed to work faster than alteplase. Reteplase appears to diffuse more quickly throughout the clot, allowing it to more efficiently lyse the clot.
- Thrombolysis with any of the agents in this class is most successful on newly formed clots. The older the clot is, the more established the fibrin *mesh* is, and the harder the clot

is to dissolve. Therefore time is of the essence when using fibrinolytics. Patients with MI appear to benefit most if they receive therapy within 6 hours of symptoms.

EVIDENCE

Thrombolytics versus Heparin or Placebo for Treatment of Acute Pulmonary Embolism

- A 2009 Cochrane review (eight trials, N = 679 participants) compared thrombolytics with placebo or heparin in patients with acute PE. The rates of mortality, PE recurrence, major hemorrhagic events, and minor hemorrhagic events were similar between thrombolytics and heparin. In one study that examined combination therapy, the use of rt-PA combined with heparin versus heparin alone reduced the need for further treatment for in-hospital events (OR 0.35).

Thrombolytics for Treatment of Ischemic Stroke

- A 2009 Cochrane review (26 trials, N = 7152 participants) compared thrombolytics with controls in patients with definite ischemic stroke. Although thrombolytics reduced the proportion of patients who were dead or dependent at 3 to 6 months after stroke (OR 0.81), they increased the risk of symptomatic intracranial hemorrhage (OR 3.49) and death by 3 to 6 months after stroke (OR 1.31).

Thrombolytics versus Angioplasty in Myocardial Infarction

- A 2003 systematic review (23 trials, N = 7739 participants) compared percutaneous transluminal coronary angioplasty (PTCA) with thrombolytics for acute STEMI. There were fewer overall deaths in the short term with PTCA compared with thrombolytics (incidence of 7% versus 9%, respectively), and also a lower incidence of nonfatal reinfarction (3% versus 7%) and stroke (1% versus 2%) with PTCA versus thrombolytics. The results for PTCA continued to be better than thrombolytics during long-term follow-up.

FYI

- Hemorrhage is a particular problem with agents displaying less specificity for newly formed thrombi (streptokinase and urokinase).
- Thrombolytics are all very expensive but have proven to be an effective method for treating acute MI.
- rt-PA is often simply called *tPA*.
- Streptokinase is produced by β-hemolytic streptococci.
- Urokinase was originally extracted from urine.

Erythropoietins

DESCRIPTION
Erythropoietins are agents that stimulate the production of red blood cells (RBCs).

PROTOTYPE AND COMMON DRUGS
- Prototype: epoetin alfa (also known as recombinant human erythropoietin, rHuEPO or simply, EPO)
- Other: darbepoetin alfa

MOA (MECHANISM OF ACTION)
- Erythropoietin is an endogenous protein that **stimulates the production of RBCs** (erythrocytes). Erythropoietin is typically released in response to hypoxia and is largely synthesized in the kidneys, with a small amount coming from the liver (Figure 16-11).

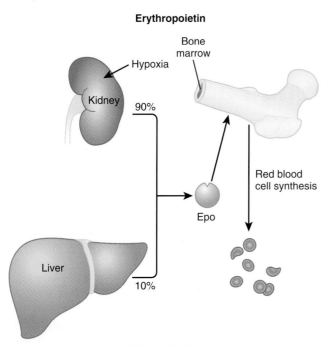

Erythropoietin

Figure 16-11.

- Patients with a deficiency of erythropoietin will be anemic. This occurs commonly in patients with renal failure.
- Once released, erythropoietin binds to a receptor on the surface of committed erythroid progenitor cells in the bone marrow. Binding to this receptor mediates a variety of intracellular effects through tyrosine kinases, including the inhibition of apoptosis. Inhibiting apoptosis prevents RBCs from dying at an early stage of development. Erythropoietin also promotes proliferation through Janus protein kinase-2 (JAK2) pathways.

PHARMACOKINETICS
- Epoetin alpha is administered parenterally by either the SC or the IV route. The elimination half-life of IV Epoetin alpha is approximately 4 to 8 hours.

- Darbepoetin alfa is a modified form of erythropoietin, with amino acid mutations that have led to a prolonged elimination half-life of approximately 24 hours.

INDICATIONS
- **Anemia:**
  - ▲ In **advanced renal failure**
  - ▲ Associated with **chemotherapy** and **acquired immunodeficiency syndrome (AIDS)**

CONTRAINDICATIONS
- **Uncontrolled hypertension:** See Side Effects.

SIDE EFFECTS
- **Iron deficiency:** If iron stores cannot keep up with erythropoiesis, patients may develop a functional iron deficiency. Patients on chronic erythropoietin therapy will likely need an iron supplement.
- **Thrombosis:** Serious thromboembolic events have been reported, particularly in patients on dialysis. It is recommended that these patients receive anticoagulant therapy as a prophylactic measure.
- **Hypertension:** Treatment with erythropoietins can lead to an increase in blood pressure. Although increased hematocrit can lead to increased blood pressure, the mechanism is believed to be more likely a result of the interaction between erythropoietin and vasoactive factors such as angiotensin II.
- **Seizures:** Seizures have been reported in dialysis patients receiving epoetin alfa.

IMPORTANT NOTES
- Some formulations of erythropoietin contain benzyl alcohol, which has been shown to be toxic to premature infants.
- A link between cancer and erythropoietin use has been proposed. Some studies in certain cancers have reported an increased risk of death and/or worsening of condition with erythropoietin use. Erythropoietin appears to act through receptors similar to those of growth factors associated with neoplasia, although these problems do not appear to be associated with all cancers.
- Hematocrit is frequently monitored during therapy with the erythropoietins. Erythrocytes have a long half-life; therefore the results of any dose adjustments made in response to hematocrit would not be seen for 2 to 6 weeks.

EVIDENCE
Recombinant Human Erythropoietin in Predialysis Patients with Anemia
- A 2005 Cochrane review (15 trials, N = 461 participants) compared the use of rHuEPO with no treatment or placebo

in *predialysis* patients with renal anemia. rHuEPO significantly improved hemoglobin and hematocrit and significantly reduced the number of patients requiring blood transfusions (relative risk [RR] 0.32). Quality of life and exercise capacity were also improved, where reported. rHuEPO did not appear to have an effect on the progression of renal disease, and there was no increase in the incidence of adverse events with rHuEPO therapy.

Recombinant Human Erythropoietin in Preventing Transfusion in Premature Infants

■ A 2006 Cochrane review (19 studies, N = 912 infants) compared rHuEPO with placebo or no treatment in reducing the use of RBC transfusions in preterm and/or low–birth-weight infants. The authors found that rHuEPO reduced the risk of having one or more transfusions (typical RR 0.66 [0.59 to 0.74]). rHuEPO also reduced the average volume of blood transfused per infant by 7 mL and the average number of transfusions per infant; however, the clinical significance of these small differences was questioned by the authors. Several hard outcomes such as mortality, hypertension, and numerous other complications were not affected by therapy.

Darbepoetin or Epoetin in Anemia Associated with Cancer Treatment

■ A 2006 Cochrane review (57 trials, N = 9353 participants) assessed darbepoetin and epoetin in the prevention or treatment of anemia in cancer patients. Both agents reduced the risk of transfusions (RR 0.64 [0.60 to 0.68]) and resulted in a requirement for an average of one less unit of blood. However, the risk of thromboembolic events was increased (RR 1.67 [1.35 to 2.06]). The authors were not able to conclude whether these agents have an impact on tumor response or overall survival.

FYI

■ The chemical structure of epoetin alfa differs slightly from that of human endogenous erythropoietin. Although this difference does not have any clinical relevance, it has proven useful in trying to detect athletes who have been using epoetin alfa for *blood doping*. This is a practice by which athletes will try to stimulate an artificial increase in hematocrit before a competition to increase the oxygen-carrying capacity of their blood, presumably enhancing performance.

Colony-Stimulating Factors

DESCRIPTION
Colony-stimulating factors (CSFs) are agents that stimulate the production of neutrophils and monocytes.

PROTOTYPE AND COMMON DRUGS
Granulocyte Colony-Stimulating Factor (G-CSF)
■ Prototype: filgrastim
■ Other: pegfilgrastim

Granulocyte-Monocyte Colony-Stimulating Factor (GM-CSF)
■ Prototype: sargramostim

MOA (MECHANISM OF ACTION)
■ Neutropenia is a common and serious side effect of cytotoxic cancer chemotherapy. Cytotoxic agents preferentially target rapidly dividing cells, including those of the bone marrow. The major complication of neutropenia is a reduced immune response, greatly increasing the probability of developing infections of both "normal" and opportunistic microbes.
■ The CSFs work by binding to receptors on myeloid progenitor cells. These are cells in the bone marrow that make RBCs, platelets, granulocytes, and monocytes. The actions of these receptors are mediated through the Janus protein kinase/signal transducers and activators of transcription (JAK/STAT) pathway.
■ G-CSFs stimulate proliferation and differentiation *only* of progenitors commited to becoming neutrophils.

■ GM-CSFs stimulate the production of *neutrophils and monocytes*, as well as the actions (phagocytosis, superoxide production, and cell-mediated toxicity) of neutrophils, monocytes, and eosinophils (Figure 16-12).

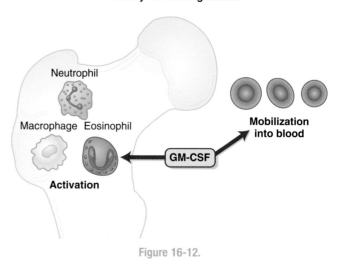

Colony stimulating factors

Figure 16-12.

PHARMACOKINETICS
■ The elimination half-life of filgrastim is 3 to 5 hours and is fairly consistent between the IV and SC routes. It is largely cleared through renal excretion.

- The addition of a polyethylene glycol (PEG) to filgrastim produced pegfilgrastim, which because of its large size is not as readily cleared by the kidneys. Pegfilgrastim therefore has an extended elimination half-life of about 40 hours, compared with filgrastim.

INDICATIONS

- Adjunct to myelosuppressive chemotherapy
- Severe chronic neutropenia
- Prevention and treatment of neutropenia in human immunodeficiency virus (HIV) infection

CONTRAINDICATIONS

- None of major significance

SIDE EFFECTS

- **Bone loss:** G-CSF increases osteoclast activity, leading to bone resorption.
- **Joint pain:** G-CSF appears to stimulate cytokine release, leading to joint pain.
- **Renal dysfunction:** G-CSF causes a transient and reversible renal impairment, believed to be caused by leukostasis (clumping of leukocytes) in the kidneys.
- **Acute respiratory distress:** G-CSF can lead to lung injury because of accumulation and activation of neutrophils in the lungs.

- **Splenomegaly or splenic rupture:** Cases of splenic rupture have been reported with G-CSF.
- **Sickle cell crises:** Sometimes fatal, sickle cell crises occur in patients with sickle cell disorders.

EVIDENCE
Colony-Stimulating Factor in Children with Acute Lymphocytic Leukemia

- A 2005 Cochrane review (six studies, N = 332 patients) looked at safety and effectiveness of adjunctive G-CSF or GM-CSF in children with acute lymphocytic leukemia (ALL). There was not enough data to assess survival. CSF significantly reduced the number of episodes of febrile neutropenia, length of hospitalization, and number of infectious disease episodes. CSF did not affect the length of neutropenia episodes or delays in chemotherapy episodes.

FYI

- The CSFs are also referred to as *myeloid growth factors*. The term *myeloid* is associated with bone marrow, which is the site of action of these agents.

B Vitamins

DESCRIPTION
B vitamins is the collective name for a series of supplements.

PROTOTYPE

- B_1: thiamine
- B_2: riboflavin
- B_3: niacin
- B_6: pyridoxine
- B_9: folic acid
- B_{12}: cyanocobalamin, hydroxocobalamin

MOA (MECHANISM OF ACTION)
Vitamin B_1

- Vitamin B_1 is converted to **thiamine** in the body and is a coenzyme in carbohydrate metabolism, including the decarboxylation of pyruvic acid. Increased pyruvic acid levels are therefore indicative of vitamin B_1 deficiency. Deficiency can lead to damage in regions of the brain, including the thalamus, midbrain, and brainstem, and this appears to be mediated, at least in part, by oxidative stress. This brain damage manifests as Wernicke-Korsakoff syndrome, a condition associated with alcoholism (Figure 16-13).

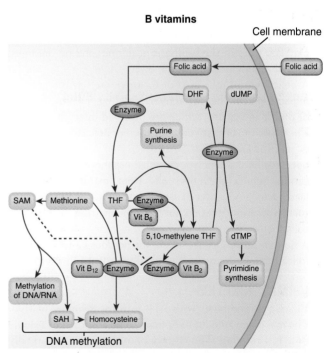

B vitamins

Figure 16-13. SAM = S-adenosylmethionine; SAH = S-adenosylhomocysteine; THF = tetrahydrofolate; dUMP = deoxyuracilmonophosphate; dTMP = deoxythyminemonophosphate

Vitamin B$_2$

- The two coenzyme forms of vitamin B$_2$ (riboflavin-5-phosphate and flavin adenine dinucleotide) play a role in adenosine triphosphate (ATP) production, through the metabolism of carbohydrates, fats, and proteins. Deficiency typically manifests as fissures in lips or cracks in the mouth, swelling of the tongue, or seborrheic dermatitis. Normochromic-normocytic anemias can also occur, as well as peripheral neuropathy.

Niacin (Vitamin B$_3$)

- Niacin is converted in vivo to nicotinic adenine dinucleotide (NAD) and nicotinamide adenine dinucleotide phosphate (NADP). These metabolites serve as coenzymes for a number of reactions involving lipid and protein metabolism, as well as anaerobic reactions in the Krebs cycle.
- Niacin binds to a G protein–coupled receptor in adipocytes and inhibits lipolysis in adipose tissue. This reduces the supply of free fatty acids, and because the liver uses free fatty acids to produce triglycerides, which are then used in very low-density lipoprotein (VLDL) synthesis, VLDL is reduced. Accordingly, niacin decreases low-density lipoprotein (LDL) and also increases high-density lipoprotein (HDL) by reducing its catabolism.

Vitamin B$_6$

- Vitamin B$_6$ is converted to the coenzyme pyridoxal-5-phosphate (PLP), which plays a role in amino acid and fatty metabolism. Of note, B$_6$ facilitates the metabolism of tryptophan to niacin, methionine to cysteine, and glutamic acid to γ-aminobutyric acid (GABA).

Vitamin B$_{12}$ and Folic Acid

- Vitamin B$_{12}$ and folic acid play key roles in **DNA synthesis**. Active forms of folic acid serve as enzyme cofactors that play key roles in the synthesis of purines and pyrimidines, as well as amino acids, in the body.
- A deficiency of folic acid or B$_{12}$ therefore has the greatest impact on cells that are actively dividing, such as the cells of the bone marrow, which are involved in erythropoiesis. Therefore the primary complication of deficiencies of these vitamins is **anemia.**
- Specifically, B$_{12}$ deficiency results in abnormal DNA replication, which prevents cells from maturing properly, leading to production of large, dysfunctional RBC precursors (*megaloblasts*) that do not leave the marrow, or abnormal cells that do leave the marrow.
- A B$_{12}$ deficiency can also affect the nervous system, causing inflammation, demyelination, and neuronal cell death.

PHARMACOKINETICS

- Vitamin B$_1$ combines with ATP to form thiamine in vivo. The maximum amount of B$_1$ that can be absorbed in a single dose is 4 to 8 mg. The absorption of thiamine is markedly reduced in alcoholics and in those with folate deficiency.
- Vitamin B$_1$ is stored in the body, in heart, liver, skeletal muscle, kidneys, and brain. It undergoes hepatic metabolism and is excreted by the kidneys. Large doses of vitamin B$_1$ may simply be renally excreted.
- Vitamin B$_2$ absorption occurs by active transport in the upper ileum, and this transport mechanism is saturable (maximum of 20 to 25 mg vitamin B$_2$ can be absorbed in a single dose). It is widely distributed to tissues, but very little is stored. Riboflavin is excreted in urine unchanged.
- Niacin (B$_3$) is converted to niacinamide in the liver. This conversion is saturable, so when patients take higher doses for an antihyperlipidemic effect, much of the niacin is not converted to niacinamide and instead is excreted unchanged in urine. Niacinamide is widely distributed and undergoes further hepatic metabolism before being excreted in urine.
- Vitamin B$_6$ absorption is not via active transport, and therefore is not saturable. It is stored, and its metabolite is excreted in urine.
- Gastric intrinsic factor facilitates the absorption of vitamin B$_{12}$, and absorption is also pH sensitive. **Intrinsic factor** is secreted by parietal cells, so patients who have had gastric surgery or some other disruption of their parietal cells may have a relative deficiency of intrinsic factor and thus a vitamin B$_{12}$ deficiency. These patients can be treated with intramuscular injections of B$_{12}$, which bypasses the need for intrinsic factor.
- After ingestion, folic acid is converted to its active form, tetrahydrofolate, by the liver.

INDICATIONS
Vitamin B$_{12}$

- Pernicious anemia
- Megaloblastic and macrocytic anemias caused by poor B$_{12}$ absorption

Folic Acid

- Megaloblastic and macrocytic anemias
- Prevention of neural tube defects in neonates
- Adjunct to methotrexate to prevent methotrexate toxicity
- Pernicious anemia (combined with B$_{12}$)

Pyridoxine

- Sideroblastic anemias (particularly those secondary to isoniazid and pyrazinamide)

Thiamine

- Prophylaxis for B$_1$ deficiency: beriberi, Wernicke's encephalopathy

Riboflavin

- No specific indication other than treatment of deficiency; typically adjunctively with other B vitamins

Niacin

- Hypercholesterolemia

CONTRAINDICATIONS

- None of major significance

SIDE EFFECTS

- The B vitamins are generally well tolerated.
- Adverse effects can be seen at high doses (15 mg daily) of folic acid, although these are well above the recommended daily intake, which is typically 1 mg or less.

Niacin

- At the recommended daily intake, niacin is well tolerated; however, when used as an antihyperlipidemic, it is often used at high doses, which can result in the following:
  - ▲ **Flushing** is caused by vasodilation of cutaneous vessels, typically accompanied by pruritus and tingling. This is believed to be caused by cutaneous PG release and can be mitigated by pretreatment with aspirin or by use of a sustained-release formulation of niacin.
  - ▲ **Hepatic dysfunction** can increase serum transaminase and cause hepatitis.
  - ▲ **GI** effects include nausea and abdominal discomfort.
  - ▲ **Reduced glucose tolerance** is an infrequent, typically reversible side effect whose mechanism has not been established.

IMPORTANT NOTES

- B_{12} preparations are available that contain intrinsic factor from animal sources. Although these might be useful initially in patients with intrinsic factor deficiency, patients typically become less responsive to the intrinsic factor, perhaps because of an antibody response launched against the animal protein.
- Folinic acid, also known as leucovorin, is a reduced form of folic acid. It is used as *rescue* therapy in patients who are being treated with **methotrexate**. Methotrexate is an *antifolate* drug, and patients who are on high doses or chronic therapy are likely to experience severe symptoms of folate deficiency unless they are treated adjunctively with leucovorin.
- Folic acid alone will not be effective in treating pernicious anemia, as it does not address the neurologic complications. If used in pernicious anemia, folic acid should be given as an adjunct to vitamin B_{12}.
- Pyridoxine is used as an antidote for overdoses. See Table 16-1.
- Although vitamin B_3 can be sourced from the diet, concentrations of niacin in foods are not high enough to have an antihyperlipidemic effect. That is why patients who are using niacin to reduce cholesterol will take high doses of niacin supplements.

EVIDENCE
Folic Acid with or without Vitamin B_{12} for Cognition

- A 2008 Cochrane review (eight studies, N = 1317 participants) examined the effects of folic acid supplementation, with or without vitamin B_{12}, on healthy elderly or demented participants, in preventing cognitive impairment or slowing its progress. The authors found no evidence that folic acid, with or without B_{12}, has a positive impact on mood and cognitive function in healthy elderly people.
- However, one trial enrolled healthy elderly people with elevated homocysteine levels and found a significant improvement in global functioning, memory storage, and information-processing speed.
- The evidence for the use of folic acid in patients with cognitive disorders is scant, with only one small study showing a benefit when combined with cholinesterase inhibitors in Alzheimer's disease.

FYI

- Cyanocobalamin and hydroxocobalamin are synthetic forms of vitamin B_{12}.
- The discovery of vitamin B_{12} as a treatment for pernicious anemia began with an experiment in the 1920s in which patients with this condition were fed large quantities of raw liver. A few years later, it was discovered that patients whose stomachs had been removed did not respond to the liver "cure." It was hypothesized that an "intrinsic factor" must be secreted by the stomach to facilitate the absorption of the yet-unnamed curative "extrinsic factor." This extrinsic factor was later isolated from the liver, and named vitamin B_{12}.
- The preferred source of B vitamins for daily supplementation is from the diet. Food sources and recommended intakes are summarized in Table 16-2.

	TABLE 16-1. Agents That Use Pyridoxine As an Antidote	
Overdose Agent	**Mechanism of Toxicity**	**Mechanism of Pyridoxine as Antidote**
Isoniazid (INH)	Seizures INH depletes pyridoxal-5-phosphate (P5P), a cofactor in conversion of glutamic acid to γ-aminobutyric acid (GABA). This leads to increased glutamic acid (excitatory) and reduced GABA (inhibitory).	Pyridoxine replenishes P5P.
Mushrooms (false morel)	Seizures Similar mechanism to INH–enhanced glutamic acid, reduced GABA because of depleted P5P.	Pyridoxine replenishes P5P.
Ethanol	Ethanol is primarily converted to acetaldehyde, a toxic metabolite.	Pyridoxine accelerates the metabolism of ethanol, reducing exposure time to acetaldehyde.

TABLE 16-2. Sources and Recommended Dietary Intakes for Various B Vitamins

Vitamin	Recommended Dietary Allowances	Sources
B_1 (thiamine)	Infants: 0.2-0.3 mg Children: 0.5-0.9 mg Adults: 1.0-1.2 mg	Fortified breads, cereals, pasta, whole grains (especially wheat germ), lean meats (especially pork), fish, dried beans, peas, and soybeans
B_2 (riboflavin)	Infants: 0.3-0.4 mg Children: 0.5-0.9 mg Adults: 1.0-1.3 mg Pregnancy: 1.4 mg Lactation: 1.6 mg	Dairy, eggs, enriched cereals and grains, meats, liver, and green vegetables (such as asparagus or broccoli)
B_3 (niacin)		Meats, fish, legumes, whole grains
B_6 (pyridoxine)	Infants: 0.1-0.3 mg Children: 0.5-1.0 mg Adults: 1.3-1.7 mg	Cereal grains, legumes, vegetables (carrots, spinach, peas), potatoes, milk, cheese, eggs, fish, liver, meats, and flour
B_9 (folate)	Infants: 65-80 mcg Children: 150-300 mcg Adults: 400 mcg (men, women over age 50) 800 mcg (women under age 50)	Asparagus, avocados, cantaloupe, strawberries, oranges, legumes, and fortified cereals and grains
B_{12} (cyanocobalamin)	Infants: 0.4-0.5 mcg Children: 0.9-1.8 mcg Adults: 2.4 mcg Pregnancy: 2.6 mcg Lactation: 2.8 mcg	Dairy, eggs, fish, liver, meats, chicken, and fortified cereals

Iron

DESCRIPTION
Iron formulations are used for treatment of iron deficiency.

PROTOTYPES AND COMMON DRUGS
Oral
- Prototype: ferrous sulfate
- Others: ferrous fumarate, ferrous gluconate, polysaccharide-iron complex

IV
- Prototype: iron dextran
- Others: Sodium ferric gluconate, iron sucrose

MOA (MECHANISM OF ACTION)
- Most iron is recycled through the body; RBCs contain the majority of iron in hemoglobin. Because the life span of an RBC is about 120 days, in 1 day about 0.8% of the RBCs are broken down, and their iron is recycled:
  - ▲ Senescent (old) RBCs are taken up by the reticular system (spleen and macrophages) and are relieved of their iron (Figure 16-14).
  - ▲ The iron is bound to **ferritin** (the main cellular *storage* protein), and a smaller amount is stored as protein deposits called **hemosiderin.**
  - ▲ Iron that is released is transported by **transferrin** (the *transport* protein).
  - ▲ Transferrin delivers the iron to either the liver for storage or to bone marrow for further hemoglobin and RBC production.

- Iron that is lost from the body must be replaced, which is usually accomplished through diet, but abnormal states overwhelm the dietary iron and supplemental iron is required.

PHARMACOKINETICS
- Ferrous iron (Fe^{2+}) is better absorbed than ferric iron (Fe^{3+}) and is absorbed in the duodenum. About 25% of ferrous iron is absorbed.
- Iron from animals (heme iron) is ferrous; iron from vegetarian foods (nonheme iron) is ferric, and so a smaller percentage is available for absorption.
- Iron should be taken on an empty stomach; many foods inhibit iron absorption. Other factors that markedly decrease absorption include antacids, H_2 blockers, proton pump antagonists, and calcium supplements.
- Most ingested iron either is not absorbed or is lost with the enterocytes when their turnover results in shedding into the lumen of the GI tract.
- Some oral compounds are combined with ascorbic acid, which is designed to enhance absorption.

INDICATIONS
- **Iron deficiency anemia:**
  - ▲ Parenteral (IV) iron is indicated for patients who are noncompliant or unable to tolerate oral iron. treatment and prevention

CONTRAINDICATION
- Anaphylaxis-like reactions to the IV formulations

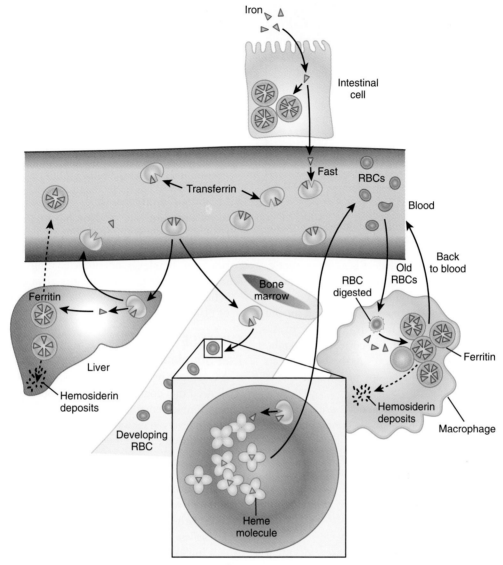

Figure 16-14.

SIDE EFFECTS
Oral Administration

- **GI symptoms** are common and dose related: nausea, epigastric discomfort, abdominal cramps, constipation, and diarrhea. These signs and symptoms can be reduced by lowering the daily dose.
- **Black stool** can confound the ability to diagnose GI bleeding.

Intravenous Administration

- **Anaphylaxis-like reactions** occur in 0.7% of patients taking iron dextran. Chest pain, wheezing, and a fall in blood pressure mandate immediate termination of the infusion and a call for the emergency medical team.
  - ▲ Iron sucrose results in a much lower incidence of anaphylaxis-like reactions.

IMPORTANT NOTES

- Free inorganic iron is extremely toxic; therefore iron is quickly bound by transferrin and subsequently stored in the body in the form of hemoglobin, myoglobin, ferritin, and, to a small degree, transferrin. Hemoglobin and myoglobin constitute about 80% of all stored iron.
- Iron deficiency is caused by the following:
  - ▲ Malnutrition
  - ▲ Any chronic blood loss
    - • Menstruation, GI bleeding
    - • Cancers
  - ▲ Increased utilization:
    - • Pregnancy
    - • Recombinant erythropoietin administration: common in patients with renal failure caused by abnormally low erythropoietin production by the peritubular capillary endothelial cells in the kidney

TABLE 16-3. Laboratory Measurements Used for Diagnosis of Iron Deficiency

Hemoglobin	Low
Serum iron: measure of iron bound to serum ferritin	Low
Ferritin: ferritin level correlates with total body iron stores	Low
Total iron binding capacity (TIBC): refers to the number of *unoccupied* binding sites on transferrin and is determined by both the iron levels and the transferrin levels	High
Transferrin percent saturation: percent of iron bound to transferrin; a calculated value based on serum iron and TIBC	Low
Bone marrow iron	Low

■ Iron deficiency results in small, pale RBCs: **microcyctic**, **hypochromic** anemia. RBC size is measured by the mean cell volume (**MCV**).

■ A number of laboratory measurements can be used for the diagnosis of iron deficiency. See Table 16-3.

■ The goal of iron therapy is twofold: to correct the anemia, and to correct the deficient iron stores in the body. It can take 6 to 12 months of oral iron therapy to correct the iron stores.

■ The hemoglobin should increase by about 2 g/dL (20 g/L) after 3 weeks of therapy in a normally responding patient.

■ Foods with high iron content include the following:
  ▲ Tofu, beans, lentils, asparagus, broccoli, eggs
  ▲ Red and white meats: pork, beef, chicken, turkey (livers are very high)
  ▲ Many seafoods: clams (highest), oysters, mussels, sardines, shrimp
  ▲ Enriched cereals, pastas, oatmeals

■ **Iron toxicity** occurs in iron storage diseases including hemochromatosis and hemosiderosis, as well as iron-loading anemias such as thalassemia.

■ **Iron toxicity** is treated with phlebotomy (removing blood) and iron chelators **deferoxamine** (parenteral), **deferasirox** (oral), and **deferiprone** (oral but not available in the United States). Phlebotomy is not indicated when the patient is anemic or being treating for anemia. Chelators are discussed further in Chapter 7.

Advanced

■ **Myelodysplastic syndrome** (a bone marrow disease resulting in abnormal blood counts) can produce a microcytic hypochromic anemia. However, iron storage measurements are not low, and this is not an iron deficiency state. It is an abnormality of iron utilization in the bone marrow.

■ **Thalassemia** is a hemoglobinopathy (hemoglobin disease) that also results in a microcytic hypochromic anemia with a normal iron profile.

■ Transferrin saturation percent is calculated as follows:

$$\text{Serum iron} \times 100 \div \text{Total iron binding capacity (TIBC)}$$

■ Hypothyroidism can lower ferritin levels; infection or states of inflammation can increase ferritin because it is an *acute phase reactant*.

■ Oral iron preparations with other additives, polysaccharide-iron complexes, or enteric coatings or sustained-release forms probably do not offer any advantages beyond those achieved by reducing the dose or timing of administration of plain ferrous salts.

EVIDENCE
Iron Supplementation in Pregnancy

■ A Cochrane review in 2009 (49 studies, N = 23,200 women) showed that compared with placebo or no treatment, daily iron supplementation was associated with increased hemoglobin levels in maternal blood both before and after birth and reduced risk of anemia at term.

FYI

■ Nomenclature:
  ▲ *Myelo* refers to bone marrow. *Dysplasia* means abnormal growth.
  ▲ *Thallasa* is Greek for the sea. Mediterranean natives have a high incidence of thalassemia.

■ Ferroxidase oxidizes iron from Fe^{2+} to Fe^{3+}; ferrireductase reduces iron from Fe^{3+} to Fe^{2+}.

■ Dextran is a branched complex polysaccharide made of glucose molecules.

■ Deferasirox is a newer treatment for iron overload.

■ *Hemosiderin-laden macrophages* are a finding seen with bronchoalveolar washing, in conditions that cause chronic bleeding in the lungs.

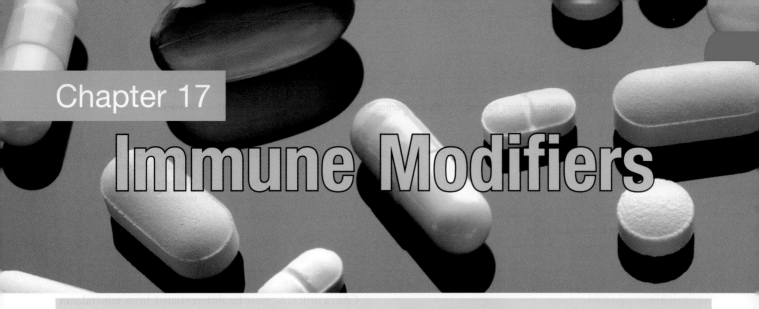

Chapter 17

Immune Modifiers

Systemic Steroids

DESCRIPTION

Steroids as used in this section refers to glucocorticoids that are administered systemically. Inhaled, topically administered, and injected steroids are described in other sections.

PROTOTYPE AND COMMON DRUGS

- Prototype: prednisone
- Others: cortisone, hydrocortisone, methylprednisolone, dexamethasone, triamcinolone

MOA (MECHANISM OF ACTION)

- Cortisol is the endogenous glucocorticoid and is synthesized from cholesterol. The hypothalamus secretes corticotropin-releasing hormone (**CRH**), which stimulates the anterior pituitary to release adrenocorticotropic hormone (**ACTH**), which acts on the adrenal glands to produce cortisol.
- Cortisol acts in the nucleus of the cell; therefore it must first diffuse through the cell membrane. It is bound in the cytoplasm with heat shock protein and other proteins and transported into the nucleus.
- Steroid receptors located in the nucleus are called **glucocorticoid receptor elements**. They regulate transcription of DNA by acting on **promoters**, which are specific DNA sites where RNA polymerase binds and starts transcription.
- Steroids exert their actions in a broad range of tissues, and therefore there are many effects of glucocorticoids:
  - ▲ Catabolism
    - **Increased serum glucose**: increased gluconeogenesis, increased lipolysis, decreased uptake of glucose into tissues, and direct inhibition of insulin via cortisone (breakdown of cortisol)
    - Mobilization of calcium from bones
    - Increased breakdown of muscle to liberate amino acids
  - ▲ Inflammatory effects
    - Increased blood neutrophil counts: increased marrow release and decreased tissue margination

- Decreasing numbers of other white blood cells: lymphocytes, eosinophils, macrophages
- Reduced function of lymphocytes and macrophages
- Reduced function of phospholipase A_2, resulting in reduced mediators of inflammation: prostaglandins and leukotrienes
- ▲ Antimitotic effects (decreased cell division)
- ▲ Water retention (because of mineralocorticoid effect)

PHARMACOKINETICS

- Cortisol is largely bound to corticosteroid-binding globulin (CBG); it is also bound to albumin but with only low affinity (Table 17-1).

INDICATIONS

- Inflammatory states:
  - ▲ Autoimmune disorders
    - Lupus, rheumatoid arthritis (RA), Crohn's disease, and many others
  - ▲ Asthma
  - ▲ Allergic responses, including anaphylaxis
- Cancer treatment
  - ▲ As one component of chemotherapy for some tumors
  - ▲ In brain tumors that are associated with swelling of the brain and increased intracranial pressure from edema secondary to the tumor
- Transplant medicine
  - ▲ Prevention of rejection
  - ▲ Graft-versus-host disease (GVHD)
- Steroid deficient states
  - ▲ Addison's disease
  - ▲ Adrenal suppression (which is caused by previous steroid administration)
  - ▲ Adrenal insufficiency during severe illness
- Maturation of fetal lungs (if preterm delivery is anticipated)
- *Pneumocystis* pneumonia co-treatment

TABLE 17-1. Steroid Potencies				
Drug	**Antiinflammatory Potency**	**Mineralocorticoid Potency**	**Biologic Half-Life (h)**	**Comments**
Hydrocortisone cortisol (endogenous)	1	1	8-10	
Cortisone	0.8	0.8	8-10	Intravenous only; three-times-a-day administration
Prednisone	4	0.3	18-36	Oral only
Methylprednisolone	5	0.3	18-36	Intravenous only
Dexamethasone	25-50	0	200	Most potent and longest acting
For Comparison with Mineralocorticoids				
Aldosterone	0.3	300	8-12	Not a clinical drug
Fludrocortisone	10	200	18-36	

CONTRAINDICATION

- Active serious infection

SIDE EFFECTS

- **Hyperglycemia** and steroid induced diabetes
- **Weight gain** and severe **swelling**, particularly in the face; caused, in part, by the mineralocorticoid effects
- **Psychiatric** symptoms including depression, mania, and psychosis; other types of cognitive dysfunction can also occur, including euphoria, insomnia, mental confusion
- **Gastric and duodenal bleeding** secondary to inflammation or ulceration
- **Infections** resulting from immunosuppression
- **Skin effects:** thin skin, violaceous striae (stretch marks), acne
- **Eyes:** cataracts and glaucoma
- **Muscular effects:** muscle wasting, myopathy
- **Adipose distribution:** buffalo hump, central obesity
- Skeletal effects:
  - ▲ Adults and children: Osteoporosis may occur.
  - ▲ Children: **Short stature** results from interference with growth plates.
  - ▲ **Avascular necrosis** (AVN) of the hips: The femoral head loses its blood supply, resulting in a devastating destruction of bone and joint. The lack of blood supply means that healing cannot occur and could necessitate joint replacement.
- **Cushing's syndrome** is a collection of signs from endogenous overproduction of cortisol. A cushingoid appearance can be produced from iatrogenic exogenous steroid:
  - ▲ Moon facies, buffalo hump (cervical fat pad), central obesity, supraclavicular fat collection, acne
- **Adrenal suppression:** Because of negative feedback loops, exogenous glucocorticoids will suppress CRH and ACTH. Rapidly terminating exogenous glucocorticoids after prolonged exposure will result in hypoadrenalism. Steroids must therefore be tapered (administration of smaller and smaller doses) before being stopped if they have been administered for more than about 1 or 2 weeks.

IMPORTANT NOTES

- The baseline secretion of cortisol in the body is 10 to 20 mg. In periods of stress (illness, trauma, inflammation, infection), the secretion increases.

- Glucocorticoids must be differentiated from **mineralocorticoids;** the prototype mineralocorticoid is aldosterone, also a steroid, which acts primarily on the kidney to regulate water and electrolyte homeostasis.
- One significant side effect of glucocorticoids is an increased white blood count (driven by an increase in neutrophils). Increased neutrophil counts are more commonly caused by infection; because steroids increase the risk of infection, it is sometimes clinically difficult to differentiate whether the increased white count is the result of a new infection (which would make the steroids relatively contraindicated) or the result of a direct effect of the steroid. The rise in white cell count can be quite dramatic when caused by steroid effect alone.
- Steroids and nonsteroidal antiinflammatory drugs (NSAIDs) are commonly coadministered for inflammatory conditions that result in pain (e.g., RA). The risk of gastrointestinal (GI) bleeding with steroids or NSAIDs alone is 2 times and 4 times (respectively) higher than baseline, but when these agents are taken together, the risk is 12 times higher than baseline.
- Because of the long list of side effects, steroids are not ideal for long-term high-dose administration. In diseases in which prolonged and substantial immunosuppression is required, steroid-sparing immunosuppressants are administered so that doses of steroids can be reduced or the steroids can be completely discontinued.

Advanced

- Prophylactic antibiotics against *Pneumocystis* pneumonia (also called *Pneumocystis jiroveci* pneumonia or *Pneumocystis carinii* pneumonia [PCP]) are administrated to patients on long-term moderate- to high-dose steroids because of the risk of acquiring this infection when immunosuppressed. Human immunodeficiency virus (HIV) infection is the most common risk factor for PCP
- In addition to being a risk factor for PCP, steroids are also coadministered to patients being **treated** for PCP because the antibiotic-mediated destruction of the pathogen generates a strong inflammatory response in the lungs, making the respiratory condition much worse. Steroids blunt this response.

EVIDENCE

The range of diseases treated with systemic steroids is too large to be summarized, but some of the more common uses of systemic steroids are presented here.

- **Systemic steroids** and **adult asthma**: A systematic review in 2009 concluded that the available studies were frequently underpowered. However, some general conclusions and recommendations were made: steroids administered in the emergency department reduce hospitalizations; steroids accelerate improvements in lung function; there was no benefit in using doses larger than 50 to 100 mg prednisone equivalent; and no benefit was seen when steroids were administered for longer than 5 to 10 days total.
- **Systemic steroids and RA**: A Cochrane review in 2007 (15 studies, N = 1414 patients) examined *radiological progression*

of disease and concluded that the proportion of benefit gained by glucocorticoids in reducing the progression of erosions from an average of all the studies over 1 year was 67.2% (confidence interval [CI] 48.9%, 85.4%) and over 2 years was 61.3% (CI 46.5%, 76.1%). Furthermore, this benefit was achieved in patients who were (mostly) already receiving disease-modifying antirheumatic drug (DMARD) treatment. It therefore represents a gain over and above any benefits from DMARDs alone.

FYI

- Memory tip: the effects of elevated cortisol in starvation would predict the metabolic effects: releasing and making available carbohydrate, fats, and proteins from body stores to be used by the body.

Introduction to Monoclonal Antibodies

Monoclonal antibodies (mAbs) belong to a broad category of agents (often called simply *biologics*) with a very large number of effects and clinical indications. The common denominator among all these drugs is the use of engineered proteins that are antibodies. There are two main categories of biologic drugs: mAbs and dimeric fusion proteins.

mAbs are produced by the body's immune system (by B lymphocytes) for the function of recognizing, binding, and subsequently destroying infectious agents that display foreign antigens. By creating antibodies that target antigens that are part of a *disease process*, the disease process can potentially be inhibited or completely destroyed.

To produce large quantities of an antibody, an animal first needs to be exposed to an antigen so that the B cells are able to produce the specific antibody. Second, a method of collecting the antibody-producing cell and enabling it to produce massive quantities is required. This is accomplished by fusing two cells together into a *hybridoma*. Antibody-producing cells (which have a limited life span) are then fused with cells that have an unlimited life span (a cancer cell, specifically a B-lymphoma cancer cell called a *myeloma*), which creates cells that can indefinitely produce antibodies. In a *batch* of these cells, there are many different cells, giving rise to many different clones of future generations (polyclonal). The isolation and growth of *single cells* that produce the desired antibody results in a *monoclonal* production of antibodies. These monoclonal hybridomas can be grown in cultures or in mice.

Newer technologies are enabling the animal (usually mouse) portion of the antibody to be less and less, so that the resulting antibody is mostly human and therefore not destroyed by the patient's own immune system for being a *foreign* antibody by **human antimurine antibodies (HAMAs)**. **Chimeric** (human-mouse combination) antibodies contain fewer mouse regions than full mouse antibodies. **Humanization** involves replacing most of the mouse antibody with equivalent human regions while keeping only the variable, antigen-specific regions intact. Humanized mAbs have more human regions than chimeric mAbs do. Finally, **fully human** mAbs that contain no mouse regions are now being created (Figure 17-1).

FUSION PROTEINS

Fusion proteins are antibodies but are engineered differently than mAbs. The antigen portion is fused to the Fc fragment. The dimeric molecule can then bind to the specific cell surface binding protein and allow the activity of the Fc portion of the antibody to be directed to the cell. For example, etanercept is a combination of tumor necrosis factor (TNF) receptor bound to the antibody Fc fragment. The drug binds TNF, and the Fc fragment results in inactivation and removal of circulating TNF.

USE OF MONOCLONAL ANTIBODIES

The list of uses for mAbs is growing, but the major categories are as follows:

- **Cancer**: Cancer cells express unique antigens that can be directly targeted for destruction. Furthermore, there are growth factors that stimulate cancer cell growth that can also be inhibited.
- **Immunosuppressants**:
  - *Inflammatory diseases*: Autoimmune diseases in which the immune system attacks *self* tissues and cells, such as lupus and RA, have been treated with mAbs that target specific components of the immune system such as TNF and many of the interleukins (ILs) in an attempt to blunt the immune response.
  - *Transplant rejection*: Organs that are transplanted in a host patient are foreign tissue and therefore will be attacked by the host; mAbs are being used to inhibit the process of rejection.

Monoclonal antibodies

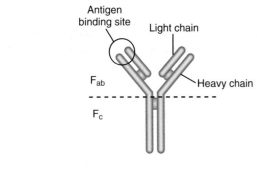

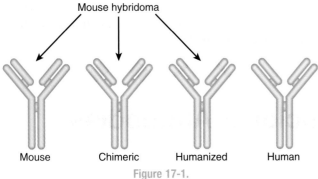

Figure 17-1.

■ **Infection treatment:** By binding specific functional proteins expressed on bacteria or viruses, the infectious agent can be suppressed or controlled.

Conjugating or combining other molecules can provide special functions to the mAb. For example, attaching **radioactive isotopes** can deliver radiation to provide highly localized radiation to kill tumor cells. An example is ibritumomab, which is a CD20 mAb bound to radioactive yttrium. Conjugating **toxins** is another approach to delivering highly targeted cytotoxicity. An example is gemtuzumab ozogamicin; the antibody-bound toxin calicheamicin dimethyl hydrazide is cleaved from the antibody inside the cell and binds to DNA, producing apoptosis.

NAMING MONOCLONAL ANTIBODIES

■ mAbs have multiple different targets (but only one each). mAbs are derived from different sources.
■ The convention for naming mAbs is as follows: target-source-*mab*.

Targets

■ *Disease processes or tissues:* immune = *lim*, ILs = *kin*, viral = *vir*, bacterial = *bac*, infectious lesions = *les*, cardiovascular = *cir*, fungal = *fung*, neurologic = *ner*, musculoskeletal = *mul*, bone = *os*, toxin as target = *toxa*
■ *Tumors:* any tumor = *tu(m)*, prostate = *pro*, colon = *col*, melanoma = *mel*, mammary = *mar*, testis = *got*, ovary = *gov*

Sources

■ Human = *u*, mouse = *mo*, humanized = *zu*, chimera = *xi*

TABLE 17-2. Monoclonal Antibodies

Name	Type	Target
Rituximab	Chimeric	CD20 on B lymphocytes
Ocrelizumab	Humanized	CD20 on B lymphocytes
Ofatumomab	Human	CD20 on B lymphocytes
Tositumomab	Mouse	CD20, bound to ^{131}I
Ibritumomab	Mouse	CD20, bound to ^{90}Y or ^{111}In
Epratuzumab	Humanized	CD22 on B lymphocytes
Alemtuzumab	Humanized	CD52 on B and T lymphocytes
Muromonab	Mouse	CD3 on T lymphocytes
Efalizumab	Humanized	CD11a on T lymphocytes
Inolimomab	Mouse	CD25 (IL-2) on T lymphocytes
Basiliximab	Chimeric	CD25 (IL-2) on T lymphocytes
Daclizumab	Humanized	CD25 (IL-2) on T lymphocytes
Gemtuzumab	Humanized	CD33 on hematopoietic cells
Bevacizumab	Humanized	Vascular-endothelial growth factor (VEGF)
Ranibizumab	Humanized	Vascular-endothelial growth factor (VEGF)
Cetuximab	Chimeric	Epidermal growth factor receptor (EGFR)
Satumomab	Mouse	Tumor-associated glycoprotein TAG-72
Capromab	Mouse	PSA (prostate), bound to ^{111}In
Omalizumab	Humanized	IgE (increased in asthma)
Eculizumab	Humanized	C5 (complement)
Palivizumab	Humanized	Fusion protein of RSV
Trastuzumab	Humanized	HER2 (EGF)
Infliximab	Chimeric	TNF-α
Adalimumab	Human	TNF-α
Certolizumab pegol	Humanized	TNF-α, bound to polyethylene glycol
Denosumab	Human	Receptor activator for nuclear factor κ B ligand (RANKL) in bone

EGF, epidermal growth factor; *HER2,* human epidermal growth factor receptor 2; ^{131}*I,* iodine-131; *IgE,* immunoglobulin E; *IL,* interleukin; ^{111}*In,* indium-111; *PSA,* prostate-specific antigen; *TNF,* tumor necrosis factor; ^{90}*Y,* yttrium-90.

Examples

■ **Abciximab:** *ci* + *xi* + *mab* = circulatory, from chimeric source
  ▲ IIb/IIIa blocker on platelets; for antiplatelet therapy
■ **Trastuzumab:** *tu* + *zu* + *mab* = tumor, from humanized source
  ▲ Human epidermal growth factor target; for breast cancer
  ▲ Trastuzumab is the first mAb to be approved for the treatment of a solid tumor.
■ **Infliximab:** *li* + *xi* + *mab* = immune, from chimera
  ▲ TNF-α blocker; antiinflammatory

NOTES

Clinical uses for each mAb are changing and thus are not specifically listed for each drug. For drugs with which there is considerable clinical experience, separate sections will discuss further details.

Table 17-2 will not be fully inclusive by the time it is published because of the rapid growth of this area of medicine. Some drugs listed may not yet be approved for use.

B-Cell Biologics

DESCRIPTION
B-cell biologics specifically target B-cell lymphocytes for either destruction or suppression.

PROTOTYPES AND COMMON DRUGS
mAbs (-**tu-mab** refers to tumor)
CD20 Target
- Prototype: ri**tu**ximab
- Others: bound to radioactive ligands: tosi**tu**momab, ibri**tu**momab

CD22 Target
- Prototype: epra**tu**zumab

MOA (MECHANISM OF ACTION)
- Drugs that target B cells cause either destruction of the cells or interference with their ability to mount an immune response.
- As a **B cell–depleting** agent (destruction of B cells):
  - ▲ CD20 is implicated in antibody-dependent cytotoxicity, complement-dependent cytotoxicity, and induction of apoptosis of B lymphocytes.
  - ▲ Through this process, CD20 blockade therapy results in depletion of mature B cells in the blood.
  - ▲ CD20 is located on 90% of B-cell neoplasms and therefore is effective at depleting these (abnormal) cell lines.
- Accelerated destruction by other anticancer drugs has also been observed when used in combination with CD20 therapy.
- As an **immunomodulator** (inhibitor of B cells):
  - ▲ B-cell depletion (through the cytotoxic actions described previously) is an effective method of blunting a pathologic inflammatory response.
  - ▲ B cells play a pivotal role in the development and progression of many autoimmune diseases. B cells must go through a series of steps before they become immunologically active, and many of these steps require cytokine binding and stimulation. Therefore blocking these cytokines can result in inhibition of the following B cell functions:
    - Maturation and differentiation
    - Memory induction (TNF)
    - Activation
    - Proliferation
- Bound to **radioactive ligands**: When bound to radioactive ligands, the mAb delivers targeted radiotherapy to the target cells and destroys the cells through close contact with the radioactive ligand.
- CD20 is expressed only on B cells and is present on all stages of B-cell differentiation except the very first and very last stages.
  - ▲ CD20 regulates early steps in the activation process for B-cell cycle initiation and differentiation.
- Rituximab is a *chimeric* mAb, and most CD20 therapy clinical experience and publications are currently based on rituximab.

PHARMACOKINETICS
- The half-life of rituximab can be variable when treating tumor. The drug will become bound and removed from circulation when a high number of CD20 receptors are present, effectively decreasing the drug concentration and half-life. Therefore at the start of cancer therapy the half-life is around 75 hours, whereas at the end of therapy it can be as long as 200 hours.
- Rituximab is usually administered every 2 weeks by intravenous infusion.

INDICATIONS
- **Tumors of B-cell lineage** (through actions that destroy the cells):
  - ▲ Multiple myeloma
  - ▲ Lymphocytic leukemias: acute (ALL) and chronic (CLL)
  - ▲ B-cell lymphomas
- **Inflammatory autoimmune diseases** (inhibiting or depleting B cells will potentially reduce inflammation and the disease process):
  - ▲ RA
  - ▲ Systemic lupus erythematosus (SLE)
  - ▲ Some types of vasculitis such as Wegener's vasculitis
  - ▲ Many other inflammatory diseases are being treated in clinical trials.
- **Transplant medicine** (inhibiting or depleting B cells will potentially reduce a response against either the transplant or the host):
  - ▲ Preventing and treating organ rejection
  - ▲ Treating GVHD

CONTRAINDICATIONS
- **Active infection**: These drugs are immunosuppressants and therefore would inhibit the body's ability to fight off an infection.
- **Latent infection**: An example would be viral hepatitis (hepatitis B or C).

SIDE EFFECTS
Early
- Infusion reactions:
  - ▲ **Common and mild**: hypotension, hypertension, chills, rash, *scratchy* sensation in the throat, and bronchospasm
  - ▲ Mucocutaneous reactions
  - ▲ **Rare and severe**: hypoxia, acute respiratory distress syndrome (ARDS), myocardial infarction, shock, death
  - ▲ Infusion reactions are most common during the **first infusion** and can be reduced by slowing down the infusion and pretreating with intravenous steroids.

Late

- **Immunosuppression resulting in infections**: Patients should be monitored closely for infection, particularly when treated with other immunosuppressive agents.
- **Progressive multifocal leukoencephalopathy** (PML) is destruction of white brain matter in a patchy distribution, believed to be caused by reactivation of the JC virus, a polyomavirus, through the process of immunosuppression. This is a rare event.

IMPORTANT NOTES

- CD20 antigen is not expressed by either plasma cells or B-lymphoid stem cells; therefore rituximab does not reduce total immunoglobulin (Ig) serum concentrations.
- After a four-dose course of rituximab therapy, B-lymphocyte counts recover in 9 to 12 months.

Advanced

- B cell–depleting and B cell–nondepleting strategies have both been used for treatment of autoimmune diseases.
- Future therapies:
  - ▲ BAFF (B-cell activating factor), also called BlyS (B-lymphocyte stimulator), prolongs the survival of B cells, stimulates maturation, and promotes survival of autoreactive B. Anti-BAFF antibodies (belimumab) or BAFF receptor fusion proteins (briobacept) are being investigated for treating RA and SLE.
  - ▲ Similarly, another receptor called APRIL (a proliferation-inducing ligand) is being targeted by a fusion protein (atacicept) that binds BAFF and APRIL. It is still under investigation.

EVIDENCE

- The diseases being treated with B cell–targeting drugs are too numerous to list, and a summary of the current evidence is beyond the scope of this text.

FYI

- Rituximab was the first mAb used for treating cancer.
- Epratuzumab, a B cell CD22 (not CD20)–targeting drug is currently being investigated in a number of phase 3 trials for treatment of lupus and lymphoma but is not yet approved in North America.
- Ocrelizumab and ofatumumab are *humanized* and *human* mAbs respectively that target CD20 but are not yet approved. Rituximab is a *chimeric* mAb.

T-Cell Biologics

DESCRIPTION

T-cell biologics specifically target T-cell lymphocytes for either destruction or suppression.

PROTOTYPE AND COMMON DRUGS

mAbs (-li-mab, -li- refers to the immune system)
CD3 Target
- Prototype: OKT3 (an early murine mAb)
- Others: Teplizumab, otelixizumab, and visilizumab

CD25 Target (IL-2 receptor)
- Prototype: daclizumab
- Others: basiliximab, inolimomab

CD11a Target (lymphocyte function–associated antigen 1 [LFA-1])
- Prototype: efalizumab

Fusion Proteins (-cept)
LFA-3 Target
- Prototype: alefacept

CD28 Target (cytotoxic T-lymphocyte antigen [CTLA4])
- Prototype: abatacept

MOA (MECHANISM OF ACTION)

- The roles and activities of T cells are extremely diverse and complicated. Their contributions to disease are currently incompletely understood, and this section is a very simplified explanation of a very complicated system. This area of medicine is changing quickly, as is the understanding of these disease processes.

CD3

- CD3 is the defining marker for T cells. Therefore, all T cells express CD3. As a result, drugs that target CD3 have the potential to influence all subtypes of T cells and are therefore nonspecific. They will influence proinflammatory as well as antiinflammatory T cells and also target activated and nonactivated T cells.
- A strong inflammatory reaction, *cytokine-release* syndrome, often occurs with the first dose of OKT3. It can be severe, resulting in a range of signs and symptoms from fever to tachycardia to meningitis (noninfectious) and adult respiratory distress syndrome (ARDS). This reaction occurs because of a massive synchronized T-cell activation.
  - ▲ Newer modified CD3 inhibitors have been designed to be *nonactivating*, thus reducing the probability of this syndrome.
- CD3 targeting drugs also induce selective apoptosis of activated T cells after binding to CD3.

Transplant Medicine

- CD3 inhibition has been used to prevent acute graft rejection.

Autoimmune Diseases

- Newer CD3 inhibitors are currently in clinical trials for diseases such as psoriatic arthritis (arthritis associated with psoriasis) and type I diabetes.

CD25 (IL-2 Receptor)

- CD25 is the IL-2 receptor. There are many roles of IL-2.

Autoimmune Diseases

- Increased CD25 (IL-2 receptor) expression has been demonstrated in many autoimmune diseases. Suppression or antagonism of IL-2 has resulted in reduced inflammation in many of these diseases.
- Important source of apparent conflict:
  - ▲ **Regulatory T cells** (T_{reg}) are very important in the control of **self-tolerance**. They play a vital role in preventing the immune system from attacking a person's own tissues and cells. They express CD25 and require IL-2 for their growth and survival; however, they *suppress* the immune system.
  - ▲ **Autoreactive** T cells are defined as T cells that attack *self* antigens (those that are present in the body), and these attacks are a major contributor to autoimmune diseases.
  - ▲ T_{reg} cells suppress the autoreactive T cells. Abnormal (low) T_{reg} levels and function are associated with many autoimmune diseases.
  - ▲ Treatment with CD25 inhibition seems clearly beneficial, so the benefits from *overall* T cell immune suppression must outweigh any specific effects on suppressing T_{reg} function.

Cancer

- Very few normal (nonactivated) cells express CD25; however, many lymphocyte malignancies express this receptor. Targeting this receptor in certain cancers with a lymphocyte lineage will deplete those cells.

Transplant Medicine

- Solid organ transplant rejection is associated with an elevated CD25 level that is linked to the activation of T cells. Inhibiting CD25 therefore blunts the immune response to transplanted organs.
- Bone marrow and stem cell transplants result in foreign white blood cells being introduced into the patient. These cells can mount an immune response against the patient, a condition called **graft-versus-host disease** (GVHD). This process can be suppressed by inhibition of CD25.

CD28 (CTLA-4)
Autoimmune Diseases

- T cells require two signals to activate them: the antigen and a second **costimulator**. Costimulatory molecules are **antigen independent**; the costimulation does not require the binding of antigen. CTLA-4 is a costimulator that regulates the immune response. It is up-regulated in activated T cells.

- CTLA-4 inhibition:
  - ▲ Interrupts the costimulatory signal, preventing and potentially reversing T-cell activation. In fact, exposure of T cells to antigen in the *absence* of costimulation *inhibits* responses to future exposure to antigen.
  - ▲ Increases the number of T_{reg} cells.

Cancer Therapy

- CTLA-4 inhibition does not deplete T cells or other leukocytes and is therefore not useful for cancer treatment.

Transplant Medicine

- Prevention of binding of the costimulator on first exposure to a new antigen (the transplanted organ) blunts the immune response against the organ and is therefore effective.

CD11a (LFA-1)

- CD11a is important for interactions between the integrin LFA-1 and cell adhesion molecule intercellular adhesion molecule 1 (ICAM-1). Integrins are proteins that facilitate the attachment of cells to other cells or to extracellular matrices. Once attached, the cell can transmigrate from the blood into the tissue, across the endothelial barrier.
- In addition to adherence, integrins also communicate signals to the inside of the lymphocyte.
- Efalizumab inhibits tight lymphocyte adhesion to inflamed endothelium; inhibiting this adhesion results in reduced lymphocyte entry into the site of inflammation and thus reduces the inflammatory response locally.
- It is currently being used to treat psoriasis.

Cancer Therapy

- LFA-1 inhibition does not deplete T cells or other leukocytes and is therefore not useful for cancer treatment.

LFA-3

- LFA-3, like LFA-1, is involved with cellular adhesion. LFA-3 is located on antigen-presenting cells (APCs).

PHARMACOKINETICS

- These drugs are administered by intravenous infusions over 30 minutes to a few hours.

INDICATIONS

- **Tumors of T-cell lymphocyte lineage** (through actions that destroy the cells)
- **Inflammatory autoimmune diseases** (inhibiting inflammatory cells such as T cells will potentially reduce inflammation and the disease process):
  - ▲ Rheumatoid arthritis (RA)
  - ▲ Systemic lupus erythematosis (SLE)
  - ▲ Some types of vasculitis such as Wegener's vasculitis
  - ▲ Many others inflammatory diseases are being treated in clinical trials.
- Transplant medicine
  - ▲ Preventing and treating rejection
  - ▲ Preventing and treating GVHD

CONTRAINDICATION

- Active infection is a contraindication to immunosuppressive therapies.

SIDE EFFECTS

- With all classes of drugs, the risk of immunosuppression leading to infection is an ever-present side effect.
- **Infusion reactions**: Nausea, vomiting, diarrhea, hypotension, shortness of breath, and headache, to name a few, can all occur.

CD3

- With OKT3 only, **cytokine release syndrome**: a massive inflammatory response caused by binding to the T cells combined with Fc receptor cross-linking.
  - ▲ The syndrome is attributed to increased serum levels of cytokines, particularly the production of TNF.
  - ▲ Symptoms usually are worst with the first dose; frequency and severity decrease with subsequent doses.
  - ▲ Signs and symptoms include the following:
    - • **Common**: fever, chills, rigor, headache, tremor, nausea, vomiting, diarrhea, abdominal pain, malaise, muscle and joint pain, and generalized weakness
    - • **Less common**: skin reactions, aseptic meningitis, and cardiorespiratory effects:
      - ▲ **Potentially fatal**: severe cardiac and/or respiratory dysfunction, namely ARDS, circulatory shock, arrhythmias, and cardiac arrest

EVIDENCE
Abatacept and Rheumatoid Arthritis

- A Cochrane review in 2009 (seven studies, 2908 patients) found that patients treated with abatacept, compared with placebo, were more likely (relative risk [RR] 2.21) to achieve clinical benefit as measured by the ACR50, an index of pain, disability, and number of affected joints. The number needed to treat (NNT) was 5. The risk of side effects was low (RR 1.05) compared with placebo, and the harms were assessed to be not significant except for increased infections assessed at 12 months.

FYI

- CD4+ T cells are depleted in acquired immunodeficiency syndrome (AIDS); drugs that target CD4 exist but are currently not in clinical practice.

Mixed Biologics

DESCRIPTION

Mixed biologics target B- and T-cell lymphocytes or their cytokine mediators for either destruction or suppression.

PROTOTYPE

mAbs (**-tu-mab** refers to tumor and **-li-mab** to the immune system)

CD52 (CAMPATH-1) Target

- Prototype: alem**tu**zu**mab**

IL-6 Receptor Target

- Prototype: toci**li**zu**mab**

MOA (MECHANISM OF ACTION)
CD52 (CAMPATH-1)

- Alemtuzumab is a *humanized* mAb against CD52.
- CD52 is present on both B- and T-cell lymphocytes, normal neutrophils, and most B- and T-cell lymphomas.
- CD52 is not expressed on CD34+ lymphocytes (which is a marker for hematopoietic progenitor cells), so hematopoietic progenitor cells are not targeted with CD52 therapy. This is important because targeting very *early* stem cells will result in destruction of multiple cell lines, which would be undesirable.
- CD52 targeted by mAbs induces tumor cell death through the following:
  - ▲ Antibody-dependent cellular cytotoxicity
  - ▲ Complement-dependent cytotoxicity
- This results in extensive lympholysis (destruction of lymphocytes) by inducing apoptosis and produces prolonged T- and B-cell depletion
- Through the depletion of T- and B-cell lymphocytes, CD52 targeted therapy has become clinically useful for the treatment of:
  - ▲ Lymphomas and leukemias, especially CLL because of its ability to destroy these cells
  - ▲ Transplant medicine (GVHD) and autoimmune disorders because of its ability to suppress B- and T-cell function, thus acting as an immunosuppressant

IL-6 Receptor

- Tocilizumab is a *humanized* mAb.
- Overproduction of IL-6 is thought to play an important role in the pathogenesis of some autoimmune diseases such as RA. IL-6 is elevated in patients with RA, and IL-6 levels correlate with disease severity
- Tocilizumab binds selectively and competitively to both soluble (in the blood) and cell surface IL-6 receptors, blocking IL-6 signal transduction.
- Blockage of IL-6 does not destroy lymphocytes, and therefore IL-6 does not deplete cell lines and is *not* used in cancer treatment.

PHARMACOKINETICS

- Tocilizumab is administered intravenously every 4 weeks.

INDICATIONS
Alemtuzumab
- Leukemia and lymphoma
- Transplant medicine
  - ▲ Prevention and treatment of rejection
  - ▲ Prevention and treatment of GVHD

Tocilizumab
- RA

CONTRAINDICATIONS
- Active infections: Immunosuppression results in a decreased ability to fight off infection.
- An existing immunodeficiency would result in an increased risk of new infection.

SIDE EFFECTS
Alemtuzumab
- Acute infusion reactions and the depletion of hematopoietic cells and T cells may occur. Patients also may develop severe pancytopenia and death.
- Opportunistic infections are a serious side effect.

Tocilizumab
- Nasopharyngitis
- Elevated cholesterol (reversible)
- Elevated liver enzymes (mild and not associated with detectable liver damage)
- Neutropenia
- Infections

IMPORTANT NOTES
- Nomenclature (-li- or -tu-) designation does not restrict the use of a drug to that class of therapy. Many drugs are used to treat both autoimmune diseases and hematologic cancers because of the roles that lymphocytes play in both.

EVIDENCE
- Beyond scope

Tumor Necrosis Factor (TNF)–α Inhibitors

DESCRIPTION
- TNF-α is an important inflammatory cytokine.

PROTOTYPE AND COMMON DRUGS
mAbs (-li-mab; -li- refers to the immune system)
- Prototype: infliximab
- Others: adalimumab, certolizumab, golimumab

Fusion Protein (-cept)
- Prototype: etanercept

MOA (MECHANISM OF ACTION)
- TNF-α is mostly produced by macrophages but is also produced by other inflammatory cells. It binds to TNF receptors (called TNFRs), which are present on many different cells of the immune system.
- It promotes inflammation and is believed to play important roles in both inflammatory reactions to infections and also, when present in abnormally high levels, in the pathogenesis of autoimmune diseases. It has been called the *master regulator* of the immune system.
- The inflammatory cascades are very complicated. TNF-α is believed to exert its proinflammatory actions by promoting:
  - ▲ The acute phase response, which occurs early in the inflammatory response and is mediated in part by the release of other proinflammatory cytokines, including IL-1, IL-6, and IL-8, resulting in fever, loss of appetite, vasodilation, and tachycardia
  - ▲ Increased expression of endothelial adhesion molecules, which results in increased migration of leukocytes into target organs
  - ▲ Apoptosis
- In summary, through inhibition of TNF-α, the inflammatory response is blunted.
- mAbs bind TNF-α *receptors*. In contrast, the fusion protein etanercept is a circulating TNF receptor that binds TNF (the ligand itself, not the receptor).

PHARMACOKINETICS
- Drugs are administered by injection, usually every 2 to 4 weeks.
- The half-lives of these drugs are in the range of 5 to 14 days. The elimination half-life of certolizumab (a PEGylated mAb) is the longest, because of the polyethylene glycol (PEG) portion, which decreases renal elimination.

INDICATIONS
- Autoimmune diseases:
  - ▲ Rheumatoid arthritis (RA)
  - ▲ Crohn's disease and ulcerative colitis (inflammatory conditions of the digestive tract)
  - ▲ Psoriasis (inflammatory disease of the dermis)
  - ▲ Ankylosing spondylitis

CONTRAINDICATIONS
- Latent TB: TB can be reactivated if the immune system is suppressed.

- Patients who are **immunocompromised**: Combination with additional immunosuppression increases the risk of infection.
- **Active infection**: The immune system must remain intact to fight the current infection before treatment with an immunosuppressant begins.

SIDE EFFECTS

- **Injection site irritation**
- **Acute inflammatory reaction**: Because of the ability of TNF to influence the immune system, extensive inflammatory reactions can occur within 24 hours (usually within 6 hours) after administration. They are characterized by fever, hypotension, tachycardia, itching, chest pain, and shortness of breath. These reactions are relatively common (10% of the time), but only rarely are they severe enough to discontinue treatment.
- **Delayed inflammatory reaction**: Signs and symptoms that occur within 2 weeks after the injection are probably mediated by antibodies to the drug. Symptoms of these reactions include fever, rash, urticaria (itching), myalgia (muscle pain), arthralgia (joint pain), jaw tightness, and edema.
- **Infection**: Because of the immune suppression, common bacterial and also opportunistic infections are more common in patients receiving TNF suppression:
  - ▲ Bacterial sepsis (widespread inflammatory response caused by bacterial infection in the blood)
  - ▲ Fungal infections
  - ▲ Latent TB (previous TB can be reactivated); patients *must* be screened for previous TB infections before starting anti-TNF therapy
  - ▲ Herpes zoster
- **Severe but rare** side effects include heart failure, liver failure, and demyelinating disorders of the central nervous system (CNS).
- **Cancer**: Another function of the immune system is to provide surveillance of early cancer cells and to destroy them early. A blunted immune system therefore can increase the potential for development of cancer.

IMPORTANT NOTES

- Anti-TNF therapy for RA is considered a *biologic* **DMARD**, which, as previously noted, stands for **disease-modifying antirheumatic drug**. DMARDs slow the progression of joint destruction. Use of DMARDs is in contrast to "symptom-only" therapy, which would include analgesics (such as acetaminophen or NSAIDs), in that symptom-only therapy does not slow the progression of the disease.
- **Antibodies to the antibody** (ATA) can occur. In this situation, the patient's immune system recognizes the mAb as a foreign antigen and generates antibodies against it, thus neutralizing it. This reaction is less common with mAb types that are more similar to human antibodies: human (3%) < humanized < chimeric (10%).

Advanced

- TNF is active when three monomers bind together into a trimeric unit and bind to two different receptors: TNFR1 and TNFR2. These receptors are also called p55 and p75, respectively.
- In contrast to infliximab and adalimumab, **certolizumab** does not contain an Fc portion and therefore does not induce complement activation, antibody-dependent cellular cytotoxicity, or apoptosis. Remember that the Fab portion is the antigen-specific region and the Fc region is important for determining the type of response that occurs *after* the Fab portion binds to the antigen.
  - ▲ The Fc portion is replaced by polyethylene glycol (PEG), which is conjugated to the Fab portion. The PEG portion results in a longer half-life and also eliminates any immune function that would have been activated by the Fc portion of the antibody.

EVIDENCE
Rheumatoid Arthritis
Monotherapy versus Methotrexate, and
Monotherapy versus Combination Therapy

- A 2008 systematic review of DMARD therapy for RA concluded that anti-TNF monotherapy was similar in efficacy to treatment with methotrexate alone, whereas the combination of an anti-TNF agent with methotrexate reduced disease activity more and slowed radiographic progression to a greater extent than did anti-TNF monotherapy or methotrexate alone. These findings were similar to those of a Cochrane review in 2009 that examined all biologic DMARDs in the treatment of RA.

Infliximab (with or without Methotrexate) versus Placebo (Plus Methotrexate)

- A Cochrane review in 2002 (two trials, 529 patients) found that after 6 months, response rates were significantly improved with all infliximab doses compared with controls. The NNT with infliximab to achieve an American College of Rheumatology (ACR) 20, 50, or 70 response (these are different measures of response based on disability, pain, and number of affected joints) in patients with refractory RA under specialist care ranged from 2.94 to 3.33 for ACR 20, up to 5.88 to 12.5 for ACR 70. Withdrawals because of adverse events and withdrawals for other reasons were not statistically significantly different in patients receiving infliximab than in controls.

Crohn's Disease
Infliximab versus Placebo

- A 2004 Cochrane review (four studies) found one randomized controlled trial (RCT) (N = 108) that provided evidence that infliximab was more effective than placebo in inducing remission of Crohn's disease (RR 8.1). The four studies were too heterogeneous for results to be combined.

Ulcerative Colitis
Infliximab versus Placebo or Steroid

- A 2006 Cochrane review showed that in the population of patients with *refractory* ulcerative colitis, infliximab was more effective in inducing clinical remission than placebo (RR 3.22); it also showed that there was no statistical difference between steroid and infliximab for the same endpoint.

FYI

- TNF-α was initially called cachexin and was described in 1975 for its ability to lyse tumors in animal models (giving rise to the name *tumor necrosis factor*).
- *Cachectic* is a term used to describe someone who has lost a lot of weight with considerable muscle atrophy, generally because of an advanced disease process.
- TNF-β (note this is beta, not alpha) is also called lymphotoxin and is produced by CD8+ T cells.

Antimetabolites

DESCRIPTION

- Antimetabolites are purine or pyrimidine analogues. This section deals with antimetabolites that are used primarily as immunosuppressants; see also the section on antimetabolites used for cancer therapy.

PROTOTYPES

- Azathioprine
- Mycophenolate (mycophenolate mofetil [MMF])

MOA (MECHANISM OF ACTION)

- Purines and pyrimidines are the two types of bases used in DNA and RNA. Purines are guanine (G) and adenine (A); pyrimidines are cytosine (C), thymine (T), and uracil (U). Uracil (U) is found only in RNA, whereas thymine (T) is only in DNA. The bases are all attached to a single phosphate group, making them monophosphates.
- Inosine monophosphate (IMP), the precursor to guanine monophosphate (GMP), is converted by **IMP dehydrogenase**.
- Mycophenolate is hydrolyzed to mycophenolic acid (MPA), which inhibits IMP dehydrogenase and thereby **prevents GMP production**. GMP is a required base for both DNA and RNA, and without it, DNA and RNA synthesis is reduced (Figure 17-2).
- Azathioprine is converted to mercaptopurine (itself a drug), which is then metabolized through more steps to **6-thio-GTP**; 6-thio-GTP can be incorporated into DNA and RNA, but because it is not a normal base, it halts further DNA and RNA synthesis. It is called a **fraudulent nucleoside**.
- Regardless of the exact mechanism of action on DNA and RNA:
  - Reduced DNA synthesis results in reduced proliferation of cells. As a general rule, rapidly dividing cells are more sensitive to drugs that influence cell division. These include the following:
    - Hematologic precursor cells in the bone marrow; lymphocyte suppression is the primary mechanism by which these drugs are immunosuppressants
    - GI tract mucosal cells
    - Cancer cells

Immune antimetabolites

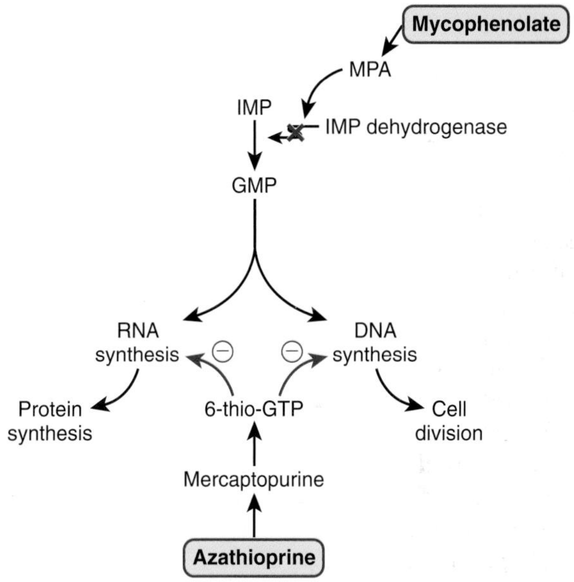

Figure 17-2.

  - Reduced RNA synthesis results in reduced protein transcription and thus reduced functional activity of cells.
    - For example, antibody-producing cells (B lymphocytes) would produce less antibody.
- Two features of antimetabolites that make them a little more specific to inhibiting the immune system include:
  - Both T and B lymphocytes depend on *de novo* (they must produce their own) synthesis of purines, whereas other cell types are able to use salvage pathways to obtain their DNA and RNA building blocks. Therefore lymphocytes are more susceptible to antimetabolites than are these other cell lines.
  - Mycophenolate reversibly inhibits the *type II* isoform of IMP dehydrogenase, which is preferentially expressed by *activated* lymphocytes.
- The similarities between mercaptopurine (the azathioprine metabolite) and the purines guanine and adenine are easily seen (Figure 17-3).

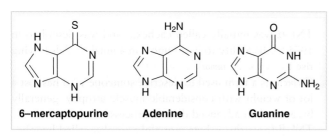

Figure 17-3.

PHARMACOKINETICS
Azathioprine

- Azathioprine is metabolized quickly (half-life of 10 minutes) but has many active metabolites; therefore blood level measurements of the parent drug do not provide useful information.
- Azathioprine is metabolized by the liver to mercaptopurine; mercaptopurine metabolism occurs via a couple different enzymes, one of which is **xanthine oxidase**, an enzyme that is important in the disease gout; **allopurinol**, a xanthine oxidase inhibitor used to treat gout, results in dramatically increased levels of active metabolites. This is an important **drug interaction**.
  - ▲ Another important enzyme that metabolizes mercaptopurine is **thiopurine methyltransferase (TPMT)**; the TPMT activity rate is very important because TPMT catalyzes a reaction to produce an *inactive* metabolite and is therefore felt to be a strong predictor for myelosuppression and hepatotoxicity. Patients with low TPMT activity develop higher levels of 6-thio-GTP and are therefore more susceptible to acute bone marrow suppression and liver damage. TPMT activity is **genetically** determined, and tests for TPMT activity levels are available.
- **Timing of efficacy:** It can take a couple of months before azathioprine exerts its effects. This is thought to be related to the long time required to generate **intracellular** levels of 6-thio-GTP.
- Because these drugs are frequently used in patients with kidney transplants and the transplanted **kidney function** is often less than the level of function of a normal kidney, it is critical to know how these drugs are metabolized and eliminated
  - ▲ Azathioprine: Although renal clearance is not the primary mode of elimination, the dose should be decreased in patients who are anuric (complete absence of renal function).

Mycophenolate

- As with azathioprine, the half-life of the parent compound is only minutes, because of conversion to active and inactive metabolites.

SIDE EFFECTS

- Most side effects are related to systems that require high cell turnover:
  - ▲ **GI:** mucositis, diarrhea, vomiting

- ▲ **Bone marrow:** leukopenia, thrombocytopenia, anemia
- ▲ **Alopecia:** hair loss caused by hair follicle suppression
- Immunosuppression-related effects include the following:
  - ▲ **Infections**
  - ▲ **Cancer risk** from decreased tumor surveillance by the immune system
  - ▲ **Dermatitis:** many different inflammatory skin diseases
- Other effects:
  - ▲ **Hepatic dysfunction:** indicated by elevated liver laboratory test results and possibly jaundice

INDICATIONS

- Prevention of cell division:
  - ▲ **Cancer**
- Decreased lymphocyte T-cell division:
  - ▲ Prevention and treatment of **transplant organ rejection**
  - ▲ Treatment of **autoimmune diseases** such as the following:
    - • RA
    - • Inflammatory bowel disease
    - • Psoriasis
    - • Lupus (especially for lupus nephritis)

CONTRAINDICATIONS

- Mycophenolate is contraindicated in pregnancy, whereas azathioprine is not.
- An active, severe infection is a contraindication.

IMPORTANT NOTES

- In treatment of autoimmune diseases, steroids are generally the first-line immunosuppressants employed because they act quickly; however, there are many side effects related to prolonged steroid use, and therefore nonsteroid immunosuppressants are generally preferred for long-term immunosuppression. Antimetabolites are used therefore for long-term "steroid-sparing" immunosuppression.
- Antimetabolites exert their immunosuppressant effects over a period of weeks, which is a slower onset than that of steroids, which become effective in about a day.

Advanced

- Azathioprine is converted to mercaptopurine; however, azathioprine is felt to be a more effective immunosuppressant than mercaptopurine because of increased intracellular uptake. *Intracellular* levels of the metabolite 6-thio-GTP need to be high for the drugs to be effective, and azathioprine appears to be taken up specifically by lymphocytes.
- Another mechanism recently suggested for the immunosuppressive effect of azathioprine involves 6-thio-GTP leading to activation of a mitochondrial pathway of **apoptosis** in lymphocytes.

EVIDENCE
Azathioprine Plus Steroid versus Steroid Alone for Treatment of Lupus Nephritis

- A Cochrane review in 2004 (3 studies, 78 patients) demonstrated that azathioprine plus steroids reduced the risk of all-cause mortality compared with steroids alone (RR 0.60) but did not alter renal outcomes. Neither therapy was associated with increased risk of major infection.

FYI

- The two drugs in this class are structurally different but do have some common features (the side-by-side rings) (Figure 17-4).
- One of the other pyrimidine antimetabolites (flucytosine) is an antifungal drug.
- When all three hematologic cell lines (white cells, red cells, and platelets) are decreased, the condition is called *pancytopenia*.

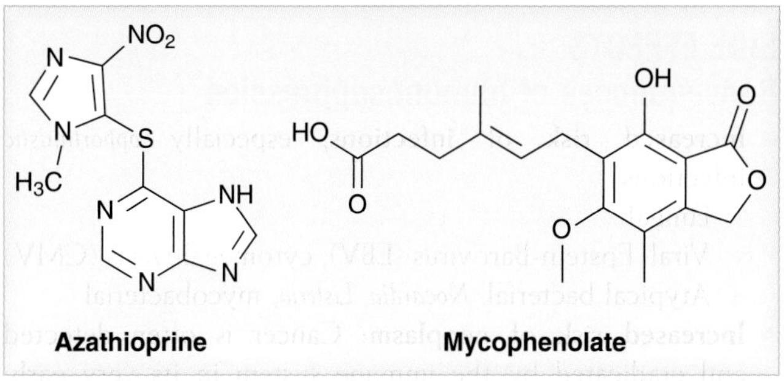

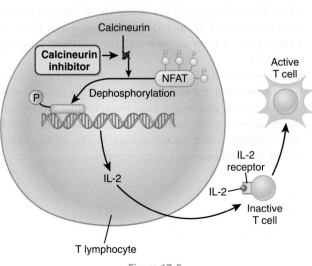

Azathioprine   **Mycophenolate**

Figure 17-4.

Calcineurin Inhibitors

DESCRIPTION

Calcineurin inhibitors are immunosuppressants.

PROTOTYPE AND COMMON DRUGS

- Prototype: cyclosporine
- Others: tacrolimus (FK506), pimecrolimus

MOA (MECHANISM OF ACTION)

- These drugs act on **T cells** (a type of lymphocyte). T cells are involved in *cell-mediated* immunity (as opposed to *humoral immunity*, which is mediated by B lymphocytes).
- Calcineurin is a protein phosphatase responsible for the transcription of IL-2, an important immune system cytokine. Calcineurin inhibitors stop the production of IL-2.
- IL-2 enables the *activation* of inactive T cells. It also plays a role in proliferation and differentiation of T cells (resulting in immunologic memory).
- A protein called nuclear factor of activated T cells (NFAT) binds T cell DNA and stimulates production of IL-2. NFAT

is activated through dephosphorylation by calcineurin (Figure 17-5).

- Therefore, calcineurin is an enzyme in T cells that results in **transcription of IL-2**.
- Through the *inhibition* of IL-2 production and thus T cell activation, proliferation, and differentiation, calcineurin inhibitors are immunosuppressants.
- Calcineurin inhibitors are not very effective at blunting the activity of T cells that have already been activated. They are more effective at *preventing* the immune response before it starts. For example, if acute rejection of a transplanted organ has already started, other immunosuppressants are required for effective treatment.

PHARMACOKINETICS

- Cyclosporine has a narrow therapeutic index. Levels must be frequently measured to help reduce the probability of side effects.
- Cyclosporine is extensively metabolized by the liver and secreted in the bile. Only 6% is secreted in the urine. Dose adjustment is required in liver failure but not in kidney failure.
  - ▲ When cyclosporine is administered to liver transplant patients, there is an important consideration if the transplanted liver is not functioning at 100%, and cyclosporine toxicity could result.
- Drugs that inhibit CYP3A will result in increased cyclosporine levels.
- Drugs that induce CYP3A will result in decreased cyclosporine levels.

INDICATIONS

- To prevent or suppress organ rejection in solid organ transplant recipients, most commonly the kidney
- To suppress inflammation in inflammatory diseases, but not as a first-line drug:
  - ▲ Psoriasis
  - ▲ RA

Calcineurin inhibitors

Calcineurin

Calcineurin inhibitor

NFAT

Dephosphorylation

P

Active T cell

IL-2

IL-2 receptor

IL-2

Inactive T cell

T lymphocyte

Figure 17-5.

SIDE EFFECTS
Consequences of Immunosuppression
- **Increased risk of infections,** especially *opportunistic* infections
  - ▲ Fungal
  - ▲ Viral: Epstein-Barr virus (EBV), cytomegalovirus (CMV)
  - ▲ Atypical bacterial: *Nocardia, Listeria,* mycobacterial
- **Increased risk of neoplasm:** Cancer is often detected and eradicated by the immune system in its very early stages.

Other
- **Nephrotoxicity:** Kidney damage is a common problem with administration of cyclosporine. This is the most important side effect. It is possibly mediated through renal arteriolar vasoconstriction. Renal damage often limits administration of cyclosporine.
- **Hypertension:** The exact mechanism is unknown, but cyclosporine has been shown to increase sympathetic nervous system activity, which would result in increased blood pressure.
- **CNS problems:** Tremors and headaches may occur, usually seen with larger doses.
- Tacrolimus only: **Hyperglycemia** (diabetes) may occur as a result of pancreatic beta cell inhibition.

Less Common
Cyclosporine Only
- **Hirsutism or hypertrichosis** (hair growth): a cosmetic problem
- Gum hyperplasia

Tacrolimus Only
- Alopecia (paradoxically, the opposite of hypertrichosis)

IMPORTANT NOTES
- In patients with kidney transplants (a population of patients who regularly receive calcineurin inhibitors), it can be diagnostically difficult to determine if declining renal function is a result of rejection (which would be managed by increasing the dose or adding immunosuppressive drugs) or of toxicity of the immunosuppressive drugs (which would be managed by lowering the dose or stopping the drugs).

Advanced
- Less common side effects include the following:
  - ▲ **Haemolytic uremic syndrome** is characterized by micro-angiopathic anemia, thrombocytopenia, and acute renal failure. Simply thought of, it is a process whereby platelets are consumed into intravascular aggregates, causing a meshwork of clots that lyse red blood cells and the floating intracellular debris plugs up the glomeruli and tubules, resulting in kidney failure.
  - ▲ **Posterior reversible encephalopathy syndrome** is an uncommon side effect with cyclosporine that is also seen with eclampsia and in the setting of severe hypertension (two conditions of extreme vasoconstriction). On brain imaging studies, there is widespread edema that predominates in the parietal and occipital regions (*posterior regions*). There is also clinical evidence of neurotoxicity (dysfunction).
- Cyclosporine versus tacrolimus side effects:
  - ▲ Tacrolimus seems to induce less nephrotoxicity and less hypertension.
  - ▲ Cyclosporine seems to induce less neurotoxicity.

EVIDENCE
Cyclosporine versus Tacrolimus in Kidney Transplants
- A Cochrane review in 2005 (20 studies, 4102 patients) found that kidney transplant loss at 6 months was significantly reduced (RR 0.56) in patients treated with tacrolimus. This effect was persistent for up to 3 years.

FYI
- Nomenclature caution:
  - ▲ Do not confuse cyclo**sporine** with another immunosuppressant, cyclo**phosphamide.**
  - ▲ Si**rolimus** and eve**rolimus** are immunosuppressives and also function to inhibit T cells, but they do not bind to calcineurin and therefore are *not calcineurin inhibitors.* Note the similarity of nomenclature to tac**rolimus.**
- Tacrolimus is in the same chemical family as macrolide antibiotics, but it is never used as an antibiotic.
- The IL-2 receptor is also called CD25. *CD* stands for cluster of differentiation and reflects a nomenclature system for defining cell surface markers on white blood cells (and now for other cells, too). There are more than 300 different CDs. The number gives no indication of the function or structure of the CD, and there is an enormous range of CDs. CD4 and CD8 are probably the most widely recognized CDs.
- Cyclosporine is not water soluble and requires bile production to be intact for oral administration. In patients with liver transplant who might have impaired bile production, the absorption of cyclosporine would be unpredictable. It was modified into a microemulsion in the 1990s, which solved this problem.

Target of Rapamycin (mTOR) Inhibitors

DESCRIPTION

mTOR inhibitors are immunosuppressant and antineoplastic agents and are classified as proliferation signal inhibitors.

PROTOTYPE AND COMMON DRUGS

- Prototype: sirolimus (also called rapamycin)
- Others: temsirolimus, everolimus

MOA (MECHANISM OF ACTION)

- mTOR (mammalian target of rapamycin) is a serine-threonine protein kinase activated by several growth factors after receptor binding.
- Sirolimus binds a protein called FKBP 12 (FKBP stands for FK506 binding protein) in the cytoplasm. The drug-protein complex then binds and inhibits mTOR (Figure 17-6).

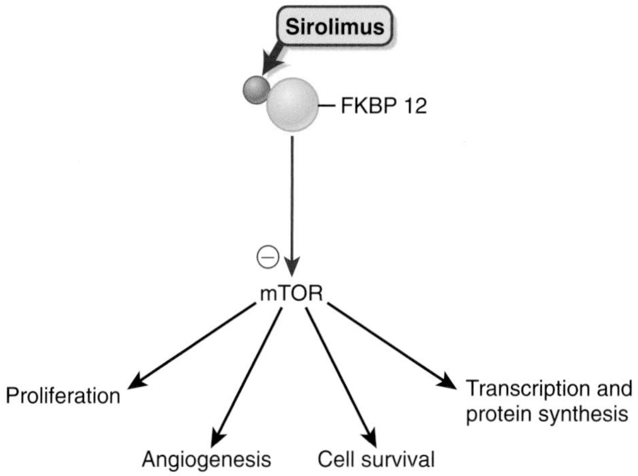

Figure 17-6.

- Inhibition of mTOR blocks cell-cycle progression at the G_1 → S phase transition.
- mTOR regulates important functions of the cell, including proliferation, angiogenesis (blood vessel formation), cell survival, protein synthesis, and transcription. It is recognized as a key point in many cellular functions.
- Through this mechanism, mTOR inhibitors:
  - ▲ Impede vascular endothelial cell stimulation by vascular endothelial growth factor (VEGF)
  - ▲ Reduce abnormally increased proliferation of endothelial and vascular smooth muscle cells, which is an important component of chronic rejection
  - ▲ Block the action of IL-2 and alter the activation of T and B lymphocytes
  - ▲ Alter the growth and proliferation of cancerous lymphocytes
- All functions of mTOR are not yet fully elucidated, and mTOR could be involved in a wider variety of biologic effects.

PHARMACOKINETICS

- Sirolimus and everolimus are administered orally, whereas temsirolimus is administered intravenously.
- Half-lives are 43 hours for everolimus and 60 hours for sirolimus.
- Metabolism is by CYP3A4, and transport is by P-glycoprotein. Temsirolimus is metabolized to sirolimus.
- Drug interaction: **Cyclosporine**, another antirejection drug used in renal transplants, increases the levels of sirolimus and everolimus; when used together with sirolimus or everolimus, drug levels must be measured.

INDICATIONS

- To prevent transplant rejection
- Drug-eluting stents: to reduce endothelial overgrowth of coronary (and other vascular) stents
- Treatment of renal cell carcinoma

CONTRAINDICATIONS

- None

SIDE EFFECTS

- Antiproliferative side effects (reduced proliferation of cells that normally proliferate quickly):
  - ▲ **Mucositis** and aphthous ulceration (oral canker sores) may occur.
  - ▲ **Anemia, thrombocytopenia, and neutropenia**: Inhibitors of mTOR should be stopped if the platelet count falls below 75 or the absolute neutrophil count (ANC) falls below 1.0.
- **Interstitial pneumonitis**
- **Infection** (resulting from immunosuppression)
- Metabolic effects: **hyperglycemia, hyperlipidemia**

IMPORTANT NOTES

- Sirolimus is not nephrotoxic, a very significant advantage over calcineurin inhibitors, especially when being used in the setting of renal transplant, when every effort is made to protect the new transplanted kidney. Calcineurin inhibitors, which are also used in renal transplant patients, are nephrotoxic.

Advanced

- Sirolimus first binds FKBP (FK506 binding protein), the protein that FK506 (tacrolimus) binds to. However, the drug-protein complex when bound to sirolimus acts differently than when bound to tacrolimus. Therefore the two drugs act on the same protein in the body but in a different way.
- Among rapamycin, cyclosporine, and tacrolimus (immunosuppressants for transplant rejection), rapamycin has the strongest antiangiogenic activity.

- ▲ It may be useful for the prevention of secondary tumors (lymphomas and squamous carcinomas) in the transplant population.
- ▲ Chronic use of cyclosporine or tacrolimus is a risk factor for secondary tumor development, as these agents suppress the tumor surveillance function of the immune system.
- **Drug interaction**: Although sirolimus is not nephrotoxic alone, coadministration with a calcineurin inhibitor (another drug used for renal transplants) results in greater **kidney damage** than with a calcineurin inhibitor alone. Therefore there is some interaction with calcineurin inhibitors that potentiates the renal damage induced by the calcineurin inhibitor, and the two drugs should *not* be coadministered.

FYI
- Important nomenclature:
  - ▲ Tacrolimus is not an mTOR inhibitor. It is a *calcineurin inhibitor*, and although it is also an immunosuppressant used for prevention of organ rejection, these drugs belong to two different classes of drug, despite the similarity of their names.
    - ▲ Sirolimus is produced by the bacterium *Streptomyces hygroscopicus*, which was isolated from **Rapa** Nui (Easter Island).
- Sirolimus is classified as a macrolide (antibiotic). However, it was initially developed as an antifungal and does have antifungal properties. It is important to note that when an infection is being treated, a strong immune system is desirable; sirolimus is an immunosuppressive and therefore is used clinically in a way, ironically, that is the polar opposite of the use for which it was originally designed.
- Sirolimus is a large cyclic molecule (as are macrolides), and the difference between sirolimus and everolimus is a single hydroxyl (-OH) group.
- Sirolimus is being investigated as:
  - ▲ An antiangiogenic agent for cancer therapy, specifically renal cell carcinoma
  - ▲ Therapy for psoriasis

Activated Protein C

DESCRIPTION
Activated protein C is part of the coagulation cascade but is used as an antiinflammatory.

PROTOTYPE
- Drotrecogin alfa (also called *activated protein* C or *APC*)

MOA (MECHANISM OF ACTION)
- The **inflammatory system** and **coagulation system** are tightly linked:
  - ▲ Activation of each system activates the other; thus inflammation causes coagulation and coagulation causes inflammation.
- Therefore, selectively inhibiting the coagulation cascade has the potential to inhibit the inflammatory response, and this is the basis for using activated protein C in severe inflammatory states known as **severe sepsis** or **septic shock**.
- Protein C is a natural anticoagulant that is a **vitamin K–dependant** protein synthesized by the liver. It becomes *activated* and works in conjunction with protein S to inhibit coagulation by:
  - ▲ Inactivating factors Va and VIIIa
  - ▲ Inhibiting release of plasminogen activator inhibitor 1 (plasminogen is converted to plasmin, which lyses clots; inhibition of an inhibitor of this process will therefore increase its activity)
  - ▲ Inhibiting activation of thrombin-activatable fibrinolysis inhibitor (TAFI) (Figure 17-7)

- In addition to its anticoagulant properties, activated protein C has also been shown to demonstrate the following antiinflammatory effects:
  - ▲ Blocks the accumulation of leukocytes at sites of inflammation
  - ▲ Modulates endothelial cell function
- Low levels of protein C are present in more than 85% of patients with severe sepsis, and therefore the ability of naturally occurring protein C to exert its antiinflammatory effects in these patients is reduced and could potentially be enhanced by supplementation of activated protein C.

PHARMACOKINETICS
- Activated protein C is metabolized by **plasma proteases**: 80% is eliminated within 13 minutes, and **98% is cleared within 2 hours**. This is important because patients with septic shock sometimes require surgery, and activated protein C needs to be discontinued 2 hours before surgery. Furthermore, if bleeding occurs while a patient is on activated protein C, then the anticoagulant effect can be reversed within 2 hours.
- Activated protein C is administered intravenously as an infusion, usually for 96 hours.

INDICATIONS
- **Severe sepsis** or **septic shock** in selected (very sick) patients

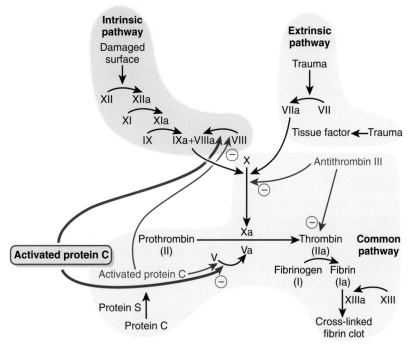

Figure 17-7.

▲ Specifically, patients with an APACHE score (measure of severity of acute illness) greater than 25

CONTRAINDICATIONS
■ Active bleeding or very high risk of bleeding (e.g., a recent stroke)

SIDE EFFECT
■ Bleeding

IMPORTANT NOTES
■ Patients who are candidates for activated protein C are very sick and are cared for in a critical care setting. Decisions to administer activated protein C are generally made by physicians specializing in critical care.

EVIDENCE
■ In two large RCTs (the PROWESS and ADDRESS studies) comparing activated protein C with placebo, a mortality benefit (absolute risk reduction of 6.1%) was demonstrated in patients who were *very sick* (APACHE score greater than 25) and treated with activated protein C. However, there was no mortality benefit in patients who were less sick (APACHE score less than 25).

FYI
■ *APACHE* stands for Acute Physiology and Chronic Health Evaluation, and the APACHE scoring system is used to describe severity of illness of patients admitted to the intensive care unit. The score ranges from 0 to 71 and is based on 17 physiologic parameters such as heart rate, white blood count, and P_{CO_2}.
■ Primitive organisms use coagulation as an immune response; to produce clot around the infection and isolate it from the rest of the circulation. This helps to defend against the advancement of the infection.
■ Other primitive organisms without a circulatory system (and thus no need to stop bleeding) still have a coagulation system to help defend against microbial invasion.
■ Activation of plasminogen to plasmin (a step that is promoted by activated protein C) results in lysis of clots; tPA, or tissue plasminogen activator, is a thrombolytic drug.

Glatiramoids

DESCRIPTION

Glatiramoids are used in the treatment of multiple sclerosis (MS).

PROTOTYPE

- Glatiramer

MOA (MECHANISM OF ACTION)

- The key pathophysiologic features of MS include mononuclear cell infiltration, demyelination, and scarring (gliosis) of the central nervous sytem, leading to significant neurologic deficits.
- The actions of glatiramer in the treatment of MS are not well understood and are believed to be mediated by multiple mechanisms, with the common theme of having an immunomodulating effect.
- Glatiramer competes for binding to major histocompatibility complex (MHC) class II molecules on APCs.
- Glatiramer also induces specific T-helper 2 (TH2)–type suppressor cells. The TH2 cells may cross the blood-brain barrier and secrete antiinflammatory cytokines and neurotropic factors that suppress surrounding inflammation (commonly referred to as *bystander suppression*).
- These neurotrophic factors may also facilitate remyelination and provide a protective effect for axons.

PHARMACOKINETICS

- Glatiramer is administered by subcutaneous injection.
- It is rapidly degraded after injection, leaving only about 10% at the site of injection after only 1 hour. Systemic plasma concentrations are therefore not detectable, nor can any be detected in the feces or urine.

INDICATIONS

- MS:
  - ▲ Relapsing-remitting
  - ▲ Clinically isolated syndrome (CIS)

CONTRAINDICATIONS

- None of major significance

SIDE EFFECTS

- **Local injection site reactions** may occur.
- **Chest pain** has been observed during clinical trials; its mechanism is unknown. The pain is transient and does not appear to be clinically harmful.
- **Postinjection reaction:** Flushing, palpitations, anxiety, dyspnea, and constriction of the throat may occur. Serious anaphylactic-type reactions are rare.
- **Infection:** Glatiramer is an immunomodulator and may impair the immune response to infection.

IMPORTANT NOTES

- CIS is characterized by a single demyelinating event, an attack that is suggestive of MS. These attacks include typical MS symptoms, such as sudden loss of vision. CIS is a recognized precursor to development of MS, although not all patients with CIS will go on to develop this disease. This has made it difficult to determine whether CIS patients should be initiated on this very expensive therapy, which includes daily injections, for an indeterminate amount of time.
- The other main agents used to treat MS are the interferons (IFNs) IFN alfa-1a and IFN beta-1b. These agents also have to be injected, and their main side effect is a flulike syndrome.

Advanced

- A new class of drugs has emerged in the fight against MS. The integrin inhibitors prevent the movement of lymphocytes from blood vessels into the brain. α4β1 Integrin is expressed on the surface of activated lymphocytes and acts on a receptor on the luminal surface of vascular endothelium, vascular cell adhesion molecule (VCAM).
- This interaction between α4β1 integrin and VCAM results in adherence of the activated lymphocyte to the vascular wall, which induces the lymphocyte to secrete proteases that enable the lymphocyte to transmigrate across the vascular endothelium and gain access to tissue.
- Natalizumab binds to α4β1 integrin, thus interfering with the interaction between it and VCAM, resulting in the inhibition of lymphocyte adherence and preventing transmigration of activated lymphocytes into tissue.
- The theory is that by preventing activated lymphocytes from gaining access to the CNS, natalizumab could reduce neuroinflammation and therefore modify the disease course.
- Natalizumab is reserved for advanced MS because of concerns over toxicity caused by an opportunistic infection of the CNS called *progressive multifocal leukoencephalopathy*.

FYI

- Protiramer, the second glatiramoid, is currently being evaluated in clinical trials for treatment of MS.
- A random sequence of amino acids is often referred to as a *polymer* by biochemists, in the same way that a polymer in chemistry is a sequence of molecules. Glatiramer is actually a polypeptide consisting of a random sequence of four amino acids: **g**lutamate, **l**ysine, **a**lanine, and **t**yrosine, hence the name *glatiramer*.

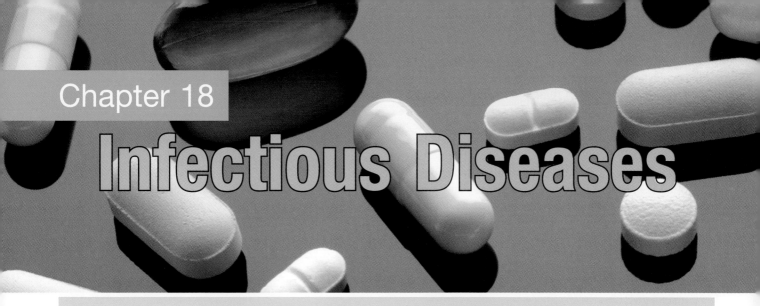

Chapter 18

Infectious Diseases

Introduction to Antibiotics

Antibiotics is the term used to describe drugs that kill or inhibit the growth of bacteria. The more general term *antiinfective* describes drugs that do the same to any type of organism that could infect humans, including viruses, parasites, and bacteria.

IMPORTANT CONSIDERATIONS

Learning about antibiotics can be overwhelming for the following reasons:

- There are many antibiotics.
- There are many, many infectious organisms.
- Every year, drug resistance patterns change.
- Geographically, drug resistance patterns are different.
- Multiple drugs are used to treat multiple different bacteria.

Therefore it might be helpful to organize your approach to learning the antibiotics. This introduction will offer some suggestions to assist you.

SUGGESTIONS

- Know which category the individual drugs belong to, and learn the category as a whole. For example, ceftriaxone is a third-generation cephalosporin. Therefore learn about cephalosporins in general, and then know the general differences among first-, second-, third-, and fourth-generation cephalosporins. In some circumstances there might be one or two extra important bits of information pertaining to individual drugs that are important to learn.
- Learn the *unique* common side effects of the drug.
  - For example, many drugs cause nausea, rash, diarrhea, and gastrointestinal (GI) upset. It is good to know these side effects, but these are common, and if a patient is experiencing these signs and symptoms, a drug should always be considered as a potential cause.
- Learn the *dangerous* (and usually rare) side effects of the drug.
  - If a side effect were dangerous *and* common, the drug would not be used. Therefore the really dangerous side

effects are usually rare and therefore easily forgotten about. *Do not forget about them.*

- Antibiotics can usually be classified in terms of the categories of bacteria they kill. These categories include the following:
  - Gram-positive organisms (which are usually cocci but sometimes rods)
  - Gram-negative organisms (which are usually rods but sometimes cocci)
  - Anaerobes
  - Atypical organisms (e.g., *Chlamydia, Rickettsia*)
  - Mycobacterial organisms (tuberculosis [TB])
- For each drug, make a small table to summarize what categories of bacteria it usually kills.
- You will have to learn "bugs" (not covered in this text) and drugs in at least **three different frameworks:**
  - Drugs: Which bugs do they kill?
    - List the bugs that are sensitive to penicillin.
  - Bugs: Which drugs kill them?
    - Methicillin-resistant *Staphylococcus aureus* (MRSA) is usually sensitive to (killed by) which drugs?
  - Clinical infections: Which bugs usually cause them, and by extension, which drugs should be used to treat them?
    - Dental abscesses are most commonly caused by…and treated with….
- To adequately study infectious disease, you will need to establish a mental framework that organizes your knowledge in the methods just described.

IMPORTANT CONSIDERATIONS

- It is *required* that you learn the **mechanism of action (MOA)** of a drug and also the **mechanism of resistance**, which enables an organism to live in the presence of the drug. This is important because when you are selecting an antibiotic, if your first choice does not work, you will have a better understanding of why it did not work and will be better educated to select a different antibiotic that will have a greater probability of killing the organism. For example, if a penicillin (a β-lactam) was given and the bug is known to produce β-lactamase, a third-generation cephalosporin (another β-lactam) might be a poor next choice.

- Make sure that the drug you select can get to the tissue in which the infection is located. Special examples include the following:
  - ▲ Gut (intraintestinal, not intraperitoneal) infections are often best treated with oral medications that *cannot* be absorbed into the body (because they remain in the gut, which is where the infection is)—for example, oral vancomycin for *C. difficile* colitis.
  - ▲ Central nervous system (CNS) infections: Some drugs do not penetrate the blood-brain barrier. These would be poor choices for treatment of bacterial meningitis.
  - ▲ Abscesses: There is no blood flow to an abscess. Therefore how can antibiotics get to the site of infection? *They cannot.* Abscesses have to be physically drained.
- The choice of antibiotic (oral versus intravenous, broad-spectrum versus narrow-spectrum agents) is usually determined by how sick the patient is and how certain you are about which bacterium is causing the infection. If you are uncertain, choose a broad-spectrum drug.
- If you can do cultures, try to do them *before the patient starts taking antibiotics*, because after you administer antibiotics the drug will be in the patient's system and will inhibit growth of specimens collected from the patient after that point in time.
- If you have positive cultures, then adjust your antibiotics to ensure proper coverage.
- Broad-spectrum drugs tend to be more expensive and more "powerful" and should be reserved for situations in which narrow-spectrum agents are not indicated. Development of resistance is a very real risk every time an antibiotic is used. Always using the powerful drugs will result in bacterial resistance to them. *Then what will you use?*

It is important to understand the MOA of a given antimicrobial because two drugs of a *different* class will have a higher probability of being **synergistic** and *making the kill* compared with two drugs that act on the same part of the bug. This does not mean that antibiotics should always be doubled up, but when they do need to be, MOA is an important consideration.

Note that **antimicrobial** means any drug that kills any living organism. Therefore antimicrobials include the following:

- ▲ Antibiotics (kill bacteria)
- ▲ Antifungals (kill fungi)
- ▲ Antiparasitics (kill parasites)

Viruses are technically not alive, so antivirals are usually not referred to as *antimicrobials*.

ADVANCED KILLING TECHNIQUES

Knowledge of pharmacokinetics is required to enable a clinician to be really good at knowing how to kill off an infection. Understanding some very important fundamental concepts are required (Figure 18-1).

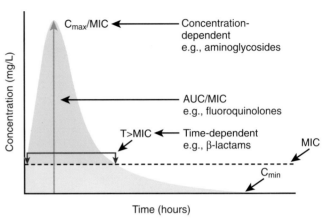

Antibiotic pharmacokinetics

Figure 18-1.

- **Minimum inhibitory concentration (MIC):** The MIC of an antimicrobial is the minimum concentration that will inhibit growth of a pathogen. Obviously, it is desirable to have the concentration in the patient's *infected tissues* to be greater than the MIC. If drug A has a lower MIC than drug B, then drug A kills the pathogen at a lower concentration of drug and would therefore be better at killing that particular pathogen, assuming all other factors are identical. When the MIC level of a drug for a given pathogen is low, the pathogen is considered *sensitive* to the drug (i.e., the drug will kill it). When the MIC is a moderate value, the pathogen's sensitivity to the drug will be *intermediate*, and when the MIC is high, the pathogen will be *resistant* to that drug. Laboratory values often report *sensitivities* as *S, I,* or *R* to report sensitive, intermediate, and resistant, respectively.

Now, exactly *how* the concentration of the antimicrobial stays above the MIC in the body is very important and is different for different drugs. The most important concepts are illustrated in Figure 18-1 and include:

- ▲ **Time dependence** is the total length of time that a drug level stays above the MIC. What matters is the total duration that the concentration is above the MIC. These drugs are called **time-dependent** antimicrobials. β-Lactams (penicillins, cephalosporins, and carbapenems) all fall into this category. Note that it does not matter if the drug level is *just barely* above the MIC or is 10 times the MIC.
- ▲ **C$_{MAX}$/MIC** is the *maximum concentration of the drug compared with the MIC.* In other words, some drugs kill better when the maximum concentration of the drug is very high. These drugs are called **concentration-dependent** antimicrobials. As a general rule, it is important to measure drug concentrations of these drugs. Vancomycin and aminoglycosides fall into this category and it is common to measure levels of both of them. Note that it does not matter how long the concentration stays above the MIC for these drugs, which is in complete contrast to the time-dependent drugs.

▲ **AUC > MIC:** This is the area under the curve (AUC), *above* the MIC. For these drugs, both time and concentration are important components (and when multiplied result in the area under the curve). Both the higher the concentration *and* the longer the concentration remains above MIC are important.

ANTIBIOTIC SPECTRA EXPLANATION

For each class of antibiotic, an abbreviated description of which bacteria are susceptible is included. The terms *very good,* *good, poor,* and *resistant* are used to describe the extent to which a given organism is susceptible to the antibiotic. *Very good* refers to very low rates of resistance, and *resistant* refers to very high rates, with *good* and *poor* being in between.

In addition to the categories of gram-positive, gram-negative, anaerobic, and commonly resistant organisms, additional *special* organisms that are susceptible to the antibiotic are also listed.

Penicillins

DESCRIPTION

Penicillins belong to a class of antibiotics known as **β-lactams**.

PROTOTYPES AND COMMON DRUGS

■ Prototypes: Penicillin G, Penicillin V

Others

■ Narrow-spectrum penicillins:
  ▲ Cloxacillin, oxacillin, nafcillin
■ Aminopenicillins:
  ▲ Ampicillin, amoxicillin
■ Broad-spectrum penicillins:
  ▲ Piperacillin, ticarcillin

MOA (MECHANISM OF ACTION)

■ Two major components are required for β-lactam activity:
  1. The first is the binding to **penicillin-binding proteins**.
  2. The second is the destruction of the bacterial cell wall.
■ All β-lactams (penicillins, carbapenems, and cephalosporins) act through this common sequence of events.

Binding

■ Virtually all bacteria contain penicillin-binding proteins.
■ Different bacteria have **different amounts and different types** of penicillin-binding proteins. For example, *Escherichia coli* has seven types, and *Staph. aureus* has four.
■ Different penicillin-binding proteins have different affinities for β-lactams, and therefore different bacteria will demonstrate different sensitivities to β-lactams.

Cell Wall Destruction

■ **Transpeptidases** are enzymes that cross-link **peptidoglycan** molecules in bacterial cell walls. Cross-linking these molecules gives strength to the cell wall.
■ β-Lactams work by **inhibiting transpeptidase**, preventing it from forming cross-links. This results in a bacterium with a structurally deficient cell wall, typically leading to bacterial lysis (Figure 18-2).

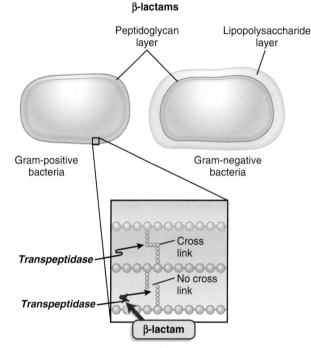

Figure 18-2.

■ **Gram-positive** bacteria have a thick peptidoglycan layer. They are therefore sensitive to β-lactams.
■ **Gram-negative** bacteria have a thinner peptidoglycan layer, but external to this layer is a **lipopolysaccharide** layer. This lipopolysaccharide layer protects the peptidoglycan layer from β-lactam activity, and therefore gram-negative bacteria are significantly more resistant to β-lactams.
■ **β-Lactamase inhibitors** are added to some β-lactam antibiotics to overcome resistance caused by β-lactamase. Although β-lactamase inhibitors do contain a β-lactam, they are not toxic to the bacteria; they merely bind to β-lactamase. Examples of β-lactamase inhibitors include the following:
  ▲ **Clavulanic acid** (added to amoxicillin)
  ▲ **Tazobactam** (added to piperacillin)

- **Narrow-spectrum penicillins** contain a larger molecule on the penicillin molecule side chain that confers steric hindrance: the inability to twist the molecule into other stereoisomers. This results in these penicillins being **resistant to β-lactamase** but at the same time restricts their spectrum of activity (thus they are said to be *narrow-spectrum* agents).
- **Aminopenicillins** have an added amino group (NH_2) that makes the molecule more hydrophilic and thus able to cross the lipopolysaccharide layer more easily. Therefore aminopenicillins have greater activity against gram-negative bacteria.
- **Broad-spectrum penicillins** are modifications of aminopenicillins: nitrogen and carbon atoms are added to the molecule. This increases the range of bacteria that are sensitive to the antibiotic. These penicillins are usually coadministered with a β-lactamase inhibitor because they are β-lactamase sensitive (a common example is "Pip/Tazo," which is piperacillin and tazobactam).

Mechanisms of Resistance

- Gram-negative bacteria, as described previously, inherently have an outer protective lipopolysaccharide layer that guards the peptidoglycan layer from attack by some β-lactams.
- The main mechanisms of resistance to β-lactams include the following:
  - ▲ **Variation of the penicillin-binding protein** leading to decreased binding of the β-lactam
  - ▲ Production of **β-lactamase**, which enzymatically destroys the four-carbon β-lactam ring
    - Genes for β-lactamase may exist on **plasmids** or on **bacterial chromosomes** and may be produced **constitutively** (all the time) or can be **induced**.
    - Genes that are on plasmids can readily be passed from one bacterium to another; thus resistance can be **transmitted** to different species.
    - There are a few different classification schemes for β-lactamases, and there are many different individual β-lactamase enzymes. Some other names of β-lactams include **penicillinase** and **carbapenemase**.
  - ▲ Changes in membrane channels called **porins** that are important in allowing influx of the antibiotic
  - ▲ Efflux pump mechanisms, which pump the drug out of the bacteria

PHARMACOKINETICS

- Eighty percent of penicillin is cleared by the kidneys within 4 hours. Therefore it is very quickly eliminated from the body, which is an undesirable characteristic if the goal is to expose the bacterial infection to prolonged concentrations of the drug.
- **Probenecid**, a uricosuric, competes with penicillin in the organic acid transporter in the kidney and therefore decreases renal clearance of penicillin, thereby prolonging *high tissue concentrations and a longer half life*. It is coadministered with penicillin.

- Most penicillins are renally cleared, and the dose must be adjusted in patients with renal dysfunction. However, **cloxacillin** is **hepatically cleared** and does not require dose adjustment in patients with renal dysfunction.

Spectra at a Glance

- **Gram-positive**: very good, especially for the narrow-spectrum penicillins
- **Gram-negative**: good for aminopenicillins and broad-spectrum penicillins
- **Anaerobes**: very good but only with *broad-spectrum* penicillins
- **Resistant organisms**:
  - ▲ **Methicillin-resistant *Staph aureus* (MRSA)**: resistant
  - ▲ **Vancomycin-resistant *Enterococcus* (VRE)**: resistant
  - ▲ ***Pseudomonas***: good, but only with *broad-spectrum* penicillins
- **Special sensitivities**:
  - ▲ *Neisseria meningitidis* (a gram-negative coccus) is an important cause of life-threatening (and reportable) meningitis and is susceptible to intravenous penicillin G.

CONTRAINDICATIONS

- Hypersensitivity (allergy)
  - ▲ Incidence is as high as 10%.
  - ▲ Signs and symptoms are as follows:
    - Maculopapular rash (mostly flat and confluent, not itchy)
    - Urticarial rash (hives)
    - Anaphylaxis
  - ▲ Cross-reactivity between penicillin allergy and other β-lactam antibiotics (cephalosporins and carbapenems) is around 1% to 10%.

SIDE EFFECTS

- **Hypersensitivity**: most commonly only a rash, but can include anaphylaxis
- Nausea and vomiting if given orally
- Diarrhea
- Stinging in the vein if given intravenously (IV)

IMPORTANT NOTES

- Methicillin is no longer used clinically, because of toxicity. It is, however, used to determine whether a staphylococcal infection is sensitive to the penicillins in its class. The term *methicillin-resistant Staph. aureus* (**MRSA**) is now commonly used to describe these organisms.
- MRSA is a huge problem. The problem of resistance will continue to get worse as continued exposure to antibiotics creates an environment for bacteria that promotes the survival of resistant strains.

FYI

- A lactam is a chemical ring. A β-lactam is a four-molecule ring (three carbons and one nitrogen) and is the *nucleus* of the penicillin molecule. The penicillin nucleus is shown in Figure 18-3. Modifications to the five-membered ring are

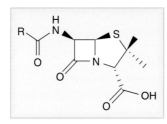

Figure 18-3.

the basis on which cephalosporins and carbapenems (two other β-lactam antibiotics) were derived.

- Penicillin was originally isolated from the mold *Penicillium*.
- Peptidoglycans are polymers of sugars and amino acids. Cross-linking of these polymers results in a rigid crystal structure.

- The clinically significant difference between amoxicillin and ampicillin is that amoxicillin is generally administered orally whereas ampicillin is generally administered IV.
- *Pip/Tazo* is a commonly used abbreviation for piperacillin plus tazobactam.
- A common dose for Pip/Tazo is 3.375 g, which means 3 g of piperacillin and 375 mg of tazobactam.
- Penicillin G, benzylpenicillin, is only given intravenously.
- Penicillin V, phenoxymethylpenicillin, is only given orally.
- It would be nice for memorization if penicillin G were given in the *gut* and penicillin V were given *IV*; unfortunately, it is the other way around.
- Uricosurics are drugs that promote the excretion of uric acid and are used in patients who have gout (high uric acid levels leading to uric acid crystal formation in joints).

Cephalosporins

DESCRIPTION

Cephalosporins are antibiotics that belong to the class of β-lactams.

PROTOTYPES AND COMMON DRUGS

- First-generation agent: cephalexin
  - Others: cefazolin, cefadroxil, cephalothin, cephapirin, cephradine
- Second-generation agents: cefaclor and cefuroxime
  - Others: cefoxitin, cefamandole, cefmetazole, cefonicid, cefotetan, cefoxitin, cefprozil, loracarbef
- Third-generation agent: ceftazidime
  - Others: ceftriaxone, cefixime, cefdinir, cefditoren, cefoperazone, cefotaxime, cefpodoxime, ceftibuten, ceftizoxime
- Fourth-generation agent: cefepime

MOA (MECHANISM OF ACTION)

- Two major components are required for β-lactam activity:
  1. The first is the binding to **penicillin-binding proteins**.
  2. The second is the destruction of the bacterial cell wall.
- All β-lactams (penicillins, carbapenems, and cephalosporins) act through this common sequence of events.

Binding

- Virtually all bacteria contain penicillin-binding proteins.
- Different bacteria have **different amounts and different types** of penicillin-binding proteins. For example, *E. coli* has seven types and *S. aureus* has four.
- Different penicillin-binding proteins have different affinities for β-lactams, and therefore different bacteria will demonstrate different sensitivities to β-lactams.

Cell Wall Destruction

- **Transpeptidases** are enzymes that cross-link **peptidoglycan** molecules in bacterial cell walls. Cross-linking these molecules gives strength to the cell wall (see Figure 18-2).
- β-lactams work by **inhibiting transpeptidase**, preventing it from forming cross-links. This results in a bacterium with a structurally deficient cell wall, typically leading to bacterial lysis.
- **Gram-positive** bacteria have a thick peptidoglycan layer. They are therefore sensitive to β-lactams.
- **Gram-negative** bacteria have a thinner peptidoglycan layer, but external to this layer is a **lipopolysaccharide** layer. This lipopolysaccharide layer protects the peptidoglycan layer from β-lactam activity, and therefore gram-negative bacteria are significantly more resistant to β-lactams.

Mechanisms of Resistance

- The main mechanisms of resistance to β-lactams include the following:
  - **Variation of the penicillin-binding protein**, leading to decreased binding of the β-lactam
  - Production of **β-lactamase**, which enzymatically destroys the four-carbon β-lactam ring
    - Genes for β-lactamase may exist on **plasmids** or on **bacterial chromosomes** and may be produced **constitutively** (all the time) or can be **induced**.
    - Genes that are on plasmids can readily be passed from one bacterium to another; thus resistance can be **transmitted** to different species.
    - There are a few different classification schemes for β-lactamases, and there are many different individual

β-lactamase enzymes. Some other names of β-lactams include **penicillinase** and **carbapenemase**.

▲ Changes in membrane channels called **porins** that are important in allowing influx of the antibiotic

▲ Efflux pump mechanisms

PHARMACOKINETICS

■ Cephalosporins are mainly renally excreted, except ceftriaxone, excretion of which is 50% hepatic.

■ Penetration to the brain through the blood-brain barrier is a very important factor for antibiotics because it will determine whether or not an antibiotic will be effective against **bacterial meningitis**. Third-generation cephalosporins have good CNS penetration.

Spectra at a Glance

■ **Gram-positive**: very good, especially the first-generation agents

■ **Gram-negative**: third-generation agents very good, second-generation agents good

■ **Anaerobes**: resistant against first-generation agents, good with second- and third-generation agents

■ **Resistant organisms**:

▲ **MRSA**: resistant

▲ **VRE**: resistant

▲ *Pseudomonas*: very good with ceftazidime (third-generation agent) and fourth-generation agents only

■ **Special sensitivities**:

▲ *N. meningitidis* (a gram-negative coccus) is an important cause of life-threatening (and reportable) meningitis and is susceptible to intravenous third-generation agents.

CONTRAINDICATIONS

■ Anaphylaxis to penicillins is an **absolute contraindication**.

■ Nonanaphylactic allergy to penicillins is a *relative contraindication*; however, the cross-reactivity is reported to be 2% to 10%, and cephalosporins have been used frequently in patients with a *penicillin allergy*.

▲ Maculopapular rash (flat confluent red rash)

▲ Urticaria (itchy hives)

▲ Eosinophilia (which is common to allergic reactions)

■ Side effects (GI upset, nausea) are sometimes called *allergies* by patients when in fact they are not allergies. *Always ask what reaction the patient experienced.* Side effects are not a contraindication.

SIDE EFFECTS

■ **Hematologic**: rare cases of bone marrow suppression resulting in a low white blood cell (WBC) count (aka neutropenia or granulocytopenia)

■ **Nephrotoxicity**: occasional interstitial nephritis and tubular necrosis

■ **Pseudomembranous colitis**: many antibiotics, including cephalosporins, can wipe out gut flora and permit the bacterium *C. difficile* to colonize, which causes this condition.

This is more common in the broad-spectrum (higher-generation) agents.

IMPORTANT NOTES

■ First-generation cephalosporins are:

▲ Good for skin infections (which are commonly *Streptococcus* or *Staphylococcus*)

▲ Commonly used as prophylactic antibiotics (preventative) given before surgery to prevent wound infections

■ Second-generation cephalosporins are:

▲ Good for *Bacteroides* infection (anaerobic), which can occur with intraabdominal infections

▲ Used less commonly for severe infections because third-generation cephalosporins are more efficacious. Second-generation cephalosporins can be used for **mild infections** in which gram-negative organisms are predicted or known

■ Third-generation cephalosporins are:

▲ Commonly used for severe infections in combination with another drug of a different class (different MOA)

■ Fourth-generation cephalosporins are:

▲ Reserved for severe nosocomial (hospital-acquired) infections, which have a tendency to be:

• Resistant to multiple other antibiotics

• More severe infections

• Commonly caused by gram-negative organisms

FYI

■ Note how the four-membered ring (the β-lactam) is the same as in penicillins; however, the *other* ring is six-membered, whereas in penicillins it is five-membered. The diagram shows the core nucleus of cephalosporins. There are currently four generations of cephalosporins (Figure 18-4).

■ Cephalosporins were first isolated from *Cephalosporium acremonium* from the sea near a sewer outlet in 1948. They were initially found to cure *Staph. aureus* infection and typhoid.

■ The suffix *-penia* means low cell counts. WBCs are granulocytes. The most abundant type of WBC is the neutrophil. Thus a low WBC count can be referred to as *granulocytopenia* or *neutropenia*.

■ Eosinophilia occurs in *drug hypersensitivity reactions* and also in other conditions. The mnemonic CHINA can help you remember the common causes of eosinophilia:

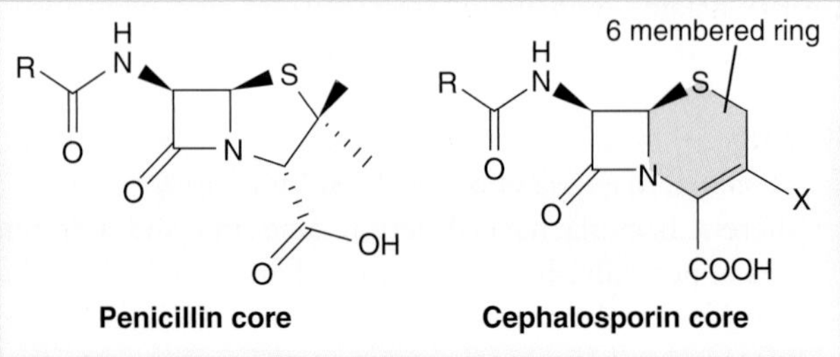

Figure 18-4.

▲ Connective tissue diseases, such as Churg-Strauss syndrome
▲ Helminthic (worm) parasitic infections
▲ Idiopathic eosinophilia
▲ Neoplastic (cancer) conditions, such as certain leukemias and lymphomas

▲ Allergic reactions, including interstitial nephritis
■ Pseudomembranous colitis is treated with antibiotics that kill *C. difficile*: metronidazole or vancomycin. Because the infection is in the gut, oral administration of these antibiotics delivers high concentrations of drug to the site of infection.

Carbapenems

DESCRIPTION
Carbapenems are antibiotics that belong to the class called *β-lactams*.

PROTOTYPE AND COMMON DRUGS
■ Prototype: imi**penem**
■ Others: mero**penem**, erta**penem**, dori**penem**

MOA (MECHANISM OF ACTION)
■ Two major components are required for β-lactam activity:
  1. The first is the binding to **penicillin-binding proteins.**
  2. The second is the destruction of the bacterial cell wall.
■ All β-lactams (penicillins, carbapenems, and cephalosporins) act through this common sequence of events.

Binding
■ Virtually all bacteria contain penicillin-binding proteins.
■ Different bacteria have **different amounts and different types** of penicillin-binding proteins. For example, *E. coli* has seven types and *S. aureus* has four.
■ Different penicillin-binding proteins have different affinities for β-lactams, and therefore different bacteria will demonstrate different sensitivities to β-lactams.

Cell Wall Destruction
■ **Transpeptidases** are enzymes that cross-link **peptidoglycan** molecules in bacterial cell walls. Cross-linking these molecules gives strength to the cell wall (Figure 18-5).
■ β-Lactams work by **inhibiting transpeptidase**, preventing it from forming cross-links. This results in a bacterium with a structurally deficient cell wall, typically leading to bacterial lysis.

Mechanisms of Resistance
■ The main mechanisms of resistance to β-lactams include the following:
  ▲ **Variation of the penicillin-binding protein,** leading to decreased binding of the β-lactam
  ▲ Production of **β-lactamase**, which enzymatically destroys the four-carbon β-lactam ring
    • Genes for β-lactamase may exist on **plasmids** or on **bacterial chromosomes** and may be produced **constitutively** (all the time) or can be **induced.**

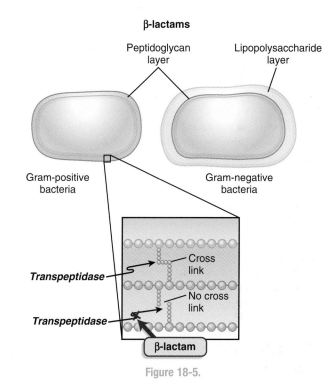

β-lactams

Peptidoglycan layer

Lipopolysaccharide layer

Gram-positive bacteria

Gram-negative bacteria

Transpeptidase — Cross link

No cross link

Transpeptidase —

β-lactam

Figure 18-5.

• Genes that are on plasmids can readily be passed from one bacterium to another; thus resistance can be **transmitted** to different species.
• There are a few different classification schemes for β-lactamases, and there are many different individual β-lactamase enzymes. Some other names of β-lactams include **penicillinase** and **carbapenemase.**
• Carbapenems are resistant to most β-lactamases but are generally not resistant to **metallo-β-lactamases.**
▲ Changes in membrane channels called **porins** that are important in allowing influx of the antibiotic
▲ Efflux pump mechanisms

PHARMACOKINETICS
■ Carbapenems are administered via IV.
■ Carbapenems are eliminated by the kidneys.
■ Imipenem is hydrolyzed by renal tubular dipeptidase. Imipenem is therefore always combined with **cilastatin**, which inhibits this breakdown. Other carbapenems do not require

coadministration with cilastatin because they are not metabolized by dipeptidase.

- Doses must be reduced in patients with renal dysfunction. With imipenem, there is increased risk for seizures in patients with renal dysfunction.
- Ertapenem has a longer half-life and can be administered once a day.

Spectra at a Glance

- **Gram-positive:** very good
- **Gram-negative:** very good
- **Anaerobes:** very good
- **Resistant organisms:**
  - ▲ MRSA: resistant
  - ▲ VRE: good to poor
  - ▲ *Pseudomonas:* very good
- **Special sensitivities:**
  - ▲ SPACEs:
    - Refers to five genera of gram-negative rods (**Enterobacteriaceae**) that are commonly resistant to β-lactams: *Serratia, Pseudomonas, Acinetobacter, Citrobacter, and Enterobacter*
  - ▲ ESBL:
    - Refers to extended-spectrum β-lactamase, which is able to deactivate third-generation cephalosporins and also confer resistance to non–β-lactam antibiotics, including aminoglycosides and fluoroquinolones

INDICATIONS

- Carbapenems are generally reserved for very severe infections.

CONTRAINDICATION

- **Seizure history:** Imipenem causes seizures in approximately 1.5% of patients. Patients with a seizure history should not receive imipenem. Other carbapenems do not share this neurotoxicity and therefore have largely replaced imipenem.

SIDE EFFECTS

- **Nausea** and **vomiting**
- **Neurotoxicity:** Imipenem can cause seizures. Meropenem and ertapenem do not.
- **Fever:** This can cause diagnostic dilemmas because carbapenems are administered to patients with suspected infections, who usually already have a fever. If the drug starts to create a fever, then it can be very difficult to know when the infection is gone (which is usually accompanied by a normalization of the patient's temperature).

IMPORTANT NOTES

- **MRSA** is an important resistant strain of *S. aureus.* It is *not* sensitive to carbapenems. It is treated with vancomycin.
- **VRE** is another important resistant strain. About 50% of VRE infections are sensitive to carbapenems.
- Carbapenems are very broad-spectrum agents. They are considered "big guns" and are used only in patients who are very sick or suspected of having resistant organisms. They are generally **not** used as first-line treatment.

Advanced

- Meropenem and ertapenem are not broken down by a renal dehydropeptidase and therefore are not coadministered with cilastatin.
- Ertapenem is not active against *Pseudomonas* or *Enterococcus.*
- Meropenem is more active against *Pseudomonas* and less active against *S. aureus* and *Enterococcus* than imipenem is.

FYI

- Carbapenems differ structurally from penicillins in that the five-membered ring that is attached to the β-lactam ring contains a carbon atom instead of a sulfur atom. The name *carbapenem* comes from **carb**on and **pen**icillin. Figure 18-6 shows the core structure of a carbapenem but does not show the side chains.

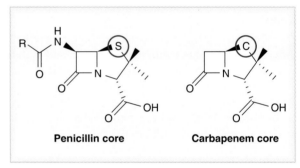

Penicillin core   **Carbapenem core**

Figure 18-6.

- The *entero-* in Enterobacteriaceae refers to enteral, or within the GI tract, which is where Enterobacteriaceae (and *Enterococcus*) colonize.
  - ▲ Enteral feeding is feeding into the GI tract (either orally or by feeding tube). Parenteral feeding is via the intravenous route (i.e., around or not directly into the GI tract); it has nothing to do with a parent feeding a child.

Glycopeptides

DESCRIPTION
Glycopeptides are antibiotics that are cell wall synthesis inhibitors.

PROTOTYPE AND COMMON DRUGS
- Prototype: Vancomycin
- Others: Teicoplanin, telavancin

MOA (MECHANISM OF ACTION)
- Glycopeptides inhibit cell wall synthesis by attaching to the end of the peptidoglycan precursor units (a short four– or five–amino acid sequence called the **D-alanyl-D-alanine [D-ALA-D-ALA] terminus**) that are required to be laid down into the matrix. This step is catalyzed by **transglycosylase**. Because the glycopeptide binds to the end of the precursor, the precursor is not released from the carrier and thus **peptidoglycan synthesis** stops (Figure 18-7).

Glycopeptides

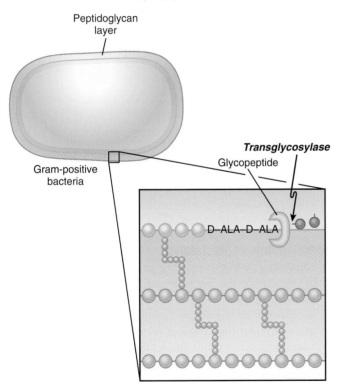

Figure 18-7.

- Glycopeptides are bactericidal in organisms that are dividing, because a dividing bacterium requires new cell wall synthesis, and the absence of the new cell wall results in death of the organism.
- As a result of targeting the peptidoglycan layer, glycopeptides are effective *only* against gram-positive organisms. This is because gram-negative bacteria possess a thick outer layer of lipopolysaccharide that covers the peptidoglycan layer.

Mechanisms of Resistance
- A change to the end of the amino acid precursor (which has a D-alanyl-D-alanine terminus) can result in the drug not binding to the precursor. This is the most common method by which *Enterococcus* becomes resistant (and is then called **VRE**, vancomycin-resistant *Enterococcus*).
- Excess cell wall production by the bacteria.
- Biofilm production: *Staphylococcus epidermidis* can produce a film that can block penetration of the antibiotic. This is a slimy way to become resistant.
- The mechanisms by which *S. aureus* develops resistance to vancomycin are still being investigated.

PHARMACOKINETICS
- The half-life of vancomycin is 6 hours, whereas the half-life of teicoplanin is much longer, as high as 100 hours (assuming normal kidney function).
- Glycopeptides are very poorly absorbed from the GI tract. If the infection that is being treated is inside the GI tract (for example, *C. difficile* colitis, also called "C diff colitis," or pseudomembranous colitis), then administering the drug orally provides the highest exposure of antibiotic to the infection.
- If the infection is anywhere other than inside the GI tract (e.g., blood, soft tissues, brain, heart), then the drug must be administered via the intravenous route—or, for teicoplanin, also intramuscularly.
- They are renally cleared, and in patients who have renal dysfunction or renal failure, the frequency of administration must be dramatically reduced (sometimes as infrequently as one dose every 2 to 3 days) and should be guided by drug levels in the blood. Because teicoplanin has a longer half-life, it can actually be administered once a week in patients without any renal function.
- Glycopeptides are cleared by dialysis. This is important because patients on dialysis usually get dialyzed three times a week. The best time to administer vancomycin would be just **after** dialysis, which would result in the drug remaining at high levels in the blood and tissues for the full 2 to 3 days until next dialysis. It would not be logical to give the drug right before dialysis.

Spectra at a Glance
- **Gram-positive**: very good
- **Gram-negative**: resistant
- **Anaerobes**: resistant
- **Resistant organisms**:
  - ▲ MRSA: very good
  - ▲ VRE: resistant

▲ *Pseudomonas:* resistant
- **Special:**
  - ▲ *C. difficile*
  - ▲ *Enterococcus* (excluding VRE)

CONTRAINDICATIONS

- None

SIDE EFFECTS

- **Flushing:** When vancomycin is administered quickly, the blood pressure can fall because of histamine release. Therefore vancomycin must be administered slowly (usually over 1 hour). The flushing caused by histamine release has been called *red man syndrome* and is not an allergy but a predictable response to rapidly administered vancomycin.
- **Ototoxicity** is very rare, unless vancomycin is administered with another ototoxic agent such as aminoglycosides.
- **Nephrotoxicity** is rare (6% to 7%), unless administered with another nephrotoxic agent such as aminoglycosides. The role of vancomycin as a nephrotoxic agent is probably overestimated, and it should probably be considered to be only *very weakly* nephrotoxic.
- **Neutropenia** (a low neutrophil [WBC] count): Vancomycin is administered in the setting of infection, and if it simultaneously weakens the immune system by lowering the WBC count, this will potentially be a very serious problem.

IMPORTANT NOTES

- Although vancomycin can kill *S. aureus* organisms that are resistant to cloxacillin (or methicillin [i.e., **MRSA**]), cloxacillin has a lower MIC than vancomycin for strains that are β-lactam susceptible. Therefore cloxacillin is a *better killer* of *S. aureus* when there is no resistance. Vancomycin is not a *stronger* antibiotic. It is simply a different but paradoxically slightly weaker one that avoids β-lactam resistance.
- An important resistant strain of bacteria is **VRE**.

FYI

- Common levels that are reported for serum vancomycin levels are *peak* (right after a dose) and trough (right before a dose). The trough should range from 15 to 25.
- VRE is currently treated with linezolid.
- MRSA is treated with vancomycin; the first MRSA strain that was resistant to vancomycin was reported in Japan in 1997.
- Teicoplanin is approved in Europe but not in North America.

Fluoroquinolones

DESCRIPTION

Fluoroquinolones are antibiotics.

PROTOTYPE AND COMMON DRUGS

- Prototype: ciprofloxacin
- Others: levofloxacin, moxifloxacin, norfloxacin

MOA (MECHANISM OF ACTION)

- DNA is normally supercoiled. Supercoiled DNA is under too much tension to be separated, so an extra step is required before replication and transcription can occur. **DNA gyrase** relaxes supercoiled DNA by cutting it, allowing rotation to occur, and then reattaching it.
- Fluoroquinolones bind to and inhibit DNA gyrase (also called **topoisomerase II**) and **topoisomerase IV**. Fluoroquinolones inhibit DNA gyrase in gram-negative organisms and topoisomerase IV in gram-positive organisms (Figure 18-8).
- The fluoroquinolones inhibit DNA gyrase after the cutting step, preventing reattachment from occurring. At high doses this leads to the release of these broken segments of DNA. It is thought that the accumulation of these DNA fragments leads to cell death, accounting for the bactericidal action of fluoroquinolones.
- Inhibiting topoisomerase IV interferes with separation of replicated chromosomal DNA into the respective daughter cells during cell division. Thus cell division is halted.
- Eukaryotes (humans) possess different forms of topoisomerase II and topoisomerase IV.

Mechanisms of Resistance

- Mutations in the genes that encode type II topoisomerase result in the enzyme not being inhibited by the fluoroquinolone.
- Alterations in membrane porins or efflux pumps that actively pump the drug out of the bacterial cell result in lower drug levels inside the bacteria.

PHARMACOKINETICS

- Fluoroquinolones can enter human cells easily and therefore are often used to treat *intracellular* pathogens.
- Fluoroquinolones are **absorbed very well from the gut.** Therefore if a person can tolerate oral medication, he or she can usually be switched from an intravenous form to an oral form.
- Most fluoroquinolones are cleared renally, and dose adjustment may be required in patients with renal impairment.

Fluoroquinolones

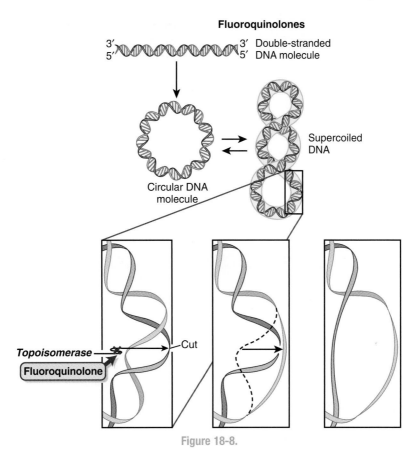

Figure 18-8.

▲ An exception is **moxifloxacin**, which is cleared by the liver and therefore contraindicated in patients with hepatic failure.

Spectra at a Glance

■ **Gram-positive:** good
■ **Gram-negative:** very good
■ **Anaerobes:** good with levofloxacin and moxifloxacin
■ **Resistant organisms:**
  ▲ **MRSA:** resistant
  ▲ **VRE:** resistant
  ▲ *Pseudomonas:* poor to good
■ **Special sensitivities:**
  ▲ **Intracellular organisms:**
    • *Chlamydia*
    • *Mycobacterium avium*

CONTRAINDICATIONS

■ Pregnancy
■ Children: Joint pain (arthralgia) and swelling has occurred, and therefore administration to children is not common.

SIDE EFFECTS

■ Generally well tolerated
■ Nausea, vomiting, diarrhea
■ Tendon ruptures (Achilles, shoulder); occur rarely. The mechanism of this complication is not well understood.

IMPORTANT NOTES

■ Originally, quinolones were mainly effective against gram-negative bacteria, but newer agents are useful against gram-positive cocci as well.
■ Drugs from a different but similarly named class called *quinolines* do not have antibacterial properties but rather are antimalarials.

Advanced

Drug Interactions

■ With NSAIDS, fluoroquinolones may potentiate CNS toxicity and cause seizures.
■ With theophylline, they will increase theophylline levels and increase risk of theophylline toxicity.

FYI

■ As the name suggests, fluoroquinolones possess a fluorine ion. They all contain two six-membered rings. Ciprofloxacin is shown in the diagram (Figure 18-9). Earlier generations of fluoroquinolones were not fluorinated and were simply called *quinolones.* They are infrequently used now.
■ An isomerase converts a molecule from one isomer to another isomer. *Topo-* refers to topographic, or surface shape. Therefore topoisomerase enzymes convert DNA molecules from one shape to another shape.
■ More than 30 different fluoroquinolones exist. Some are used for veterinary purposes only.

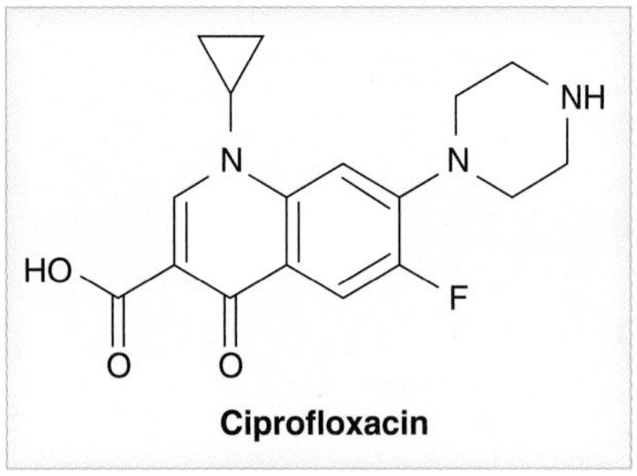

Ciprofloxacin

Figure 18-9.

- Many fluoroquinolones have been withdrawn from the market because of side effects:
  - ▲ Gatifloxacin: hyperglycemia
  - ▲ Trovafloxacin: acute liver failure and death
  - ▲ Temafloxacin: hemolytic anemia
  - ▲ Grepafloxacin: long QT syndrome and sudden death
  - ▲ Fleroxacin: phototoxicity

Aminoglycosides

DESCRIPTION

Aminoglycosides are a form of antibiotics that are derived from bacteria.

PROTOTYPE AND COMMON DRUGS

- Prototype: gent**amicin**
- Others: tobr**amycin**, amik**acin**, ne**omycin**, strepto**mycin**, kan**amycin**, parom**omycin**

MOA (MECHANISM OF ACTION)

- The production of proteins from mRNA is called **translation**; this step requires **ribosomes**, transfer RNA (**tRNA**), and messenger RNA (**mRNA**) (Figure 18-10).
- mRNA contains the sequencing code based on DNA; tRNA contains single amino acids and binds to a three-base sequence of mRNA; ribosomes are like *assembly line* processing machinery, bringing the mRNA and tRNA together to assemble sequences of amino acids.
- The ribosomes are different sizes:
  - ▲ Prokaryotes (bacteria) have 70S ribosomes made of a small (30S) and a large (50S) subunit.
    - The 50S subunit is composed of a 5S and a 23S subunit plus 34 other proteins.
  - ▲ Eukaryotes (humans) have 80S ribosomes, composed of a small (40S) and a large (60S) subunit.
- Ribosomes have different binding sites, named:
  - ▲ **Aminoacyl (A):** Incoming tRNA binds to this site.
  - ▲ **Peptidyl (P):** This is where the existing amino acid chain (connected to tRNA) is elongated when the incoming amino acid is transferred to it through the action of **peptidyl transferase.**
  - ▲ **Exit or egress (E):** After the tRNA gives up the amino acid chain, it must leave so that new tRNA can take its place.
- There are two theories about how aminoglycosides work:
  1. Aminoglycosides are protein synthesis inhibitors. They *irreversibly* bind the 30S **ribosomal subunit (RSU)**. At

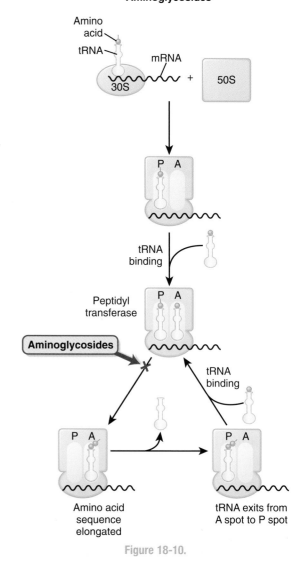

Aminoglycosides

Figure 18-10.

low concentrations they cause **misreading** of the mRNA by ribosomes, leading to synthesis of proteins with incorrect amino acid sequences. At higher concentrations they **halt** protein synthesis, trapping the ribosomes at the AUG start codon. Accumulation of these abnormal initiation complexes halts translation.

2. Recent experimental studies show that the initial site of action is the outer bacterial membrane. The cationic antibiotic molecules create fissures and pores in the outer cell membrane, resulting in leakage of intracellular contents and enhanced antibiotic uptake.
   - This rapid action at the outer membrane probably accounts for most of the bacteri*cidal* activity.
   - Energy is needed for aminoglycoside uptake into the bacterial cell. Anaerobes have less energy available for this uptake; therefore aminoglycosides are less active against anaerobes.

■ Aminoglycosides are particularly effective against gram-negative bacteria.

■ Many other *protein synthesis inhibitors* are bacteriostatic (only inhibit replication of bacteria versus killing bacteria). The action of aminoglycosides on the outer bacterial membrane, in addition to its protein synthesis inhibition, is thought to be the reason that aminoglycosides are bactericidal.

Mechanisms of Resistance

■ Three mechanisms of resistance have been recognized:
  ▲ Ribosome alteration
  ▲ Decreased permeability
  ▲ Inactivation by aminoglycoside modifying enzymes

■ The third mechanism is of most clinical importance, because the genes encoding aminoglycoside-modifying enzymes can be disseminated by plasmids, which are segments of DNA that are outside of the chromosome.

PHARMACOKINETICS

■ Penetration of biologic membranes is poor because of the drug's polar structure. Therefore all aminoglycosides are **poorly absorbed in the GI tract** and are not administered orally, and intracellular concentrations are usually low.
  ▲ The exception to this rule is the **proximal tubule in the kidney**. Aminoglycosides accumulate inside these kidney cells, and this is the basis for **nephrotoxicity** of this drug.

■ The most common route of administration is the intravenous route, but tobramycin can be inhaled (for treatment of severe pneumonia), and some aminoglycosides are available as topical drops for the ears or eyes.

■ Aminoglycosides are rapidly excreted by glomerular filtration in the kidney, resulting in a plasma half-life of 2 hours in a patient with *normal* renal function, but up to 30 to 60 hours in patients who have nonfunctioning kidneys. **Therefore repeat doses in patients with renal dysfunction will lead to very high levels in the body and will cause toxicity.**

▲ Kidney function in all patients receiving aminoglycosides must be measured **before** administration and **monitored throughout** treatment.

■ Aminoglycosides have a narrow therapeutic index. Toxicity occurs at a serum concentration just slightly higher than the therapeutic concentration.

■ Paromomycin is effective against GI parasites and is poorly absorbed in the GI tract. Administering this aminoglycoside results in high levels of drug inside the GI tract (where the parasite exists) with negligible systemic absorption.

Spectra at a Glance

■ **Gram-positive:** poor, unless in combination with other antibiotic active against gram-positive organisms
■ **Gram-negative:** very good
■ **Anaerobes:** resistant
■ **Resistant organisms:**
  ▲ **MRSA:** resistant
  ▲ **VRE:** resistant
  ▲ *Pseudomonas:* good
■ **Special sensitivities:**
  ▲ **Multidrug-resistant organisms:** amikacin
  ▲ **Intestinal parasites** (*Entamoeba,* *Cryptosporidium*): paromomycin
  ▲ **TB:** streptomycin

CONTRAINDICATION

■ **Renal dysfunction:** Patients starting with poor functioning kidneys can experience a further decline in kidney function if exposed to aminoglycosides.

SIDE EFFECTS

■ **Ototoxicity** (damage to the inner ear)
  ▲ Occurs in about 10% of patients
  ▲ Is caused by inhibition of *human* mitochondrial ribosomes, damaging the hair cells of the inner ear
  ▲ Symptoms can include the following:
    - Decreased hearing
    - Tinnitus (ringing in the ear)
    - Vertigo (a spinning type of dizziness)
■ **Nephrotoxicity**
  ▲ Occurs in up to 10% of patients and in up to 25% of patients who are critically ill
  ▲ Drug accumulates in proximal tubule cells, leading to mitochondrial poisoning and cell membrane disruptions. If the **serum creatinine starts to rise** during administration, then there must be a very high suspicion that kidney damage secondary to the aminoglycoside is occurring. The **aminoglycoside should be immediately stopped.**
  ▲ Nephrotoxicity is usually mild and reversible if the drug is stopped.
  ▲ Elevated "trough" levels (the lowest serum concentrations, just before a dose) are correlated with toxicity. Peak levels (the highest serum concentrations, just after a dose) are not correlated to toxicity.

▲ Risk factors for nephrotoxicity include the following:
  • Low perfusion states (heart failure or septic shock)
  • Advanced age
  • Preexisting renal disease
  • Failure to monitor creatinine and drug trough levels

IMPORTANT NOTES

▪ Serum levels of aminoglycosides **must** be monitored. Peak and trough levels help determine required doses.
▪ Doses **must** be adjusted according to the patient's renal function (creatinine clearance).
▪ Amikacin is particularly effective when used against bacteria that are resistant to other aminoglycosides, because its chemical structure makes it less susceptible to inactivating enzymes.

Advanced

▪ **Neuromuscular blockade** occurs because of a reduction in acetylcholine release. These drugs do not paralyze patients, but under anesthesia in patients who are already receiving a neuromuscular blocking drug (such as rocuronium or vecuronium), the duration of blockade can be longer than normal. Other conditions in which neuromuscular blockade could become problematic are:
  ▲ Myasthenia gravis (weakness caused by antibodies to the ACh receptors in the neuromuscular junction)
  ▲ Hypocalcemia (causes weakness)
▪ In patients on dialysis, about 65% to 75% of a given dose will be removed by a single treatment of dialysis. The objective with antibiotics is to maintain a concentration in the blood that will kill bacteria (and not be toxic to the patient); if the drug is immediately removed after it is administered, this objective will not be met. Common sense dictates, therefore, that the drug should be given *after* a dialysis run and not before.

FYI

▪ Nomenclature:
  ▲ The suffix *-mycin* is for drugs that are derived from *Streptomyces*, a genus of bacteria commonly found in soil. Streptomycin is named after *Streptomyces*, but it is no longer commonly used.
  ▲ The suffix *-micin* is for drugs that are derived from *Micromonospora*, also a genus of bacteria found in soil.
  ▲ The suffix *-mycin* is a common antibiotic suffix. Be aware of confusion with names:
    • Vancomycin is **not** an aminoglycoside. It is a glycopeptide.

• Erythromycin, clarithromycin, and azithromycin are **not** aminoglycosides. They are macrolides.
▲ Amikacin **is** an aminoglycoside, even though its name does not exactly follow the pattern of other aminoglycosides.
▪ The *S* in 50S and 23S refers to Svedberg units. A Svedberg unit is a measurement of time and equals 10^{-13} seconds. It is used to describe speed of sedimentation during centrifuging. Combining two molecules (30S + 50S) and predicting the combined Svedberg units is not simply an *additive* process because the surface area changes. Thus in the bacterial ribosome, 30S + 50S = 70S (and not 80).
▪ Glycosides are molecules produced in nature that contain sugar molecules. Therefore aminoglycosides contain amino groups connected to sugar molecules. Gentamicin, with three sugar molecules and five amino groups, is shown in Figure 18-11.

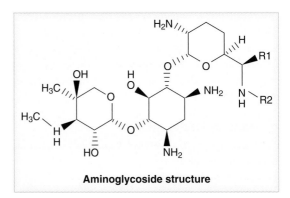

Aminoglycoside structure

Figure 18-11.

▪ The first aminoglycoside was streptomycin and was discovered in 1943.
▪ Gentamicin, the most commonly used aminoglycoside, was discovered in 1963.
▪ Neomycin is used only in creams or drops (for the ear). It is not administered systemically.
▪ Tobramycin is available in an inhaled form and is used for patients with cystic fibrosis who develop chronic gram-negative infections (particularly *Pseudomonas*). Inhaled administration increases the dose of drug delivered to the site of infection.
▪ Digoxin, is also a glycoside, but it is not an antibiotic. It is used for cardiac purposes and is derived from a purple flowered plant called foxglove.

Lincosamides

DESCRIPTION
Lincosamides are antibiotics that inhibit the 23S bacterial ribosome.

PROTOTYPE AND COMMON DRUGS
- Prototype: clindamycin
- Others: lincomycin

MOA (MECHANISM OF ACTION)
- The production of proteins from mRNA is called **translation**; this step requires **ribosomes, tRNA,** and **mRNA.**
- mRNA contains the sequencing code based on DNA; tRNA contains single amino acids and binds to a three-base sequence of mRNA. Ribosomes are like "assembly line" processing machinery, bringing the mRNA and tRNA together to assemble sequences of amino acids (Figure 18-12).
- The ribosomes are different sizes:
  - ▲ Prokaryotes (bacteria) have 70S ribosomes made of a small (30S) and a large (50S) subunit.
    - The 50S subunit is composed of a 5S and a 23S subunit plus 34 other proteins.
  - ▲ Eukaryotes (humans) have 80S ribosomes, composed of a small (40S) and a large (60S) subunit.
- Ribosomes have different binding sites, named:
  - ▲ **Aminoacyl (A): Incoming** tRNA binds to this site.
  - ▲ **Peptidyl (P):** This is where the existing amino acid chain (connected to tRNA) is elongated when the incoming amino acid is transferred to it through the action of **peptidyl transferase.**
  - ▲ **Exit or egress (E):** After the tRNA gives up the amino acid chain, it must leave so that new tRNA can take its place.
- Lincosamides bind the **23S** rRNA molecule of the 50S RSU and inhibit **peptidyl transferase,** blocking the transfer of the new amino acid onto the growing chain.
- Inhibition of protein synthesis does not typically kill bacteria cells, so these agents are generally **bacteriostatic** but in high concentrations can be bactericidal.
- Clindamycin, because of its action on protein synthesis, has been postulated to be beneficial in **toxin-producing infections;** most bacterially produced toxins are proteins, so an added benefit of a protein synthesis inhibitor is reduced toxin production, in addition to slowed bacterial growth.

Mechanisms of Resistance
- **Mutation of the ribosomal receptor site** or modification of the receptor by a **methylase** enzyme results in decreased binding to the 50S subunit.
- Enzymatic inactivation of clindamycin occurs.
- Some bacteria possess an efflux-based pump mechanism (which lowers bacterial intracellular drug levels and confers

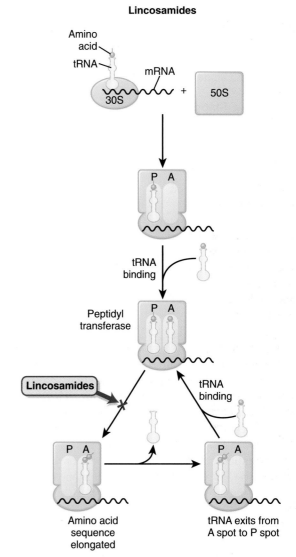

Lincosamides

Figure 18-12.

resistance) to other ribosomal inhibitors, such as macrolides. However, bacteria that are resistant to macrolides because of the presence of these efflux pumps are *not* resistant to clindamycin. Even though these drugs act very similarly, they are chemically different, and clindamycin is unaffected by the pump.
  - ▲ However, resistance to clindamycin usually implies cross-resistance also to macrolides.

PHARMACOKINETICS
- Clindamycin is well absorbed orally and is metabolized by the liver. Dose adjustments are not required in patients with renal dysfunction but are required in those with severe hepatic dysfunction.

■ Clindamycin penetrates bone well and is therefore effective for dental infections that might have bony involvement.

■ Clindamycin does not penetrate into the brain very well; therefore, it should **not** be used for CNS infections.

■ Coadministration of two different antibiotic classes that *both* bind the 50S subunit (e.g., lincosamides, oxazolidinones, macrolides) is not recommended because although the drugs bind different sites on the subunit, they can displace each other and result in being less effective than if administered alone.

Spectra at a Glance

■ **Gram-positive:** good
■ **Gram-negative:** resistant
■ **Anaerobes:** very good, especially for oral anaerobes
■ **Resistant organisms:**
  ▲ MRSA: poor to good
  ▲ VRE: resistant
  ▲ *Pseudomonas:* resistant
■ **Special sensitivities:**
  ▲ In combination with other bactericidal drugs for severe gram-positive infections

CONTRAINDICATIONS

■ None

SIDE EFFECTS

■ **Pseudomembranous colitis** (aka *C. difficile* colitis or "C diff" colitis) may occur. Bacterial flora of the colon changes with antibiotic administration. Some antibiotics (clindamycin is the worst offender) wipe out the normal flora and enable pathologic flora to grow, resulting in inflammation of the colon and diarrhea. This is a major problem and requires a second antibiotic (usually metronidazole or vancomycin) to be used to treat the diarrhea, which can be moderate to severe in intensity. *C. difficile* infections can sometimes be very difficult to eradicate.

IMPORTANT NOTES

■ Although a very effective antibiotic for gram-positive infections, the extremely high incidence of *C. difficile* colitis severely limits the use of clindamycin when other, alternative antibiotics can be used effectively.

■ Clindamycin is commonly used in infections in and around the oral cavity because of the high preponderance of anaerobic bacteria causing these infections.

■ Lincomycin has been essentially replaced by clindamycin.

■ **Toxic shock syndrome** is an inflammatory response resulting from a *Staphylococcus* or *Streptococcus* infection by a strain of bacteria that produces proteins that function as *superantigens* and trigger a full-blown inflammatory response. Clindamycin is thought to be helpful with these infections because it inhibits the production of the superantigen protein.

■ **Necrotizing fasciitis** is also called **flesh-eating disease** and is caused by **group A streptococci (GAS)**. GAS is also a toxin-producing strain and produces a superantigen that can cause a dramatic, amplified, and virtually unregulated inflammatory cascade resulting in life-threatening illness. In addition, the infection causes severe necrosis of soft tissues and spreads faster than antibiotics can treat (because blood vessels are destroyed in the area of the infection and intravenous antibiotics cannot actually be delivered to the site of the infection). Management requires surgical removal of the infected tissue (sometimes limb amputation) and high-dose antibiotics.

FYI

■ The *S* in 50S and 23S refers to Svedberg units. A Svedberg unit is a measurement of time and equals 10^{-13} seconds. It is used to describe speed of sedimentation during centrifuging. Combining two molecules (30S + 50S) and predicting the combined Svedberg units are not simply an *additive* process because the surface area changes. Thus in the bacterial ribosome, 30S + 50S = 70S (and not 80).

Tetracyclines

DESCRIPTION

Tetracyclines are antibiotics, chemically composed of four rings.

PROTOTYPE AND COMMON DRUGS

■ Prototype: tetra**cycline**
■ Others: doxy**cycline**, mino**cycline**, demeclo**cycline**, tige**cycline**

MOA (MECHANISM OF ACTION)

■ The production of proteins from mRNA is called **translation**; this step requires **ribosomes**, transfer RNA (**tRNA**), and messenger RNA (**mRNA**) (Figure 18-13).

■ mRNA contains the sequencing code based on DNA; tRNA contains single amino acids and binds to a three-base sequence of mRNA; ribosomes are like "assembly line" processing machinery, bringing the mRNA and tRNA together to assemble sequences of amino acids.

■ The ribosomes are different sizes:
  ▲ Prokaryotes (bacteria) have 70S ribosomes made of a small (30S) and a large (50S) subunit.
    • The 50S subunit is composed of a 5S and a 23S subunit plus 34 other proteins.
  ▲ Eukaryotes (humans) have 80S ribosomes, composed of a small (40S) and a large (60S) subunit.

■ Ribosomes have different binding sites, named:

Tetracyclines

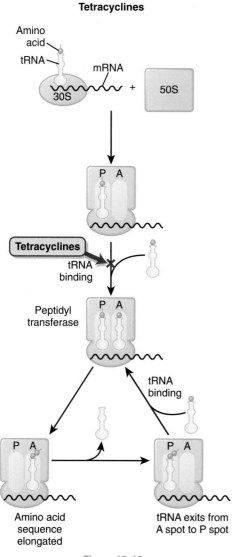

Figure 18-13.

▲ **Aminoacyl (A): Incoming** tRNA binds to this site.
▲ **Peptidyl (P):** This is where the existing amino acid chain (connected to tRNA) is elongated when the incoming amino acid is transferred to it through the action of **peptidyl transferase.**
▲ **Exit or egress (E):** After the tRNA gives up the amino acid chain, it must leave so that new tRNA can take its place.

■ Tetracyclines must first enter the microorganism before they can exert their antimicrobial effects. Microbes that actively take in tetracycline develop increased susceptibility to the drug because intracellular levels of the drug are high.
■ Tetracyclines bind reversibly to the **16S** subunit of the **30S** RSU and inhibit translation (protein synthesis). Binding of tetracycline to the ribosome weakens the **ribosome-tRNA** interaction; this prevents addition of amino acids to the growing peptide. This is in contrast to antibiotics that bind the 23S subunit and inhibit the *initiation* of translation.

■ Because tetracyclines stop protein synthesis, they are **bacteriostatic.** When drug levels fall, the protein synthesis can continue.
■ Mammalian cells lack the active transport system that bacteria use to take up tetracycline; this provides part of the basis of selectivity of tetracyclines on microbes and not the host. Different ribosome shapes and sizes also confer selectivity of bacterial versus human ribosome binding.
■ **Demeclocycline** has a further action, which is to inhibit the binding of antidiuretic hormone (ADH) to its receptor. This is clinically important and is the basis for using this drug for treatment of a condition in which ADH levels are too high.

Mechanisms of Resistance
■ There are three commonly recognized mechanisms by which tetracycline resistance is conferred to organisms:
  1. **Efflux** by tetracycline-specific pumps: The drug is actively pumped out of the bacterial cell (the drug is unchanged). The newer drug **tigecycline** is not a substrate for these pumps, and therefore microbes that are resistant to other tetracyclines by this method are **still sensitive** to tigecycline.
  2. **Ribosomal protection:** Despite high levels of drug inside the bacterial cell, the ribosome is still able to function because of complex interactions with other proteins that are produced by the bacteria. These other proteins interfere with the binding of tetracycline to the ribosome and impart some degree of protection against it.
  3. **Enzymatic inactivation:** The drug is broken down inside the cell. This is a less common mechanism of resistance.

PHARMACOKINETICS
■ Tetracyclines are bound and inactivated by divalent cations such as calcium and magnesium, and co-ingestion of these agents (e.g., in the form of calcium supplements or antacids) interferes with the effectiveness of tetracyclines. Therefore, tetracyclines should be taken on an empty stomach.
■ Tigecycline is not well absorbed and therefore is administered only via the intravenous route.
■ All tetracyclines are excreted in urine and bile; doses should be reduced in patients with advanced renal dysfunction. Doxycycline is less dependent on renal excretion, because a lower fraction is excreted renally.

Spectra at a Glance
■ **Gram-positive:** good
■ **Gram-negative:** good
■ **Anaerobes:** poor to good
■ **Resistant organisms:**
  ▲ **MRSA:** resistant
  ▲ **VRE:** resistant
  ▲ *Pseudomonas:* resistant
■ **Special sensitivities:**

▲ **Intracellular** organisms: *Chlamydia, Mycoplasma,* and *Rickettsia*
▲ Spirochetes (syphilis and borreliosis)
▲ Malaria
▲ *Stenotrophomonas* (minocycline only)

CONTRAINDICATIONS
■ Pregnancy and lactation
■ Children under 8 years old, because of tooth discoloration (see Side Effects)

SIDE EFFECTS
■ **GI**: Significant nausea, vomiting, and diarrhea are caused by direct irritation to the GI tract. This is more of a problem with tetracycline than the other tetracyclines.
■ **Mottling of teeth**: Because of binding with calcium, this is a particular problem in newborns; therefore it is contraindicated in pregnancy and lactation. Furthermore, it can permanently stain teeth in children whose adult teeth are still being formed and is therefore contraindicated in children under the age of 8.
■ **Photosensitivity**: This results in skin damage caused by sunlight (ultraviolet-A in particular). It resembles an exaggerated sunburn and can involve blistering. The exact mechanism is not fully elucidated. Absorbed photons are converted into chemical energy, such as oxygen free radicals. These species then result in chemical damage to nearby tissues. Of particular interest is the fact that tetracycline is used for malaria prophylaxis, and many regions in which malaria is endemic are very sunny.
■ **Superinfection**: Superinfection is a rare but serious side effect. Because of the wide spectrum of activity, tetracyclines can wipe out normal flora, which provides an opportunistic environment in which pathogens can grow. This complication is more common in patients who are also immunocompromised.
■ **Diabetes insipidus**: Demeclocycline blocks ADH and therefore can cause diabetes insipidus (water wasting in the urine because of impaired water reabsorption in the collecting duct) if it is used in patients who do not have syndrome of inappropriate ADH secretion (SIADH).
■ **Liver damage**: Liver enzymes can be elevated from tetracyclines. Significant hepatic dysfunction and damage are very rare.
■ **Kidney damage**: Acute tubular necrosis is a rare complication.

IMPORTANT NOTES
■ Important clinical uses for tetracyclines include the following:
▲ Treatment of acne (for role of eradication of bacteria)
▲ Malaria prophylaxis
▲ Treatment of intracellular or *atypical* infections
■ Although **demeclocycline** is classified as an antibiotic, its clinical use is pretty much limited to treating patients diagnosed with **SIADH**. Remember that a diuretic produces increased urine volume, so ADH works to decrease urine volume (via reabsorption of water).

■ **Tigecycline** is a new tetracycline and is classified as a **glycylcycline**; antibiotics of this class are derivatives of tetracyclines and were designed to overcome the two primary methods of resistance—namely, efflux pumps and ribosomal protection.
■ Tetracycline **spontaneously degrades** over time (before it is ingested). Ingesting **outdated tetracycline is dangerous** because the degradation products are nephrotoxic and can cause a condition called **Fanconi's** syndrome, which is characterized by damage to the proximal tubules, resulting in impaired reabsorption of glucose, amino acids, and other compounds from the ultrafiltrate within the tubule.

Advanced
■ Porphyria cutanea tarda is a form of porphyria that affects the skin. Porphyria is a group of diseases caused by enzyme deficiencies resulting in accumulation of porphyrins, which are precursors to heme. Tetracycline can cause a rare form of phototoxicity that mimics porphyria and is called *pseudoporphyria* (but does not involve porphyrins).
■ Four other ribosomal proteins (S3, S8, S14, and S19) are important for tetracycline binding, but these are *low affinity* binding.
■ *Stenotrophomonas* is a genus of bacteria that was originally classified as *Pseudomonas*. It is usually susceptible to sulfa antibiotics, but if it is resistant to sulfa antibiotics it is sometimes susceptible *only* to minocycline.
■ With respect to mechanisms of resistance, there are at least 23 genes for energy-dependent efflux proteins, 11 genes for ribosomal protection proteins, three genes for an inactivating enzyme, and one gene with an unknown mechanism of resistance.
■ *Proteus* and *Pseudomonas* constitutively produce an efflux pump for which *all* tetracyclines are substrates; therefore these microbes are **universally resistant** to all tetracyclines.

FYI
■ The class of tetracyclines was first discovered in the 1940s, but tetracycline itself was not the first drug in this class.
■ Chlortetracycline was the first tetracycline (and thus the true prototype). However, it is no longer used clinically.
■ A modification of tetracyclines has resulted in a new class of antibiotic called glycylcyclines (tigecycline). These chemicals contain an N-O-N group added to the tetracycline. They were introduced in 2006, and this class of antibiotics can overcome some forms of tetracycline resistance.
■ Humans carry a 30S ribosome subunit within their mitochondria. However, the side effects of tetracyclines do not involve the mitochondria.
■ Tetracycline is produced by *Streptomyces* bacteria. Some tetracyclines are natural, and some are modified or synthetic.

■ The *S* in 50S and 23S refers to Svedberg units. A Svedberg unit is a measurement of time and equals 10^{-13} seconds. It is used to describe speed of sedimentation during centrifuging. Combining two molecules (30S + 50S) and predicting the combined Svedberg units are not simply an *additive* process because the surface area changes. Thus in the bacterial ribosome, 30S + 50S = 70S (and not 80).

Macrolides

DESCRIPTION

Macrolides are antibacterial agents that contain a large macrolide ring.

PROTOTYPE AND COMMON DRUGS

■ Prototype: ery**thromycin**
■ Others: azi**thromycin**, clari**thromycin**

MOA (MECHANISM OF ACTION)

■ The production of proteins from mRNA is called **translation**; this step requires **ribosomes**, transfer RNA (**tRNA**), and messenger RNA (**mRNA**) (Figure 18-14).
■ mRNA contains the sequencing code based on DNA; tRNA contains single amino acids and binds to a three-base sequence of mRNA; ribosomes are like *assembly line* processing machinery, bringing the mRNA and tRNA together to assemble sequences of amino acids.
■ The ribosomes are different sizes:
   ▲ Prokaryotes (bacteria) have 70S ribosomes made of a small (30S) and a large (50S) subunit.
      • The 50S subunit is composed of a 5S and a 23S subunit plus 34 other proteins.
   ▲ Eukaryotes (humans) have 80S ribosomes, composed of a small (40S) and a large (60S) subunit.
■ Ribosomes have different binding sites, named:
   ▲ **Aminoacyl (A):** Incoming tRNA binds to this site.
   ▲ **Peptidyl (P):** This is where the existing amino acid chain (connected to tRNA) is elongated when the incoming amino acid is transferred to it through the action of **peptidyl transferase.**
   ▲ **Exit or egress (E):** After the tRNA gives up the amino acid chain, it must leave so that new tRNA can take its place.
■ Macrolides bind the **23S** rRNA molecule of the 50S RSU and inhibit **peptidyl transferase**, blocking the transfer of the new amino acid onto the growing chain.
■ Inhibition of protein synthesis does not typically kill bacteria cells, so these agents are generally **bacteriostatic**, but in high concentrations they can be bactericidal.
■ Macrolides are phagocytosed by macrophages, which is a benefit because WBCs preferentially travel to sites of infection, thereby theoretically delivering the drug to the site at which it is needed. *This is very convenient.*

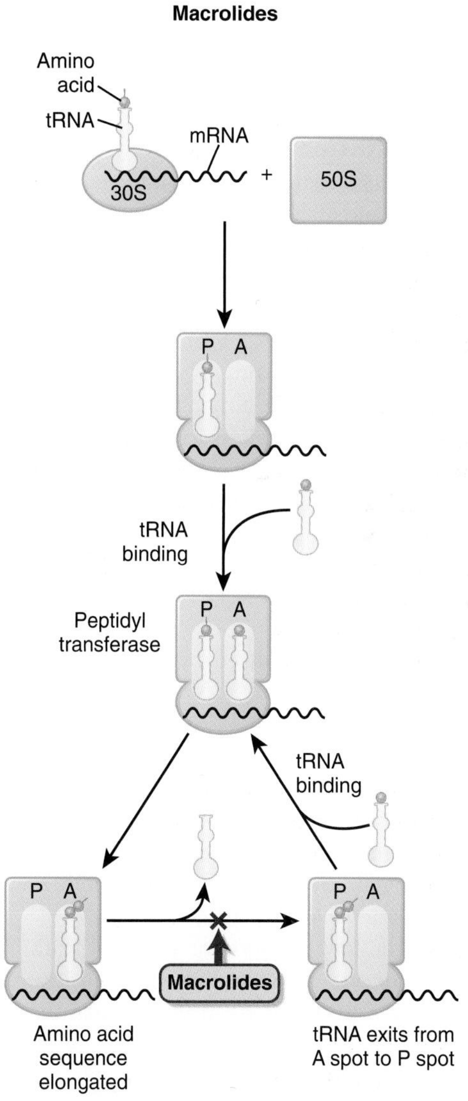

Figure 18-14.

Motility

■ Erythromycin also stimulates motilin receptors on the GI smooth muscle. This results in increased GI muscular activity, leading to increased forward transit of GI contents.

Mechanisms of Resistance

- Modification of the **RSU binding** site either by chromosomal mutation or through methylation via **methylase** greatly decreases the efficacy of macrolides; bacterial methylase can be produced *constitutively* (all the time) or can be *induced*.
- Reduced intracellular concentrations are found within the bacterium, through either reduced permeability of cell membrane to macrolides or, probably more important, **increased efflux** of macrolides via active pumps.
- A third, and maybe least prominent, method of resistance is through the production of esterases that hydrolyze macrolides; this is more common with gram-negative enteric bacteria (bacteria that colonize the GI tract).
- Cross-resistance is complete among all macrolides; if a bacterium is resistant to one, it will be resistant to all others in this class.

PHARMACOKINETICS

- Half-lives of erythromycin, clarithromycin, and azithromycin are 1.5, 6, and 68 hours, and administration is four times daily, twice daily, and once daily, respectively. At high doses, clarithromycin is sometimes administered once a day.
- Azithromycin contains an additional nitrogen molecule in the macrolide ring to make it a 15-atom ring. This imparts increased stability of the ring. A very high amount of drug is distributed *intracellularly*; although distribution into tissues is excellent, it is *not distributed into* CNS (and therefore is not useful for CNS infections). The intracellular distribution contributes to its long half-life.
- Erythromycin and clarithromycin are significant CYP450 enzyme inhibitors and are metabolized by the liver. Drug interactions with other CYP450 inhibitors should be monitored.
- Azithromycin is metabolized by the liver but is not an enzyme inhibitor.
- Erythromycin is *unstable* in gastric acid and therefore must be administered with salts or esters or via enteric-coated tablets when administered orally.
- The addition of a methyl group to erythromycin creates clarithromycin, and the addition of a methylated nitrogen to erythromycin creates azithromycin; both are stable in gastric acid and very well absorbed orally.
- Because of the long duration of action of azithromycin, a 5-day, oral, once-a-day course for most sensitive infections is considered a treatment of adequate duration.

Spectra at a Glance

- **Gram-positive**: very good (but resistance to erythromycin has developed)
- **Gram-negative**: very good
- **Anaerobes**: resistant
- **Resistant organisms**:
  - MRSA: resistant
  - VRE: resistant
  - *Pseudomonas*: resistant
- **Special sensitivities**:

  - Atypical bacteria (many of which are intracellular organisms): *Mycoplasma*, *Rickettsia*, *Chlamydia*, *Legionella*

INDICATIONS

- In addition to antibacterial activity, erythromycin specifically is used to enhance **GI motility**. Through direct stimulation of the GI tract, this mechanism is responsible both for the enhanced motility that is of benefit in patients who have dysmotility and also, unfortunately, for the GI *intolerance* (side effects) in patients who have normal motility.
  - Examples of conditions associated with dysmotility include diabetes (gastroparesis), scleroderma, and ileus.
- Clarithromycin and azithromycin are commonly used in sexually transmitted infections when chlamydia or gonorrhea is suspected and are also commonly used for treatment of pneumonias.

CONTRAINDICATION

- Previous liver complications with a macrolide are likely to recur and therefore should be considered a contraindication to macrolide use.

SIDE EFFECTS
Erythromycin

- **GI**: Significant GI upset because of increased gut motility
- **Acute cholestatic hepatitis**: Likely hypersensitivity-related, this side effect can lead to fever, jaundice, and impaired liver function. Abdominal pain, especially right upper quadrant pain, should lead to the suspicion of liver involvement.

Azithromycin and Clarithromycin

- These agents are better tolerated but can also cause liver impairment.

IMPORTANT NOTES

- The short duration of treatment, good oral absorption, once-a-day administration, and low side effect profile are all favorable characteristics for an antibiotic and have contributed to azithromycin's popularity.
- Scleroderma results in severe esophageal disease that frequently leads to acid reflux; increasing motility helps to empty the stomach and reduce (in part) reflux of acid and stomach contents into the esophagus.
- **Gastroparesis** (decreased motility or even paralysis of the stomach) in diabetes is a result of autonomic dysfunction. This occurs because small nerves become glycosylated in patients with diabetes, leading to neuropathy.

FYI

- A macrolide ring is a 12-, 14-, or 16-atom ring made of 11 carbon and three oxygen molecules. Two sugar molecules are attached to the macrolide ring. Erythromycin is shown in Figure 18-15.
- Nomenclature of macrolides is similar to that of aminoglycosides (gentamicin) except that for macrolides, *thro* precedes the *mycin*.

- Tacrolimus is technically also a macrolide, but it is not an antibiotic. It is an immunosuppressive.
- Erythromycin is produced by *Saccharopolyspora erythraea* bacteria. The 14-member ring is difficult to synthesize. It was isolated in the Philippines in 1949.
- The GI motility profile was discovered through the observation of the multitude of GI side effects.

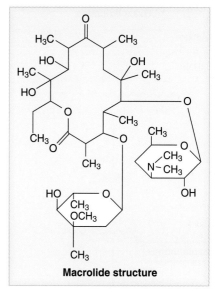

Macrolide structure

Figure 18-15.

Oxazolidinones

DESCRIPTION

Oxazolidinones form a newer class of antibiotics that are ribosomal inhibitors.

PROTOTYPE

- Linezolid

MOA (MECHANISM OF ACTION)

- The production of proteins from mRNA is called **translation**; this step requires **ribosomes**, transfer RNA (**tRNA**), and messenger RNA (**mRNA**) (Figure 18-16).
- mRNA contains the sequencing code based on DNA; tRNA contains single amino acids and binds to a three-base sequence of mRNA; ribosomes are like *assembly line* processing machinery, bringing the mRNA and tRNA together to assemble sequences of amino acids.
- The ribosomes are different sizes:
  - Prokaryotes (bacteria) have 70S ribosomes made of a small (30S) and a large (50S) subunit.
    - The 50S subunit is composed of a 5S and a 23S subunit plus 34 other proteins.
  - Eukaryotes (humans) have 80S ribosomes, composed of a small (40S) and a large (60S) subunit.
- Ribosomes have different binding sites, named:
  - **Aminoacyl (A):** Incoming tRNA binds to this site.
  - **Peptidyl (P):** This is where the existing amino acid chain (connected to tRNA) is elongated when the incoming

amino acid is transferred to it through the action of **peptidyl transferase.**
  - **Exit or egress (E):** After the tRNA gives up the amino acid chain, it must leave so that new tRNA can take its place.
- Linezolid blocks the translocation step of protein synthesis by binding the **23S** rRNA of the 50S RSU.
- It is therefore bacteriostatic.
- Mitochondrial and bacterial ribosomes are similar, and therefore bacterial ribosomal suppression can also result in human mitochondrial suppression. Linezolid is therefore a mitochondrial inhibitor, which is probably the cause of some rare but very serious side effects.

Mechanism of Resistance

- Mutation of the 23S binding site

PHARMACOKINETICS

- Linezolid has 100% oral bioavailability, so the oral and intravenous doses are the same.
- Linezolid is a weak monoamine oxidase inhibitor (MAOI); this could result in increased sensitivity to sympathomimetic drugs.   .

Spectra at a Glance

- **Gram-positive:** very good
- **Gram-negative:** resistant

Oxazolidinones

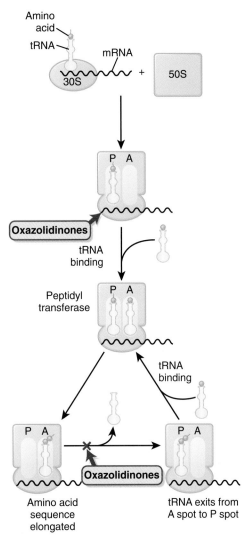

Figure 18-16.

- **Anaerobes:** resistant
- **Resistant organisms:**
  - ▲ MRSA: very good
  - ▲ VRE: very good
  - ▲ *Pseudomonas:* resistant
- **Special sensitivities:**
  - ▲ *Mycobacterium tuberculosis*

CONTRAINDICATIONS
- None of significance

SIDE EFFECTS
- The side effects, although very serious, are rare.
- **Serotonin syndrome** is a condition characterized by high levels of serotonergic activity in the brain. It occurs in patients who are taking drugs that increase the amount of available serotonin in the brain. Drugs in the selective serotonin reuptake inhibitor (SSRI) class of antidepressants are the most common offenders, but drugs that possess MAOI activity can also produce the syndrome.
- **Hyperlactatemia and metabolic acidosis** are probably caused by mitochondrial inhibition. The lactate is produced by the cells that cannot undergo aerobic metabolism because of the mitochondrial suppression, and the accumulation of lactate, which is an acid, produces metabolic acidosis.
- **Nerve damage:** Central and peripheral neuropathies have been reported. The nerve damage has occurred at the same time as the lactic acidosis and therefore could also be mediated by mitochondrial suppression.
- **Hematologic:** Bone marrow suppression (myelosuppression) characterized by low blood counts (platelets, RBCs, or WBCs) has been reported in patients treated with linezolid for at least 21 days. It is usually mild and is reversible within 4 weeks of stopping the drug. It is not common and usually occurs around 1 month after a patient begins to take the drug.

IMPORTANT NOTES
- Linezolids were approved in 2000, and linezolid resistance was first reported in 2001. New drugs often have low rates of resistance, but over time, increased evolutionary pressure from exposure of the drug to bacteria results in increased levels of resistance.
- Currently their use is generally limited to infections caused by multidrug-resistant gram-positive bacteria. Liberal use of antibiotics is associated with resistance, and therefore antibiotics that are effective against resistant organisms should not be used against organisms that are still sensitive to other antibiotics:
  - ▲ VRE
  - ▲ MRSA

Advanced
- Patients who are on long-term treatment with linezolid may develop optic neuropathy (in other words, a peripheral neuropathy), resulting in symmetric painless decreased vision.
- Myelosuppression risk is 1/750 in exposed patients, specifically those with the following:
  - ▲ Low platelet count (thrombocytopenia)
  - ▲ Low RBC count (anemia)
  - ▲ Pancytopenia (all three blood cell lines)

Sulfonamides and Other Folate Synthesis Inhibitors

DESCRIPTION

The sulfonamides are antibacterial agents that are inhibitors of folate synthesis. They are frequently also referred to as *sulfa* antibiotics.

PROTOTYPE AND COMMON DRUGS

- Prototype: **sulfa**methoxazole
  - ▲ Others: **sulfa**diazine, **sulfa**nilamide, **sulfa**cytine, **sulfa**methizole
- **Topical**: silver **sulfa**diazine, **sulfa**cetamide
- Nonsulfas: trimethoprim, pyrimethamine

MOA (MECHANISM OF ACTION)

- Most bacteria must synthesize their own folate for survival; they cannot use external sources. In contrast, humans do not synthesize folate but rather obtain it through the diet.
- Sulfonamides are **inhibitors of folate synthesis**.
- A few steps are required in the synthesis of folate. Specifically, **sulfonamides** are competitive inhibitors with *p*-aminobenzoic acid (**PABA**) in the **first reaction** of the folate synthesis pathway, catalyzed by the enzyme **dihydropteroate synthase**. Inhibiting the synthesis of tetrahydrofolate (THF) results in **reduced DNA synthesis**, which stops bacterial growth (a bacteriostatic effect).
- **Trimethoprim** inhibits the **last reaction** of folate synthesis (catalyzed by **dihydrofolate reductase**) and is commonly administered in conjunction with sulfonamides for greater antibiotic efficacy. Inhibition of the folate synthesis pathway at two different steps results in a **bactericidal** action and is the reason why trimethoprim and sulfamethoxazole (TMP-STP) are combined and commonly used clinically for many infections.

Mechanisms of Resistance (Figure 18-17)

- Bacteria that do not synthesize their own folate (similar to humans) are inherently completely resistant to sulfonamides.
- **Overproduction of PABA** by bacteria can overcome the action of competitive inhibition of sulfas.
- **Enzyme mutation** of dihydropteroate synthase leads to reduced affinity for sulfas and results in resistance.
- **Lower levels of drug** inside bacterial cells because of either decreased membrane permeability to sulfas or active efflux of the drug also confer resistance to organisms.
- An **alternative metabolic pathway** for synthesis of folate within bacteria has also been postulated as a method of resistance.

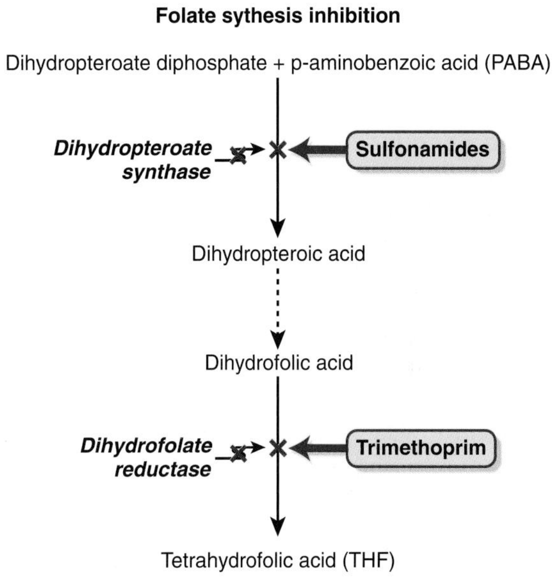

Folate sythesis inhibition

Figure 18-17.

PHARMACOKINETICS

- Metabolism of sulfonamides is via the liver and excretion by the kidney. In patients with advanced renal dysfunction, doses should be reduced.
- Sulfadoxine has a long half-life (7 to 9 days), whereas the half-life of sulfamethoxazole, a commonly prescribed sulfa drug, is 10 to 12 hours.

Spectra at a Glance

- **Gram-positive**: good
- **Gram-negative**: good
- **Anaerobes**: resistant
- **Resistant organisms**:
  - ▲ **MRSA**: resistant
  - ▲ **VRE**: resistant
  - ▲ *Pseudomonas*: resistant
- **Special sensitivities**:
  - ▲ *Pneumocystis jiroveci* causes *P. jiroveci* pneumonia (**PJP**) (the older name is *Pneumocystis carinii* pneumonia or PCP)
  - ▲ *Toxoplasma*
  - ▲ *Nocardia*
  - ▲ *Stenotrophomonas*

CONTRAINDICATIONS

- Allergy to *sulfa* antibiotics
- Glucose-6 phosphate dehydrogenase deficiency (a rare enzyme deficiency)

SIDE EFFECTS

- **Precipitation in urine:** Sulfa molecules might precipitate at neutral or acidic pH, leading to **crystalluria** (crystals in the urine), and possibly **hematuria** (blood in urine secondary to reaction from crystals).
- **Nausea, vomiting, diarrhea**
- **Photosensitivity**
- **Hypersensitivity:** Cross-reactivity can occur with other sulfone-containing drugs, including hydrochlorothiazide and sulfonylureas. There is little evidence to support cross-reactivity, which is usually not severe and limited to rash.

Rare and Serious

- **Stevens-Johnson syndrome** is a rare but very serious (life-threatening) hypersensitivity reaction involving skin and mucous membranes.
- **Blood cell problems** include hemolytic anemia (red cell destruction), aplastic anemia (absence of red cell production), granulocytopenia, and thrombocytopenia.
  - ▲ A rare condition glucose-6—phosphate dehydrogenase deficiency increases the risk of hemolytic anemia
- **Kernicterus:** Sulfa antibiotics compete with bilirubin binding sites on albumin, leading to increased free bilirubin and jaundice in the newborn.

IMPORTANT NOTES

- TMP-SMX is a very common preparation used clinically.
- Common clinical infections treated by sulfonamides include the following:
  - ▲ **Urinary** tract infections (UTIs)
  - ▲ **Respiratory** tract infections (including community-acquired pneumonia)
  - ▲ PJP prophylaxis and treatment
    - *Pneumocystis* is a fungus, and although technically only one organism infects humans, it was originally thought to be a different species and so is referred to by two names:
      - ○ *P. jiroveci* (the proper name) and *P. carinii* (the original name)
      - ○ Pneumonia caused by *Pneumocystis* is therefore abbreviated as both **PJP** and **PCP.**
    - PJP only occurs in patients who are **immunocompromised.**
  - ▲ Topical application for infection prevention:
    - Burns
    - Severe blistering diseases of the skin (pemphigus)
- Sulfasalazine contains a sulfa component but is used clinically as an antiinflammatory (because of the salicylate component) for the GI tract (because it is very poorly absorbed

and thus has exposure only to the GI tract). It is described in the section on salicylates.

Advanced

- Other drugs that contain a sulfone group include the following:
  - ▲ Sulfonylureas (oral hypoglycemics)
  - ▲ Thiazides (diuretics)
  - ▲ Sumatriptan (for migraines)
  - ▲ Sulfasalazine (an antiinflammatory salicylate)
  - ▲ Probenecid (a uricosuric drug used for treatment of gout and for prolonging the half-life of penicillin)

FYI

- A sulfone is an O=S=O group connected to two R groups. A sulf**onamide** is created when one of the R groups is an amide (NH$_2$). Sulfonamides are also called *sulfa drugs*.
- Sulfonamides are technically derivatives of *p*-aminobenzene **sulfonamide** (Figure 18-18).

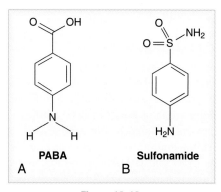

Figure 18-18.

- Sulfa drugs were discovered in the 1930s and were the only antibiotics available before penicillin. They were therefore the first antibiotics.
- Other drugs that interfere with the folate synthesis pathway include:
  - ▲ Methotrexate (used for cancer therapy and treatment of autoimmune diseases)
- PABA was found in sunscreens but has been replaced largely by padimate O, a derivative of PABA. It is interesting that the sulfonamides increase the risk of photosensitivity and that PABA was used to protect the skin, despite their similar chemical structures.
- Folate deficiency causes megaloblastic anemia: big RBCs (contrast this with iron deficiency, which causes microcytic anemia: small RBCs). The cells cannot divide in the absence of folate, but they can continue to produce RNA and protein; hence they grow large, but their numbers are low.

Metronidazole

DESCRIPTION

Metronidazole is an antibiotic that is a member of the *imidazoles*, a class of drug usually associated with antifungals. However, the antiinfective activity of metronidazole is limited to anaerobic bacteria and protozoa but **not** fungi.

PROTOTYPE

- Metronidazole

MOA (MECHANISM OF ACTION)

- Metronidazole is a prodrug. The nitrogen group must be reduced (addition of electron) before the chemical obtains its antiinfective function. It is reduced by a nitroreductase enzyme called a **ferredoxin** (an iron- and sulfur-containing enzyme). The extra nitrogen side chain is reduced in this reaction.
- With *aerobic* bacteria the electron transport chain does not require these special enzymes because oxygen is the terminal electron acceptor; therefore the prodrug is not converted to the active form of the drug. However, with **anaerobic** bacteria, with which oxygen is absent, these special enzymes are present. Therefore metronidazole is not activated with aerobic bacteria but is particularly effective against anaerobic bacteria.
- Reduction of the prodrug metronidazole results in the production of toxic products (hydroxylamine) and other free radicals that damage DNA.

Mechanisms of Resistance

- Some bacteria are *facultatively anaerobic* (can live with or without oxygen) or are *microaerophiles* (can live in the presence of very little oxygen). In these bacteria, the genes required to produce ferredoxin can be switched off; this would result in metronidazole not becoming reduced, and therefore it would remain in the inactive prodrug state.

PHARMACOKINETICS

- Oral administration results in nearly complete absorption.
- Metronidazole is metabolized by the liver. Dose adjustments are not required in patients with renal dysfunction but are required in those with hepatic dysfunction.

Spectra at a Glance

- **Gram-positive**: poor (if aerobic)
- **Gram-negative**: poor (if aerobic)
- **Anaerobes**: very good (for both gram-positive and gram-negative organisms)
  - ▲ **Microaerophilic bacteria** (limited activity): *Propionibacterium, Actinomyces*
- **Resistant organisms**:
  - ▲ **MRSA**: resistant
  - ▲ **VRE**: resistant
  - ▲ *Pseudomonas*: resistant

- **Special sensitivities**:
  - ▲ *C. difficile*
  - ▲ **Protozoa**: (*Trichomonas, Giardia, Entamoeba*)

CONTRAINDICATIONS

- **Ethanol**: Metronidazole can have a disulfuram-like effect: ingestion with alcohol can lead to severe nausea and vomiting. This results from inhibition of the enzyme acetaldehyde dehydrogenase, leading to increased levels of acetaldehyde, which are toxic.
- **Pregnancy (first trimester in particular)**: Metronidazole causes tumor growth in laboratory rats and readily crosses the placenta. It should be used only in extreme situations in pregnancy, after risks have been weighed against benefits.

SIDE EFFECTS

- **GI**: nausea
- **Metallic taste**: common, harmless
- **CNS toxicity**: rare, manifests as ataxia, encephalopathy, or seizure.
- **Rare**:
  - ▲ Neutropenia
  - ▲ Pancreatitis
  - ▲ Peripheral neuropathy
  - ▲ Hepatitis

IMPORTANT NOTES

- For treatment of *C. difficile* infection, oral administration is the preferred route because the infection is inside the GI tract.

FYI

- Metronidazole contains the five-member imidazole ring (three carbons + two nitrogen atoms), but there is a nitrogen side chain; it is therefore a *nitro*imidazole. It is in a drug category all on its own (Figure 18-19).

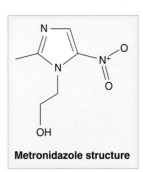

Metronidazole structure

Figure 18-19.

- Imidazole rings are present in a number of biologically important molecules, including:

- ▲ Histamine
- ▲ Theophylline (airway medication)
- ▲ Antifungals
- ■ The first ferredoxin enzyme was isolated from *Clostridium* (a genus of anaerobic bacteria) in 1964.

- ■ Metronidazole causes mutation in bacteria and is tumorigenic in laboratory animals, suggesting that large doses over long periods of time might be associated with a risk of cancer.

Introduction to Antimycobacterials

A tubercle is a nodule or wartlike projection, depending on the context in which the term is being used. Therefore the name *tuberculosis* means a condition of having nodules. One of the many chest x-ray findings of TB is the presence of nodules (round shadows) in the lungs.

TB is hard to kill because it grows very slowly. Effective treatment requires multiple antibiotics for prolonged periods of time, up to as long as 12 months and even longer for resistant strains.

The main anti-TB drugs and their abbreviations include the following:
- ▲ **First-line agents**
  - Ethambutol (EMB or E)
  - Isoniazid (INH or H)
  - Pyrazinamide (PZA or Z)
  - Rifampin (RMP or R)
  - Streptomycin (STM or S)
- ▲ **Second-line agents** (in preferred order)
  - Aminoglycosides: kanamycin, amikacin
  - Polypeptides: capreomycin, viomycin, enviomycin
  - Fluoroquinolones: moxifloxacin
  - Thioamides: ethionamide, prothionamide
  - Cycloserine
  - *p*-Aminosalicylic acid (PAS or 4-ASA)

Second-line agents are either less effective or more toxic than first-line agents. Other drugs are even less effective against TB than second-line agents. They are sometimes called *third-line drugs*. They are not listed here.

There are now many resistant strains of TB, including multidrug-resistant tuberculosis (MDR-TB) and extensively drug-resistant tuberculosis (XDR-TB).
- ▲ **Criteria for MDR-TB:**
  - Isoniazid resistant **and**
  - Rifampin resistant
- ▲ **Criteria for XDR-TB:**
  - Isoniazid resistant **and**
  - Rifampin resistant **and**
  - Aminoglycoside resistant **and**
  - Fluoroquinolone resistant

MDR-TB and XDR-TB should be treated with five drugs simultaneously (excluding the drugs to which they are resistant). Resistant TB strains should be treated by physicians who are experienced in the treatment of TB. Treatment for MDR-TB must be given for a **minimum of 18 months** and

cannot be stopped until the patient has been *culture negative* for a minimum of 9 months. **Some patients have been treated for longer than 2 years.**

MUTATION RATE

- ■ The rate of mutations in TB resulting in drug resistance is:
  - ▲ 3 in 10^7 for EMB (relatively high)
  - ▲ 2.5 in 10^8 for STM and INH
  - ▲ 2 in 10^{10} for RMP (quite low)
- ■ Severe, advanced pulmonary TB has approximately 10^{12} bacteria in the body, resulting in approximately:
  - ▲ 10^5 EMB-resistant bacteria
  - ▲ 10^4 STM-resistant bacteria
  - ▲ 10^4 INH-resistant bacteria
  - ▲ 10^2 RMP-resistant bacteria
- ■ The mutations occur independently of one another. Chances of harboring a bacterium that is resistant to:
  - ▲ INH **and** RMP is 1 in 10^6
  - ▲ All four drugs is 1 in 10^{11}
- ■ The high rate of mutations and the low probability of bacteria with resistance to four drugs is the rationale for using multiple drugs in the treatment of TB.

STANDARD REGIMEN

- ■ Treatment involves an induction phase (high dose, more drugs) followed by a maintenance phase (fewer drugs).
- ■ Abbreviations are used to denote drugs, duration of treatment, and frequency of administration: (months)(single letter drug abbreviations)(times per week). For example:
  - ▲ The current standard regimen is **2HREZ/4HR**, which means:
    - 2 months of isoniazid + rifampin + ethambutol + pyrazinamide
    - Followed by 4 months of isoniazid + rifampin
    - When there is no subscript *times per week*, the drugs are to be taken daily.
  - ▲ 2SHRZ/4HR is an alternate to the standard regimen (replaces streptomycin for ethambutol).
  - ▲ **If patients are still culture positive 2 months after finishing the full regimen** (about 15% of patients), then another 6HR is required (6-month extension of the maintenance portion), and testing for resistance is also required in case the drugs being used are no longer effective.

Ethambutol

DESCRIPTION

Ethambutol is a first-line drug for treatment of TB. It is used in combination with other antituberculous drugs.

PROTOTYPE

■ Ethambutol

MOA (MECHANISM OF ACTION) (Figure 18-20)

■ The mycobacterial cell wall is composed of a peptidoglycan–arabinogalactan–mycolic acid structure.
■ Ethambutol disrupts formation of the tuberculous cell wall by blocking **arabinosyl transferases**. These enzymes attach the arabinose residue of arabinogalactan to mycolic acid.
■ Ethambutol is bacteriostatic; it suppresses the growth of TB but does not kill TB.

Mechanisms of Resistance

■ The emb (A, B, and C) genes code for arabinosyl transferases. Mutations in these genes affect binding of ethambutol and can result in ethambutol being ineffective.
■ Resistance to ethambutol develops quickly when the drug is used as a solo medication; therefore it is always used in combination with other agents.

PHARMACOKINETICS

■ Ethambutol is cleared primarily by the kidneys, and doses need to be adjusted downward in patients with moderate to severe renal dysfunction.

INDICATION

■ TB: first-line drug, given in combination with other anti-TB medications

CONTRAINDICATION

■ **Age <5**: It is difficult to test vision in young children, and therefore toxicity relating to vision cannot be assessed in these patients.

SIDE EFFECTS

■ In general, ethambutol is minimally toxic (<2% incidence of side effects)
■ Neurologic:
  ▲ **Optic neuritis**: <1% occurrence. Inflammation of the optic nerve results in decreased visual acuity (blurred vision). Recovery usually occurs after discontinuation of the drug. This is a dose-related effect and occurs more commonly with higher doses. One theory for the MOA of ocular toxicity is related to its zinc chelating effect, but the mechanism has not been fully established.
    • **Permanent blindness** can occur if the drug is not stopped early enough.

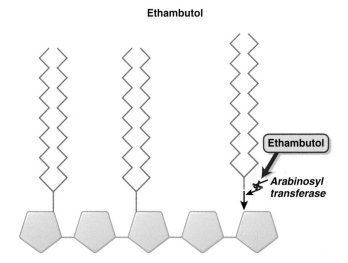

Ethambutol

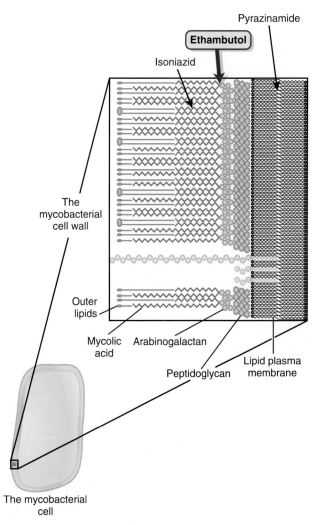

Figure 18-20.

▲ Red-green color blindness can also occur.
▲ **Peripheral neuropathy** causes numbness and tingling of fingers and feet.
■ **Rash**
■ **Fever**

IMPORTANT NOTES

■ Vision tests for acuity and color discrimination should be performed at the start of administration of ethambutol and should be repeated periodically, or immediately if visual problems are reported.
■ Renal dysfunction leads to increased levels of ethambutol; therefore patients with renal dysfunction should be monitored more closely for visual changes.

Advanced

■ Ethambutol can result in increased urate in the urine. This makes it a uricosuric drug, which is beneficial to patients with elevated blood uric acid but detrimental to patients with a tendency to form renal stones.

FYI

■ Ethambutol is abbreviated as *EMB* or simply *E.*

Isoniazid

DESCRIPTION

Isoniazid is a first-line anti-TB drug. It is used in combination with other anti-TB drugs.

PROTOTYPE

■ Isoniazid

MOA (MECHANISM OF ACTION) (Figure 18-21)

■ Isoniazid passively enters mycobacterial cells and kills rapidly dividing cells.
■ In short, isoniazid inhibits mycobacterial cell wall synthesis.
■ The chemical steps are a bit complicated; the following is a simplified version:
   ▲ Isoniazid is a prodrug activated by the mycobacterial enzyme **katG.**
   ▲ The activated compound reacts with nicotinamide adenine dinucleotide (NAD) to form an INH-NAD complex.
   ▲ The INH-NAD complex inhibits one of the final steps of **mycolic acid synthesis** via the enzyme that is abbreviated **InhA.**
   ▲ The net results are accumulation of long-chain fatty acids, decreased production of mycolic acid, and cellular death.

Mechanisms of Resistance

■ As a result of the MOA being multistepped, there are many opportunities for TB to develop isoniazid resistance:
   ▲ Mutation leading to *over*expression of InhA (the enzyme that needs to be inhibited)
   ▲ Mutation leading to *under*expression of katG (the enzyme that converts the prodrug to the active form)

PHARMACOKINETICS

■ Isoniazid is distributed in serum, in cerebrospinal fluid (CSF), and within caseous granulomas (which often surround TB). *Caseous* means having a cheeselike consistency.
■ Isoniazid is metabolized in the liver via acetylation.
   ▲ There are two forms of acetylation enzymes. Therefore some patients metabolize INH faster than others.
■ Isoniazid is a **hepatic enzyme inducer.** It will decrease the serum levels of other drugs that are hepatically cleared.

SIDE EFFECTS

■ **Hepatitis,** which can be initially asymptomatic and detected only by hepatic enzyme elevation. Significant enzyme elevation might mandate that isoniazid be discontinued in that patient. Note that the term *hepatitis* here does not refer to viral hepatitis, but rather a noninfectious inflammation of the liver that is directly drug induced.
■ **Peripheral neuropathy**—dysesthesia (tingling), hyperesthesia (pain), or anesthesia (loss of sensation) commonly present in the hands or feet—is believed to be mediated by a drug-induced vitamin B_6 deficiency, which is prevented by administering pyridoxine (vitamin B_6).
■ Mild CNS effects may occur.
■ Rash may be present.

IMPORTANT NOTES

■ Baseline measurements of hepatic enzymes are required because of the risk of hepatitis. Repeat measurements as follows:
   ▲ At regular intervals
   ▲ If baseline results are abnormal
   ▲ If the patient has signs or symptoms of hepatitis

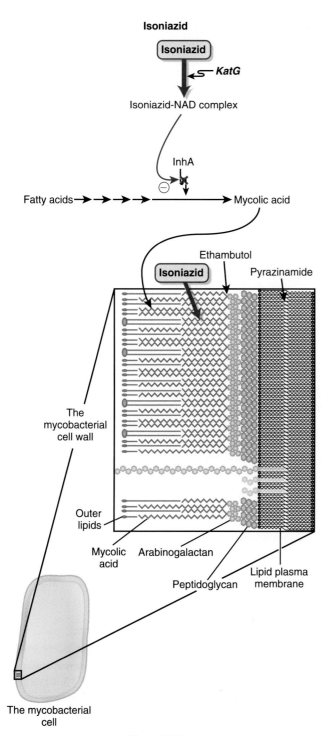

Figure 18-21.

Advanced

- *Deficiency* mutations cause loss of an enzyme. Therefore if two genes (one normal and one mutated) are present, the mutated gene will be recessive because the normally functioning gene will replace the missing enzyme. Recessive INH-resistant genes include *katG, ndb, msh,* and *nat.*
- *Overexpression* mutations cause too much enzyme. Therefore if two genes (one normal and one mutated) are present, the mutated gene will be dominant because the mutated gene will continue to pump out excessive enzyme even in the presence of the normal gene. Dominant INH-resistant genes include InhA, which is inhibited by INH-NAD. It is more difficult to inhibit an enzyme that is produced in high quantity.
- There are more mechanisms of isoniazid resistance not listed here.

FYI

- Isoniazid was the first anti-TB drug and was discovered in 1952. The name *isoniazid* is derived from **isoni**cotinic acid hyd**razid**e.
- Isoniazid is often abbreviated as *INH* or simply *H.*
- Isoniazid is a pyridine (five carbon plus one nitrogen ring). Pyridine is a component of nicotinamide, which in turn is a component of nicotinamide adenine dinucleotide (NAD).
- Nicotinamide is the amide of nicotinic acid.
  - ▲ Nicotinic acid is incorporated into NAD.
  - ▲ Nicotinic acid is also known as *niacin* (vitamin B$_3$), a drug used to lower cholesterol.

Pyrazinamide

DESCRIPTION

Pyrazinamide is an antituberculous drug. It is an analog of nicotinamide. It is abbreviated *PZA* or simply *Z.*

PROTOYPE

- Pyrazinamide

MOA (MECHANISM OF ACTION) (Figure 18-22)

- Pyrazinamide is a prodrug. It must first be converted to pyrazinoic acid by a mycobacterial enzyme called *pyrazinamidase.*

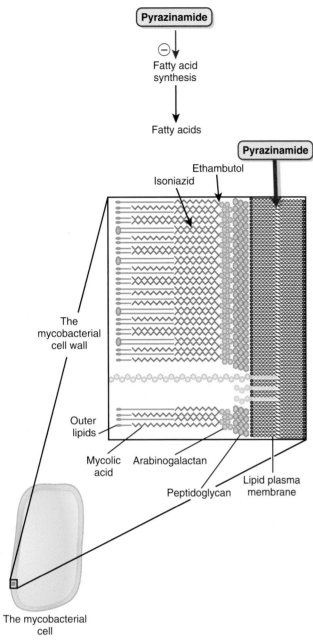

Figure 18-22.

- Pyrazinoic acid *probably* exerts its antituberculous activity via inhibition of an enzyme called **fatty acid synthase I** that is involved in cell wall synthesis.
- Fatty acid synthase I activity is required for fatty acid synthesis, but the exact role that it plays in mycobacterial growth and structure is not fully elucidated.

- Pyrazinamide is active only if the bacterium is in an acidic environment; pyrazinoic acid appears to accumulate in higher levels.

INDICATIONS
- The only use for pyrazinamide currently is part of a multi-drug treatment of *M. tuberculosis* infection.
- It is not effective against other strains of *Mycobacteria*.
- It is **never used as a single drug**; resistance develops very quickly when it is used alone.

CONTRAINDICATION
- Preexisting hepatic dysfunction

SIDE EFFECTS
Serious
- **Hepatic injury**: Drug-induced hepatitis is the most serious side effect of PZA.
  - ▲ Hepatic enzymes must be measured while patients are taking PZA.
  - ▲ If signs or symptoms of hepatitis occur, then the drug must be stopped immediately.

More Common (Less Serious)
- **Arthalgia** (joint pain) occurs in approximately 1% of patients.
- **Increased uric acid**: PZA inhibits the excretion of urate (uric acid salt) and therefore increases the probability of precipitating **gout** (which causes joint pain and inflammation via deposition of uric acid crystals in joints, especially the great toe).
- **Anorexia** (loss of appetite): This effect is not to be confused with anorexia nervosa, which is a psychiatric condition. Anorexia (not the psychiatric type) can occur with many diseases and in fact can be a symptom of hepatic disease.
- **Nausea and vomiting** are also signs of hepatic disease but can be isolated side effects of PZA.

IMPORTANT NOTES
- The dose of PZA used to be higher (40 to 50 mg/kg, whereas it is now 15 to 30 mg/kg). The incidence of hepatic injury *used to be* as high as 15%, with 2% to 3% of patients demonstrating jaundice and with deaths from liver disease also being reported.

FYI
- PZA is structurally similar to vitamin B_3 but is not itself a vitamin.
- A pyrizine molecule is a six-membered ring with two nitrogens at opposite ends, producing a symmetrical molecule.
- Pyraz**amide** also has an amide group attached to the side chain, hence its name.
- Note the common denominator of nicotinamide among INH and PZA.

Rifamycins

DESCRIPTION

Rifamycins are antibiotics that are well known for their anti-TB activity. They are also active against other bacteria.

PROTOTYPE AND COMMON DRUGS

- Prototype: **rifa**mpin (also known as **rifa**mpicin)
- Others: **rifa**butin, **rifa**pentine

MOA (MECHANISM OF ACTION) (Figure 18-23)

Rifamycin

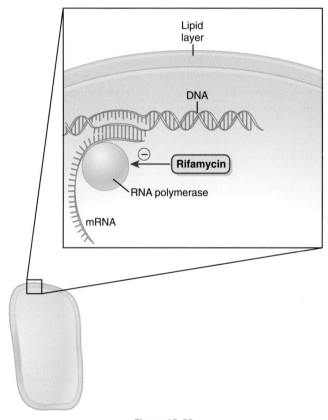

Figure 18-23.

- RNA polymerase *reads* DNA to produce an mRNA copy of the genetic code. Without RNA, protein synthesis cannot occur.
- Rifampin **inhibits bacterial RNA synthesis** by binding prokaryotic (bacterial) **RNA polymerase**. It prevents *initiation* of RNA synthesis (but not *elongation* of RNA).
- Rifampin does *not* bind human RNA polymerase, so its action on RNA synthesis is limited to bacterial RNA, which serves to limit its side effects.
- Rifampin is **bactericidal** for extracellular and intracellular bacteria, but despite this, it is **not** commonly used as a **solo agent** for treatment of established infections because of the high rates of resistance that develop.

- Rifampin is **highly lipophilic**. This is extremely important because it confers the property that the drug can easily cross lipophilic membranes:
  - ▲ **Mycobacterial** cell walls contain mycolic acids, which are long fatty acids and therefore lipids. Rifampin therefore easily and readily enters mycobacterial cells.
  - ▲ **Biofilms** (inert films that bacteria can live in) created by some bacteria generate a barrier that antibiotics generally cannot enter. However, rifampin can enter the biofilms because of its lipophilic nature.
  - ▲ **CNS distribution** is high (and therefore rifampin is effective for CNS infections such as bacterial meningitis).
  - ▲ Rifampin enters **phagocytic cells** and therefore can kill organisms that are poorly accessible to many other drugs, such as **intracellular** organisms and organisms inside abscesses, which do not have good blood supplies.

Mechanisms of Resistance

- Mutations to the gene rpoB, which gives rise to bacterial RNA polymerase, confer resistance to rifampin.
- Resistance occurs in about 1 in 10^6 bacteria, and therefore when rifampin is used **as a solo agent**, resistant strains are preferentially selected for and **resistance is quickly established**.

PHARMACOKINETICS

- Rifamycins are primarily metabolized by the liver and eliminated in the bile. Dose adjustments are not required in liver or renal dysfunction.
- Rifamycins are potent inducers of a number of CYP enzymes. Therefore patients on drugs broken down by CYP enzymes will require higher doses of these drugs. Important examples include warfarin, an anticoagulant; human immunodeficiency virus (HIV) medications (protease inhibitors and nonnucleoside reverse transcription inhibitors); and methadone.
  - ▲ HIV medications and methadone are relevant because patients who are HIV positive or abusers of intravenous narcotics have a higher likelihood of contracting mycobacteria and requiring rifampin.
- Aminosalicylic acid may delay the absorption of rifampin and cause inadequate plasma concentrations. If both drugs need to be administered, it is important to space out administration by as many hours as possible.
- Rifampin is distributed widely in body fluids and tissues, and adequate CSF concentrations are achieved, but only in the presence of meningeal inflammation (which occurs with bacterial meningitis).

Spectra at a Glance

- **Gram-positive**: good
- **Gram-negative**: moderate

- **Anaerobes**: resistant
- **Resistant organisms**:
  - ▲ MRSA: good
  - ▲ VRE: resistant
  - ▲ *Pseudomonas:* moderate
- **Special sensitivities**:
  - ▲ Mycobacteria (TB)
  - ▲ *N. meningitidis*

CONTRAINDICATIONS

- None of major significance

SIDE EFFECTS
Common and Mild

- **Discoloration of secretions**: Because of its lipophilic nature, it enters secretions readily and **colors them orange or red.** Such secretions include tears, urine, sweat, stool, sputum, and saliva. Contact lenses can be stained. Patients should be warned about this so that they do not become unnecessarily alarmed when it happens.
- **Cholestatic jaundice and hepatitis**: Levels of liver enzymes such as aspartate aminotransferase (AST), alanine amino-transferase (ALT), and bilirubin can be elevated. Elevations in bilirubin usually resolve after 10 days. Rifampin blocks bilirubin excretion, and liver enzyme production increases to compensate. Isolated mild elevations in bilirubin are not an indication to stop treatment.
- Rash occurs rarely.

Rare but Serious

- **Acute interstitial nephritis (AIN)**: inflammation of the renal interstitium caused by an allergic-type reaction
- **Thrombocytopenia**: a decreased platelet count

IMPORTANT NOTES

- *Staphylococcal* infections (*S. epidermidis* and *S. aureus*) are commonly associated with biofilm production. Because of the lipophilic nature of rifampin, it absorbs into and crosses biofilms and can be more effective against these infections.

- Rifampin is commonly **coadministered** for the following serious infections:
  - ▲ Meningitis
  - ▲ Osteomyelitis
  - ▲ TB
  - ▲ Endocarditis
  - ▲ Joint hardware (joint replacement) infections (poor access because of no blood supply)
  - ▲ Resistant strains of *S. aureus* (MRSA)
- Rifampin is indicated as a **prophylactic measure** in the case of exposure to a patient with meningitis caused by *N. meningitidis.*

Advanced

- Many guidelines recommend rifampin as a second drug to be used in combination for some staphylococcal and strep-tococcal infections. However, a meta-analysis found that only orthopedic infections (bone, joint, or joint hardware) with *Staphylococcus* showed a significant improvement in cure rates with combination treatment.
- Rifampin is an inducer of the P-glycoprotein (Pgp) transport system. This can result in decreased efficacy of other drugs that are transported by the Pgp system.
- Examples of clinically relevant interactions (reduced levels because of P-450 enzyme induction) demonstrated by recent reports include (in addition to the drugs mentioned previously) everolimus, atorvastatin, rosiglitazone and pio-glitazone, celecoxib, clarithromycin, caspofungin, and lorazepam.
- Rifampin is a strong inducer of the enzyme UGT1A1 and can thus reduce levels of the HIV agents atazanavir and raltegravir. This is clinically relevant because patients with HIV often develop infections that are treated with rifampin.

FYI

- Rifamycin B was the first rifamycin to be introduced commercially.
- Mycobacterial cell walls are very lipophilic because of the mycolic acid content and therefore *hydrophilic attacks* by hydrophilic antibiotics are ineffective, thereby making mycobacteria difficult to kill.

CCR5 Antagonists

DESCRIPTION

CCR5 antagonists are a newer class of drugs that inhibit HIV by preventing its entry into human cells.

PROTOTYPE

- Prototype: maraviroc

MOA (MECHANISM OF ACTION)

- Several steps are involved in the replication of HIV. The virus must fuse to the host cell, uncoat, enter and be tran-

scribed by reverse transcriptase, become incorporated into the host genome, and be transcribed to viral RNA, which is then translated into polyproteins (Figure 18-24).
- Entry of HIV into the host cell begins with the attachment of the **HIV envelope glycoprotein (gp120)** to the CD4 T-cell receptor. This interaction produces a conformational change in gp120 that allows it to **bind to a chemokine co-receptor, either CCR5 or CXCR4.**
- Once gp120 is bound to either CCR5 or CXCR4, further conformational changes occur that allow the HIV envelop

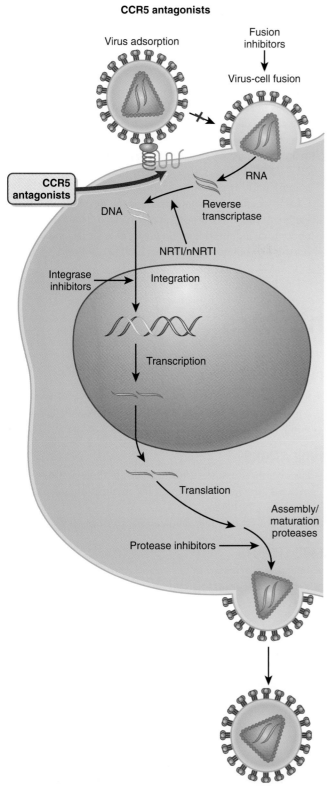

CCR5 antagonists

Virus adsorption

Fusion inhibitors

Virus-cell fusion

CCR5 antagonists

RNA

DNA

Reverse transcriptase

NRTI/nNRTI

Integrase inhibitors

Integration

Transcription

Translation

Assembly/ maturation proteases

Protease inhibitors

Figure 18-24. (Modified from Pommier Y, Johnson AA, Marchand C: Integrase inhibitors to treat HIV/AIDS, *Nat Rev Drug Discov* 4(3):236, 2004. Reprinted by permission from Macmillan Publishers.)

gp41 fusion peptide to insert into the cell membrane, causing the virion to fuse with the cell membrane.

■ The CCR5 antagonists block the interaction of gp120 with CCR5, thus **preventing viral entry.**

■ Some patients express CCR5, some express CXCR4, and some express a mixture of the two ("dual-mixed"). The CCR5 antagonists are typically reserved for patients expressing CCR5. Use of CCR5 antagonists in dual-mixed patients leads to selection of CXCR4 and resistance.

Mechanisms of Resistance

■ Switching of CCR5 to CXCR4 or dual-mixed population of CCR5 and CXCR4

PHARMACOKINETICS

■ Maraviroc is eliminated primarily by hepatic metabolism.

■ Maraviroc is a CYP3A4 substrate and a substrate for Pgp. However, it does not appear to either inhibit or induce CYP3A4.

■ With the exception of tipranavir and ritonavir, concomitant use with protease inhibitors will require a maraviroc dose reduction because of their ability to act as CYP inhibitors.

INDICATION

■ HIV-1 in patients in whom prior therapies have failed with evidence of CCR5 tropism

CONTRAINDICATIONS

■ None of major significance

SIDE EFFECTS

■ Antiretrovirals are typically administered in combination regimens, which can make it unclear how each individual drug contributes to side effects.

■ **Postural hypotension and syncope:** Caution is advised in patients taking antihypertensives or who have a history of syncope. The mechanism is not established.

Rare

■ **Hepatotoxicity:** There were more hepatic adverse events with maraviroc-treated patients during clinical trials. The mechanism was not established.

■ **Cardiovascular events:** Myocardial ischemia and infarction were reported in clinical trials, although infrequently. The mechanism was not established.

IMPORTANT NOTES

■ In clinical trials, virologic failure typically occurred in patients exhibiting a switch in HIV-1 from CCR5 to CXCR4 or dual-mixed. However, once patients had discontinued maraviroc, they typically reverted back to CCR5.

■ The switching of HIV-1 to CXCR4 after therapy with CCR5 antagonists has prompted the search for CXCR4 antagonists. These agents have not been successfully brought to market yet, because of concerns over toxicity and lack of response.

Advanced

- There is a theoretical concern that CCR5 antagonism may interfere with the body's response to infection and predispose patients to cancer. To date, there is no obvious indication from clinical trials that maraviroc increases the incidence of infection or cancer versus placebo.

Pregnancy

- Typical of antiretroviral agents, the safety of maraviroc in pregnancy has not been established. Animal studies do not indicate any obvious potential harm; however, these data cannot be reliably generalized to humans.

Lactation

- Maraviroc is secreted into breast milk in animals, but this observation has not been established in humans.

FYI

- The development of CCR5 antagonists was inspired by the observation that individuals who did not express CCR5 because of a gene deletion were resistant to HIV infection.
- The name *chemokine* comes from the ability of these agents to act as chemotaxic cytokines. Chemokines induce chemotaxis in responding cells and thus direct the movements of various cells within the body. Once a chemokine binds to a chemokine receptor, that cell begins to migrate toward a site of injury or maturation. Certain viruses, including HIV, also bind to chemokine receptors, as a means for gaining entry into host cells.
- CCR5 receptors are targets of drug development for a variety of other indications involving an inflammatory component, including cancer, rheumatoid arthritis, and chronic obstructive pulmonary disease (COPD).

Fusion Inhibitors

DESCRIPTION

Fusion inhibitors block fusion of the HIV virus to the human cell and thereby reduce entry of the virus into the CD4 cell. They are also called *entry inhibitors*.

PROTOTYPE AND COMMON DRUGS

- Prototype: enfuvirtide
- Others: PRO 140, ibalizumab

MOA (MECHANISM OF ACTION) (Figure 18-25)

- Several steps are involved in the replication of HIV. The virus must fuse to the host cell, uncoat, enter and be transcribed by reverse transcriptase, become incorporated into the host genome, and be transcribed to viral RNA, which is then translated into polyproteins.
- Enfuvirtide mimics the HIV machinery required to fuse to the CD4 cell. It competes with the HIV proteins and prevents entry of the virus into the CD4 cell:
  - ▲ Glycoprotein gp120 binds HIV and *activates* gp41.
  - ▲ Glycoprotein gp41 changes conformation and creates an entry channel (pore) into the cell.
  - ▲ Specifically, enfuvirtide binds gp41 and prevents conformation change.

PHARMACOKINETICS

- Enfuvirtide is injected only. It is an amino acid sequence and therefore would be enzymatically degraded if taken orally.

INDICATIONS

- Fusion inhibitors are used in multiple-drug–resistant HIV patients, already on multiple HIV medications, as part of a combination therapy.
- These are *not* first-line medications to treat HIV.

SIDE EFFECTS

- Injection site irritation
- Peripheral neuropathy (can cause pain, numbness, or weakness in extremities)

IMPORTANT NOTES

- When added to an existing drug regimen in patients who had high HIV levels and had already been treated for many years, enfuvirtide resulted in lower HIV levels.

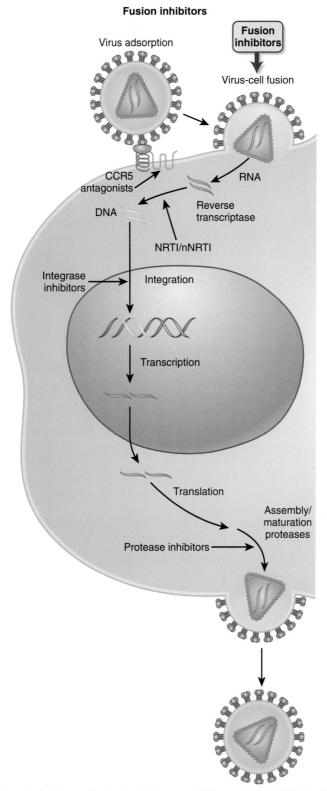

Figure 18-25. (Modified from Pommier Y, Johnson AA, Marchand C: Integrase inhibitors to treat HIV/AIDS, *Nat Rev Drug Discov* 4(3):236, 2004. Reprinted by permission from Macmillan Publishers.)

Integrase Inhibitors

DESCRIPTION

Integrase inhibitors are a newer class of drugs for HIV infection that inhibit HIV by preventing the virus from incorporating its DNA into the host genome.

PROTOTYPE

■ Prototype: raltegravir

MOA (MECHANISM OF ACTION)

■ Several steps are involved in the replication of HIV. The virus must fuse to the host cell, uncoat, enter and be transcribed by reverse transcriptase, become incorporated into the host genome, and be transcribed to viral RNA, which is then translated into polyproteins (Figure 18-26).

■ The **integrase enzyme incorporates viral DNA into the host genome.**

■ Specifically, integrase binds to viral DNA and joins it with host DNA. The divalent cations in the catalytic core of integrase enable it to form covalent bonds with DNA. This is followed by cellular repair activities that seal the viral DNA into the chromosome.

■ Integrase inhibitors prevent the formation of covalent bonds with host DNA. This prevents incorporation of HIV into the host genome.

Mechanisms of Resistance

■ Raltegravir is considered to have a low genetic barrier to resistance, as a single point mutation in HIV can lead to a change in sensitivity of integrase to inhibition.

■ Cross-resistance among integrase inhibitors may occur, but there is not yet enough experience with these agents to confirm this.

PHARMACOKINETICS

■ The main route of elimination for raltegravir is hepatic; however, dose adjustments are not required in patients with mild to moderate hepatic impairment. Adjustments in severe hepatic impairment have not been studied. Because renal elimination plays a relatively minor role, no adjustments are required in patients with renal impairment.

■ Raltegravir is not a substrate for CYP450 enzymes. It also does not inhibit or induce CYP450 enzymes. It is primarily metabolized by glucuronidation (UGT1A1), and it is a Pgp substrate.

INDICATION

■ HIV-1 infection in patients who have tried other therapies with continued viral replication and multidrug resistance

CONTRAINDICATIONS

■ None of major significance

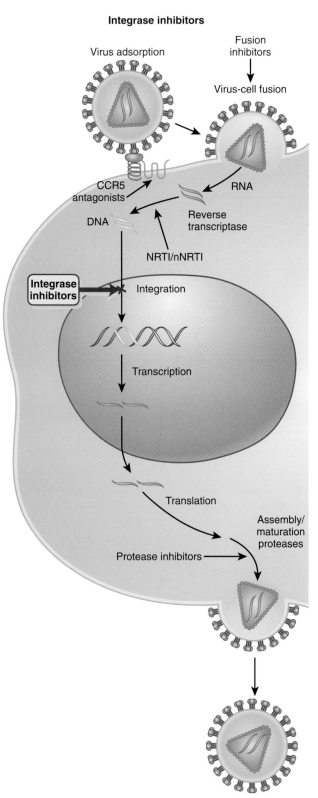

Integrase inhibitors

Figure 18-26. (Modified from Pommier Y, Johnson AA, Marchand C: Integrase inhibitors to treat HIV/AIDS, *Nat Rev Drug Discov* 4(3):236, 2004. Reprinted by permission from Macmillan Publishers.)

SIDE EFFECTS

- Because the antiretrovirals are typically administered in combination regimens, it is difficult to determine the side effects that are associated with a specific class or drug within that class.
- **Generally well-tolerated**: In controlled trials, raltegravir did not elicit more adverse effects than placebo.

IMPORTANT NOTES

- At present, integrase inhibitors are active against HIV-2.
- During clinical trials, there was a slight, non–statistically significant increase in the incidence of cancer in patients treated with raltegravir versus placebo-treated patients. Although these differences were not statistically significant and raltegravir is not considered to be a carcinogen, rates of cancer are being monitored closely in the postmarketing period.

Advanced
Drug Interactions

- Atazanavir is a UGT1A1 inhibitor, and concomitant administration of raltegravir and atazanavir has been shown to elevate raltegravir levels.
- Rifampin is a strong inducer of UGT1A1; therefore concomitant administration of these two agents can significantly reduce raltegravir levels.

Pregnancy

- As with most antiretrovirals, the safety of integrase inhibitors in pregnancy has not been established.

FYI

- An assay (PhenoSense Integrase Assay) has been developed to measure the susceptibility of HIV-1 to integrase inhibitors.

Nucleoside Reverse Transcriptase Inhibitors (NRTIs)

DESCRIPTION

- Nucleoside reverse transcriptase inhibitors (NRTIs) are agents used in the treatment of HIV infection that inhibit HIV by preventing its transcription.

PROTOTYPE AND COMMON DRUGS

- Prototype: zidovudine
- Others: didanosine, lamivudine, stavudine, zalcitabine, emtricitabine
- **Nucleotide reverse transcriptase inhibitor**: tenofovir

MOA (MECHANISM OF ACTION)

- Several steps are involved in the replication of HIV. The virus must fuse to the host cell, uncoat, enter and be transcribed by reverse transcriptase, become incorporated into the host genome, and be transcribed to viral RNA, which is then translated into polyproteins.
- Reverse transcriptase is an enzyme that **transcribes viral RNA into viral DNA** (hence the term *reverse*).
- Once they have entered the host cell, NRTIs are converted to nucleotides by host cell kinases. These nucleotides then **compete with endogenous nucleosides** for incorporation into **viral DNA** in the reaction catalyzed by reverse transcriptase (Figure 18-27).
- NRTIs therefore act as **competitive inhibitors of reverse transcriptase**. Once they incorporate themselves into DNA, NRTIs cause termination of the DNA chain, in a manner analogous to that seen with the nucleoside analogues such as acyclovir. Chain termination halts the process of viral replication.

- NRTIs also inhibit host cell DNA polymerase, although this likely contributes more to their toxic effects than their efficacy. Inhibition of DNA polymerase in mitochondria leads to depletion of mitochondrial DNA and subsequent depletion of mitochondrial RNA and peptides involved in oxidative phosphorylation. This leads to mitochondrial dysfunction, and this is believed to be the cause of several of the important toxicities associated with drugs of this class.
- Unlike nonnucleoside reverse transcriptase inhibitors (nNRTIs), in which binding to the reverse transcriptase is very specific, NRTIs indirectly inhibit reverse transcriptase and are therefore **not specific for HIV-1**. nNRTIs act specifically on the HIV-1 strain and lack activity against HIV-2.

Mechanisms of Resistance

- Mechanisms of resistance include mutations in reverse transcriptase.
- Stavudine, didanosine, and zidovudine have the same resistant mutations.

PHARMACOKINETICS

- Zidovudine can be given orally or IV, whereas the rest of the NRTIs are available only in oral dosage forms.
- Zidovudine and didanosine are metabolized by the liver, whereas the others rely on the kidneys for their elimination, therefore dose adjustments for these agents should be considered in patients with renal impairment.
- The NRTIs have a short elimination half-life ($t_{1/2}$); however, their intracellular $t_{1/2}$ tends to be a lot longer. Early in

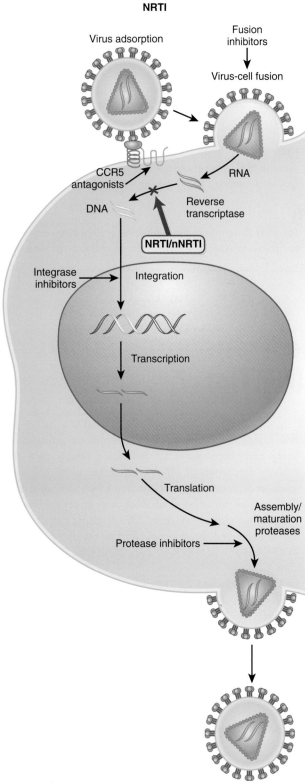

NRTI

Virus adsorption

Fusion inhibitors

Virus-cell fusion

CCR5 antagonists

RNA

DNA

Reverse transcriptase

NRTI/nNRTI

Integrase inhibitors

Integration

Transcription

Translation

Assembly/ maturation proteases

Protease inhibitors

Figure 18-27. (Modified from Pommier Y, Johnson AA, Marchand C: Integrase inhibitors to treat HIV/AIDS, *Nat Rev Drug Discov* 4(3):236, 2004. Reprinted by permission from Macmillan Publishers.)

the history of NRTIs, before a more complete understanding of their pharmacokinetics, this led to overdoses of NRTIs.

- Food also decreases the bioavailability of didanosine, so it should be administered on an empty stomach. Because most protease inhibitors must be taken with food, this complicates the use of these combinations.

INDICATION

- HIV
  - ▲ Treatment of infection
  - ▲ Prevention of transmission from mother to child
  - ▲ Postexposure prophylaxis

CONTRAINDICATIONS

- Avoid in patients with history of pancreatitis or neuropathy: particularly true with didanosine, stavudine, and zalcitabine (see later).

SIDE EFFECTS

- **Myalgia:** One of the most common and earliest side effects associated with NRTIs, myalgia was also the first indication of the mitochondrial toxicity that has become associated with these agents. The mitochondrial toxicity is believed to be caused by the inhibition of DNA polymerase by the NRTI.
- **Headache**
- **Diarrhea** is most associated with didanosine, likely as a result of the buffers used in oral formulations, some of which contain magnesium, a known laxative.

Serious

- **Lactic acidosis:** The impairment of mitochondrial function leads to a reliance on anaerobic metabolism, which produces excessive amounts of lactate.
- **Lipodystrophy** is most associated with stavudine.
- **Peripheral neuropathy (didanosine, stavudine, zalcitabine)** is likely caused by mitochondrial toxicity. Typically this effect will improve or resolve completely as long as the drug is stopped as soon as the symptoms appear.
- **Pancreatitis (didanosine, stavudine, zalcitabine)** is a rare but potentially fatal adverse effect, likely caused by mitochondrial toxicity. It is more common with didanosine and particularly common when two of these agents are combined.
- **Hepatotoxicity (didanosine, zidovudine)** is rare but potentially fatal.
- **Bone marrow suppression** is likely the result of toxic effects on erythroid stem cells.

Unique

- **Hypersensitivity (abacavir),** characterized by fever, GI problems including abdominal pain, rash, malaise, and fatigue may occur. If fever, abdominal pain, and rash occur within 6 weeks of initiation of therapy, the drug should be discontinued.

- **Acute renal failure (tenofovir)** is a rare side effect, and although tenofovir is an antiviral nucleotide like cidofovir and adefovir, it is not believed to share their nephrotoxic effects.
- **Stomatitis and oral ulcers (zalcitabine):** Zalcitabine may be toxic to rapidly dividing cells, but the mechanism is unclear.

IMPORTANT NOTES

- Lamivudine, emtricitabine, and tenofovir are also active against hepatitis B virus. This presents an opportunity to treat two indications (HIV and hepatitis B) with one drug, but also means that care must be taken when withdrawing these agents from hepatitis B co-infected patients. These patients may experience a rebound and worsening of hepatitis B.
- Lamivudine and abacavir do not share many of the serious mitochondrial toxicities associated with other NRTIs. This is thought to result from the fact that they are weak DNA polymerase inhibitors.
- Antiretrovirals are typically used in combination with one another, referred to as **highly active antiretroviral therapy (HAART)**. The most common combinations are an NRTI with an nNRTI, and an NRTI with a ritonavir-boosted protease inhibitor. Two NRTIs are typically used in these regimens.

ADVANCED
Pharmacogenetics

- The hypersensitivity reaction to abacavir is more common in those with the HLA-B*5701 allele. This allele is more common in Caucasians and to a lesser extent Hispanics.

Drug Interactions

- Didanosine is easily degraded in an acidic environment and is therefore formulated with buffers such as calcium carbonate and magnesium hydroxide. Agents that bind to divalent cations (e.g., calcium and magnesium) should be administered separately from didanosine. Examples of these agents include fluoroquinolones such as ciprofloxacin. The same is true for agents whose dissolution is pH dependent, such as itraconazole.
- Stavudine and zidovudine compete for intracellular phosphorylation and should not be used in combination with each other.

FYI

- A few NRTIs share the same nomenclature (i.e., end in -vir) as the protease inhibitors.
- Individual antiretrovirals are commonly referred to by three letter or digit acronyms. Aside from the fact that the abbreviation of drug names can lead to dispensing errors, the acronyms typically reflect the chemical rather than the generic name of the drug and are thus very confusing. See examples in Table 18-1.

TABLE 18-1. Origins of the Abbreviations for Various Antiretrovirals

Generic Name	Chemical Name	Abbreviation
Zidovudine	Azidothymidine	AZT
Lamivudine	3-Thiacytidine	3TC
Emtricitabine	Fluorothiacytidine	FTC
Didanosine	Dideoxyinosine	ddI

Nonnucleoside Reverse Transcriptase Inhibitors (nNRTIs)

DESCRIPTION

nNRTIs, used in the treatment of HIV infection, inhibit HIV by preventing its transcription.

PROTOTYPE AND COMMON DRUGS

- Prototype: nevirapine
- Others: delavirdine, efavirenz
- Second-generation: etravirine

MOA (MECHANISM OF ACTION)

- Several steps are involved in the replication of HIV. The virus must fuse to the host cell, uncoat, enter and be transcribed by reverse transcriptase, become incorporated into the host genome, and be transcribed to viral RNA, which is then translated into polyproteins (Figure 18-28).
- Reverse transcriptase is an enzyme that **transcribes viral RNA into viral DNA** (hence the term *reverse*).
- The nNRTIs bind to a site distant from the active site of the reverse transcriptase, and induce a conformational change in the enzyme. This conformational change greatly reduces the activity of the enzyme.
- Unlike the NRTIs, the nNRTIs have **no activity against DNA polymerase.**
- Also, because the binding of nNRTIs to the reverse transcriptase is very specific, nNRTIs **act specifically on the HIV-1 strain** and lack activity against HIV-2. Conversely, the NRTIs indirectly inhibit reverse transcriptase and are therefore not specific for HIV-1.

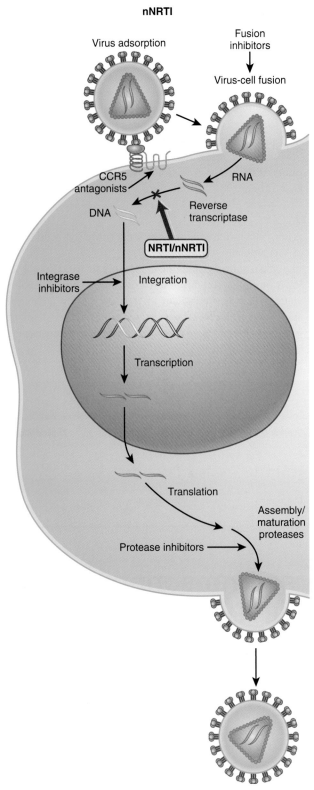

nNRTI

Virus adsorption

Fusion inhibitors

Virus-cell fusion

CCR5 antagonists

RNA

DNA

Reverse transcriptase

NRTI/nNRTI

Integrase inhibitors

Integration

Transcription

Translation

Assembly/ maturation proteases

Protease inhibitors

Figure 18-28. (Modified from Pommier Y, Johnson AA, Marchand C: Integrase inhibitors to treat HIV/AIDS, *Nat Rev Drug Discov* 4(3):236, 2004. Reprinted by permission from Macmillan Publishers.)

Mechanisms of Resistance

- Mutations occur in the binding site on the reverse transcriptase.
  - ▲ A single amino acid change can make the virus resistant to nNRTIs; thus this class as a whole tends to be **more susceptible to drug resistance.**

Pharmacokinetics

- Nevirapine crosses the placenta and is therefore recommended for prevention of mother-child transmission of HIV.
- The nNRTIs are all metabolized in the liver.
- Because nevirapine is both a substrate and an inducer of CYP3A4, it is able to induce its own metabolism. This means that the dose of nevirapine typically must be adjusted upward after 2 weeks of therapy.
- Optimal absorption of delavirdine is achieved at low pH (<2); thus administration of agents that raise the pH (antacids, proton pump inhibitors, H_2 antagonists) may interfere with absorption.

INDICATION

- HIV-1
  - ▲ Treatment of infection
  - ▲ Prevention of transmission from mother to child
  - ▲ Postexposure prophylaxis

CONTRAINDICATIONS

- **Pregnancy (efavirenz):** Of all the antiretrovirals, efavirenz carries the clearest risk in pregnancy, as it has demonstrated teratogenicity in primates.

SIDE EFFECTS

- **Rash:** Macular or papular rash, often pruritic and also self-limiting, may occur with continued drug administration. In a minority of individuals, rash can progress to more serious **Stevens-Johnson syndrome.**

Serious

- **Hepatitis** can be severe and fatal; it is more common in female patients, especially during pregnancy. Most cases are the result of a hypersensitivity reaction. Delavirdine has not been associated with fatal hepatitis.
- **Neutropenia** is a rare effect.

Unique

- **CNS (efavirenz):** The mechanism has not been established. These side effects are typically transient, resolving after a few hours or up to several weeks.
  - ▲ Dizziness
  - ▲ Impaired concentration
  - ▲ **Psychiatric:** dysphoria, vivid dreams, psychosis, insomnia

IMPORTANT NOTES

- The nNRTIs do not inhibit DNA polymerase and therefore do not exhibit the same mitochondrial toxicities as the

NRTIs. Inhibition of DNA polymerase in mitochondria leads to depletion of mitochondrial DNA and subsequent depletion of mitochondrial RNA and peptides involved in oxidative phosphorylation. This leads to mitochondrial dysfunction, and this is believed to be the cause of several of the important toxicities associated with the NRTIs.

■ Etravirine is the first of the second-generation nNRTIs. It was developed through rational drug design, by testing a variety of compounds against known mutations of the HIV-1 reverse transcriptase. This means that etravirine was designed to exhibit minimal cross-resistance with existing nNRTI mutants. However, unique resistant mutations to etravirine have developed.

Combination Therapy

■ The nNRTIs as a class are particularly prone to resistance (see MOA for explanation). Therefore it is important that the nNRTIs be given in combination with other antiretrovirals in order to reduce the development of resistance.

■ Antiretrovirals are typically used in combination with one another (HAART). The most common combinations are an NRTI with an nNRTI, and an NRTI with a ritonavir-boosted protease inhibitor. Two NRTIs are typically used in these regimens.

Advanced
Drug Interactions

■ **Many of the nNRTIs are CYP3A4 substrates** (nevirapine, delavirdine, efavirenz, and etravirine). Given the number of CYP3A4 inducers and inhibitors, these drugs might be more likely to have their metabolism inhibited or induced by other drugs.

■ CYP450 inducers:
  ▲ Efavirenz, nevirapine, and etravirine are moderate inducers of CYP3A4.

■ CYP450 inhibitors:
  ▲ Delavirdine (CYP3A4)
  ▲ Etravirine (CYP2C9 and CYP2C19)

FYI

■ Efavirenz was the first once-daily drug approved for HIV. Now once-daily formulations are commonplace and are an expectation of new agents.

Protease Inhibitors

DESCRIPTION

Protease inhibitors treat HIV infection by inhibiting a key enzyme involved in the maturation of the virus.

PROTOTYPE AND COMMON DRUGS

■ Prototype: saqui**navir**
■ Others: indi**navir**, nelfi**navir**, rito**navir**, ataza**navir**, fosampre**navir**, ampre**navir**, lopi**navir**, daru**navir**

MOA (MECHANISM OF ACTION)

■ Several steps are involved in the replication of HIV. The virus must fuse to the host cell, uncoat, enter and be transcribed by reverse transcriptase, become incorporated into the host genome, and be transcribed to viral RNA, which is then translated into **polyproteins** (Figure 18-29).

■ These polyproteins are then cleaved into smaller viral proteins by **proteases** as they are released from the cell. This process is called **viral maturation**. These smaller viral proteins perform important functions, either structural or acting as enzymes such as reverse transcriptase, integrase, or protease itself.

■ Protease inhibitors bind to these proteases and prevent them from performing this important step in viral maturation. This results in the production of **immature, noninfectious virus particles.**

■ The selective toxicity of the protease inhibitors is based on structural differences between human proteases and viral proteases.

Mechanisms of Resistance

■ Mutations in the viral protease
  ▲ The protease inhibitors are **more prone to developing resistance** than the NRTIs, for a reason similar to that of the nNRTIs (i.e., they directly target an enzyme). However, they are less prone to resistance than the nNRTIs because they require mutations at both the active site of the enzyme and a secondary site before sensitivity is lost.

PHARMACOKINETICS

■ Indinavir absorption is also affected by pH; therefore agents that raise pH such as antacids should not be administered simultaneously.

■ Fosamprenavir is a prodrug of amprenavir.

■ The protease inhibitors are all extensively metabolized by CYP450 enzymes, most commonly via CYP3A4. Nelfinavir is metabolized primarily by CYP2C19, with CYP3A4 taking a secondary role.

■ The protease inhibitors are also are CYP inhibitors; thus they have significant potential for drug interactions.

■ Ritonavir is by far the most potent CYP3A4 inhibitor and is **purposely combined with other protease inhibitors** that are substrates of CYP3A4 in order to prolong the half-life of these agents.

Protease inhibitors

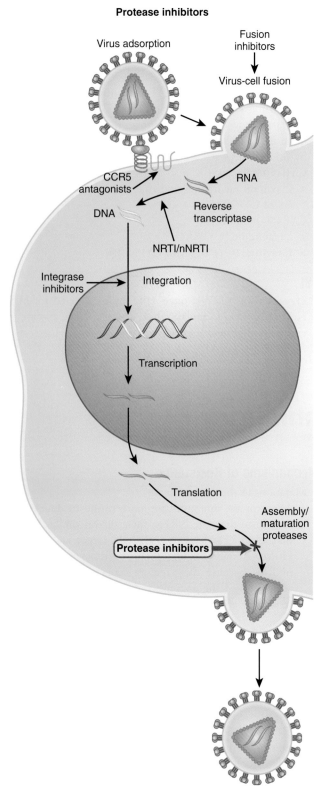

Figure 18-29. (Modified from Pommier Y, Johnson AA, Marchand C: Integrase inhibitors to treat HIV/AIDS, *Nat Rev Drug Discov* 4(3):236, 2004. Reprinted by permission from Macmillan Publishers.)

INDICATION

■ HIV
  ▲ Treatment of infection
  ▲ Prevention of transmission from mother to child
  ▲ Postexposure prophylaxis

CONTRAINDICATIONS

■ **Drug interactions (CYP3A4)**: Ritonavir is such a potent CYP3A4 inhibitor that its use is contraindicated with drugs that are highly dependent on CYP3A4 for their elimination, and where elevated plasma levels of these agents would lead to unacceptable toxicity.

SIDE EFFECTS

■ **GI (nausea, vomiting, diarrhea)**: Diarrhea in particular is a common and troublesome adverse effect of protease inhibitor therapy. The mechanism is not established and is complicated by the fact that diarrhea is a complication of HIV infection.
■ **Hyperlipidemia**: A side effect common to all protease inhibitors, hyperlipidemia might occur less frequently with atazanavir. Protease inhibitors appear to stimulate lipogenesis in hepatocytes.
■ **Lipodystrophy**: Fat redistribution is a problem in HIV that appears to be exacerbated with the use of protease inhibitors. The nature of the fat redistribution may depend to an extent on the total body fat at baseline as well as energy balance.
■ **Hyperglycemia, insulin resistance**: Protease inhibitors appear to inhibit the activity of the glucose transporter (GLUT-4), inhibiting insulin-stimulated glucose uptake by cells. Atazanavir may be less likely to cause this side effect compared with other protease inhibitors.
■ **Rash** is most common with amprenavir.

Unique

■ **Crystalluria, nephrolithiasis (indinavir)**: Indinavir has poor solubility and precipitates easily. Patients are advised to increase fluid intake while on indinavir.
■ **Hyperbilirubinemia (atazanavir)** is not considered to be a serious side effect or sign of hepatotoxicity.

IMPORTANT NOTES

■ Although ritonavir has antiviral activity versus HIV-1, its use as a single protease inhibitor is limited by significant GI toxicity seen at therapeutic doses. Therefore ritonavir is now used in lower doses to **boost the activity** of other protease inhibitors by inhibiting their metabolism (see Pharmacokinetics). The combination of lopinavir and ritonavir has been one of the most commonly used therapies in management of HIV. Lopinavir is available only in combination with ritonavir.
■ The capsule and solution formulations of ritonavir contain alcohol, so drugs such as metronidazole and disulfuram should be avoided in patients taking ritonavir.

Advanced

- The absorption of the protease inhibitors is generally not affected by food, with the exception of indinavir, which should be taken either on an empty stomach or with a low-fat meal, and atazanavir, which should be taken with food.

FYI

- Nelfinavir has gained both a positive and a negative reputation with respect to cancer. After observations of anticancer effects in vitro, it is now being investigated as a new anti-

cancer agent. Conversely, ethyl methanesulfonate, an excipient found in many formulations of nelfinavir, has recently been identified as a carcinogen in animals.

- When protease inhibitors first came out, they were hailed as an additional, unique weapon in the armamentarium against HIV. With time though, the drugs quickly became known for their high pill burden and unpleasant side effects, including GI and disfiguring side effects such as lipodystrophy. Protease inhibitors soon fell out of favor and out of HIV drug regimens. With the advent of newer, more tolerable once-daily protease inhibitors, this class is making a comeback.

Uncoating Inhibitors

DESCRIPTION

Uncoating inhibitors are a group of antivirals that are used in the management of influenza A and Parkinson's disease.

PROTOTYPE AND COMMON DRUGS

- Prototype: amantadine
- Others: rimantadine

MOA (MECHANISM OF ACTION)

- The life cycle of a virus has several stages. Virsuses first attach to the host cell, enter the cell, uncoat, and release their nucleic acid content. The viral genome is enclosed in a capsid, and uncoating is a process where the viral capsid degrades enough to release viral nucleic acids so that they may be transcribed into mRNA, which are then translated on host ribosomes (Figure 18-30).
- Uncoating is mediated by the actions of an M2 protein, a proton channel that facilitates the dissociation of the RNA-protein complex. This dissociation is a pH-dependent event, so when uncoating inhibitors prevent the influx of protons through M2, they prevent this dissociation from occurring.
- It is still unclear how these agents inhibit the activity of the M2 proton channel.
- In addition to inhibition of uncoating, an early stage in viral replication, these agents might also inhibit a late step in viral assembly, although it is unclear as to what extent this mechanism contributes to efficacy.

Mechanisms of Resistance

- Alterations in the structure of M2 prevent its inhibition by the uncoating inhibitors. This mechanism exhibits cross-resistance between rimantadine and amantadine.

Parkinson's Disease

- The CNS actions of amantadine are still poorly understood. It appears to alter dopamine release and is believed to have anticholinergic properties. These actions on dopamine and/or acetylcholine may account for its efficacy in Parkinson's disease. Evidence also suggests that amantadine is an

Uncoating inhibitors

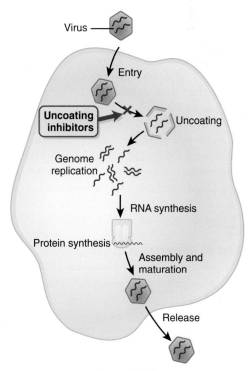

Figure 18-30.

N-methyl-D-aspartate (NMDA) antagonist, and this could also contribute to efficacy in Parkinson's disease.

PHARMACOKINETICS

- Amantadine undergoes minimal metabolism (<10% is metabolized), whereas rimantadine is extensively metabolized (approximately 75%). The elimination half-life of amantadine may therefore be increased significantly in patients with renal impairment, requiring a dose adjustment.
- Rimantadine is less lipophilic and does not cross the blood-brain barrier as readily as amantadine. Therefore it is less

prone to CNS side effects (see later) but is also not used in the treatment of Parkinson's disease.

INDICATIONS
- Influenza A
  - ▲ Treatment and prevention
- Parkinson's disease (amantadine)

CONTRAINDICATIONS
- None of major significance

SIDE EFFECTS
- **CNS**: nervousness, light-headedness, difficulty concentrating, insomnia—Amantadine, specifically, has several effects on the CNS and is used in the treatment of Parkinson's disease.
- **Loss of appetite**: The mechanism is not established but may be related to the CNS effects.
- **Nausea**: The mechanism is not established, but this is a common side effect with agents that increase dopamine release.

IMPORTANT NOTES
- Amantadine is only minimally efficacious in Parkinson's disease; therefore its actions in the CNS primarily limit its tolerability as an antiviral.
- The uncoating inhibitors are often used for the **prevention** rather than the treatment of influenza. They can be particularly useful for reducing the impact of outbreaks in institutionalized settings. Like the neuraminidase inhibitors, the uncoating inhibitors have also demonstrated an ability to reduce the duration and severity of illness in those infected.

EVIDENCE
Prevention of Influenza A in Children
- A 2008 Cochrane review (12 trials, N = 2400 participants) found that amantadine can prevent influenza A in children,

with a number needed to treat (NNT) of 14 to prevent one case over a 14- to 28-week treatment period. No trials were found in elderly patients. The efficacy of rimantadine in preventing influenza A has not been established in children or the elderly. Rimantadine did affect fever, abating fever by the third day of treatment versus 4 to 8 days without drug.
- Because of the small number of trials, no conclusions could be drawn about the safety of amantadine. The authors concluded that rimantadine was safe.

Prevention of Influenza A in Adults
- A 2006 Cochrane review (21 trials, N = 12,600 participants) found that amantadine prevented 25% of cases of influenza-like illness and 61% of influenza A cases and reduced duration of fever by 1 day. The results for rimantadine were not statistically significant, but the authors noted that there were fewer trials of rimantadine, and the numeric results were comparable to those for amantadine.
- Amantadine and rimantadine both elicited considerable GI adverse effects. CNS adverse effects and withdrawals were significantly more common with amantadine versus rimantadine.

FYI
- Amantadine is used off-label to treat fatigue in MS patients.
- Overuse of amantadine by Chinese farmers during an outbreak of bird flu (H5N1) in chickens is believed to have accelerated development of resistance to amantadine, rendering the drug useless in many parts of the world. In an effort to save their livestock, farmers in China are believed to have given amantadine to their chickens, introducing resistant strains into the human food chain.

Neuraminidase Inhibitors

DESCRIPTION
Neuraminidase inhibitors are a group of antivirals used in the treatment of Influenza.

PROTOTYPE AND COMMON DRUGS
- Prototype: zanamivir
- Others: oseltamivir, peramivir

MOA (MECHANISM OF ACTION)
- Influenza viruses possess two important surface glycoproteins: **hemagglutinins** and **neuraminidase**. Changes in these

glycoproteins confer the ability to evade our immune systems and result in the potential for new diseases to appear year after year.
- Hemagglutinins are responsible for **binding and uptake** of virus. They bind to **sialic acid residues** on the host cell.
- Neuraminidases **cleave** the sialic acid residues that are bound to the viral hemagglutinin and thus result in **release** of new virus from cells.
- Neuraminidase inhibitors thus block the cleavage of sialic acid residue and **prevent release** of new virus from early infected cells (Figure 18-31).

- Replication of influenza virus peaks at 24 to 72 hours; therefore drugs such as the neuraminidase inhibitors that act at the stage of viral replication must be administered as early as possible in order to be effective.
- Development of influenza A resistance to neuraminidase inhibitors has been rare but the H1N1 outbreak in 2009 has resulted in resistance to oseltamivir.

Mechanisms of Resistance

Neuraminidase inhibitors

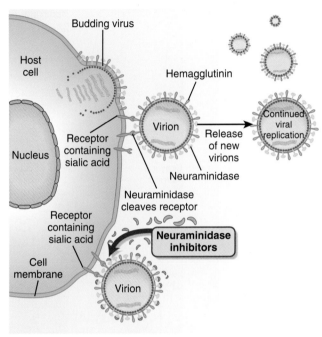

Figure 18-31.

- For oseltamivir binding to occur, the amino acids within neuraminidase must undergo a **conformational change** to accommodate oseltamivir's hydrophobic sidechain; mutations that prevent this change may lead to resistance.

- Zanamivir is more structurally similar to the natural substrate of neuraminidase and fits directly into the active site without a conformational change required. Therefore mutations that prevent the rearrangement· do not bring about resistance to zanamivir.

PHARMACOKINETICS

- Neuraminidase inhibitors are orally administrated.

INDICATIONS

- For **treatment** of influenza infection in patients younger than 1 year old who have had symptoms for less than 2 days
- For **prevention** of influenza infection in select populations

CONTRAINDICATIONS

- None of significance

SIDE EFFECTS

- Possible worsening of respiratory symptoms, including bronchospasm, may occur.
- **GI**: Nausea, vomiting, and abdominal pain may occur.
- Unusual dreams have been rarely reported.

IMPORTANT NOTES

- Early initiation of treatment appears to be the most important determinant of treatment efficacy. This is because viral replication and releases new viral particles from infected cells; stopping this process *before* it occurs reduces viral burden in the patient.
- When taken early for treatment of influenza, neuraminidase inhibitors can shorten the duration of illness by 1 to 4 days.
- When neuraminidase inhibitors are taken as **prophylaxis** against getting influenza, infection rate is reduced by about 70% to 90%.

FYI

- Neuraminidase inhibitors were recommended therapy for the H1N1 (swine flu) pandemic that occurred in 2009.

Nucleoside Analogues

DESCRIPTION

Nucleoside analogues are a group of antivirals that have a structural similarity to guanosine.

PROTOTYPE AND COMMON DRUGS

- Prototype: **acyclovir**
- Others: vala**cyclovir**, pen**ciclovir**, fam**ciclovir**, gan**ciclovir**, cidofovir

MOA (MECHANISM OF ACTION)

- The nucleoside analogues act as DNA polymerase inhibitors, thereby reducing DNA synthesis and viral replication. They are guanosine analogs.

- The life cycle of a virus has several stages. Virsuses first attach to the host cell, enter the cell, uncoat, and release their nucleic acid content. An important step in the viral life cycle is the synthesis of viral DNA.
- Viral and host cell kinases convert the nucleoside analogues (acyclovir depicted in Figure 18-32) to active nucleoside triphosphates.
- These nucleoside triphosphates compete with viral DNA polymerase for incorporation into the primer strand of viral DNA.
- Some nucleoside analogues (acyclovir, valacyclovir) cause **chain termination** when incorporated into the DNA strand, as they lack the 3'-OH group that attaches to the next

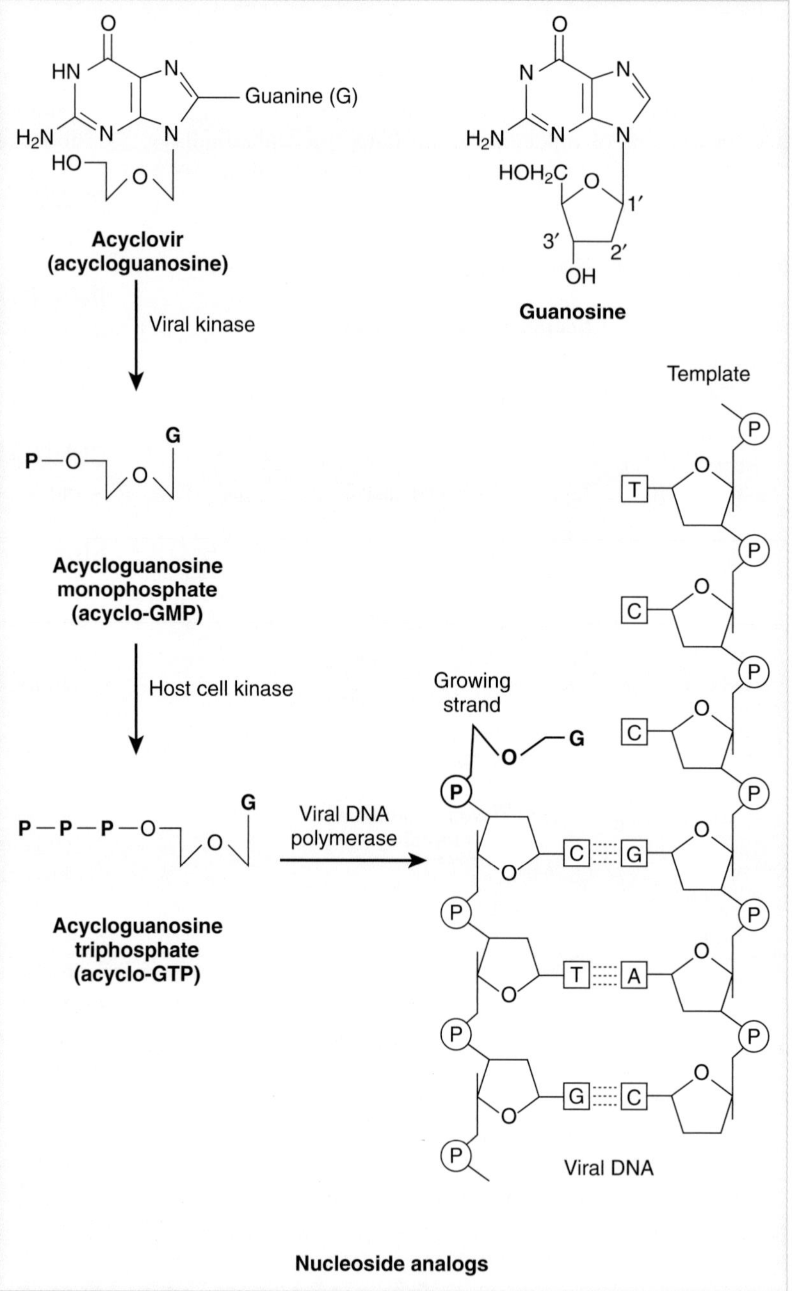

Figure 18-32.

nucleoside. Other nucleoside analogues (penciclovir) work by the same mechanism but because they have a 3'-OH group do not cause chain termination and **instead inhibit DNA elongation**.

- The selective toxicity of these agents is based on the following:
  - ▲ Affinity for herpes simplex virus (HSV) thymidine kinase ("viral kinase" in Figure 18-32), is about 200× greater than that for the human version of this enzyme.
  - ▲ Greater affinity for viral versus human DNA polymerase

Mechanisms of Resistance

- Absence or partial production of viral thymidine kinase
- Phosphorylation of thymidine instead of acyclovir by thymidine kinase
- Alterations in viral DNA polymerase

PHARMACOKINETICS

- The low oral bioavailability of acyclovir is overcome by the prodrug valacyclovir, which is rapidly converted to acyclovir after oral administration.

- Acyclovir is widely distributed, including to CSF and breast milk. It is largely eliminated unchanged in the urine through tubular secretion, and therefore metabolic drug interactions are not an issue. However, because it is eliminated renally, dose adjustment should be considered in patients with renal impairment.
- The oral bioavailability of penciclovir is also low, and thus it also has a prodrug form, famciclovir.
- Penciclovir is also largely excreted in the urine unchanged, via both filtration and tubular secretion. Again, metabolic drug interactions are not an issue.
- Ganciclovir also has low oral bioavailability, and a prodrug, valganciclovir, has been developed to improve bioavailability.
- Acyclovir is available in oral, intravenous, and topical routes. Cidofovir is the only nucleoside analogue that is available for only the intravenous route, penciclovir is available for only topical use, and trifluridine (a uridine analog) is available as topical eye drops.
- A sustained-release intraocular implant of ganciclovir is available for use in patients with cytomegalovirus (CMV) retinitis.

INDICATIONS
- **Herpes simplex**:
  - ▲ Cold sores and oral (mucocutaneous) infections
  - ▲ Genital herpes
  - ▲ Bell's palsy (cranial nerve VII paralysis)
  - ▲ Herpetic whitlow (finger infection)
  - ▲ Rarer but serious infections:
    - • Herpes encephalitis
    - • Herpes pneumonitis or pneumonia
    - • Ophthalmic herpes (keratitis)
- **Varicella zoster virus (VZV)**
  - ▲ Chickenpox
  - ▲ Herpes zoster (shingles)
- **CMV**
  - ▲ Systemic infections in solid organ transplant patients
  - ▲ Retinitis
- **Human herpesvirus 8** (causes **Kaposi's sarcoma** in immunocompromised patients)

CONTRAINDICATIONS
- None of major significance

SIDE EFFECTS
- **Nausea, diarrhea**: mechanism not established
- **Rash**: mechanism not established
- **Headache**: mechanism not established

Rare
- **CNS: Confusion, hallucinations, and tremor** have been reported with both acyclovir and valacyclovir, with a higher incidence in patients with renal failure. After many years, the mechanism has not been determined, although metabolites of acyclovir may play a role.

- **Nephrotoxicity** has been reported mainly with acyclovir and valacyclovir. The mechanism may be related to tubular cell death and/or crystal deposits leading to obstruction. Predisposing factors include bolus intravenous administration and dehydration. Cidofovir is associated with severe nephrotoxicity.

Unique (Ganciclovir)
- **Hematologic**: leukopenia, thrombocytopenia
- **Reproductive**: aspermatogenesis

IMPORTANT NOTES
- Although acyclovir is a more potent inhibitor of viral DNA polymerase than penciclovir and famciclovir, penciclovir and famciclovir achieve higher intracellular concentrations for longer periods of time than acyclovir, and thus they have a prolonged antiviral effect.
- Cidofovir is associated with nephrotoxicity to a much greater extent than other drugs in this class. It binds to a transporter and accumulates in the renal cortex; therefore it is given with probenecid, a drug that competes for tubular secretion with cidofovir. This reduces the rate of cidofovir accumulation in the cortex, mitigating the damage inflicted by this agent.
- Viral infections are more common in immunosuppressed and immunocompromised patients; rare but serious herpesvirus infections must be considered in these patient populations.

EVIDENCE
Acyclovir in Children with Chickenpox
- A 2005 Cochrane review found only three moderate- to poor-quality studies comparing acyclovir with placebo in otherwise healthy children with chickenpox. Acyclovir reduced the duration of fever by 1 day and reduced the maximum number of lesions. Results were inconclusive regarding the number of days with no new lesions and relief from itchiness. Overall, the clinical importance of acyclovir treatment in otherwise healthy children remains uncertain.

Antiviral Prophylaxis for Recurrent Genital Herpes in Pregnancy
- A 2008 Cochrane review (seven trials, N = 1249 patients) compared acyclovir (five trials) and valacyclovir (two trials) with placebo or no treatment. There were no cases of symptomatic neonatal herpes in either the treatment or placebo groups; therefore the effect of antepartum antiviral prophylaxis could not be determined. Women who received antiviral prophylaxis were less likely to have HSV detected at delivery. Women who received prophylaxis were also less likely to have recurrence of genital herpes at delivery and less likely to have a caesarean delivery as a result of genital herpes.

Various Interventions for Dendritic or Geographic Herpes Simplex Virus Epithelial Keratitis

- A 2008 Cochrane review (99 trials, N = 5363 patients) compared various agents (vidarabine, trifluridine, acyclovir, ganciclovir, and interferon). There were no significant differences in efficacy between antivirals or interferon alone. Interferon was very effective when *combined* with another antiviral agent, such as trifluridine. The topical application of antivirals resulted in a high proportion of patients healing within 1 week.

Prevention of Cytomegalovirus Disease in Solid Organ Transplant Recipients

- A 2008 Cochrane review (34 studies, N = 3850 patients) included studies comparing acyclovir, ganciclovir, or valacyclovir with placebo or no treatment. The authors found that prophylaxis reduced risk of CMV disease (relative risk [RR] 0.42, 19 studies), CMV infection (RR 0.61, 17 studies) and all-cause mortality (RR 0.63, 17 studies). The reduction in mortality was largely attributable to reduced CMV deaths. Prophylaxis did not reduce the risk of acute organ rejection or loss. In seven studies, ganciclovir was more effective than acyclovir (RR 0.37) in preventing CMV disease.

FYI

- Acyclovir was the first nucleoside analogue. Its name reflects the fact that the major difference between its chemical structure and that of guanosine is the lack of a third ring (**a**-cyclo).
- Memory tip: Many antivirals contain the three letters *vir* at the end of their name.
- *Solid organ* transplant includes kidney, liver, lung, heart, and pancreas. Bone marrow transplants are not solid and therefore are not included as solid organ transplants. These patients have different risks and problems and so are often considered separately.

Azoles

DESCRIPTION

The azoles are a class of antifungals named for their chemical structure.

PROTOTYPE AND COMMON DRUGS

- Prototype: flu**conazole**
- Others: keto**conazole**, itra**conazole**, clotri**mazole**, mic**onazole**
- Second-generation agent: Vori**conazole**

MOA (MECHANISM OF ACTION)

- Ergosterol is an integral part of the fungal cell membrane.
- Azoles inhibit fungal wall synthesis via inhibition of **ergosterol synthesis**, which is catalyzed by a CP450 enzyme called *14α-demethylase.*
- **14α-Demethylase** converts lanosterol to ergosterol in fungi (Figure 18-33).

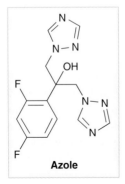

Azole

Figure 18-33.

- Azoles are direct CP450 enzyme inhibitors.
- In humans, 14α-demethylase converts lanosterol to cholesterol. The human enzyme is less effected than the fungal enzyme, which is why the drug can be used safely but is also the mechanism through which some side effects are created.

PHARMACOKINETICS

- **Drug interactions** are a major factor with these agents, given their MOA (CP450 inhibitors).
- Clotrimazole and miconazole are both used topically, whereas the remainder are available in oral or intravenous form.

INDICATIONS

- **First-generation azoles:**
  - ▲ **For superficial fungal infections:**
    - Oral, vaginal, and esophageal *Candida*
    - Dermatophytes
  - ▲ For **uncomplicated systemic infections** in immuno*competent* patients:
    - *Candida*
      - ▲ Excluding *Candida glabrata* and *Candida krusei* (these two species are usually resistant)
    - *Cryptococcus*
    - Blastomycosis, coccidioidomycosis, histoplasmosis
    - *Aspergillus*

CONTRAINDICATIONS

- None of significance

SIDE EFFECTS
- Relatively nontoxic
- **GI**: mild GI side effects have been reported
- **Hepatotoxicity** (has occurred rarely)

IMPORTANT NOTES
- Dermatophytes are fungi that infect skin, hair, and nails and are able to obtain nutrients from keratin, which is abundant in these tissues. Dermatophytes include *Microsporum, Epidermophyton,* and *Trichophyton.* Dermatophytes usually do not invade into living tissue but rather live only on the outer layers of skin.
- Fungal systemic infections can be difficult to diagnose because they can mimic bacterial infections; as a result, drugs targeting bacteria are started and the infection persists. Delayed therapy is not uncommon with these types of infections and is particularly true with pneumonia.
- Fungal systemic infections are more common in patients with a weakened immune system, including patients with acquired immunodeficiency syndrome (AIDS) and patients on immunosuppression.

FYI
- An azole is a five-membered ring that includes at least one noncarbon atom. Triazoles have three nitrogens. Fluconazole is pictured in Figure 18-33 and shows two triazole rings.
- Aromatase inhibitors (they block the synthesis of estrogen) are also triazoles but have no antifungal properties.
- Ketoconazole is the true prototype but is no longer used clinically very much and therefore was replaced as the prototype. Fluconazole is probably the most commonly used azole today.
- Many of the drugs in this class are available without a prescription, particularly those used topically.

Echinocandins

DESCRIPTION
Echinocandins are a class of antifungals that target fungal cell walls.

PROTOTYPE AND COMMON DRUGS
- Prototype: caspo**fungin**
- Others: anidula**fungin**, mica**fungin**

MOA (MECHANISM OF ACTION)
- Fungal cells have both an outer cell wall and a cell membrane. It is believed that the cell wall provides structural rigidity to the fungal cell, in the same way that cell walls provide rigidity for bacteria.
- Chitin and β-(1,3)-glucan help to provide structural rigidity to the **cell wall** of many fungi (Figure 18-34).

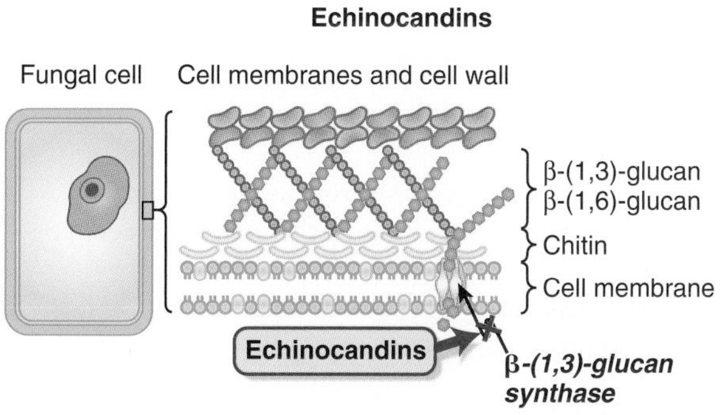

Echinocandins

Figure 18-34.

- β-(1,3)-glucan is synthesized by an enzyme called **β-(1,3)-glucan synthase.**

- The echinocandins inhibit this enzyme, thus inhibiting synthesis of β-(1,3)-glucan, which in turn weakens the cell wall. This eventually results in lysis of the cell.
- The echinocandins might also have a secondary mechanism. By disrupting the cell wall, they expose β-glucan, exposing additional antigens for antibody deposition and recognition by the immune system.

PHARMACOKINETICS
- The echinocandins have poor oral absorption and are therefore all administered IV.
- Caspofungin and micafungin undergo hepatic metabolism; however, the role of CYP450 enzymes in this metabolism is believed to be minimal. Anidulafungin is degraded almost entirely in the plasma, not the liver. None of the echinocandins require dose adjustments in patients with renal impairment.

INDICATIONS
- Severe invasive fungal infections
  - ▲ *Candida*
  - ▲ *Aspergillus*

CONTRAINDICATIONS
- None of major significance

SIDE EFFECTS
- Generally well tolerated
- **GI**: Nausea, vomiting, and diarrhea have been observed infrequently.
- **Infusion reactions**: Swelling and rash occur and may be an allergic-type reaction mediated by histamine.

■ **Elevated liver enzymes:** This side effect occurs mainly in patients receiving both cyclosporine and caspofungin. Cyclosporine is an immunosuppressant, and patients who are immunosuppressed are more likely to develop fungal infections and therefore are more likely to be treated with antifungals.

IMPORTANT NOTES

■ The echinocandins are the first antifungals to target the fungal cell wall. Virtually all of the other antifungals target the fungal cell membrane. Because the differences between cell membranes in humans and those in fungi are subtle, some of the antifungals that target cell membranes are quite toxic (e.g., amphotericin).

■ Humans do not have a cell wall; therefore targeting the fungal cell wall is thought to be an important advance in treating fungal infections while minimizing toxicity.

■ There appears to be a synergistic effect from combining echinocandins with either amphotericin B or the azole antifungals. This is likely because the combination targets both the cell wall (echinocandins) and cell membrane (amphotericin B and azoles).

■ The echinocandins are fungistatic for *Aspergillus* and fungicidal for *Candida* species.

Advanced
Drug Interactions

■ The pharmacokinetics of micafungin do not appear to be affected by other drugs; however, micafungin has been shown to increase levels of amphotericin B. Because of their complementary MOA, these two antifungal agents might be combined.

FYI

■ The echinocandins also have demonstrated activity against *P. jiroveci*, but they have not been pursued further for this indication.

■ *P. jiroveci* is an opportunistic infection seen in HIV patients. It causes pneumonia, and the causative organism was originally thought to be *P. carinii*.

Griseofulvin

DESCRIPTION
Griseofulvin is an antifungal used for dermatophytes.

PROTOTYPE
■ Griseofulvin

MOA (MECHANISM OF ACTION)
■ Griseofulvin is deposited in **keratin precursor** cells. It is subsequently taken up by fungal cells and binds to microtubular proteins and **tubulin**. Tubulin is required for separation of dividing chromosomes, and therefore it inhibits mitosis in dividing fungal cells.

■ As a result of its distribution in the body, new skin and hair growth is subsequently resistant to fungal invasion.

PHARMACOKINETICS
■ Griseofulvin is a hepatic enzyme inducer. It therefore reduces the half-life of other drugs that are metabolized by CYP3A4.

■ The half-life of griseofulvin is about 24 hours.

INDICATIONS
■ **Tinea:** dermatophyte infections of the skin and hair. *Trichophyton* is the most common fungal species, followed by *Microsporum* and *Epidermophyton*.

CONTRAINDICATIONS
■ Pregnancy: Griseofulvin is a potential teratogen.

SIDE EFFECTS
Common and Not Severe
■ **CNS:**
  ▲ **Headache:** can sometimes be very severe and force discontinuation of the drug
  ▲ **Peripheral neuropathy:** tingling of the hands and feet
  ▲ Sleep disturbances and fatigue
■ **Dermatologic:**
  ▲ **Skin rashes:** Remember that the drug is in high concentrations in the keratin. Different rash types can include the following:
    • Urticaria (hives)
    • Lichen planus (*pruritic, planar, purple, polygonal papules*)
    • Erythema (red rash)
    • Erythema multiforme (red rash with target appearance)
    • Photosensitivity (rash from sun exposure)
    • Angioedema (swelling of the skin from edema)

Rare but Severe
■ Neutropenia: a decreased neutrophil count

IMPORTANT NOTES
■ Blood counts must be measured weekly for the first month to screen for neutropenia.
■ Griseofulvin is not effective in nail or subcutaneous infections. It is useful only for superficial infections.

EVIDENCE
Griseofulvin versus Other Antifungals for Tinea Capitis (Ringworm)
- A Cochrane review in 2007 (21 studies, 1812 participants) revealed that among multiple comparisons there were no differences in cure rates (griseofulvin versus terbinafine, itraconazole, or fluconazole) for infections involving *Trichophyton* species. However, compared to griseofulvin, treatment with the other 3 (newer) agents required shorter durations of treatment (2 to 4 weeks shorter) but were more expensive than griseofulvin.

Griseofulvin versus Other Antifungals for Tinea Pedis (Athlete's Foot)
- A Cochrane review in 2001 (12 studies, 700 participants) compared griseofulvin with terbenifine and itraconazole

and found that terbenifine worked faster, was more effective and cost more than griseofulvin. Terbenifine and itraconazole were both superior to placebo.

FYI
- Colchicine, a drug used in gout, and vinca alkaloids, drugs used in cancer, have similar MOAs in that they all bind different regions of the microtubular apparatus and inhibit mitosis.

Polyenes

DESCRIPTION

The polyenes are a class of antifungals.

PROTOTYPE AND COMMON DRUGS
- Prototype: **Amphotericin B** (commonly abbreviated as "Ampho B")
- Others: Nystatin

MOA (MECHANISM OF ACTION)
- Polyenes bind sterols (steroid + alcohol). Cholesterol and ergosterol are two examples of sterols. **Ergosterol** is an integral part of the fungal cell membrane; it is not present in human cells. Its counterpart in the human is cholesterol.
- Polyenes have multiple C=C bonds; this creates long straight hydrophobic segments that bind to the hydrophobic rings of steroids through van der Waal's forces (Figure 18-35).
- Polyene exposure to fungi results in binding of the polyene to ergosterol, which results in the development of pores within the fungal membrane through which H^+ and K^+ ions leak out, killing the cell. See Figure 18-35.
- Polyenes also bind to cholesterol but to a much lesser degree than to ergosterol. The binding to sterols *in humans* is the basis for their toxicity.

Mechanisms of Resistance (Amphotericin B)
- Alteration in amount of ergosterol in membrane
- Modification of structure to reduce drug binding

PHARMACOKINETICS
- **Nystatin** is too toxic for parenteral administration and is poorly absorbed from the skin, mucous membranes, and GI tract. Therefore it is used only **topically** (cream, ointment, suppository) or as an oral rinse (swish and swallow).

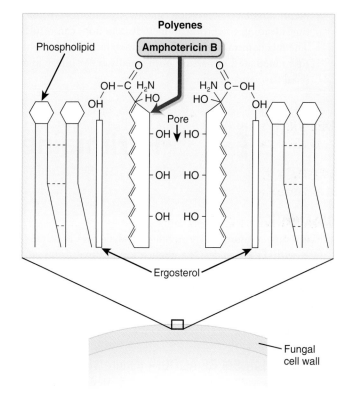

Figure 18-35.

- Amphotericin B is administered only IV. Different formulations of amphotericin B have been manufactured to try to reduce the risk of nephrotoxicity. These preparations include liposomal amphotericin and amphotericin B lipid complex.
- The terminal half-life of amphotericin is 15 days.

INDICATIONS
Nystatin
- Noninvasive candidal infections
  - ▲ Oropharyngeal thrush
  - ▲ Vaginal candidiasis
  - ▲ Intertriginous candidal infections

Amphotericin B
- Serious invasive or systemic fungal infections:
  - ▲ Examples include (but are not limited to) *Candida, Aspergillus, Coccidioides, Histoplasma,* and *Blastomyces.*

CONTRAINDICATIONS
- Nystatin
  - ▲ None of significance
- Amphotericin B
  - ▲ **Renal dysfunction,** because amphotericin B is nephrotoxic

SIDE EFFECTS
- **Amphotericin B** (nystatin is not administered systemically because of high toxicity)
  - ▲ Nephrotoxicity: Reversible kidney dysfunction, sometimes leading to chronic kidney dysfunction, can result. The mechanism is incompletely understood but thought to be mediated in part by both renal tubular injury and renal vasoconstriction.
  - ▲ **Infusion reactions:** Fever, chills, hypotension, vomiting, dyspnea, and headaches may occur. The mechanism of these reactions is unknown.
  - ▲ **Electrolyte abnormalities:** Because of increases in the distal tubular permeability, potassium and magnesium wasting, leading to hypokalemia and hypomagnesemia, can occur.

FYI
- An *ene* is a C=C bond. Polyenes have multiple C=C bonds. The antifungals in this category contain a 38-atom ring structure; within this ring are seven alternating C=C bonds.
- *Amphoteric* means having the ability to exist as or react with either an acid or a base. *Amphipathic* (not related to this discussion) means both hydrophobic and hydrophilic.
- Amphotericin B was first isolated from *Streptomyces nodosus* in 1955.
- Amphotericin A also exists. It is not used because it is less effective in vivo.
- As a result of the large list of side effects, amphotericin B has the nickname *amphoterrible.*
- *Intertriginous* refers to areas where skin contacts skin (i.e., between fat folds).
- Cholesterol is required for the integrity and function of cell membranes; it maintains membrane fluidity. The steroid and the hydrocarbon chain are embedded within the membrane.

Pyrimidine Antifungals

DESCRIPTION
- Pyrimidine antifungals are pyrimidine analogues that interfere with DNA and RNA replication. Other drugs are pyrimidine analogues but are not antifungals; they are used for anticancer therapy.

PROTOTYPE
- Flucytosine

MOA (MECHANISM OF ACTION) (Figure 18-36)
- Flucytosine was originally developed as an antimetabolite for cancer but is only used for antifungal therapy.
- Flucytosine (5-FC) is taken up by fungi by **cytosine permease,** which is not present on mammalian cells and is the basis for its selectivity.
- Although they are similar, there are two distinct mechanisms of action:
  1. 5-FC is converted to 5-fluorouracil (5-FU) and then to further 5-fluorodeoxyuridylic acid monophosphate (5-FDUMP), which is an irreversible inhibitor of **thymidylate synthase,** resulting in **termination of DNA synthesis.**

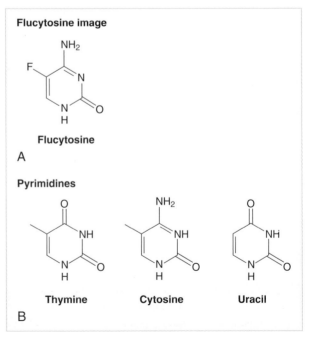

Figure 18-36.

2. 5-FU can also be converted into 5-fluorouridine triphosphate, which is incorporated into fungal **RNA**, thereby preventing protein synthesis.

PHARMACOKINETICS

- Flucytosine is administered orally, and in Europe an intravenous preparation is available.
- It is renally eliminated, and dose adjustments are required in patients with renal dysfunction.

INDICATIONS

- *Cryptococcus* infections
- *Candida* infections
- Other fungal infections

CONTRAINDICATION

- Pregnancy is a contraindication because of the conversion to 5-FU, which is an antimetabolite for human DNA and a potential teratogen.

SIDE EFFECTS

- There is a risk of infection. Avoid treating patients with nonfungal infections.
- **GI**: Abdominal pain, nausea, vomiting, and diarrhea may occur.

Rare

- **Liver damage** can rarely occur. Liver enzymes should be routinely measured.
- **Bone marrow suppression**: Anemia, low WBC count, and low platelet counts can occur. This is due to inhibition of rapidly dividing cells, as 5-DUMP can inhibit DNA synthesis
- **Toxic epidermal necrolysis** is a severe skin reaction with a mortality rate around 30%.

IMPORTANT NOTES

- By itself, flucytosine is not very effective at killing fungi. It is always used as an adjuvant and it is synergistic with amphotericin B.
- *Cryptococcus neoformans* infections are known to cause meningitis in patients with AIDS. However, meningitis can occur in immunocompetent patients as well.

FYI

- *Cryptococcus* means hidden seed.
- *Cryptococcus* is not a bacterium, although many bacterial names do have the ending *-coccus* (e.g., *Streptococcus, Staphylococcus,* and *Enterococcus*).

Terbinafine

DESCRIPTION

Terbinafine is an allylamine antifungal used for fungal infections of nails.

PROTOTYPE

- Terbinafine

MOA (MECHANISM OF ACTION)

- Ergosterol is an integral component of fungal cell membranes.
- Terbinafine inhibits conversion of squalene to lanosterol via inhibition of squalene monooxidase.
- Lanosterol is the precursor for ergosterol (Figure 18-37).
- Terbinafine is fungicidal.
- Mammalian squalene monooxidase is inhibited only at very high concentrations of terbinafine (4000 times higher than the fungal enzyme).

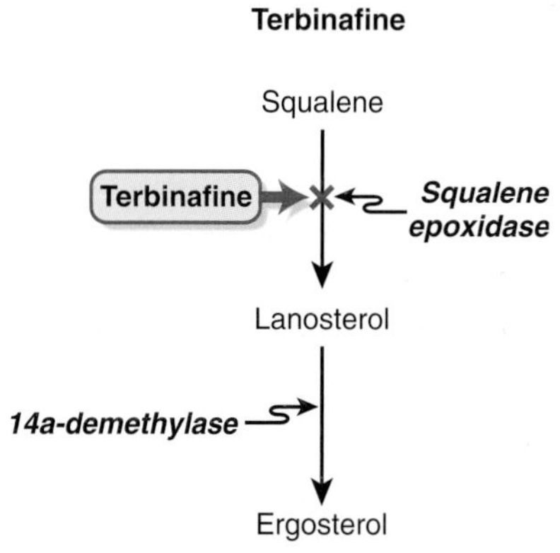

PHARMACOKINETICS

- Terbinafine is metabolized by the liver.
- Terbinafine has an initial half-life of 12 hours and a steady state half-life of 200 to 400 hours.
- Terbinafine is lipid soluble and readily distributes into skin, nails, and fat; the slow release of drug from these tissues accounts for its long steady state half-life.

Terbinafine

Squalene

Terbinafine ➡ ✕ ⬅ *Squalene epoxidase*

Lanosterol

14a-demethylase ⬅

Ergosterol

Figure 18-37.

INDICATION

- Onychomycosis (fungal infections of nails or nail beds)

SIDE EFFECTS
Rare but Serious

- **Stevens-Johnson syndrome** is a life-threatening condition whereby the dermis and epidermis separate. It is commonly caused by drugs (there is a long list). It is mediated by a hypersensitivity reaction. It occurs in about 2 to 3 per million people per year.

- **Toxic epidermal necrolysis** is a less severe form of Stevens-Johnson syndrome.
- **Liver failure**
  - ▲ Liver enzymes must be measured before patients start terbinafine.
  - ▲ Liver enzymes increase to abnormal in 3.3% of patients, compared with 1.2% in patients taking placebo.
  - ▲ Liver failure resulting in death or liver transplant has occurred. This is *extremely* uncommon, but case reports exist.
  - ▲ If symptoms of liver disease occur, the drug must be stopped immediately and tests for liver damage and liver function must immediately be performed. These symptoms can include the following:
    - • Nausea and vomiting, fatigue, anorexia (loss of appetite), jaundice (yellow skin), bilirubinuria (dark urine because of bilirubin), and right upper quadrant pain
  - ▲ Liver damage is usually reversible if the drug is discontinued.
- Systemic lupus erythematosus exacerbation
- **Neutropenia and lymphopenia:** Neutrophil and lymphocyte counts can be severely decreased. The drug should be discontinued if the counts are very low. The effect is reversible.

IMPORTANT NOTES

- The cure rate of onychomycosis is reported to be about 70% to 75%. The relapse (reinfection) rate is 15%.
- Terbinafine is usually taken for 12 weeks. Noncompliance and forgetting to take medications might contribute to failure of cure.

FYI

- Stevens-Johnson syndrome was named after two American pediatricians who described this condition in 1922.
- *Trichophyton* is the most common fungal organism to cause onychomycosis.
- **Dermatophytes** are fungal organisms that infect skin.
- **Tinea** is a fungal skin infection. The second word describes the nature or location of the tinea:
  - ▲ Tinea nigra: hyperpigmented skin
  - ▲ Tinea versicolor: hyperpigmented and hypopigmented skin
  - ▲ Tinea pedis: foot infection also called *athlete's foot*
  - ▲ Tinea capitus: scalp infection
  - ▲ Tinea cruris: perineal infection, also called *jock itch*

Quinolines

DESCRIPTION

The quinolines are a class of antimalarials that are distinct from the quinolones, which are a class of antibiotics. Certain quinolines are also used to treat disorders of the immune system.

PROTOTYPE AND COMMON DRUGS

- Prototype: chloro**quine**
- Others: prima**quine**, amodia**quine**, hydroxychloro**quine**, quinine

MOA (MECHANISM OF ACTION)

- The transmission of malaria begins with a bite from an infected mosquito, which injects *Plasmodium* sporozoites into the bloodstream of the host. The sporozoites travel to the liver, where they multiply to form schizonts, which then divide to form merozoites. This process of division to create merozoites is referred to as *exoerythrocytic schizogony* and is an asymptomatic process.
- These merozoites are then released from the liver back into the blood, where they infect erythrocytes. This process is referred to as *erythrocytic schizogony*. The infection of erythrocytes involves binding to specific ligands on the surface of the erythrocyte (Figure 18-38).
- When erythrocytes rupture periodically and merozoites are released, the patient experiences fever. These merozoites then proceed to infect other erythrocytes, propagating the cycle.

- Chloroquine, hydroxychloroquine, mefloquine, and quinine appear to act at the erythrocytic schizogony stage, perhaps by inhibiting synthesis or function of nucleic acids, although the mechanism is still unclear. Another theory as to the mechanism involves the handling of heme.
- In the erythrocyte, malaria parasites feed on hemoglobin, and one of the byproducts of hemoglobin consumption is the highly reactive heme molecule. The parasite sequesters heme so that it does not cause it harm. It is believed that chloroquine and related drugs interfere with heme sequestration, thus unleashing this highly toxic substance within the parasite, killing it.

Mechanisms of Resistance

- The actions of chloroquine and related agents on heme occur at the food vacuole, and the main theory regarding resistance centers around the ability of chloroquine and others to access the food vacuole. Malaria may limit this through various mutations that either prevent access to the vacuole or pump drug out of the vacuole. One strategy being investigated to overcome resistance is to inhibit the activity of this efflux pump using another drug.

Immune- or Inflammation-Related Conditions

- As with the use of these drugs in malaria, their mechanism in immune- or inflammation-related conditions has not been established; however, the quinolines appear to inhibit prostaglandin synthesis and, as noted earlier, affect nucleic acids.

Quinolines

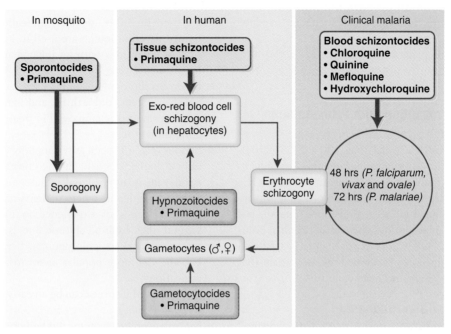

Figure 18-38.

PHARMACOKINETICS
■ Chloroquine is partially metabolized by the liver but is mostly (70%) excreted unchanged in the urine. It is an inhibitor of CYP2D6.
■ Mefloquine has a very long elimination half-life of approximately 20 days, on average. It is metabolized by the liver.
■ Primaquine undergoes extensive hepatic metabolism.

INDICATIONS
■ Malaria
■ Autoimmune diseases:
  ▲ Rheumatoid arthritis
  ▲ Lupus

Spectra at a Glance
■ See Table 18-2.

CONTRAINDICATIONS
Mefloquine
■ **Seizure disorder**: Mefloquine lowers the seizure threshold.

TABLE 18-2. Antimalarial Spectra	
Agent	**Organism**
Chloroquine hydroxychloroquine	*Plasmodium vivax* *Plasmodium ovale* *Plasmodium malariae* *Plasmodium falciparum*
Mefloquine	*Plasmodium vivax* *Plasmodium falciparum*
Primaquine	*Plasmodium vivax* *Plasmodium ovale*

■ **Schizophrenia or other psychotic disorders**: Mefloquine can cause psychosis.

Primaquine
■ **Patients at risk for granulocytopenia**, such as those with lupus and rheumatoid arthritis, should not take primaquine.
■ **Myelosuppressants**: Avoid concomitant administration of agents that suppress bone marrow.

SIDE EFFECTS
■ GI effects
■ Headache
■ Pruritus

Serious
■ **Retinopathy**: Damage to the retina leading to deterioration of vision may occur and typically is seen only at higher doses. The mechanism is still unclear, but the condition may be caused by accumulation of drug in melanin or by degradation of photoreceptors.
■ **Ototoxicity** occurs much less frequently than retinopathy; the mechanism may be similar.
■ **CNS**: Seizures and psychosis may occur and typically are seen only at higher doses or during rapid parenteral administration.
■ **Cardiovascular**: Arrhythmia (QT prolongation) and even cardiac arrest may occur at higher doses. Hypotension is seen with malaria but can also be exacerbated by quinolines.

Primaquine
■ **Hemolytic anemia** is potentially fatal but typically only a concern in patients who are glucose-6-phosphate

dehydrogenase (G6PD) deficient or in patients with other risk factors. G6PD maintains content of reduced glutathione (GSH) in erythrocytes, and primaquine tends to reduce GSH levels.

■ **Methemoglobinemia** may occur.

EVIDENCE
Malaria Relapse Prevention with Primaquine in *Plasmodium vivax*

■ A 2007 Cochrane review (nine trials, N = 3423 participants) compared various primaquine regimens for prevention of relapse in patients with *P. vivax* infection. The combination of 5-day primaquine and chloroquine was no better than chloroquine alone at preventing relapse, but 14-day primaquine plus chloroquine was better than chloroquine (odds ratio [OR] 0.24, six trials and 1071 participants). These results were confirmed by two trials that compared these two regimens head to head.

Prevention of Malaria in Pregnancy

■ A 2006 Cochrane review (16 trials, N = 12638 participants) assessed drug therapy for malaria prevention in pregnant women living in endemic areas. Antimalarials reduced antenatal parasitemia (two trials) and placental malaria (three trials) but did not have an impact on perinatal deaths (four trials). In women in their first or second pregnancy, antimalarials reduced severe antenatal anemia, antenatal parasitemia, and perinatal deaths.

Chloroquine versus Prednisone for Treatment of Lupus

■ A 1998 Cochrane review found a single trial that compared prednisone to chloroquine treatment. The results of this study suggested that the effectiveness of these two agents is similar.

IMPORTANT NOTES

■ Aside from their use in malaria, several drugs in this class are used for other, distinct, indications. Hydroxychloroquine and chloroquine are used in lupus and in a number of skin conditions with an inflammatory and/or immunologic component.

■ Hydroxychloroquine is also used as a disease-modifying agent in rheumatoid arthritis and likely works by a similar mechanism to that employed in treating inflammatory skin conditions.

■ Serious toxicities such as retinopathy are typically observed only at higher doses or during chronic therapy. The latter is relevant in nonmalarial indications such as rheumatoid arthritis and lupus, where patients may be on therapy for years. Decades of experience in using the two agents suggest that hydroxychloroquine is less likely to cause retinopathy than chloroquine; hence the former has become the more popular agent for use in these chronic indications.

■ Deposits in the cornea can be an early sign of hydroxychloroquine toxicity.

■ Malaria prophylaxis typically begins 1 to 2 weeks before a malaria area is entered and continues for 4 to 8 weeks after the area has been left.

Advanced
Pharmacogenetics

■ Chloroquine-induced pruritus has been linked to genetic markers.

FYI

■ Travelers who are taking antimalarials for prophylaxis should be advised to purchase their entire supply before travelling overseas, as reliable supplies of these agents are often not available in developing countries.

Anthelmintics

DESCRIPTION
Anthelmintics are agents that kill intestinal worms (*helminths*).

PROTOTYPE AND COMMON DRUGS
■ **Benzimidazoles:** mebendazole
  ▲ Others: thiabendazole, albendazole
■ **Others:**
  ▲ Praziquantel
  ▲ Levamisole
  ▲ Piperazine
  ▲ Diethylcarbamazine
  ▲ Ivermectin
  ▲ Niclosamide

MOA (MECHANISM OF ACTION)

■ Helminths are worms that invade human hosts. There are three types of helminths: nematodes (roundworms), trematodes (flukes), and cestodes (tapeworms).

Benzimidazoles

■ The benzimidazoles disrupt the biochemistry of worms in several different ways.

■ Their primary mechanism appears to be **binding to β-tubulin**. The polymerization of tubulin leads to formation of microtubules. Therefore benzimidazoles disrupt microtubule formation, which in turn impairs glucose uptake.

Basis for Selective Toxicity

■ Structural differences in β-tubulin between humans and parasites

Mechanisms of Resistance

■ Mutations in β-tubulin that prevent binding of drug

Others

■ The primary site of action for **praziquantel** is the tegument (skin equivalent), where it appears to increase calcium influx. This causes increased muscle contraction and eventual paralysis followed by death. At higher doses, praziquantel damages the tegument itself, which may liberate antigens that subsequently stimulate a host immune response against it.
■ **Levamisole** blocks **nicotinic receptors** at the neuromuscular junction, which results in paralysis.
■ **Piperazine** also causes paralysis by acting at the neuromuscular junction, likely by promoting the **actions of γ-aminobutyric acid (GABA)**.
■ The mechanism of **diethylcarbamazine** is unclear, but it may somehow make the organism more susceptible to the host immune system.
■ **Ivermectin** causes paralysis by enhancing the inhibitory effects of GABA or by activating a glutamate chloride channel.
■ **Niclosamide** may interfere with oxidative phosphorylation or may activate ATPases.

PHARMACOKINETICS

■ These agents typically have very limited solubility in water, and coadministration with a fatty meal can often enhance their absorption.
■ Albendazole is a prodrug, extensively metabolized in liver and possibly intestine to an active metabolite, albendazole sulfoxide. CYP450 enzymes contribute to its metabolism. Its elimination half-life varies widely.
■ Praziquantel has considerable variation in the rate of absorption. It undergoes extensive first-pass metabolism in the liver, with significant involvement of CYP450 enzymes.
■ Ivermectin is lipophilic, is widely distributed, and has a very long elimination half-life of 55 to 60 hours. It is extensively metabolized by CYP3A4 and is primarily excreted in feces.
■ Ivermectin absorption may be impaired in patients with disseminated strongyloidiasis. These patients may be treated with parenteral ivermectin; however, a parenteral version has not been approved in most jurisdictions.

INDICATIONS

■ Treatment of infestation with various helminths (Table 18-3)

CONTRAINDICATIONS

Praziquantel

■ **Ocular cysticercosis:** The type of reaction described later in the discussion of neurocysticercosis can be irreversible if it occurs in the eye.

TABLE 18-3. Anthelmintic Spectra

Agent	Susceptible Organisms
Mebendazole	Pinworms, roundworms, whipworms, hookworms
Praziquantel	Flukes
Piperazine	Roundworms, pinworms
Diethylcarbamazine	Roundworms
Levamisole	Roundworms
Ivermectin	Roundworms

SIDE EFFECTS

■ **Generally well tolerated.** Attributing side effects to drug can be challenging, as many side effects are consistent with the host response to dead or dying parasites rather than the drug itself.
■ **GI side effects** may be experienced, although in some cases these may be largely the result of passage of the worm.

Mebendazole
Serious and Rare

■ **Agranulocytosis, alopecia, and elevated hepatic enzymes** have been reported at high doses, although mechanisms have not been established for any of these side effects.

Praziquantel
Serious and Rare

■ **CNS effects (seizures, changes in mental status, intracranial hypertension)** may occur in the treatment of neurocysticercosis. These effects are believed to be caused by inflammatory reactions that occur because of the dead parasites. Corticosteroids may be coadministered with praziquantel to reduce inflammation.

Piperazine

■ **Urticaria**
■ **Bronchospasm**

Rare

■ **CNS effects:** dizziness, paresthesias, vertigo, incoordination

IMPORTANT NOTES

■ Many different intestinal worms affect humans. Pinworms (*Enterobius vermicularis*) are a type of roundworm and are relatively small (approximately 1 cm length). Pinworms live in the colon and do not typically migrate to other regions of the body.
■ Hookworms (*Ancylostoma duodenale* and *Necator americanus*) are also nematodes, and they reside in the small intestine of the host. Hookworms also do not tend to migrate, but they do suck blood from the intestine, which may lead to anemia in the host.
■ Whipworms (*Trichuris trichiura* or *Trichocephalus trichiuris*) invade the large intestine and are also roundworms. These worms are slightly larger (5 to 10 cm) and look like whips, with a widening at one end. These worms invade the wall

of the large intestine and can cause bloody diarrhea with enough blood loss to induce anemia.

- Flukes (trematodes) are flat worms. There are several different types of flukes (e.g., *Fasciolopsis buski*, *Heterophyes*, and *Gastrodiscoides hominis*). Humans acquire them through consumption of raw fish and plants.

Advanced

- Neurocysticercosis is a parasitic infection of the CNS. It is caused by a pork tapeworm. Humans typically acquire the eggs via the fecal-oral route; these ova are digested in the stomach, and oncospheres released from them reach the bloodstream. It is from the blood that they invade various organs, including the brain and the eyes.

Pregnancy

- Mebendazole and albendazole have each demonstrated teratogenic effects in animals. They are used in pregnancy, but only after a careful risk-benefit assessment.

EVIDENCE
Anthelmintics in Children

- A 2007 Cochrane review (34 trials) examined the effects of deworming drugs on growth and school performance in children. Deworming drugs increased weight after a single dose by an average of 0.34 kg across nine trials (N = 2448 children). However, in multiple-dose trials no effect on weight was shown. No significant impact on cognition or school performance was shown.

FYI

- Ivermectin was originally used as a veterinary drug and is still used for this purpose. It was derived from a fungus found in soil.

Antiprotozoals

DESCRIPTION
Antiprotozoals are used to treat protozoal infections.

PROTOTYPE AND COMMON DRUGS
- Diamidines: pentamidine
  - ▲ **Others:** diminazene
- Melarsoprol
- Nifurtimox

MOA (MECHANISM OF ACTION)
Diamidines

- Protozoa are unicellular eukaryotic organisms such as amoeba that move around using tails called *flagella*.
- Pentamidine may act by multiple modes of action, although the primary mechanisms and relative importance based on organism has not been established.
- Pentamidine, a positively charged compound, appears to interact with negatively charged compounds, including nucleic acids. It also appears to **inhibit topoisomerase II**, which would also disrupt DNA. Topoisomerase is an enzyme that cuts and reseals DNA strands, a process that is essential for DNA synthesis.
- It also appears to interfere with RNA and may also interfere with the synthesis of polyamines. Polyamines are compounds found in cells that have two or more amino (-NH_2) groups. Their exact role is unclear; however, when their synthesis is inhibited, cell growth stops.

Mechanisms of Resistance

- Pentamidine enters cells via a transporter, and alterations in the structure, including the complete loss of the transporter, can lead to resistance.

- However, because the **drug is taken up by a variety of different transporters**, this redundancy appears to have prevented widespread resistance to this older, widely used drug.

Melarsoprol

- Melarsoprol is metabolized to melarsen oxide, which **reacts with sulfhydryl (-SH) groups on proteins**. Therefore it can interfere with the activity of various enzymes, disrupting the biochemistry of the protozoan cell.
- It has an uptake transporter, much like pentamidine, that actively concentrates it within the cell; otherwise its effects tend to be fairly nonspecific, leading to a variety of toxicities.

Mechanisms of Resistance

- Similar to pentamidine, alterations in the structure, including the complete loss of the transporter, can lead to resistance. This leads to cross-resistance between it and pentamidine.
- Unlike pentamidine, melarsoprol relies more heavily on a single transporter; thus is **more prone to development of resistance**, because it lacks the redundancy seen with pentamidine.

Nifurtimox

- Nifurtimox generates **reactive oxygen species**, such as the superoxide anion, which then react with cells, disrupting cell membranes, inactivating enzymes, and damaging DNA.

PHARMACOKINETICS

- Pentamidine has low oral bioavailability and is therefore administered by injection. Intramuscular injections are preferred because of the hypoglycemia that occurs with intravenous administration (see Side Effects). It is highly ionized at physiologic pH and therefore does not penetrate the CNS.

■ Melarsoprol is a poorly water soluble prodrug that must be dissolved in propylene glycol to facilitate injection, which is always performed via the intravenous route. It is metabolized to melarsen oxide in vivo. It is able to penetrate the CNS in small amounts and is therefore useful against trypanosomes that have invaded the CNS.

INDICATIONS
■ Trypanosomiasis
■ *P. jiroveci*

CONTRAINDICATIONS
■ Although these agents have some significant toxicities, the seriousness of the infections they treat usually outweighs any contraindications to their use. In many regions of the developing world, these infections are a major source of mortality and morbidity.

SIDE EFFECTS
Pentamidine
■ **Cardiovascular:** Severe hypotension and tachycardia can occur, particularly with intravenous administration.
■ **Glucose abnormalities:** Pentamidine can induce either hypoglycemia or hyperglycemia, and it is toxic to the pancreas. Some patients have developed type 1 diabetes mellitus as a result of this toxicity.
■ **Renal dysfunction:** Nephrotoxicity occurs in up to 25% of patients.
■ **Hepatic dysfunction:** Pentamidine can elevate liver enzymes.

Melarsoprol
■ **Nausea, vomiting:** These effects may be mitigated by administering the drug on an empty stomach and by having the patient in a supine position during administration.

■ **Abdominal pain**
■ **Peripheral neuropathy**
■ **Arthralgia**
■ **Thrombophlebitis:** Melarsoprol is dissolved in propylene glycol (see Pharmacokinetics), which irritates tissues.

Serious
■ **Reactive encephalopathy** occurs in 5% to 10% of patients and is fatal in half of these cases. This effect may be caused by the drug or by the body's reaction to substances (likely antigens) released from dying parasites.

Nifurtimox
■ **Nausea and vomiting** can lead to discontinuation of the drug if patient begins to lose significant weight.
■ **CNS:** Weakness, myalgia, and peripheral neuropathy are common after prolonged treatment. Less common effects include psychic disturbances and CNS excitability. The mechanism has not been established.

Serious
■ Hypersensitivity reactions

IMPORTANT NOTES
■ Prednisolone is often coadministered with melarsoprol in order to reduce the incidence of hypersensitivity reactions and reactive encephalopathy.

FYI
■ Diamidines were originally developed as synthetic analogues of insulin, in the belief that hypoglycemia would either control or eradicate trypanosome infections in humans. Although this likely contributes little to the efficacy of these agents, hypoglycemia is one of the key and most serious side effects associated with this class.

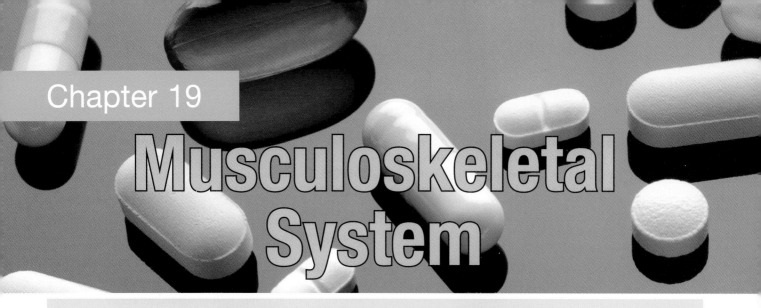

Chapter 19

Musculoskeletal System

Bisphosphonates (BPs)

DESCRIPTION
Bisphosphonates are agents that prevent the breakdown of bone.

PROTOTYPES AND COMMON DRUGS
Aminobisphosphonates
- Prototype: alen**dronate**
- Others: rise**dronate**, pami**dronate**

Non-Aminobisphosphonates
- Prototype: eti**dronate**
- Others: clo**dronate**, tilu**dronate**, zole**dronate**

MOA (MECHANISM OF ACTION)
- The structural integrity of bone is determined to a large extent by the balance between the activity of osteoclasts, which break down bone (*resorptive*), and the activity of osteoblasts, which build bone.
- Bisphosphonates (BPs) inhibit osteoclast activity through a variety of mechanisms, some better understood than others (Figure 19-1).
- Inside the osteoclast the aminobisphosphonates disrupt the mevalonate pathway, a pathway involved in the posttranslational modification of proteins that are involved in cellular signaling. Disruption of the mevalonate pathway interrupts osteoclast function and leads to apoptosis of the osteoclast.
- The non-aminobisphosphonates work by increasing the accumulation of cytotoxic metabolites within osteoclasts, interfering with their function and possibly leading to osteoclast cell death.
- The *clawlike* chemical structure of BPs facilitates their attachment to bone. The multiple oxygen atoms around the perimeter of the BP molecule bind to divalent cations such as Ca^{2+} within bone matrix. The BPs remain within the matrix until the acids released by the osteoclasts break down the matrix and liberate the BPs. Ironically, the activity of the osteoclasts seals their own fate!

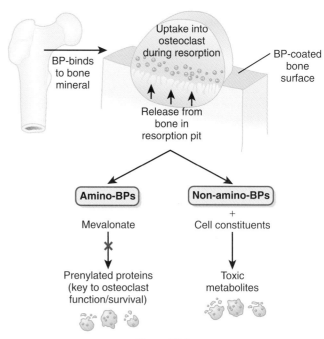

Bisphosphonates

BP-binds to bone mineral → Uptake into osteoclast during resorption — BP-coated bone surface

Release from bone in resorption pit

Amino-BPs → Mevalonate ✗ → Prenylated proteins (key to osteoclast function/survival)

Non-amino-BPs + Cell constituents → Toxic metabolites

Figure 19-1.

- Osteoclasts contribute further to their demise by devouring the BP molecules after liberating them.
- BPs have a variety of other cellular effects, inhibiting vitamin D production, intestinal Ca^{2+} transport, cell growth, metabolic changes in bone cells, and changes in acid and alkaline phosphatases.

PHARMACOKINETICS
- BPs have very low oral bioavailability (<10%), and their absorption is further reduced by food and by divalent cations such as calcium. It is therefore recommended that BPs be taken on an empty stomach, with plain water.

- The BPs that are absorbed are highly bound to bone, and are not metabolized, nor do they inhibit or induce metabolizing enzymes. They are eliminated by the kidney.
- The oral BPs are typically administered once daily. A higher dose of alendronate is also available as a once weekly formulation.

INDICATIONS
- Osteoporosis
- Paget's disease of the bone (results in enlarged, deformed bones)
- Hypercalcemia:
  - ▲ Malignancy
  - ▲ Primary hyperparathyroidism (continuous parathyroid hormone [PTH] release causes bone demineralization)
- Bone metastasis causing osteolysis:
  - ▲ Multiple myeloma
  - ▲ Bone metastases of malignant tumors

CONTRAINDICATIONS
- **Hypocalcemia:** BPs have exhibited decreases in serum calcium, so it is recommended that any deficiencies in calcium be addressed before initiation of therapy.
- **Poor renal function:** BPs are eliminated renally, so patients with creatinine clearance <30 mL/min may experience accumulation of these agents. Patients with poor renal function who begin to take BPs should be monitored closely.

SIDE EFFECTS
All
- **Gastrointestinal:** nausea, dyspepsia

Serious
- **Esophagitis or esophageal erosion** is more commonly seen with the aminobisphosphonates. It may result from a direct irritant effect from tablets lodged in the esophagus or from reflux of gastric acid including the acidic form of the BP. Patients are advised to avoid reclining for at least 30 minutes after taking a BP, reducing the chance of tablet staying in the esophagus or reflux.
- **Osteonecrosis of the jaw** is typically only seen at higher doses. The mechanism has not been established; however, the fact that BPs alter bone turnover is thought to play a role. Jaw bone may have a higher rate of turnover than other areas of the body, perhaps explaining why this side effect is localized to this area.

Aminobisphosphonates
- **Fever, flulike symptoms** are a transient, typically first-dose phenomenon seen with intravenous administration. They are believed to be caused by release of proinflammatory cytokines.

IMPORTANT NOTES
- The non-aminobisphosphonates were the original members of this drug class, whereas the aminobisphosphonates are newer, more potent agents.

- BPs have an established history as adjuncts in cancer therapy. They have demonstrated ability to reduce bone pain secondary to metastases and prevent treatment-induced bone loss.
- Etidronate can cause bone demineralization; therefore unlike the other BPs, which are typically taken once daily, etidronate is typically administered in 90-day cycles, with 14 days on treatment and 76 days off treatment. During the off-treatment period, calcium tablets are typically administered, and this 90-day treatment cycle (etidronate followed by calcium) is marketed in one kit.
- Estrogens appear to have a role in decreasing bone resorption; therefore one of the benefits of hormone replacement therapy in postmenopausal women is to maintain integrity of bone, hopefully leading to fewer fractures.
- Nonpharmacologic strategies for preventing osteoporosis include smoking cessation and weight-bearing exercise. Smoking is known to reduce bone mineral density (BMD), and weight-bearing exercise has been shown to substantially reduce fracture risk.

Advanced
Pregnancy
- The use of BPs in pregnancy has not been well studied, but they are believed to cross the placenta, based on animal studies. Given their effects on bone, a very careful assessment of risk versus benefit should be performed before these agents are used.

EVIDENCE
Risedronate versus Placebo or Calcium and Vitamin D or Both in Postmenopausal Osteoporosis
- A 2008 Cochrane review (7 trials, N = 14,049 females) found no statistically significant effects for risedronate with respect to primary prevention of vertebral and nonvertebral fractures. For secondary prevention, risedronate demonstrated statistically significant relative risk reductions (RRRs) of vertebral fractures (39%), nonvertebral fractures (20%), and hip fractures (26%). The corresponding absolute risk reductions were small: 5%, 2%, and 1%, respectively. No statistically significant differences were found for adverse events.

Etidronate versus Placebo and/or Calcium and Vitamin D in Postmenopausal Osteoporosis
- A 2008 Cochrane review (11 trials, N = 1248 females) found no statistically significant effects of etidronate with respect to primary prevention of any fractures. A statistically significant RRR of 47% was found for secondary prevention of vertebral fractures but not for nonvertebral, hip, or wrist fractures. No statistically significant differences were found for adverse events.

BPs versus Placebo or No Treatment in Myeloma
- A 2002 Cochrane review (11 trials, N = 2183 patients) found that BPs prevented pathologic vertebral fractures (number needed to treat [NNT] = 10) and relieved pain

(NNT = 11). BPs did not affect mortality, nonvertebral fractures, or hypercalcemia. No significant adverse events were associated with the BPs.

FYI

- One of the earliest indications that the BPs had potential in the treatment of bone diseases was the observation that they inhibit the dissolution of hydroxyapatite crystals.
- Because of their ability to localize in bone, one of the early uses for BPs was as bone scanning agents, used in the detection of malignancies and other skeletal lesions.

- The bisphosphonates are so named because of the two phosphate (P) groups that form the backbone of these molecules.
- The BPs have a *clawlike* chemical structure. This is a good way to remember that they attach themselves to bone matrix for long periods of time.
- The aminobisphosphonates such as alendronate have an amino (NH_2-) group.

Vitamin D Replacement

DESCRIPTION

Vitamin D replacement consists of vitamin D and its derivatives.

PROTOTYPE AND COMMON DRUGS

- Prototype: calcitriol
- Others: ergocalciferol (vitamin D_2), calcipotriene, doxercalciferol, paricalcitol

MOA (MECHANISM OF ACTION)

- The two major forms of vitamin D replacements are vitamin D_2 and vitamin D_3.
- Vitamin D is an important regulator of calcium and phosphate homeostasis and bone metabolism. It works in conjunction with PTH. The overall effect of vitamin D is to **increase serum calcium concentrations**. These effects are mediated via the following:
  - ▲ Increased calcium absorption from the intestine
  - ▲ Regulation of bone resorption and formation
    - This occurs via stimulation of both osteoblastic and osteoclastic processes. Osteoblasts form bone, and osteoclasts dissolve bone.
  - ▲ Increased calcium reabsorption in the distal renal tubules (Figure 19-2)
- Vitamin D results in a negative feedback loop and decreases transcription and secretion of PTH.
  - ▲ The overall effect of PTH is to increase serum calcium levels, so increased vitamin D inhibits the actions of PTH so that both mechanisms do not drive up calcium levels too high.
- Vitamin D is lipophilic (it is one of the fat-soluble vitamins—A, D, E, and K) and thus freely crosses the cytoplasmic membrane.
- Intracellularly, it binds vitamin D receptors (VDRs) and binds DNA, where it regulates transcription of genes in the intestine, bone, kidney, and parathyroid gland.
- Vitamin D also has actions in macrophages and T cells and in proliferation and differentiation of a large number of

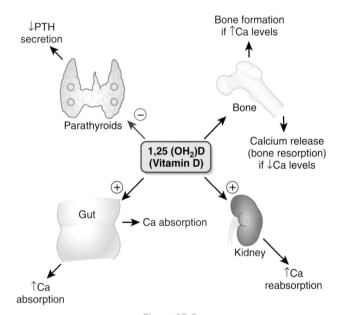

Calcitriol actions

Figure 19-2.

cells, including cancer cells. Through these actions, it has immunomodulating and potentially, anticancer actions. Also, these actions are the basis of the mechanism whereby it is effective in psoriasis.

PHARMACOKINETICS

- Calcitriol is available in oral and intravenous formulations. It is a lipid-soluble vitamin and therefore can accumulate and cause toxicity (see later).

INDICATIONS

- Osteoporosis
- Hyperparathyroidism
- Osteomalacia
- Rickets

CONTRAINDICATIONS

■ None

SIDE EFFECTS

■ Side effects are related to long-term overadministration of vitamin D supplementation. Symptoms are primarily induced by hypercalcemia, which include gastrointestinal pain, renal stones, and psychiatric disturbances.

IMPORTANT NOTES

■ Vitamin D is synthesized in the skin, liver, and kidney. Vitamin D supplementation is therefore frequently required in patients with renal failure.
■ **Rickets** is a childhood disease characterized by impeded growth and deformity (curvature) of the long bones caused by vitamin D deficiency. The fortification of milk with vitamin D has dramatically reduced the incidence of rickets in developed countries.
■ **Osteomalacia** is a condition of bone softening resulting from abnormality in the mineralization of the organic portion of the bone matrix called *osteoid*. It can be caused by vitamin D deficiency and is like an adult form of rickets. It is characterized by proximal muscle weakness, pain, and bone fragility.
■ **Osteoporosis** is characterized by reduced bone mineral density (BMD) and increased bone fragility. It is caused by abnormal osteoblastic and osteoclastic activity. The bone is porous, hence the name of the disease.

Advanced

■ Vitamin D supplements are sometimes used in the treatment of psoriasis, a common skin condition involving rapid turnover and inflammation of the skin. The evidence for this use, however, is not strongly conclusive.
■ The various forms of vitamin D are referred to by several different names, summarized in Table 19-1.

EVIDENCE

Vitamin D Alone and Bone Fractures in the Elderly

■ A meta-analysis in 2008 showed that vitamin D *alone* in the elderly was unlikely to be effective in preventing hip fractures (9 trials, N = 24,749 participants), vertebral fractures

TABLE 19-1. Various Forms of Vitamin D

Common Name	Drug Name	Abbreviation
Vitamin D$_2$	Ergocalciferol	D$_2$
1-Hydroxyvitamin D$_2$	Doxercalciferol	1(OH)D$_2$
Vitamin D$_3$	Cholecalciferol	D$_3$
25-Hydroxyvitamin D$_3$	Calcifediol	25(OH)D$_3$
1,25-Dihydroxyvitamin D$_3$	Calcitriol	1,25(OH)$_2$D$_3$
24,25-Dihydroxyvitamin D$_3$	Secalcifediol	24,25(OH)$_2$D$_3$

(5 trials, N = 9138 participants), or any new fracture (10 trials, N = 25,016 participants).

Vitamin D Plus Calcium and Bone Fractures in the Elderly

■ The same meta-analysis in 2008 showed that vitamin D *plus calcium supplements* do reduce hip fractures in the elderly (8 trials, N = 46,658 participants, relative risk [RR] 0.84). Hypercalcemia is significantly more common in people receiving vitamin D or an analogue, with or without calcium (18 trials, N = 11,346 participants, RR 2.35). There is a significant but modest increase in gastrointestinal symptoms (RR 1.04) and a small but significant increase in renal disease (RR 1.16).

FYI

■ The concept that vitamin D comes from the sun is inaccurate; the inert precursor (7-dehydrocholesterol) is present in the skin, and exposure to ultraviolet light converts it to cholecalciferol, which is then isomerized to vitamin D$_3$. Reduced exposure to sunlight is one cause of vitamin D deficiency.
■ Calcitonin is another hormone secreted by the thyroid gland. It has the opposing action of PTH: it "tones down" (lowers) the serum calcium levels.
■ Vitamin D is a secosteroid: this is a steroid with one of the rings (the B ring) broken. Vitamin D$_2$ is from ergosterol, whereas vitamin D$_3$ is from cholesterol. Ergosterol is not produced in vertebrates, and therefore vitamin D$_2$ is not produced in humans.

Parathyroid Hormone

DESCRIPTION

This agent (teriparatide) is a recombinant form of naturally occurring PTH.

PROTOTYPE

■ Prototype: teriparatide

MOA (MECHANISM OF ACTION)

■ PTH is released from the parathyroid gland. It regulates calcium and phosphate flux across cell membranes in bone and kidney. The key effects of PTH are as follows:
  ▲ Increased serum calcium
  ▲ Decreased serum phosphate
  ▲ Increased osteoclast activity in bone

- The effects on osteoclasts are indirect. PTH increases activity of the RANK (receptor activator of nuclear factor κ) ligand (RANKL). RANKL regulates osteoclast activity (see the discussion of RANKL inhibitors in this chapter). Increasing the activity of RANKL in turn stimulates an increase in the activity and number of osteoclasts.
- The stimulation of osteoclasts increases bone remodeling. PTH increases both bone resorption and formation; however, the net effect of excess PTH is to **increase bone resorption** (Figure 19-3).

Parathyroid hormone

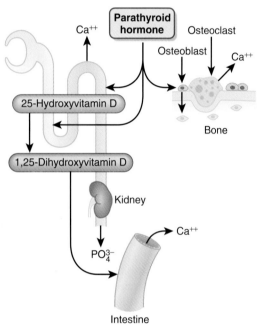

Figure 19-3.

- Low levels of **intermittent PTH,** however, can enhance **bone formation.** The actions of PTH are largely mediated through the PTH-1 receptor. The anabolic effects are mediated by direct effects of PTH on osteoblasts, increasing their number and inhibiting their apoptosis. PTH also stimulates insulin-like growth factor (IGF-1) in osteoblasts, and IGF-1 also has anabolic effects on bone.
- It is still not clear why high, sustained PTH has a catabolic effect, whereas low, intermittent administration has an anabolic effect on bone.
- In addition to these factors, PTH has several effects on the kidney:
  - ▲ Increased reabsorption of Ca^{2+} and Mg^{2+}
  - ▲ Decreased reabsorption of phosphate, amino acids, bicarbonate, Na^+, Cl^-, and sulfate
  - ▲ Stimulation of production of 1,25 dihydroxyvitamin D

PHARMACOKINETICS

- Teriparatide is administered as a subcutaneous injection once daily.

- It is both rapidly absorbed and rapidly eliminated, with plasma concentrations reaching their peak at 30 minutes postinjection and falling to undetectable levels after 3 hours.
- The metabolism of teriparatide is poorly understood, but enzymes are thought to be involved.

INDICATIONS

- **Osteoporosis**
  - ▲ Typically reserved for severe osteoporosis and/or patients in whom previous therapies, including the BPs, have failed
- **Osteoporosis secondary to corticosteroid use**

CONTRAINDICATIONS

- **Children or young adults with open epiphysis:** The safety and efficacy of teriparatide has not been studied in pediatrics, and its significant impact on bone remodeling is a concern in this population
- **Hypercalcemia:** PTH already raises Ca^{2+} levels.
- **Active Paget's disease of bone.**
- **Skeletal metastases or skeletal malignant conditions:** risk of osteosarcoma (see Important Notes).
- **History of radiation to the skeleton:** risk of osteosarcoma (see Important Notes).
- **Pregnancy and lactation:** The effects of teriparatide have not been studied in pregnancy. Given its significant effects on bone remodeling, deleterious effects on fetal bone development are possible.

SIDE EFFECTS

- **Hypercalcemia (mild):** PTH increases serum calcium. This can be managed by reducing Ca^{2+} and vitamin D intake or by adjusting teriparatide dose from daily to every other day.
- **Leg cramps** may occur.
- **Nausea** may occur.
- **Orthostatic hypotension:** PTH infusions have a vasodilatory effect in animals. Hypotension has been observed within 4 hours of infusion in clinical trials.

IMPORTANT NOTES

- The greatest safety concern associated with teriparatide is **osteosarcoma** (malignant bone cancer). However, this concern is based on observations in rodents exposed to prolonged high doses and on the ability of teriparatide to stimulate osteoblasts. So far, there does not appear to be an elevated risk of osteosarcoma with teriparatide use in humans.
- Because of the concerns over osteosarcoma, use of teriparatide is limited to 1.5 to 2 years. The reason for this cutoff is that the safety of teriparatide has not been assessed beyond 2 years in clinical trials.
- Most of the agents used to manage osteoporosis are antiresorptive and work by *inhibiting* bone turnover. Teriparatide works by *promoting* bone turnover; thus there is concern that patients switching from antiresorptive agents, particularly

potent agents such as BPs, might experience reduced efficacy with teriparatide. Therefore some clinicians suggest that there should be a washout period when switching from the BPs to teriparatide. The benefits of a washout should be balanced against the risk of no treatment, particularly in patients with severe disease.

EVIDENCE
Bisphosphonates or Teriparatide in Postmenopausal Women
■ A 2005 systematic review (90 trials) compared all BPs and teriparatide with calcium, calcium plus vitamin D, calcitriol, hormone replacement therapy, exercise, and placebo or no treatment. They found that only teriparatide and risedronate reduced the risk of nonvertebral fracture in women with severe osteoporosis and adequate calcium intake.

FYI
■ Teriparatide is supplied as prefilled injectable *pens*, which make it easier for patients to self-administer subcutaneous injections.

RANKL Inhibitors

DESCRIPTION
RANKL inhibitors regulate osteoclast activity and modify bone structure.

PROTOTYPE
■ Denosumab

MOA (MECHANISM OF ACTION)
■ RANK stands for *receptor activator of nuclear factor kappa*; RANKL stands for RANK ligand.
■ RANKL is a cytokine member of the tumor necrosis factor (TNF) superfamily and is an important regulator of osteoclast activity.
■ The primary function of osteoclasts is to break down bone; their counterparts are osteoblasts, which function to build up bone.
■ The binding of RANKL to RANK results in increased bone resorption through the differentiation, activation, and prolonged survival of osteoclasts.
■ Osteoclast activity is an important factor in the development of osteoporosis and is also strongly implicated in bone destruction associated with rheumatoid arthritis, metastatic cancer, multiple myeloma, and sex hormone deprivation (menopause, aromatase inhibitor therapy, and androgen deprivation therapy).
■ Denosumab is a new fully humanized monoclonal antibody that binds RANKL and through binding causes inhibition of RANKL and thus inhibits osteoclast activity.

PHARMACOKINETICS
■ Denosumab has a very long half-life and is administered once every 6 months via subcutaneous injection. The time to maximum concentration is 26 days.

INDICATION
■ Osteoporosis

CONTRAINDICATIONS
■ None of significance

SIDE EFFECTS
■ **Eczema** (small increase in risk)

IMPORTANT NOTES
■ Osteoporosis can be evaluated through plain x-ray films of bones, but the gold standard is dual-energy x-ray absorptiometry (DXA).
  ▲ DXA fires two different x-ray beams and through advanced calculation techniques subtracts the signal from soft tissue and then compares the absorption of the two different beams through the bone.
■ From the imaging studies, bone mineral density (BMD) scores are calculated.
■ Bones with decreased BMD are at increased risk for fracture. A score of less than 2.5 (standard deviations below normal) is the diagnostic criterion for osteoporosis.

Fractures in Osteoporosis
■ A double-blind randomized controlled trial (RCT) in 2009 (N = 7868) compared denosumab with placebo with regard to fractures over a 3-year period in *women with mild to moderate osteoporosis aged 60 to 90 years* and found an incidence of the following:
  ▲ Vertebral fractures: 2.3% (denosumab) versus 7.2% (placebo)
  ▲ Risk of hip fracture: 0.7% (denosumab) versus 1.2% (placebo)
  ▲ Nonvertebral fracture: 6.5% (denosumab) versus 8.0% (placebo)

FYI
■ As per naming convention for monoclonal antibodies (mAbs), the *-os-* refers to bone and the *-u-* refers to fully humanized.

- Densoumab has recently been approved (June 2010) with the U.S. Food and Drug Administration (FDA).
- *Osteopenia* is the term for a mild reduction in BMD. *Osteoporosis* is the term for a more advanced reduction in BMD.

The suffix *-penia* usually refers to a low cell count (e.g., *thrombocytopenia* means a low thrombocyte or platelet count); therefore *osteopenia* is somewhat of a misnomer when used in this setting when referring to BMD.

Colchicine

DESCRIPTION

Colchicine is used to treat *crystal-associated* arthritis, most commonly gout (a disease caused by uric acid crystal deposition in joints).

PROTOTYPE

- Colchicine

MOA (MECHANISM OF ACTION)

- Most of the pharmacologic effects of colchicine result from colchicine binding to tubulin (Figure 19-4). Tubulin is required for microtubule assembly, and colchicine prevents microtubule assembly. Microtubules are important components of the cytoskeleton and are involved with the following cellular functions:
  - ▲ Cellular structural support
  - ▲ Mitosis (the spindle apparatus composed of tubulin pulls the chromosomes into each new half of the dividing cell)
  - ▲ Vesicular transport

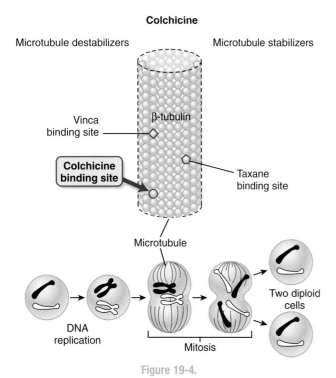

Figure 19-4.

- **Gout** is a disease that occurs when uric acid levels in the blood are elevated and uric acid crystals precipitate in

joints; the crystals induce an intense inflammatory response resulting in arthritis, a condition referred to as *crystal-induced arthritis.*
- Colchicine is also known to suppress many immune functions in the setting of crystal-induced arthritis:
  - ▲ Decreased neutrophil chemotaxis
  - ▲ Decreased neutrophil adhesion
  - ▲ Decreased release of multiple inflammatory mediators
  - ▲ Decreased phagocytosis of urate crystals by neutrophils

PHARMACOKINETICS

- The half-life of the tubulin-colchicine complex is 20 to 30 hours. The **long half-life** increases the risk of drug accumulation.
- Although clearance is primarily via the liver, renal clearance accounts for about 20%, and **renal insufficiency** is a very strong risk factor for toxicity. Doses must be reduced in patients with renal insufficiency.

INDICATIONS

- Gout
  - ▲ Acute attacks
  - ▲ Long-term prevention of recurrent attacks as an adjuvant to uric acid–lowering therapies

CONTRAINDICATION

- Renal failure: increased risk of toxicity

SIDE EFFECTS

- Colchicine has a **narrow therapeutic index.**
- **Gastrointestinal:** Diarrhea is virtually a guaranteed side effect when colchicine is given in doses suitable for acute attacks of gout and occurs in many patients treated for prevention (preventative doses are lower than those for acute attacks).
- **Bone marrow suppression:** Antimitotics preferentially target rapidly dividing cells, such as those found in the bone marrow. This explains why bone marrow function, which relies on rapid cell turnover, is suppressed.
- **Myopathy** may occur.
- **Neuropathy** may occur.

IMPORTANT NOTES

- Gout is a common disorder of uric acid metabolism whereby uric acid levels in the blood are elevated, which results in uric acid crystals being deposited into joints, causing inflammation and intense pain. The great toe is the joint most commonly affected.

- Colchicine, because of its high risk of toxicity, is *not* a first-line therapy for gout. It should be reserved for situations in which first-line therapy (nonsteroidal antiinflammatory drugs [NSAIDs]) is contraindicated or ineffective. Other drugs used to treat gout include uricosurics (drugs that increase elimination of renal uric acid) and xanthine oxidase inhibitors (which decrease uric acid formation).
- Although doses are not routinely described in this textbook, overdose of colchicine can be fatal, and therefore it is important to highlight that there are **maximum dose recommendations**.
- **Multisystem failure and death**: One study showed that eight of nine overdoses over a 15-year period resulted in death.
- The FDA reported 33 deaths associated with intravenous colchicine from 1985 to 1997. The manufacture of intravenous colchicine in the United States was halted in February 2008.

Advanced
Drug Interactions
- Because of the risk of toxicity, it is important to recognize drug interactions that could increase colchicine levels in the body. Metabolism is via CYP3A4, and therefore drugs that inhibit CYP3A4 will increase colchicine levels.
- P-glycoprotein (Pgp) influences absorption, distribution, and elimination, and therefore coadministered drugs that modulate or inhibit Pgp function carry risk of increasing toxicity also.

EVIDENCE
Acute Gout Pain
- A Cochrane review in 2006 (one RCT, N = 43), compared with placebo, colchicine demonstrated an absolute reduction of 34% for pain scales and a 30% reduction for tenderness, swelling, redness, and pain. The NNT to reduce pain was three. All participants treated with colchicine experienced gastrointestinal side effects (diarrhea and/or vomiting), and the number needed to harm (NNH) with colchicine versus placebo was one. Note: The sample size was very small, and only one study met inclusion criteria in this review.

FYI
- Colchicine is an alkaloid isolated from *Colchicum autumnale*, also called *autumn crocus* or *meadow saffron*.
- Hippocrates advocated the use of a plant extract (containing colchicine) for gout and concluded that "the best natural relief for [arthritis] is an attack of dysentery."

Nonsteroidal Antiinflammatory Drugs (NSAIDs)

DESCRIPTION
NSAIDs are antiinflammatory drugs that do not possess a steroidal structure (*nonsteroidal*).

PROTOTYPE AND COMMON DRUGS
Nonselective
- Prototype: ibuprofen
- Others:
  - **Propionic acid derivatives:** naproxen, fenoprofen, ketoprofen, flurbiprofen
  - **Acetic acid derivatives:** diclofenac, ketorolac, indomethacin, etodolac, sulindac, piroxicam, meloxicam, nabumetone, tolmetin, mefenamic acid, meclofenamate, flufenamic acid

Cyclooxygenase (COX)-2 selective
- Prototype: celecoxib
- Others: rofecoxib, valdecoxib

MOA (MECHANISM OF ACTION)
- Cyclooxygenase (COX) is an enzyme that catalyzes the conversion of arachidonic acid to prostaglandin (PG) G (PGG) and PGH. These intermediaries are then converted to a variety of important PGs as well as thromboxane A_2 (TxA_2).
- Each of these eicosanoids binds to its respective receptor, mediating the physiologic effects summarized in Figure 19-5.

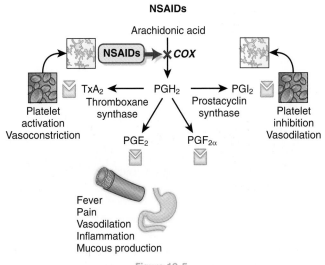

Figure 19-5.

- There are actually two major isoforms of the COX enzyme: COX-1 and COX-2. **COX-1 is a constitutive enzyme,** meaning that its levels remain relatively constant, and it is distributed widely throughout the body. COX-1 is thus believed to play a maintenance or protective role, responsible for production of cytoprotective mucus in the stomach and for platelet aggregation (clotting).
- **COX-2 is an inducible enzyme,** meaning that its levels and activity can increase rapidly and significantly in response to a stimulus. The main stimuli for COX-2 induction are inflammatory mediators, and thus COX-2 is typically associated with inflammation.
- The theory behind selective inhibition of COX-2 enzymes is therefore to preserve the gastric cytoprotective effects mediated through COX-1 while maximizing the antiinflammatory effects mediated through COX-2.
- An unanticipated consequence of selective COX-2 inhibition is a **pro-platelet effect.** TXA_2 and prostacyclin (PGI_2) have opposite effects on platelets: TXA_2 activates platelets, and PGI_2 inhibits platelet activation. Of the two enzymes, COX-1 is primarily responsible for generating TXA_2, whereas COX-2 is responsible for generating PGI_2. Therefore, selective COX-2 inhibition removes this "check" on the platelet-activating actions of TXA_2.

PHARMACOKINETICS

- Most NSAIDs are well absorbed, and food has little effect on their bioavailability.
- Most NSAIDs undergo extensive hepatic metabolism, many through either the CYP3A or CYP2C families.
- Many nonselective COX inhibitors have short to intermediate half-lives (2 to 12 hours), requiring frequent administration. The newer COX-2 selective inhibitors typically have longer half-lives and are administered once daily. One exception is celecoxib, which is administered twice daily.
- Many NSAIDs are available in topical dosage forms, including ophthalmic preparations of diclofenac, flurbiprofen, ketorolac, suprofen.
- Indomethacin is also available as a rectal suppository.

INDICATIONS

- Pain
- Inflammation
- Fever

CONTRAINDICATION

- Active peptic ulcer

SIDE EFFECTS
Nonselective

- **Gastrointestinal** effects occur because of the inhibition of COX-1–mediated production of cytoprotective mucus in the stomach.
- **Edema:** PGs inhibit the reabsorption of Na^+ and the activity of ADH, so PG inhibition leads to salt and water retention. This can lead to edema and can be problematic in patients with conditions such as congestive heart failure.

- **Acute renal failure:** Renal PGs often play a protective role in high-risk patients by counteracting the effects of vasoconstrictors such as angiotensin 2 and vasopressin. When PGs are reduced, glomerular afferent vasoconstriction activity is unopposed, reducing renal blood flow and function.

COX-2 Selective

- **Cardiovascular:** The mechanism is not confirmed, but cardiovascular effects are thought to be a result of disruption of the balance between the platelet-activating effects of COX-1 and the platelet-inhibiting effects of COX-2.

All

- **Central nervous system (CNS): Confusion, dizziness, depression, and hallucinations** may occur. The mechanism is not confirmed, but COX-2 is the most abundant COX isoform in the CNS, and COX-2 may play a role in neurotransmission. The frequency of CNS side effects appears to be higher with COX-2–selective inhibitors and possibly with indomethacin. These reactions are uncommon.

IMPORTANT NOTES

- Indomethacin is considered to be a particularly potent COX inhibitor with very strong antiinflammatory effects. However, this enhanced efficacy is balanced with an increased severity of adverse effects, particularly gastrointestinal effects. Indomethacin is therefore typically reserved for use in more severe inflammatory conditions rather than everyday analgesia.
- Diclofenac is marketed in a fixed-dose combination with the PGE analogue misoprostol. The theory is that adding a PGE analogue helps to replace the PGE that is lost through COX inhibition.
- The extent of selectivity of COX-2 inhibitors varies significantly, and the distinction between COX-2 selective and nonselective inhibitors is not as clear as one would expect. Rofecoxib is by far the most COX-2 selective among currently marketed agents, with approximately 10 times the selectivity of celecoxib. Diclofenac and etodolac are also relatively selective for COX-2, whereas ketorolac is a relatively selective COX-1 inhibitor.
- Acetylsalicylic acid (ASA; aspirin) is a nonselective COX inhibitor with all the key features of other NSAIDs (antipyretic, analgesic, antiinflammatory activity), but it is often classified separately. Reasons include the fact that it **irreversibly** inhibits the COX enzyme and as a result has prolonged antiplatelet activity.
- The antiplatelet effects of ASA are observed at doses much lower than required for antiinflammatory or other activities. This is thought to be the case because the antiplatelet effects are mediated by the irreversible inhibition of COX-1 by the parent ASA. Salicylic acid, the metabolite of ASA, is a reversible inhibitor of COX, just like the other NSAIDs. Because the antiplatelet effects of ASA are not affected by first pass, a much lower dose can be used to achieve platelet inhibition.

Advanced

■ A potential role for COX inhibitors in the treatment of cancer has been under investigation for many years. The COX-2 enzyme, which may stimulate cell division, has been selectively targeted in indications such as colon cancer. Inhibition of COX-2 may promote apoptosis, inhibit angiogenesis, and inhibit cell growth.

EVIDENCE

Alone or in Combination with Opiates for Treatment of Cancer Pain

■ A 2005 Cochrane review (42 trials, N = 3084 patients) found that NSAIDs were more effective than placebo for cancer pain. No conclusions could be drawn about the efficacy of NSAIDs relative to one another. The combination of opiates and NSAIDs was slightly and statistically better than either agent alone in 9 of 14 trials and was no different in 4 of 14 trials. The authors noted that the generalizability of the findings was limited by the short term of the studies.

Versus Opiates for Treatment of Acute Renal Colic

■ A 2006 Cochrane review (20 trials, N = 1613 patients) compared NSAIDs with opiates for treatment of renal colic. Results of the trials were too heterogeneous to perform a meta-analysis. The authors concluded that both NSAIDs and opiates can significantly relieve pain in acute renal colic. Opiates appeared to cause more adverse effects, particularly vomiting, and particularly pethidine.

FYI

■ Ibuprofen and naproxen are available without a prescription in many jurisdictions.

■ The antiplatelet effects of aspirin were first identified in the 1940s, after a physician noted increased bleeding in children who chewed aspirin gum after tonsillectomy. Speculating that a "blood-thinning" effect could reduce cardiovascular risk, he began giving aspirin to high-risk patients. Despite claims of success, the FDA did not accept the antiplatelet effects of aspirin until 1980.

■ The use of COX-2 inhibitors in cancer led to one of the largest drug withdrawals in the history of pharmaceutical development. During a very large trial in cancer prevention, it was discovered that there was a **higher incidence of cardiovascular events** in the rofecoxib-treated group versus placebo. The study was halted, the news hit the media, and this top-selling drug was withdrawn from the market.

Uricosurics

DESCRIPTION

Uricosurics lower uric acid levels in blood as a treatment for gout.

PROTOTYPE AND COMMON DRUGS

■ Prototype: Probenecid
■ Others: Sulfinpyrazone

MOA (MECHANISM OF ACTION)

■ Gout is a condition whereby uric acid crystals precipitate in joints and the crystals induce an intense inflammatory reaction within the synovial space, leading to severe pain. Uric acid is an organic acid and a byproduct of purine metabolism.

■ Uric acid levels in the blood are elevated in gout, and one treatment strategy is to lower uric acid levels by enhancing uric acid excretion, which is what uricosurics do.

■ Uric acid is freely filtered at the glomerulus and is also both reabsorbed and secreted in the proximal tubule. The amount excreted usually is about 10% of that filtered.

■ In the proximal tubule, a transporter that exchanges urate for either an organic or an inorganic anion is the channel responsible for uric acid reabsorption; uricosuric drugs compete with urate for this brush-border transporter, thereby inhibiting its reabsorption. Probenecid is completely reabsorbed by the proximal tubule (Figure 19-6).

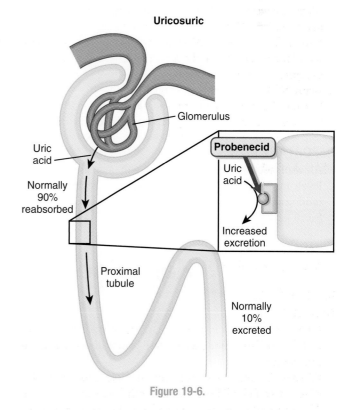

Figure 19-6.

- As the urinary excretion of uric acid increases, the amount of urate in the body decreases, although the plasma concentration may not be greatly reduced.
- With the increase in uric acid excretion, a predisposition to renal stone (urate stone) formation is increased. Therefore the urine volume should be maintained at a high level to help reduce urate concentrations in the urine and to promote flow, both acting to minimize precipitation within the renal system.
- Logically, patients with renal failure will be unresponsive to uricosurics.

PHARMACOKINETICS

- One uricosuric drug may either add to or inhibit the action of another. The biphasic effect may be seen within the normal dosage range with some drugs such as salicylates.
- Twice-a-day and up to four-times-a-day administration has resulted in probenecid being used by fewer patients compared with another class of gout therapies, the xanthine oxidase inhibitors, which decrease uric acid synthesis.

INDICATIONS

- Gout

CONTRAINDICATIONS

- **Renal insufficiency** (creatinine clearance <50 mL/min) is a contraindication.
- **Urolithiasis** (renal stones or calculi) is a contraindication because increased uric acid is excreted into the urine, where it can then precipitate and cause calculi.
- **Peptic ulcer** is a contraindication, because uricosurics could exacerbate preexisting lesions.

SIDE EFFECTS

- Probenecid is well tolerated.
- **Gastrointestinal irritation** is usually mild.
- Allergic reactions usually are mild and occur in 2% to 4% of patients. Serious hypersensitivity is extremely rare.

IMPORTANT NOTES

- Alcohol and high protein intake will increase uric acid levels in the blood. Therapy for gout must include dietary modification.

- Paradoxically, an acute attack can occur in up to 20% of gouty patients treated with probenecid *alone*. Therefore concomitant NSAIDs are indicated early in the course of therapy to avoid precipitating an attack of gout.
- Low-dose aspirin causes net retention of uric acid. It should not be used for analgesia in patients with gout.
- Fenofibrate (lipid-lowering agent) and losartan (angiotensin receptor blocker) both have uricosuric properties.
- Transport across the urate transporter is bidirectional, and depending on dose, a uricosuric drug may either decrease or increase the excretion of uric acid. Decreased excretion usually occurs at a low dose, whereas increased excretion is observed at a higher dose.
- In 2006 fewer than 5% of patients treated for gout were treated with probenecid in the United States. The low rate of use of this drug was speculated to be a result of the availability of other medications for gout, the lack of efficacy in patients with renal dysfunction, and the propensity for renal calculi.

Advanced

- **Drug interactions:** Probenecid inhibits the tubular secretion of a number of drugs and increases their serum concentrations; these drugs include the following:
  - NSAIDs
  - Methotrexate
  - Clofibrate
  - Rifampin
  - Penicillin and cephalosporins (probenecid was originally developed to prolong penicillin blood levels)

FYI

- *Tophaceous* means stonelike. Tophaceous gout is a condition in which large stony deposits of uric acid accumulate around the joint.
- Benzbromarone, a potent uricosuric drug, was introduced in the 1970s. It was registered in many jurisdictions throughout Asia, South America, and Europe. In 2003 the drug was withdrawn after reports of serious hepatotoxicity, but it is still marketed in several countries by other drug companies.
- Probenecid is given with penicillin to reduce penicillin excretion and to prolong its half-life.

Xanthine Oxidase Inhibitors

DESCRIPTION

Xanthine oxidase inhibitors decrease uric acid synthesis and are used in gout.

PROTOTYPE AND COMMON DRUGS

- Prototype: Allopurinol
- Others: Febuxostat

MOA (MECHANISM OF ACTION)

- Allopurinol is a purine analogue of hypoxanthine and is a substrate for, and inhibitor of, the enzyme **xanthine oxidase.**
- Xanthine oxidase converts hypoxanthine to xanthine to uric acid; inhibition therefore **reduces the production of uric acid** (Figure 19-7).

Uric acid production pathway

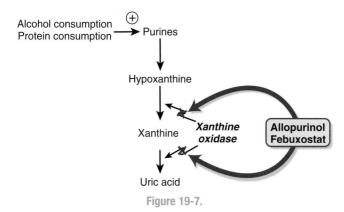

Figure 19-7.

- Allopurinol's primary metabolite, **oxypurinol,** also inhibits xanthine oxidase. Oxypurinol has a long half-life in tissues and is responsible for much of the pharmacologic activity of allopurinol.
- Allopurinol competitively inhibits xanthine oxidase at low concentrations and is a noncompetitive inhibitor at high concentrations.
- Allopurinol also results in the accumulation of **xanthine** and **hypoxanthine;** these molecules can cause feedback inhibition of purine synthesis.
- The net effect of xanthine oxidase inhibition is a lower production of uric acid and a decrease of total body uric acid (including dissolved and precipitated uric acid).
- Xanthine oxidase inhibitors facilitate the dissolution of tophi (nodular crystal deposits) and prevent the development or progression of chronic gouty arthritis by lowering the uric acid concentration in plasma below the limit of its solubility.
- Febuxostat is a new nonpurine inhibitor of xanthine oxidase. A significant difference from allopurinol is that being a nonpurine, it does not inhibit purine or pyrimidine synthesis, while allopurinol does.

PHARMACOKINETICS

- Allopurinol increases the half-life of probenecid and enhances its uricosuric effect, whereas probenecid increases the clearance of oxypurinol, thereby increasing dose requirements of allopurinol. The clinical relevance of this interaction is that both drugs are used to treat gout and therefore are potentially coadministered.
- Mercaptopurine, azathioprine, and theophylline are metabolized by xanthine oxidase, and coadministration with allopurinol will dramatically increase levels of these drugs. Coadministration should be avoided or should be performed with great caution and should include **large dose reductions** (down to 25% of the normal dose). Clinical relevance of this interaction is in the treatment of transplant patients because they are treated with immunosuppressants such as mercaptopurine and azathioprine.

INDICATIONS

- **Gout:**
  - ▲ Recurrent gout attacks not prevented by or amenable to treatment with uricosuric agents
  - ▲ Tophaceous gout (*tophaceous* refers to nodular masses of crystal deposition)
- **Renal stones** composed of uric acid
- *Complicated* hyperuricemia secondary to:
  - ▲ Increased cell turnover from **increased blood cell production:**
    - • Polycythemia vera, myeloid metaplasia, other blood dyscrasias
  - ▲ **Acute tumor lysis syndrome** (occurs when treated cancer cells break open and release contents, which are metabolized to uric acid)
  - ▲ Inborn errors of uric acid metabolism:
    - • Lesch-Nyhan syndrome (rare)
- Because of its possible serious side effects, allopurinol is not indicated in the treatment of asymptomatic hyperuricemia.

CONTRAINDICATION

- Previous hypersensitivity reactions to allopurinol

SIDE EFFECTS
Allopurinol

- **Skin reactions:** Both mild and severe reactions can occur.
  - ▲ The rash is predominantly a pruritic, erythematous, or maculopapular eruption (itchy, red, flat or slightly raised).
  - ▲ Rarely, **toxic epidermal necrolysis** or **Stevens-Johnson syndrome** occurs, which can be fatal. These are *very severe* skin reactions. The risk for Stevens-Johnson syndrome is probably limited to within the first 2 months of treatment.
  - ▲ Because the rash may precede severe hypersensitivity reactions, **patients who develop a rash should discontinue allopurinol.**
  - ▲ Incidence of rash is increased in patients receiving concurrent allopurinol and ampicillin.
- **Liver reactions:** Severe hepatic reactions including elevations of liver enzymes, fever, eosinophilia, and rash may occur. Allopurinol should be stopped immediately if a hypersensitivity reaction is suspected.
- **Renal insufficiency:** Decreased renal function has been seen after initiation of allopurinol, but the mechanism of this side effect has not been established.
- The risk of severe reactions (skin or liver reactions) from allopurinol is estimated to be 1 in 1000 to 1 in 5000.

Febuxostat

- Febuxostat appears to not produce the hypersensitivity reactions that occur with allopurinol.
- Compared with allopurinol, there is a small increase in the risk of myocardial infarction, stroke, and cardiovascular death with febuxostat.

IMPORTANT NOTES

- Paradoxically, urate-lowering therapy can cause a flare-up of gout in the early months of treatment. Therefore:
  - ▲ Allopurinol is started at a low dose (below the typical maintenance dose) and slowly increased weekly, titrated to serum uric acid levels.
  - ▲ Colchicine and NSAIDs are coadministered to help suppress acute attacks. Once excess tissue stores of uric acid are reduced, the incidence of acute attacks decreases and colchicine can be discontinued (usually at around 6 months).
- Because allopurinol has no antiinflammatory effects, it has no role in the treatment of acute gouty arthritis.
- Complete blood counts, liver function test results, and renal function test results should be assessed periodically, especially during the first few months of treatment, to monitor for liver and renal injury.
- The development of a skin rash mandates immediate assessment by a physician; a mild rash can be a precursor to a severe skin reaction.

- Lack of effectiveness of allopurinol is generally attributed to inadequate dose or duration of treatment, meaning that patients are treated with a dose that is too small or for too short a time to be effective. Precipitation of acute gout attacks early in the course of therapy is a common cause of discontinuation.

FYI

- Allopurinol initially was synthesized as a candidate antineoplastic agent but was found to lack antineoplastic activity. Subsequent testing showed it to be an inhibitor of xanthine oxidase that was useful clinically for the treatment of gout.
- Eosinophilia (increased eosinophil count in the blood) is a common marker of allergic reactions and is a hallmark of hypersensitivity-mediated drug-induced organ injury. It also occurs in parasitic infections.
- Febuxostat was approved by the FDA in February 2009. It is the first new drug for gout in many decades. It is far more expensive than allopurinol.

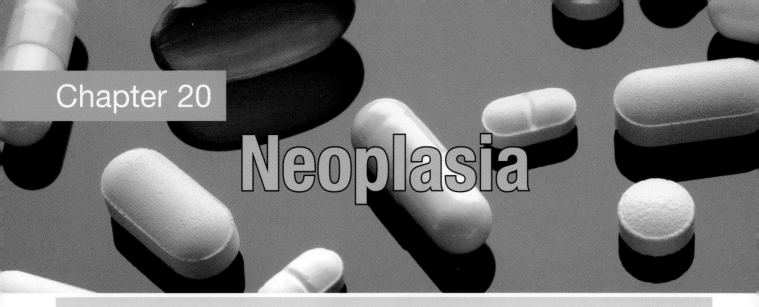

Chapter 20

Neoplasia

Alkylators

DESCRIPTION
Alkylators are chemotherapy agents used primarily in the treatment of cancer.

PROTOTYPES AND COMMON DRUGS
Nitrosoureas
- Prototype: car**mustine**
- Others: lo**mustine**, se**mustine**, benda**mustine**

Bis(chlorethyl)amines
- Prototype: cyclophosphamide
- Others: mechlorethamine, chlorambucil, melphalan, ifosfamide

Aziridines
- Prototype: thiotepa
- Others: triethylenemelamine

Alkyl Sulfonate
- Prototype: busulfan
- Others: treosulfan

MOA (MECHANISM OF ACTION)
- The alkylating agents transfer alkyl (*chemical*) groups to DNA. DNA alkylation in the nucleus leads to the **death of the cell.**
- Once in the cell, the alkylating agents undergo a structural rearrangement that results in the formation of an unstable intermediate, an ethylene immonium ion.
- This ion either directly, or via another intermediate, a carbonium ion, transfers alkyl groups to nucleic acids such as guanine or to other cellular constituents.
- **Alkylation of guanine or other bases results in abnormal base pairing** as well as the excision of these bases, which in turn leads to strand breakage.

- Alkylating agents are considered to be cell cycle phase **nonspecific**, with cells in G_1 and S phases being most susceptible (Figure 20-1).

Alkylators

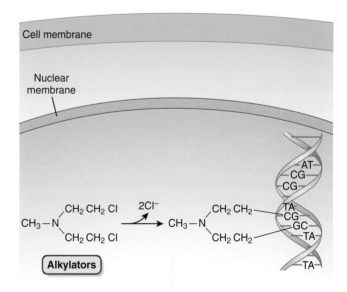

Figure 20-1.

- The connection between DNA alkylation and death of the cancer cell has not been established; however, one of the likely mechanisms is damage to DNA that is sufficient to activate proapoptotic proteins such as p53, leading to cell death.
- Nitrosoureas have an additional mechanism of action. Nitrosoureas undergo another reaction, referred to as car-

bamoylation, with lysine residues of proteins. Carbamoylation is the transfer of carbamoyl (NH_2CO) groups to an amino group, such as that found in amino acids.
- The product of this reaction is referred to as a *carbamoylated protein*, and this process appears to limit the ability of the cancer cell to repair DNA. This unique mechanism of action limits cross-resistance between nitrosoureas and other members of this class.

Mechanisms of Resistance
- Mechanisms of resistance include the following:
  - ▲ DNA repair
  - ▲ Decreased entry of drug into the cell
  - ▲ Inactivation of the alkylating agent by glutathione
- Cross-resistance is common among the various subclasses of alkylating agents, with the exception of the nitrosoureas.

PHARMACOKINETICS
- Oral dosage forms are available for cyclophosphamide, melphalan, chlorambucil, and busulfan. Lomustine is available only in oral dosage forms. The rest are all intravenous.
- Nitrosoureas are highly lipid soluble and readily cross the blood-brain barrier; therefore they are useful in the treatment of brain tumors.
- With the exception of cyclophosphamide and ifosfamide, the alkylating drugs have short half-lives, the most extreme example being mechlorethamine, which has a half-life of 10 minutes.

INDICATIONS
Cyclophosphamide
- Lymphomas
- Leukemias
- Multiple myeloma
- Mycosis fungoides
- Neuroblastoma (disseminated)
- Retinoblastoma
- Cancers of the lung, breast, ovary
- Immunosuppression

Melphalan
- Multiple myeloma
- Ovarian (epithelial) carcinoma

Chlorambucil
- Chronic lymphocytic leukemia
- Non-Hodgkin's lymphomas

Carmustine
- Malignant lymphomas
- Multiple myelomas
- Cancers of the brain, gastrointestinal (GI) tract, skin (melanoma)

Lomustine
- Hodgkin's disease
- Cancers of the breast, brain, lung, skin (melanoma)

Bendamustine
- Chronic lymphocytic leukemia

CONTRAINDICATIONS
Cyclophosphamide
- **Severe leukopenia, thrombocytopenia** will be exacerbated (see side effects).
- **Pregnancy:** Like other cytotoxic agents, cyclophosphamide can cause fetal harm.
- **Lactation:** Cyclophosphamide is excreted in breast milk, so breastfeeding should be avoided.

Melphalan, Chlorambucil
- **Radiation:** should not be administered with radiation therapy or within 4 weeks of radiation therapy (chlorambucil). Radiation also damages DNA and may impair DNA repair mechanisms in healthy cells, leaving them more susceptible to the DNA-damaging effects of alkylating agents.

Lomustine
- Severe leukopenia and/or thrombocytopenia is a contraindication.
- **Lactation:** It is not known whether lomustine is excreted in breast milk, but breastfeeding is not advised during treatment.

SIDE EFFECTS
- **Nausea, vomiting:** These are common side effects with cytotoxic agents, which tend to target rapidly dividing cells, including those of the GI tract.
- **Alopecia:** Cytotoxic chemotherapy agents tend to target tissues with rapidly dividing cells, such as those in hair follicles. This effect is seen most often with cyclophosphamide.

Serious
- **Myelosuppression:** Typical of cytotoxic agents, alkylators tend to target cells that are actively dividing, such as those found in the bone marrow.
- **Pulmonary toxicity (nitrosoureas and busulfan):** Interstitial lung disease may occur.
- **Nephrotoxicity** is seen most often with cyclophosphamide and ifosfamide.
- **Bladder toxicity** is seen most often with cyclophosphamide and ifosfamide.
- **Hemorrhagic cystitis (cyclophosphamide and ifosfamide)** is caused by **acrolein**, a metabolite of cyclophosphamide and ifosfamide. This effect can be managed by increasing fluid intake and by administering sulfhydryl donors such as *N*-acetylcysteine or mesna (an antioxidant). These agents bind with acrolein and form a nontoxic compound.

- **Leukemia (rare):** The alkylating agents work by damaging DNA. If they damage DNA in healthy cells, this may lead to mutations in the genome that rarely result in development of malignancies, particularly leukemia.

IMPORTANT NOTES

- A number of the alkylating agents (cyclophosphamide, ifosfamide, estramustine, melphalan, and chlorambucil) are also known as *nitrogen mustards*. These agents are related to *mustard gas*, a biologic warfare agent used during World War I.
- Cyclophosphamide has a significant effect on lymphocytes; therefore it is also used as an immunosuppressant to prevent rejection of transplanted organs, as well as in conditions such as rheumatoid arthritis and nephrotic syndrome. Cyclophosphamide has a *steroid-sparing* effect, meaning that it can reduce the need for use of corticosteroids.
- Estramustine is a combination of estrogen and a mustine called chlormethine. Accordingly, it has both cytotoxic and hormonal actions and is used primarily in prostate cancer.

- Patients with defective DNA repair mechanisms (ataxia-telangiectasia, Fanconi's anemia, Bloom's syndrome, and xeroderma pigmentosa) are more sensitive to DNA-damaging agents.
- The nitrosoureas (lomustine, carmustine) tend to be more lipid soluble and therefore readily cross the blood-brain barrier and are useful for tumors of the brain and meninges.

FYI

- The first rationally designed anticancer agent was a nitrosourea (methyl nitrosourea), developed in 1898.
- The U.S. Army played a role in the development of nitrogen mustards, deriving the prototype to this class (mechlorethamine) from the mustard gases used in the first World War. After an accidental exposure, it was discovered that nitrogen mustard produced lymphopenia, inspiring its use in malignant proliferative disorders.

Anthracyclines

DESCRIPTION

Anthracyclines are cytotoxic anticancer agents that work by damaging DNA and by generation of free radicals. This class is also grouped under a larger class of antitumor antibiotics (but are never used as antibiotics).

PROTOTYPE AND COMMON DRUGS

- Prototype: doxo**rubicin**
- Others: dauno**rubicin**, ida**rubicin**, epi**rubicin**, acla**rubicin**, mitoxantrone

MOA (MECHANISM OF ACTION)

- The anthracyclines are believed to exert their cytotoxic effects through a variety of mechanisms.
- Topoisomerase II (Top II) plays a key role during DNA synthesis, nicking and resealing the DNA helix so that it does not become tangled during replication.
- The anthracyclines **prevent the resealing step** from occurring by intercalating into and inhibiting the DNA–topoisomerase II complex after the nicking phase. This results in a large number of DNA fragments, eventually prompting the cancer cell to undergo apoptosis (Figure 20-2).
- As a secondary mechanism, anthracyclines **produce free radicals**, and these free radicals in turn damage cell membranes, proteins, and lipids. The generation of free radicals is also believed to mediate an important toxicity associated with this class (see Side Effects).
- In addition anthracyclines are DNA intercalators, meaning that they insert themselves into DNA structure, inhibiting transcription and replication.

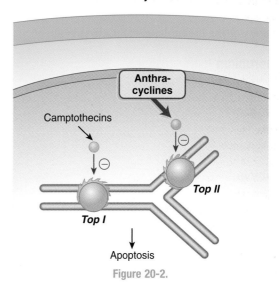

Anthracyclines

Figure 20-2.

Mechanisms of Resistance

- Drug efflux through P-glycoprotein (Pgp-170) or multidrug-resistant (MDR) gene
- Altered topoisomerase II levels
- Mutations in topoisomerase II
- Increased glutathione (a free radical scavenger)
- Increased glutathione peroxidase activity
- Decreased concentration of glucose-6-phosphate (G6P) dehydrogenase

PHARMACOKINETICS
- Doxorubicin is a prodrug, and idarubicin is the active metabolite.
- Doxorubicin was the first anthracycline to be encapsulated in liposomes to facilitate targeted delivery of the drug and therefore avoid cardiotoxicity (see Side Effects). One of the key mechanisms for this targeted delivery relies on the fact that the liposomes readily extravasate in tissues that have a disrupted vasculature, such as that found in tumors. Blood vessels in tumors tend to be "leaky" owing to the constant angiogenesis that is taking place. Conversely, the liposomes have difficulty exiting vessels in tissues such as the myocardium.
- The anthracyclines are eliminated through hepatic metabolism, through a variety of routes. Because of the toxicities associated with these agents, dose adjustments should be considered in patients with significant hepatic impairment.
- Idarubicin is the only anthracycline that can be given orally; the rest are available only in intravenous formulations.

INDICATIONS
Doxorubicin
- Acute leukemias
- Hodgkin's disease
- Non-Hodgkin's lymphoma
- Sarcomas
- Cancers of the breast, lung, stomach, thyroid

Daunorubicin
- Acute leukemia

Idarubicin
- Acute leukemia
- Breast cancer

Epirubicin
- Lymphoma
- Cancers of the lung, breast, ovary, stomach

Mitoxantrone
- Prostate cancer
- Non-Hodgkin's lymphoma

CONTRAINDICATIONS
- **Severe cardiac disease:** Anthracyclines should be used only with extreme caution and after a careful risk-benefit assessment in these patients. See Side Effects.
- **Lactation:** Patients should not breastfeed while using these agents.

SIDE EFFECTS
- **Nausea and vomiting** are common side effect with cytotoxic agents, which tend to target rapidly dividing cells, including those of the GI tract.
- **Alopecia:** Cytotoxic chemotherapy agents tend to target tissues with rapidly dividing cells, such as those in hair follicles. The hair loss is reversible.
- **Mucositis or stomatitis** is an inflammatory condition of the mouth. Cytotoxic chemotherapy agents tend to target tissues with rapidly dividing cells, such as those in the oral mucosa.
- **Soft tissue necrosis:** If the anthracyclines become extravascular, they can damage surrounding tissue. Infusions should be carried out slowly to reduce the risk of extravasation.

Serious
- **Cardiotoxicity:** The free radicals generated by the anthracyclines cause peroxidation of the cardiac sarcoplasmic reticulum, leading to a Ca^{2+}-dependent **cardiac necrosis.** The reason this toxicity is selective for cardiac tissue is that **catalase**, able to neutralize these free radicals, is not found in cardiac tissue.
- **Myelosuppression:** Cytotoxic chemotherapy agents tend to target tissues with rapidly dividing cells, such as those of the bone marrow. The bone marrow suppression is reversible but does predispose the patient to major complications such as infection while receiving treatment.

IMPORTANT NOTES
- **Cardiotoxicity** associated with anthracyclines can occur both acutely and chronically. Acute toxicity is characterized by abnormal electrocardiograms (ECGs) and reductions in systolic function. Chronic toxicity is cumulative and dose related. It manifests as congestive heart failure, and once it has reached this point it has a very high mortality rate. This chronic cardiotoxicity is of greater concern, and it is addressed using a number of strategies, including limitations on doses used, as well as use of liposomal formulations and adjuvant agents, as described later.
- **Mitoxantrone** has a chemical structure that is distinct from that of the anthracyclines, and it is believed to be less cardiotoxic than the anthracyclines. It does not generate free radicals.

Advanced
- Strategies to **minimize cardiotoxicity** include the use of a cardioprotective drug such as **dexrazoxane.** The generation of free radicals by anthracyclines is iron dependent. Dexrazoxane chelates iron that is bound in anthracycline complexes, and this prevents the formation of the free radicals that damage the myocardium. Dexrazoxane does not appear to impair the antitumor activity of the anthracyclines.

Drug Interactions
- It appears that the cardiotoxic effects of anthracyclines may be worsened by concurrent administration of trastuzumab. Trastuzumab is a monoclonal antibody that is used in the treatment of breast cancers expressing the HER2/neu receptor. A number of anthracyclines are used in treating breast cancer.

FYI

■ The anthracyclines were originally derived from the bacterium *Streptomyces peucetius* var *caesius*, and that is why they fall under a larger class of antitumor antibiotics. Other antitumor antibiotics include mitomycin and bleomycin.

Antimetabolites

DESCRIPTION

Also known as *DNA synthesis inhibitors*, antimetabolites work by inhibiting the actions of enzymes that are involved in the synthesis of DNA precursors and bases.

PROTOTYPES AND COMMON DRUGS
Folate Analogues

■ Prototype: methotrexate

Pyrimidine Analogues

■ Prototype: fluorouracil
■ Others: raltitrexed, pemetrexed, cytarabine, gemcitabine

Purine Analogues

■ Prototype: mercaptopurine
■ Others: fludarabine, pentostatin, cladribine, thioguanine

MOA (MECHANISM OF ACTION)
Folate Analogues

■ Tetrahydro**folate** (THF) is an essential cofactor in the transformation of 2'-deoxyuridylate (dUMP) to 2'-deoxythymidylate (dTMP). This is a required step in the synthesis of purines and thus DNA.
■ THF is synthesized by the actions of **dihydrofolate reductase** (DHFR). Methotrexate has a high affinity for DHFR and **competitively inhibits DHFR** (Figure 20-3).

Mechanisms of Resistance

■ Reduced transport across cell membranes
■ Changes in the conformation of the DHFR enzyme

■ Increased concentrations of DHFR
■ Increased drug efflux

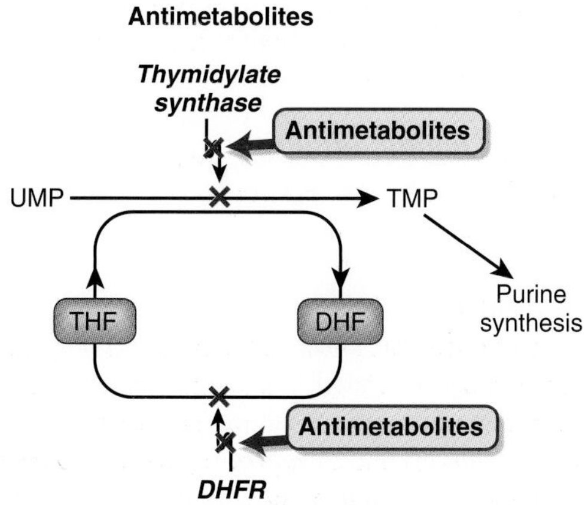

Pyrimidine Analogues

■ **Fluorouracil** is a **uracil analogue.** It is converted to FdUMP (**fluoro**deoxyuridine monophosphate) and although it interacts with thymidylate synthetase, it cannot be converted to dTMP because of the fluoro component and therefore results in a deficiency of dTMP. Without dTMP, DNA synthesis cannot occur. It is considered to be a *fraudulent* nucleotide.
■ Inhibitors of other enzymes important in dTMP synthesis include **raltitrexed** (thymidylate **synthetase** inhibitor) and **pemetrexed** (thymidylate **transferase** inhibitor).
■ **Cytarabine**, also known as cytosine arabinoside, is an analogue of 2'-deoxycytidine (essentially, cytosine). On entering the cell, it is converted to cytosine arabinoside triphosphate by the same phosphorylation reaction that 2'-deoxycytidine undergoes. The cytosine arabinoside triphosphate competitively **inhibits DNA polymerase**, inhibiting both DNA synthesis and repair.

Mechanisms of Resistance

■ Reduced enzymatic activation or increased enzymatic deactivation

Purine Analogues

■ **Fludarabine** inhibits DNA polymerases, leading to inhibition of DNA synthesis and repair. It also incorporates into DNA and may also promote apoptosis by an undetermined mechanism.
■ **Pentostatin** inhibits adenosine deaminase, an enzyme that transforms adenosine to inosine. This leads to accumulation of intracellular adenosine and deoxyadenosine, which can block DNA synthesis by inhibiting ribonucleotide reductase. Ribonucleotide reductase catalyzes the formation of deoxyribonucleotides from ribonucleotides. Deoxyribonucleotides are used in the synthesis of DNA.
■ **Mercaptopurine** is incorporated into RNA and DNA, halting further DNA and RNA synthesis.

Mechanisms of Resistance

■ Mechanisms of resistance include reduced apoptosis secondary to deficiency of p53, a proapoptotic protein, or up-regulation of bcl-2, an antiapoptotic protein. Drugs that have activity against bcl-2 may be synergistic in combination with purine analogues.

Antimetabolites

Thymidylate synthase

Antimetabolites

UMP → TMP

THF   DHF

Purine synthesis

Antimetabolites

DHFR

Figure 20-3.

PHARMACOKINETICS

- Methotrexate can be administered orally, intravenously, intramuscularly, or intrathecally. It is not able to cross the blood-brain barrier, so entry into the central nervous system (CNS) can be achieved only by intrathecal administration.
- Only a small fraction of methotrexate is metabolized; most of it is eliminated unchanged in the urine. Because of its potential for nephrotoxicity, dose adjustments must be considered in patients with renal impairment.
- The purine analogues mercaptopurine and thioguanine are available in oral dosage forms. They are metabolized by the liver. One of the enzymes responsible for mercaptopurine metabolism is xanthine oxidase; therefore inhibitors of this enzyme, such as allopurinol, can lead to toxicity. The elimination half-life of mercaptopurine is relatively short (<1 hour).
- Fludarabine and cladribine can be administered intravenously or orally, and pentostatin is administered intravenously. All are primarily eliminated by renal excretion. Dose adjustments should be considered in patients with renal impairment.
- Cytarabine is administered intravenously or subcutaneously, and 5-fluorouracil is administered intravenously or topically. Cytarabine (cytarabine triphosphate) and 5-fluorouracil (5-fluorodeoxyuridine monophosphate and triphosphate) are converted to active metabolites in the body. Both are largely metabolized by the liver, and dose adjustments should be considered in patients with hepatic impairment.

INDICATIONS
Methotrexate
- Rheumatoid arthritis
- Acute lymphoblastic leukemia
- Severe psoriasis
- Non-Hodgkin's lymphoma
- Osteosarcoma
- Cancers of the breast, head and neck, ovary, bladder

Pemetrexed
- Mesothelioma
- Non–small cell lung cancer

Thioguanine, Mercaptopurine
- Leukemia

Fludarabine, Cladribine, Pentostatin, Cytarabine
- Leukemia
- Lymphoma

5-Fluorouracil
- Cancers of the breast, colon and rectum, stomach, head and neck, skin (noninvasive)
- Actinic keratoses

Gemcitabine
- Cancers of the pancreas, lung (non–small cell cancer), ovary, bladder, esophagus, head and neck

CONTRAINDICATION
- **Pregnancy:** Most of the antimetabolites are teratogenic in animals.

SIDE EFFECTS
Folate Analogues
- **Myelosuppression:** Conventional chemotherapy agents work by targeting rapidly dividing cells. This nonspecific effect can also target rapidly dividing cells in other areas of the body, including bone marrow and the GI tract.
- **Damage to GI epithelium:** See previous entry.
- **Stomatitis:** Severe oral ulcers can develop.
- **Pneumonitis** may occur.
- **Nephrotoxicity** is caused by precipitation of drug in the renal tubules.
- **Alopecia:** Cytotoxic chemotherapy agents tend to target tissues with rapidly dividing cells, such as those in hair follicles.
- **Dermatitis** can develop.
- **Defective oogenesis or spermatogenesis** results from targeting of rapidly dividing cells.
- **Hepatic:**
  - ▲ **Acute:** reversible elevations in liver enzymes
  - ▲ **Chronic:** cirrhosis

Purine Analogues
- **Myelosuppression** develops more gradually than with the folate analogues. It tends to be worse with thioguanine.
- **Nausea and vomiting** are caused by GI epithelial damage.
- **Hepatotoxicity** occurs with long term use of mercaptopurine.
- **CNS (fludarabine):** Altered mental status and seizures may occur.

Pyrimidine Analogues
- **Myelosuppression:** Cytarabine is a particularly potent bone marrow suppressant.
- **GI** effects are caused by irritation of GI epithelium.
- **Stomatitis** may occur.
- **Hepatotoxicity:** Reversible elevations in liver enzymes may develop.
  - **CNS:** CNS effects are usually seen only with intrathecal administration or high plasma levels. They manifest as cerebellar (ataxia) or cerebral (seizures, dementia, coma) effects.

Pemetrexed-Specific Effects
- **Rash:** A red, itchy rash is very common with this agent.

IMPORTANT NOTES
- High-dose regimens of methotrexate may require *rescue* with folinic acid, also known as *leucovorin*. Folinic acid is a reduced form of folic acid. Methotrexate is an "antifolate" drug, and patients who are taking high doses or receiving chronic therapy are likely to experience severe symptoms of folate deficiency unless they are treated adjunctively with leucovorin.

- The drug interaction between mercaptopurine and allopurinol is particularly relevant because patients taking conventional chemotherapy are predisposed to development of uric acid crystals, also known as *gout*. Allopurinol is one of the key drugs used for treating gout, thus increasing the likelihood that these agents may be administered simultaneously.
- Gemcitabine is an analogue of cytarabine, with fewer side effects.

Advanced
Pharmacogenetics
- Thiopurine methyltransferase (TPMT) plays a role in the metabolic inactivation of mercaptopurine. Approximately 15% of Caucasians have reduced activity of this enzyme, and these individuals are at greater risk for toxicity. TPMT genotyping is now readily available, and genotype-based dosage recommendations are available.

- Dihydropyrimidine dehydrogenase (DPD) is one of the enzymes involved in the metabolic inactivation of 5-fluorouracil. Korean patients tend to have higher DPD activity, whereas African Americans tend to have lower activity, predisposing them to toxicity.

Drug Interactions
- Tubular secretion plays a role in the excretion of methotrexate, so agents that compete for secretion at the proximal tubule, such as aspirin, may reduce methotrexate clearance.

FYI
- The folic acid analogues were one of the first successful classes of chemotherapeutic agents, dating back to their use in the 1950s and 1960s.
- Cytarabine is also known by its full name, *cytosine arabinoside*, or *Ara-C*.

Bleomycin

DESCRIPTION
Bleomycin belongs to a family of glycopeptides that exert a cytotoxic effect by damaging DNA.

PROTOTYPE
- Prototype: bleomycin

MOA (MECHANISM OF ACTION)
- Bleomycin is a DNA intercalator. An intercalator is a molecule that binds DNA and inserts itself into DNA structure.
- Bleomycin binds to Fe^{2+}, and this complex leads to free radical formation when oxygen is added. These free radicals then intercalate between DNA strands, which produces single- and double-stranded breaks in DNA (Figure 20-4).
- When sufficient damage has been done to DNA, the cell dies.
- Once in the cell, bleomycin either translocates to the nucleus or is broken down by bleomycin hydrolase, an enzyme that is found in both normal and malignant cells but is found in decreased concentrations in lung and skin. It is believed that the toxicities seen in lung and skin with these agents are the result of the **lack of hydrolase activity** in these regions.

Mechanisms of Resistance
- Increased hydrolase activity, which leads to increased inactivation of bleomycin

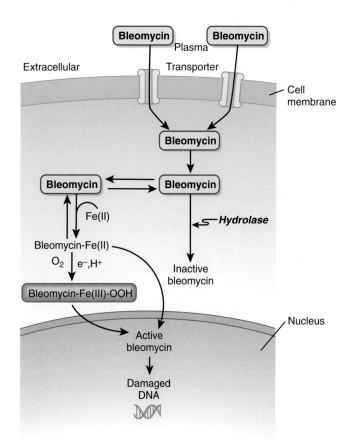

Figure 20-4.

- Decreased uptake of bleomycin into cancer cells
- Repair of DNA strand breaks
- Inactivation of bleomycin

PHARMACOKINETICS

- Bleomycin is a large cation and therefore has difficulty penetrating cell membranes. It enters cells through a special membrane binding protein.
- It is administered parenterally, either intravenously or by the intramuscular or subcutaneous route. Bleomycin can also be instilled directly into the bladder to treat bladder cancer. It can also be given intrapleurally (into the pleural space) to treat pleural effusions.
- Bleomycin is largely eliminated by the kidneys, and dose adjustments should be considered in patients with renal impairment.

INDICATIONS

- Lymphoma
- Cancers of the head and neck, cervix, testicles, bladder

CONTRAINDICATION

- **Pregnancy:** Like all cytotoxic agents, bleomycin carries the risk of fetotoxicity.

SIDE EFFECTS

- **Cutaneous** side effects appear to be more common than with other conventional cytotoxic agents, likely because of the **lack of hydrolase** activity and relative buildup of bleomycin in skin:

  - ▲ Hyperpigmentation
  - ▲ Hyperkeratosis
  - ▲ Erythema
  - ▲ Ulceration
- **Nausea, vomiting:** Cytotoxic agents tend to target rapidly dividing cells, including those of the GI tract, contributing to irritation of the GI tract.

Serious

- **Interstitial pneumonitis or fibrosis:** This is a very serious complication that results in a fatal outcome in 1% of patients who take bleomycin. Risk increases with higher doses, as well as with advanced age (>70 years) and preexisting pulmonary disease.
- **Hypersensitivity reaction:** An anaphylaxis-like reaction that is characterized by hypotension and hyperthermia, as well as cardiorespiratory collapse, may occur. Patients should be monitored closely after receiving their dose, especially when therapy is first being initiated.

IMPORTANT NOTES

- Unlike most cytotoxic agents, bleomycin causes **minimal bone marrow suppression.** The fact that it does not cause myelosuppression makes it a good candidate for combining with other cytotoxic agents that have this toxicity.

FYI

- Bleomycin is actually an antibiotic that was derived from the bacterium *Streptomyces verticillus.* However, bleomycin is never used to treat infection.

Platinum Compounds

DESCRIPTION

Platinum compounds are cytotoxic agents that work by damaging DNA and are used in the treatment of cancer.

PROTOTYPE AND COMMON DRUGS

- Prototype: cis**platin**
- Others: carbo**platin**, oxali**platin**

MOA (MECHANISM OF ACTION)

- Platinum (Pt) compounds are named for their central Pt ion, surrounded by chloride (Cl^-) atoms and ammonia groups.
- The platinum compounds **cross-link DNA strands,** thereby inhibiting DNA synthesis and function. If the DNA is damaged enough, the cell will undergo apoptosis (Figure 20-5).
- The platinum compounds enter cells through an active transporter.
- On entering the cell, the Cl^- ions dissociate, leaving behind a reactive complex that interacts with DNA.
- The dissociation of Cl^- ions is favored at low intracellular concentrations of chloride. Higher concentrations of chloride within the cell tend to stabilize the drug.

Mechanisms of Resistance

- DNA repair mechanisms
- Efflux transporter:
  - ▲ Platinum compounds enter cells through copper transporters. When copper efflux transporters become overexpressed, more drug is pumped out of the cancer cell, leading to an increased chance of therapeutic failure.

PHARMACOKINETICS

- The platinum compounds are dependent on the kidneys for their elimination. Given the toxicity associated with anticancer agents, dose adjustments must be considered in patients with renal impairment.

INDICATIONS

- Cancers of the testes, ovary, bladder, head and neck, lung

CONTRAINDICATIONS

- None of major significance, although as noted, extreme caution must be exercised in patients with renal impairment.

Platinum

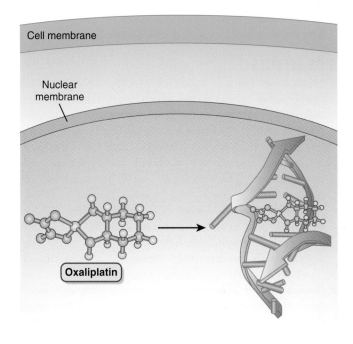

Cell membrane

Nuclear membrane

Oxaliplatin

Figure 20-5.

SIDE EFFECTS

■ **Nausea and vomiting** can be severe. Cytotoxic anticancer drugs target actively dividing cells, such as those found in the GI tract, leading to GI side effects.
■ **Nephrotoxicity** is believed to be primarily mediated by mitochondrial toxicity. Preventive measures such as generous hydration with normal saline to promote diuresis should be undertaken. Nephrotoxicity is more of a problem with cisplatin than with the other agents in this class.

■ **Myelosuppression** is less severe than with other conventional anticancer drugs. Conventional anticancer drugs target actively dividing cells, such as those found in the bone marrow, leading to bone marrow suppression.
■ **Tinnitus and hearing loss** result from promotion of apoptosis in cochlear cells and appear to be less severe with oxaliplatin.
■ **Peripheral neuropathy:** The mechanism has not been established. Neurotoxicity manifests as both acute (shortly after infusion, lasting for a few days) and chronic. The chronic neurotoxicity may be caused by cumulative damage to cells in the dorsal root ganglion.
■ **Hyperuricemia** is likely secondary to the nephrotoxicity noted previously.
■ **Hypersensitivity** may occur.

IMPORTANT NOTES
■ The 5-HT$_3$ antagonists (e.g., ondansetron) have proven effective in managing the nausea and vomiting associated with this drug class.
■ Compared with cisplatin, carboplatin (a derivative of cisplatin) causes more myelosuppression but less nephrotoxicity, neurotoxicity, ototoxicity, nausea, and vomiting.
■ Neurotoxicity seen with platinum compounds tends to be both dose and duration dependent. The longer the patient is on therapy and/or the higher the dose, the more likely he or she is to experience these side effects.
■ Infusions of calcium and magnesium before and after oxaliplatin treatment is one strategy used to mitigate neuropathies such as paresthesia and dysesthesia.

FYI
■ The discovery of platinum compounds as anticancer agents began with the observation that passing electricity through platinum electrodes caused filamentous growth in bacteria, considered to be a sign of inhibited DNA synthesis.
■ Cisplatin was considered to be a major advance in the treatment of testicular cancer, improving cure rates for metastatic disease from 5% to 15% to 70% to 90%.

Taxanes

DESCRIPTION
Taxanes are a group of naturally derived cytotoxic chemotherapy agents that work by inhibiting mitosis.

PROTOTYPE AND COMMON DRUGS
■ Prototype: pacli**taxel**
■ Others: doce**taxel**

MOA (MECHANISM OF ACTION)
■ The taxanes are microtubule inhibitors.
■ Microtubules perform several important functions in the cell, the key being the segregation of chromosomes during mitosis.

■ Microtubules are composed of tubulin, a heterodimer composed of a-tubulin and ß-tubulin. The polymerization of tubulin leads to formation of microtubules.
■ Microtubules are in a dynamic equilibrium with the intracellular pool of α-tubulin and β-tubulin. Microtubules are constantly growing and shortening, and this process, known as *dynamic instability*, leads to the polar movement of chromosomes during anaphase.
■ The taxanes bind to β-tubulin, stabilizing the microtubule and preventing its disassembly. This stabilization interferes with the segregation of chromosomes during mitosis, which leads to cell death. This is believed to be the main mechanism for the cytotoxic effects of taxanes (Figure 20-6).

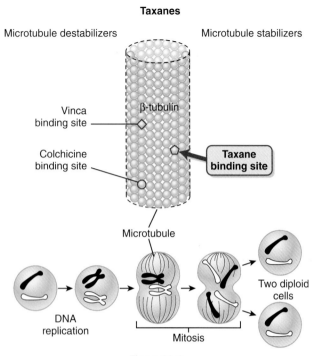

Taxanes

Microtubule destabilizers   Microtubule stabilizers

Vinca binding site — β-tubulin

Colchicine binding site

Taxane binding site

Microtubule

DNA replication

Mitosis

Two diploid cells

Figure 20-6.

- Vinca alkaloids are also microtubule inhibitors, and they also bind to β-**tubulin**; the difference is that they prevent polymerization of β-tubulin into microtubules and thus destabilize the microtubule.
- Taxanes, specifically paclitaxel, are also used in drug-eluting vascular stents (often for coronary artery disease) to reduce the incidence of restenosis. Restenosis occurs, in part, because of the growth of new cells in the area of the stent. The taxanes inhibit cell division, thus preventing the growth of these new cells.

Mechanisms of Resistance

- One mechanism of resistance is increased expression of MDR efflux pumps, which pump drug back out of the cell.
- Tumor cells can overexpress a mutated isoform of β-tubulin, preventing binding of taxanes. These cells may be more sensitive to the effects of vinca alkaloids, if the vinca alkaloids are better able to bind to the mutated β-tubulin.

PHARMACOKINETICS

- Docetaxel is administered orally, whereas paclitaxel is given intravenously.
- Paclitaxel and docetaxel both rely on the liver for their elimination. Dose adjustments should be considered in patients with severe hepatic impairment.
- The drug-eluting stents release drug from a matrix contained within the stent. This allows for a continual local low dose release of drug over time.

INDICATIONS

- Cancers of the breast, ovary, lung, head and neck, prostate (hormone-refractory)
- Prevention of restenosis after angioplasty

CONTRAINDICATIONS

- **Pregnancy**: embryotoxic and fetotoxic in animals
- **Lactation**
- **Severe hepatic impairment**: eliminated by the liver, therefore severe toxicity expected with accumulation

SIDE EFFECTS

- **Myelosuppression** is a side effect commonly seen with conventional chemotherapy, which targets rapidly dividing cells, including those in the bone marrow.
- **Neurotoxicity**: Microtubules are believed to play an important role in neuronal function, and this is the likely reason why microtubule inhibitors are associated with neurotoxicity. This manifests itself as a variety of neuropathies:
  - ▲ **Sensory**: typically loss of all modalities in feet
  - ▲ **Motor**: mild weakness in foot muscles
  - ▲ **Reflexes**: reduced ankle reflexes
  - ▲ Neuropathy occurs more frequently with paclitaxel, which is an older, less potent drug.
- **Resistant fluid retention**: Pretreatment with oral dexamethasone tends to mitigate the fluid retention. Docetaxel tends to produce more edema than the other agents in this class.
- **Hypersensitivity** is likely to happen with either agent, and therefore pretreatment with corticosteroids and antihistamines is recommended. This effect results not from the agents themselves but from the solvents (polyoxyethylated castor oil or polysorbate) that each drug has to be dissolved in because of its low solubility.

IMPORTANT NOTES

- Other microtubule binding agents include the cytotoxic vinca alkaloids and colchicine, which is most commonly used for gout.
- Paclitaxel is more likely to elicit a hypersensitivity reaction than docetaxel. This is again believed to occur because of the solvents used for these two agents, which differ slightly.

Advanced

- Paclitaxel is mainly metabolized by CYP2C8 with some contribution from CYP3A4. Docetaxel is metabolized primarily by CYP3A4 and CYP3A5. Inhibitors or inducers of these isozymes may alter the efficacy or toxicity of paclitaxel or docetaxel.

EVIDENCE
For Adjuvant Treatment of *Early* Breast Cancer

- A 2007 Cochrane review (12 studies, N = 18,304 women) compared taxane-containing with non–taxane-containing regimens as adjuvant treatment for premenopausal or postmenopausal women with early breast cancer. Overall survival (Hazard ratio [HR] 0.81) was improved with taxane-based regimens, as was disease-free survival (HR 0.81).

For Treatment of *Metastatic* Breast Cancer

- A 2005 Cochrane review (12 studies, N = 3643 women) compared taxane-containing with non–taxane-containing regimens in women with metastatic breast cancer. The authors found that overall survival was improved with taxane-based regimens versus nontaxane regimens (HR 0.93), although this difference was not statistically significant when taxane regimens were used first line. Time to progression was also improved (HR 0.92), as was overall response (odds ratio [OR] 1.34), although with considerable heterogeneity for overall response.

Docetaxel versus Vinca Alkaloids for Treatment of Advanced Non–Small Cell Lung Cancer

- A 2007 systematic review (7 trials, N = 2867 participants) compared docetaxel with vinca alkaloid–based chemotherapy regimens (both are tubulin inhibitors) for treatment of advanced non–small cell lung cancer. Vinorelbine was the comparator in six trials, and vindesine in the remaining trial. The authors found improved overall survival with docetaxel (HR 0.89). The incidence of neutropenia was significantly reduced with docetaxel compared with the vinca alkaloids (OR 0.59), as was the incidence of febrile neutropenia (OR 0.57). There were also fewer serious adverse events with docetaxel compared with the vinca alkaloids.

FYI

- Paclitaxel is derived from the bark of the Pacific yew tree. Originally used in its natural form, it can now be produced semisynthetically, using a precursor found in yew leaves, or can be synthesized completely from scratch.
- New taxanes that are orally available are in clinical development.
- Other microtubule inhibitors include the vinca alkaloids and colchicine, which is used for gout.

Topoisomerase Inhibitors

DESCRIPTION

Topoisomerase inhibitors include two classes of drugs that are derived from natural sources and exert their cytotoxic effects by interfering with DNA. Their mechanism is analogous to that of the fluoroquinolone class of antibiotics.

PROTOTYPES AND COMMON DRUGS

Camptothecins

- Prototype: topotecan
- Others: irinotecan

Podophyllotoxins

- Prototype: etoposide
- Others: teniposide

MOA (MECHANISM OF ACTION)

- The camptothecins are **topoisomerase I inhibitors**, whereas the podophyllotoxins are **topoisomerase II inhibitors**. Topoisomerase is an enzyme that cuts and reseals DNA strands, a process that is essential for DNA synthesis.
- During the process of DNA replication or transcription, a significant amount of torsional strain is placed on the DNA helix. The strain is analogous to twisting a rubber band or a telephone cord.
- The torsional strain is relieved by breaks in DNA strands that are created by the enzymes topoisomerase I (single-stranded DNA) and topoisomerase II (double-stranded DNA). The analogy would be relieving the strain in a twisted rubber band by making small breaks in the band, allowing the band to untwist, then resealing the breaks. The

Topoisomerase inhibitors

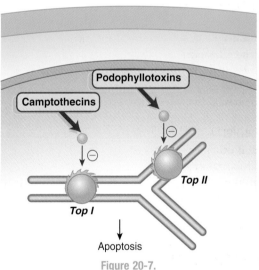

Figure 20-7.

topoisomerase enzymes also reseal the breaks after the tension has been relieved (Figure 20-7).

- Topoisomerase inhibitors **block the resealing step**, leading to large amounts of fragmented DNA. This destabilizes the cell, leading to cell death.

Mechanisms of Resistance

- Inadequate accumulation of drug in tumor
- Alterations in the topoisomerase binding

- Altered cellular response to formation of DNA fragments (i.e., enhanced expression of antiapoptotic proteins such as bcl-2)

PHARMACOKINETICS

- All topoisomerase inhibitors are available in intravenous formulations. Etoposide and topotecan are also available in an oral formulation.
- Topotecan is eliminated renally; therefore dose adjustments may be required in patients with renal impairment. The elimination half-life is 2 to 3 hours.
- Irinotecan is metabolized by the liver; therefore dose adjustments may be required in patients with hepatic impairment. The parent is metabolized by CYP3A4, and it also has an active metabolite, SN-38. SN-38 has much greater antitumor activity than the parent compound, and it is metabolized by glucuronidation via UGT1A1.
- Etoposide is cleared both by renal and nonrenal means.
- Routes of elimination for teniposide have not been well characterized. Renal excretion accounts for about 10% of clearance. Drug interactions have been observed with agents that are known to affect hepatic enzymes; therefore hepatic metabolism is likely.

INDICATIONS
Topotecan
- Cancers of the ovary, lung (small cell)

Irinotecan
- Colorectal cancer

Etoposide
- Lymphoma
- Cancers of the lung, testes

Teniposide
- Neuroblastoma
- Non-Hodgkin's lymphoma
- Acute lymphocytic leukemia

CONTRAINDICATIONS
- **Pregnancy and lactation**: Embryotoxic and teratogenic effects have been observed. Typical of chemotherapy agents, women should be discouraged from becoming pregnant during treatment and advised of the unfavorable risk-benefit profile with respect to breastfeeding.

Topotecan
- Severe bone marrow suppression
- Severe renal impairment

Irinotecan
- Concomitant administration of potent CYP3A4 inhibitors such as ketoconazole should be avoided, as this can lead to significantly increased toxicity.

- Severe leukopenia, thrombocytopenia
- Severe hepatic and/or renal impairment

SIDE EFFECTS
- **Nausea, vomiting:** Cytotoxic agents tend to target rapidly dividing cells, including those of the GI tract, contributing to irritation of the GI tract.
- **Alopecia:** Cytotoxic chemotherapy agents tend to target tissues with rapidly dividing cells, such as those in hair follicles.

Serious
- **Bone marrow suppression** may lead to severe neutropenia, thrombocytopenia, and/or anemia. These have caused fatalities. The mechanism is the same as that seen with other cytotoxic chemotherapy agents, namely destruction of actively dividing cells in the marrow.
- **Interstitial lung disease** can be fatal. Signs and symptoms include cough, fever, dyspnea, and/or hypoxia. More common with topotecan than irinotecan.

Irinotecan
- **Diarrhea** can be either early onset or late onset with irinotecan. Late-onset diarrhea can be particularly severe and life-threatening. Early onset diarrhea is caused by cholinergic activation (irinotecan is a cholinesterase inhibitor) and can therefore be managed with atropine. Late-onset diarrhea must be treated promptly with loperamide.

Etoposide, Teniposide
- **Hypersensitivity and anaphylaxis** are seen with intravenous administration, including acute fatal reactions.
- **Hypotension** is transient and occurs after intravenous administration. On rare occasions it has lead to sudden death as a result of arrhythmia or hypotension.

IMPORTANT NOTES
- Although topoisomerase inhibitors are used as anticancer treatments, topoisomerase inhibition has been linked to promoting some cancers, particularly leukemia. The reason is that some of the cells with fragmented DNA survive. The fragmented DNA in these surviving cells can recombine, forming mutations that may then lead to development of neoplasms.

Advanced
Pharmacogenetics
- Patients with the UGT1A1*28 polymorphism may have reduced activity of this enzyme, reducing their ability to metabolize SN-38, the active metabolite of irinotecan. This polymorphism is seen in approximately 10% of North Americans, and patients with it may be at greater risk of serious toxicities, including fatal hematologic toxicities such as neutropenia.

FYI

- Podophyllotoxins are derived from *Podophyllum peltatum,* more commonly known as the *mayapple* or *mandrake* plant.

- The camptothecin analogues are inspired by the campto-thecin alkaloid found in *Camptotheca acuminate.* This natural alkaloid actually has relatively weak antitumor activity compared with its synthetic analogues.

Vinca Alkaloids

DESCRIPTION

Vinca alkaloids are cytotoxic anticancer agents that work by inhibiting mitosis.

PROTOTYPE AND COMMON DRUGS

- Prototype: vincristine
- Others: vinblastine, vindesine, vinorelbine

MOA (MECHANISM OF ACTION)

- The vinca alkaloids are microtubule inhibitors.
- Tubulin exists in the cell as a heterodimer consisting of one molecule of α-tubulin and one molecule of β-tubulin. The polymerization of tubulin leads to formation of microtu-bules, which play an important role in spindle formation. Formation of the mitotic spindle is a key step in the segre-gation of chromosomes.
- When the vinca alkaloids **bind β-tubulin,** they inhibit its polymerization into microtubules, preventing spindle for-mation in dividing cells. This prevents chromosomes from aligning as they normally do, resulting in a disordered dis-persion of chromosomes throughout the nucleus. This causes cell cycle **arrest at metaphase,** and apoptosis (Figure 20-8).
- Other cellular activities that involve microtubules are also inhibited by these agents, including leukocyte phagocyto-sis and chemotaxis, as well as axonal transport in neurons.
- Taxanes are also microtubule inhibitors, and they also bind to β-tubulin; the difference is **that** they stabilize the micro-tubule, preventing it from disassembling. The vinca alka-loids prevent polymerization of β-tubulin into microtubules, and this destabilizes the microtubule.

Mechanisms of Resistance

- Intracellular levels are reduced secondary to drug efflux through the Pgp transporter. Calcium channel blockers have been used to counteract this mechanism of resistance.
- Mutations in β-tubulin prevent binding of drug.

PHARMACOKINETICS

- The vinca alkaloids have long elimination half-lives (24 to 48 hours). They are administered intravenously. The main route of elimination for the vinca alkaloids is hepatic, and dose adjustments should be considered in patients with hepatic impairment.

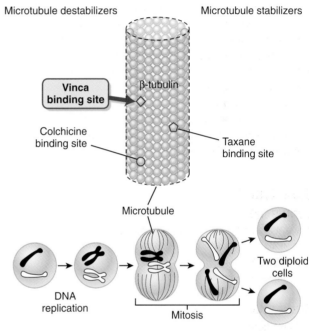

Vinca alkaloids

Microtubule destabilizers   Microtubule stabilizers

Vinca binding site — β-tubulin

Colchicine binding site — Taxane binding site

Microtubule

DNA replication   Mitosis   Two diploid cells

Figure 20-8.

- Vincristine and vinblastine are metabolized by CYP3A4; therefore caution should be used when administering known CYP3A4 inhibitors, as severe toxicity may result. Concomitant administration of CYP3A4 inducers may lead to therapeutic failure.
- A liposomal formulation of vincristine is available; it is eliminated more slowly and has a greater volume of distri-bution. This formulation may be less neurotoxic.

INDICATIONS

- Leukemias
- Lymphomas
- Testicular cancer

Vinorelbine

- Lung cancer
- Breast cancer

CONTRAINDICATIONS

- **Neurologic diseases** that might be worsened by the neurotoxic effects of the vinca alkaloids, particularly vincristine, are contraindications.
- **Intrathecal administration**: The intrathecal route (into the cerebral spinal fluid via a spinal injection) is fatal.
- **Severe bone marrow suppression**: The vinca alkaloids cause bone marrow suppression (see Side Effects) and would be expected to worsen preexisting bone marrow suppression. This is particularly the case with vinblastine, which causes the most bone marrow suppression of the group.
- **Pregnancy**: The vinca alkaloids are fetotoxic and embryotoxic in animals and should not be used in pregnancy.

SIDE EFFECTS

- **Myelosuppression**: Conventional chemotherapy agents tend to target rapidly dividing cells, such as those found in the bone marrow.
- **Alopecia**: Conventional chemotherapy agents also tend to target rapidly dividing cells found in hair follicles, leading to hair loss.
- **Peripheral neuropathy** may be caused by inhibition of microtubules in long peripheral nerves.
- **Nausea, vomiting**: Cytotoxic agents tend to target rapidly dividing cells, including those of the GI tract, contributing to irritation of the GI tract.
- **Topical**: The vinca alkaloids can cause blistering and other skin damage if the infusions extravasate and leak onto the skin, or if injections are mistakenly given by the intramuscular or subcutaneous route.

IMPORTANT NOTES

- Vincristine is less likely to cause bone marrow suppression and is therefore useful in combination regimens in treating leukemia and lymphoma. Vinblastine has less neurotoxicity, whereas vinorelbine is intermediate in terms of both bone marrow suppression and neurotoxicity.

EVIDENCE
Docetaxel versus Vinca Alkaloids in Advanced Non–Small Cell Lung Cancer

- A 2007 systematic review (seven trials, N = 2867 participants) compared docetaxel with vinca alkaloid–based chemotherapy regimens (both are tubulin inhibitors) in advanced non–small cell lung cancer. Vinorelbine was the comparator in six trials, and vindesine in the remaining trial. The authors found improved overall survival with docetaxel (HR 0.89). The incidence of neutropenia was significantly reduced with docetaxel compared with the vinca alkaloids (OR 0.59), as was the incidence of febrile neutropenia (OR 0.57). There were also fewer serious adverse events with docetaxel compared with the vinca alkaloids.

FYI

- The vinca alkaloids are derived from Madagascar periwinkle. They were originally investigated for use in diabetes mellitus, but researchers noted toxicities such as bone marrow suppression in animal studies.

Gonadotropin-Releasing Hormone (GnRH) Analogues

DESCRIPTION
Gonadotropin-releasing hormone (GnRH) analogues are agents that modulate GnRH activity.

PROTOTYPE AND COMMON DRUGS
Agonists
- Prototype: goserelin
- Others: buserelin, leuprolide, triptorelin, gonadorelin, nafarelin, histrelin, deslorelin

Antagonists
- Prototype: abarelix
- Others: cetrorelix, ganirelix

MOA (MECHANISM OF ACTION)
- GnRH is synthesized in the hypothalamus and controls the release of follicle-stimulating hormone (FSH) and luteinizing hormone (LH) from the anterior pituitary. FSH and LH stimulate the gonads (ovaries in females, testes in males), leading to the production of androgens in males.
- Important effects of LH:
  - ▲ Female: production of estrogen
  - ▲ Male: production of testosterone
- Important effects of FSH:
  - ▲ Female: growth of graafian follicles to maturation
  - ▲ Male: spermatogenesis
- GnRH is released in a pulsatile manner. This intermittent release is crucial for the proper synthesis and release of FSH and LH (Figure 20-9).
- *Pulsatile* (physiologic) release of GnRH results in *increased* gonadotropin release. *Continuous* administration of GnRH results in *suppression* of gonadotropin release via downregulation of GnRH receptors, a process called **desensitization**.

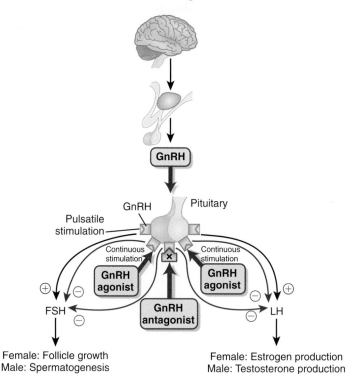

GnRH analogues

GnRH

Pulsatile
stimulation

GnRH   Pituitary

Continuous   Continuous
stimulation   stimulation

GnRH   GnRH
agonist   agonist

GnRH
antagonist

⊕   ⊖   ⊖   ⊕

FSH   LH
⊖   ⊖

Female: Follicle growth   Female: Estrogen production
Male: Spermatogenesis   Male: Testosterone production

Figure 20-9.

▲ GnRH agonists can be administered via pulsatile or continuous fashion, depending on the desired effect (stimulation or suppression of gonadotropins respectively).

■ GnRH *antagonists* simply block the GnRH receptor, resulting in reduced release of FSH and LH.

PHARMACOKINETICS

■ Goserelin as a depot injection provides continuous release of drug over a 29-day period.

■ Leuprolide depot is available in formulations that can be administered every month, 3 months, 4 months, or 6 months.

■ Buserelin is available as both a nasal spray and an injection formulation.

INDICATIONS

■ Conditions that benefit from **hypoestrogen** states (continuous administration):
  ▲ Cancers: breast, ovarian, and endometrial
  ▲ Endometriosis, dysfunctional uterine bleeding, uterine fibroids
  ▲ Precocious puberty

■ Conditions that benefit from **hypotestosterone** states (continuous administration):
  ▲ Prostate cancer

■ Conditions that benefit from *increased* GnRH (pulsatile administration):
  ▲ Kallmann syndrome (very rare—congenital absence of GnRH)

■ As one component of infertility treatment (variable administration)

CONTRAINDICATIONS

■ **Pregnancy:** The effects of GnRH analogues on the fetus have not been well studied; however, given the important role GnRH plays in gonadal development, it is assumed that their use in pregnancy should be avoided.

■ **Undiagnosed vaginal bleeding** is a contraindication (cancer could be the diagnosis).

SIDE EFFECTS
Related to Androgen Deprivation

■ Decreased libido
■ Flushing
■ Gynecomastia
■ Weight gain
■ Loss of bone mass
■ Loss of muscle mass

Related to Estrogen Deprivation

■ Hot flashes
■ Vaginitis
■ Sweating
■ Change in breast size

Rare, Serious

■ **Ovarian hyperstimulation syndrome (OHSS):** Through extensive luteinization (transformation of a follicle into a corpus luteum), estrogen, progesterone, and cytokine levels increase, resulting in leaky capillaries and in fluid shifts from the vascular compartment to the extravascular compartments. This can result in edema, ascites, and intravascular hypovolemia.

Antagonists Only

■ **Allergic reactions:** Severe, systemic, rapid onset allergic reactions were observed in trials of abarelix. The mechanism is believed to be a result of the release of histamine from mast cells after binding of active peptides to cell membranes.

IMPORTANT NOTES

■ The use of GnRH agonists results in an initial increase in testosterone release, commonly referred to as a *flare*. This flare can last anywhere from days to weeks. Once the receptors have become desensitized, GnRH is inhibited, and the antiandrogenic effects of the drug are seen. The flare can result in a temporary worsening of the clinical condition before benefits are seen.

■ One potential advantage of GnRH antagonists over GnRH agonists is that because they antagonize the GnRH receptor, this flare does not occur.

■ Another difference between GnRH agonists and antagonists is that antagonists consistently block **both FSH and LH** secretion, whereas FSH levels tend to rise after a period of time with agonist therapy. The clinical significance of this difference is not known.

■ Prostate cancer tends to be a very hormone-dependent cancer, growing under the stimulation of androgens. The growth stimulating effects of androgens can be reduced in two ways, by either surgical (removal of both testes) or "medical castration." Medical castration is essentially androgen deprivation therapy.

Advanced

■ Elevated prolactin levels decrease GnRH activity.
■ The elimination half-life of goserelin varies between genders: 2 hours in females and 4 hours in males.
■ Triptorelin is eliminated by both liver and kidneys. Renal and/or hepatic impairment extends the elimination half-life of triptorelin.

EVIDENCE
Preoperative GnRH Analogues in Treatment of Uterine Fibroids

■ A 2001 Cochrane review (26 trials) evaluated the role of pretreatment with GnRH analogues before hysterectomy or myomectomy for uterine fibroids. The authors found that the use of GnRH analogues for 3 to 4 months before fibroid surgery reduced uterine volume and fibroid size. The authors also found that midline incisions could be avoided because of a reduction in the size of the uterus.

GnRH Agonists versus Antagonists for Assisted Conception

■ A 2006 Cochrane review (27 trials) evaluated the efficacy of GnRH antagonists compared with the standard long protocol of GnRH agonists for controlled ovarian hyperstimulation in assisted conception. The pregnancy rate was lower with antagonist therapy (OR 0.84), but there was a reduction in the incidence of severe OHSS (OR 0.61).

FYI

■ *Leutin* is Latin, meaning yellow. The corpus luteum is yellow endocrine tissue released from the graafian follicle in the ovary.
■ *Myo-* refers to muscle. *Myome-* refers to myometrium, the middle muscular layer of the uterus. Myomectomy is surgical removal of a fibroid (which is composed of myometrium).
■ Fibroids can bleed when they get large enough, and this can cause anemia.
■ A third human gonadotropin is human chorionic gonadotropin (hCG), present during pregnancy and with some cancers
■ The *-relin* suffix can be a memory tip for *releasing hormones.*
■ The *-relix* suffix is found in GnRH *antagonist* names; the "x" can help you remember that these drugs are against the physiology activity.

Angiogenesis Inhibitors

DESCRIPTION
Angiogenesis inhibitors are agents that inhibit the growth of new blood vessels (angiogenesis).

PROTOTYPE AND COMMON DRUGS
■ Prototype: bevacizumab
■ Others: ranibizumab

MOA (MECHANISM OF ACTION)
■ Angiogenesis is essential to the growth of solid tumors. Neoplastic tissue, which is highly metabolically active, must have access to the nutrients in blood in order to continue growing.
■ It is believed that complete blockade of angiogenesis will not only prevent the growth of new vessels, but also promote instability and degradation of existing vessels within the tumor.
■ Angiogenic growth factors promote angiogenesis. Numerous angiogenic growth factors are found in the body, and each has the potential to play a role in promoting vascular-

ization of neoplastic tissue. Many of these angiogenic growth factors also promote the growth of other tissues.

Vascular Endothelial Growth Factor
■ Vascular endothelial growth factor (VEGF) has become the most frequent target of angiogenesis inhibitors. Bevacizumab and ranibizumab **bind to VEGF-A**, preventing it from binding to its receptor (Figure 20-10).

PHARMACOKINETICS
■ Bevacizumab is administered by intravenous infusion.
■ The metabolism of bevacizumab is unusual in that instead of being cleared by the liver or kidneys, it relies on proteolysis throughout the body, including within endothelial cells.
■ Ranibizumab is administered by intra*vitreal* injection (into the vitreus of the eye).

INDICATIONS
Bevacizumab
■ Colorectal cancer
■ Breast (HER2-negative) cancer
■ Lung (non–small cell) cancer

Angiogenesis inhibitors

Angiogenesis

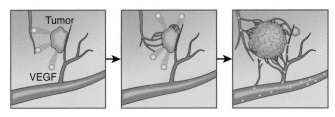

Inhibition of angiogenesis

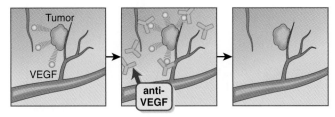

Figure 20-10.

Ranibizumab

- Age-related macular degeneration

CONTRAINDICATIONS
Ranibizumab

- **Suspected ocular infections:** Ranibizumab is administered by intravitreal injection and carries a risk of a very serious eye infection called endophthalmitis.

SIDE EFFECTS
Bevacizumab

- **GI perforation:** VEGF blockade may lead to ischemia in regions of the GI tract, promoting perforation.
- **Hemorrhage,** particularly pulmonary hemorrhage, may be fatal in some cases. This is because of the nonspecific destabilization of blood vessels secondary to VEGF blockade.
- **Hypertension:** VEGF tends to have a vasorelaxant effect, and it is believed that blockade of VEGF leads to elevation in blood pressure, which becomes clinically significant in some patients.
- **Thrombosis:** VEGF blockade prevents the renewal of endothelial cells and promotes endothelial dysfunction, which in turn promotes the development of thromboses.
- **Wound healing:** Angiogenesis plays a key role in proper wound healing, so blockade of VEGF prevents efficient healing of wounds.

Ranibizumab

- Ranibizumab is administered locally; therefore the risk of the previously noted systemic side effects should be minimal.

Serious, Rare

- **Endophthalmitis** may occur because of infection secondary to intraocular injection. Risk is minimal if proper aseptic injection technique is used.

IMPORTANT NOTES

- Bevacizumab is being used off-label in many jurisdictions for the management of age-related macular degeneration. Because it is typically administered in large doses systemically for cancer, small doses of bevacizumab administered locally are much cheaper than ranibizumab.
- Because of its effects on wound healing, bevacizumab should not be initiated within 4 weeks after surgery, and it should be discontinued at least 6 weeks before surgery.
- Ranibizumab was specifically designed to be used in age-related macular degeneration and is not used in cancer. It is administered locally, by intravitreal injection, and therefore lacks many of the side effects of bevacizumab.
- Verteporfin photodynamic therapy (PDT) is another approach used to treat age-related macular degeneration (AMD) and in fact was the favored new therapy before the approval of the angiogenesis inhibitors. This drug was administered intravenously and activated by a laser shone into the eye. The laser stimulated the production of free radicals, which then damaged blood vessels. This was an early antiangiogenic therapy, although it was primitive compared with the newer angiogenesis inhibitors.

EVIDENCE
Age-Related Macular Degeneration

- A 2008 Cochrane review (five trials, N = 2500 participants) investigated anti-VEGF therapies for age-related macular degeneration and included three trials of ranibizumab. Efficacy was measured by the ability to prevent a reduction in visual acuity of 15 letters or more, and ranibizumab prevented vision loss versus verteporfin PDT (number needed to treat [NNT = 3]) and sham (NNT = 3); the combination of ranibizumab and verteporfin PDT prevented vision loss versus verteporfin alone (NNT = 4). Ranibizumab also improved vision by 15 letters or more versus each of these agents.

Metastatic Colorectal Cancer

- A 2009 Cochrane review investigated the efficacy and toxicity of targeted antiangiogenic therapies in addition to chemotherapy in patients with metastatic colorectal cancer. The authors found five trials of bevacizumab (N = 3101 patients). The combination of bevacizumab and first-line chemotherapy significantly improved overall survival (HR 0.81) and progression-free survival (HR 0.61) versus first-line chemotherapy alone. The results for combining bevacizumab with second-line chemotherapy were not conclusive owing to significant heterogeneity.

FYI

- One of the most notorious drugs ever developed, thalidomide, is an angiogenesis inhibitor. When it first came out in the 1950s, it was marketed as an antinauseant for pregnant women. Tragically, thalidomide turned out to be one of the worst teratogens ever developed and caused countless birth defects. Many babies were born with malformed limbs; this was a result of impaired vascular development, an effect of thalidomide that was not known at the time of its development.

Tyrosine Kinase Inhibitors

DESCRIPTION

Tyrosine kinase inhibitors are a heterogeneous group of anti-cancer agents that work by inhibiting the effects of a variety of growth factors.

Monoclonal Antibodies

Human Epidermal Growth Factor Receptor (HER2)
- Prototype: trastuzumab

Epidermal Growth Factor Receptor (EGFR)
- Prototype: cetuximab
- Others: panitumumab

PROTOTYPE AND COMMON DRUGS
Small Molecules
EGFR
- Prototype: erlotinib
- Others: gefitinib

BCR-ABL/src
- Prototype: imatinib
- Others: dasatinib, nilotinib

Multikinase Inhibitors
- Prototype: sorafenib
- Others: sunitinib

Dual Kinase Inhibitors: EGFR/HER2
- Prototype: lapatinib

MOA (MECHANISM OF ACTION) (Figure 20-11)

- Phosphorylation is a process whereby a protein **kinase** transfers a phosphate group from adenosine triphosphate (ATP) or guanosine triphosphate (GTP) to free hydroxyl groups of amino acids. In doing so, they modify protein function. Most protein kinases phosphorylate serine and threonine residues, but a subset of protein kinases phosphorylate **tyrosine** residues.
- The protein tyrosine kinases are subdivided into **receptor** tyrosine kinases (RTKs) and **nonreceptor** (cytoplasmic) tyrosine kinases.
- **Tyrosine kinase receptors** regulate growth and cell differentiation. Therefore ligands for these receptors include several **growth factors**, and they play an important role in neoplasia. The RTK family includes growth factor receptors such as **epidermal growth factor receptor** (EGFR).
- Under normal circumstances, frequent binding of growth factors to these tyrosine kinase receptors leads to receptor **down-regulation**. This blunts the activity of these growth factors, preventing abnormal growth from occurring. In cancer, **mutation** of these receptors prevents this down-

Tyrosine kinase inhibitors

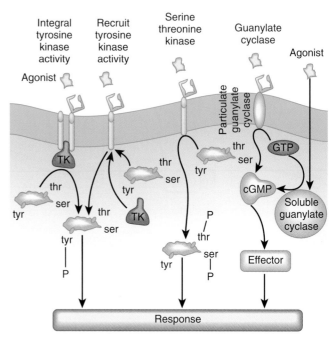

Figure 20-11.   *TK*, Tyrosine kinase; *tyr*, tyrosine; *thr*, threonine, *ser*, serine.

regulation, removing an important check on uncontrolled growth.

EGFR/HER

- The epidermal growth factor (EGF) pathway plays an important role in neoplasia. Four receptors belong to the EGF pathway: EGFR and human epidermal growth factors (HER2, HER3, HER4).
- When not bound by ligand, EGFR remains in a closed conformation. When growth factors bind, the receptor "opens" into a conformation that is able to dimerize with other receptors. Once the growth factor binds to this receptor, cell growth is stimulated.
- Trastuzumab antagonizes the HER2 receptor. The HER2 receptor is overexpressed in many breast cancers. Binding of trastuzumab to HER2 appears to inhibit cancers by promoting apoptosis and by reducing cell proliferation.

BCR-ABL/src

- Chronic myelogenous leukemia (CML) is most frequently caused by a chromosomally abnormal hematopoietic stem cell. The BCR (**b**reak **p**oint **c**luster) gene of one chromosome and the ABL (**Ab**elson) gene of another chromosome translocate, moving from separate chromosomes onto the same chromosome, fusing to become one gene, known as BCR-ABL. BCR-ABL is referred to as a *fusion oncoprotein,* because these two genes, when joined together, are associated with the development of cancer.

■ Important to drug therapy, ABL codes for tyrosine kinase receptors. BCR-ABL creates a tyrosine kinase receptor that is constitutively active, meaning that it is **continually active**. Tyrosine kinase receptors are growth factor receptors, meaning that their continual activation leads to dysregulated growth of myeloid cells.

Other Kinases

■ Drugs that inhibit multiple kinases were originally thought to be disadvantageous because of an increased likelihood of side effects. Instead, it is now believed that targeting multiple kinases addresses the redundancy that is found among signaling pathways, perhaps leading to enhanced efficacy. Sorafenib and sunitinib are examples of multikinase inhibitors, and their targets include:
  ▲ VEGF receptor (VEGFR)
  ▲ Platelet-derived growth factor receptor (PDGFR)
    ● FMS-like tyrosine kinase (FLT3), which is part of the PDGF family of growth factor receptors
  ▲ Oncogenes: Kit

PHARMACOKINETICS

■ The small molecule tyrosine kinase inhibitors used in cancer are all orally administered. The monoclonal antibodies are administered by intravenous infusion.

■ The bioavailability of sorafenib is reduced with a high-fat meal; therefore it is recommended that it either be taken on an empty stomach or with a low- or moderate-fat meal.

■ Sunitinib and its active metabolites have a long elimination half-life (40 to 60 and 80 to 110 hours, respectively).

■ Sunitinib, sorafenib, imatinib, dasatinib, and erlotinib are all metabolized by CYP3A4. Interactions with known inhibitors or inducers of these isozymes are to be expected, and concomitant use should be avoided if possible. Because these agents are primarily eliminated by hepatic metabolism, no dose adjustments are required in patients with renal impairment.

INDICATIONS
Imatinib, Dasatinib

■ Chronic myelogenus leukemia (CML)
■ Philadelphia chromosome–positive (Ph+) acute lymphoblastic anemia (ALL)
■ GI stromal tumor (GIST)

Gefitinib, Erlotinib

■ Non–small cell lung cancer

Sorafenib

■ Hepatocellular carcinoma
■ Renal cell (clear cell) carcinoma

Sunitinib

■ Metastatic renal cell (clear cell) carcinoma
■ GIST

Lapatinib

■ Breast cancer

Trastuzumab

■ Breast cancers overexpressing HER2

Cetuximab

■ Cancers of the colon and rectum, head and neck

Panitumumab

■ Colorectal cancer

CONTRAINDICATIONS

■ See Advanced section for information on use in pregnancy.

SIDE EFFECTS

■ **Diarrhea**
■ **Rash**: common with EGFR inhibitors, likely because of inhibition of epidermal turnover

Serious
Sorafenib, Sunitinib

■ **Hypertension**: VEGF inhibition reduces factors involved in vascular compliance.

Sorafenib, Imatinib

■ **Left ventricular dysfunction**: Cardiotoxicity with imatinib may be caused by mitochondrial dysfunction. Cardiomyocytes are highly energy dependent. The mechanism is not clear with sorafenib, but because the drug is a multikinase inhibitor, it might be inhibiting a kinase involved in myocardial function.

Dasatinib, Imatinib

■ **Bone marrow suppression (thrombocytopenia, neutropenia, anemia)**: The mechanism for this effect is not established, but it may be the result of inhibition of progenitor cells. Usually it is of concern only at higher doses
■ **Hemorrhage** from thrombocytopenia may occur.
■ **Fluid retention**: The mechanism for this effect has not been established.

Sorafenib, Sunitinib, Dasatinib

■ **QT prolongation** occurs, possibly because of interactions with a specific potassium ion channel. This channel facilitates the rapid component of myocardial repolarization and is associated with congenital long QT syndrome.

Gefitinib, Erlotinib

■ **Interstitial lung disease**: This side effect appears to be closely associated with the mechanism of action (EGFR blockade), as populations in which tumors respond well to these agents appear to be at higher risk of this side effect.

Erlotinib

■ **Hepatotoxicity**: Rare cases of hepatotoxicity, including liver failure, have been reported with erlotinib.

Trastuzumab

- **Cardiotoxicity**: Ventricular dysfunction and heart failure have been observed. The mechanism has not been established, although the impact of HER2 blockade on protein synthesis and cell survival pathways is one possibility.
- **Hypersensitivity reactions** are typically seen with monoclonal antibodies.
- **Pulmonary toxicity**: Pneumonitis and pleural effusions, among others, have been observed rarely. The mechanism is unknown.

Cetuximab, Panitumumab

- **Cardiopulmonary arrest** is a rare side effect seen in trials in head and neck cancer.
- **Hypomagnesemia** is a common side effect. The mechanism is not established, but it may be a result of alterations in renal transporters for magnesium.

IMPORTANT NOTES

- The tyrosine kinase inhibitors are collectively referred to as *targeted* therapies, a reflection of the fact that they target growth factors that are active only in cancer. The theoretical advantage of targeted therapies is enhanced selective toxicity and avoidance of disabling side effects such as GI effects, myelosuppression, and alopecia. It is important to note, though, that these side effects still occur with many of these targeted therapies but at a lower incidence than with conventional chemotherapy.
- Although the multikinase inhibitors both attack similar targets, sunitinib appears to have stronger binding affinity for many of these targets and therefore enhanced efficacy over sorafenib.

Advanced
Drug Interactions

- Dasatinib absorption may be decreased by antacids, so they should be administered at least 2 hours apart.

Pharmacogenetics

- Dasatinib is one of the first examples of a drug that was specifically designed to target mutations that had developed to the drug of choice for this indication, imatinib.

Pregnancy

- The extent of risk for all the tyrosine kinase inhibitors in pregnancy is approximately the same. Because they inhibit growth factors, in many cases angiogenic growth factors, there is serious concern about their effects on fetal development. These agents are therefore not recommended in pregnancy unless the withdrawal of therapy represents unacceptable risk to the mother.

FYI

- The Abelson (ABL) in BCR-ABL is named for the Abelson virus, which can cause leukemia.
- The translocation that results in the formation of the BCR-ABL fusion oncoprotein is called the *Philadelphia chromosome*. It was named after the city in which it was discovered.
- The tyrosine kinase inhibitors ending in -*nib* (e.g., erlotinib, imatinib) are often referred to as *small-molecule* tyrosine kinase inhibitors to distinguish them from the tyrosine kinase inhibitors that are monoclonal antibodies. Because monoclonal antibodies are proteins, they have a much larger structure.
- The tyrosine kinase receptors are known by several names, making it very confusing. For example, HER2 (human epidermal growth factor receptor 2) and ERBB2 are names for the same receptor. *HER2/neu* is the gene for HER2, so this receptor is also referred to as *HER2/neu*.

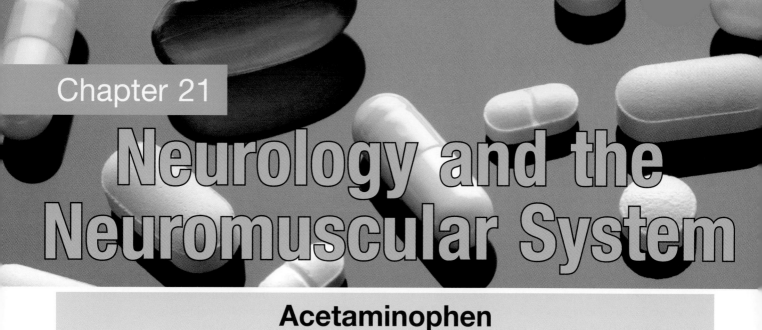

Chapter 21

Neurology and the Neuromuscular System

Acetaminophen

DESCRIPTION
Acetaminophen is an analgesic and antipyretic.

PROTOTYPE AND COMMON DRUGS
- Prototype: acetaminophen (also called *paracetamol*)
- Antidote: *N*-acetylcysteine (NAC)

MOA (MECHANISM OF ACTION) (Figure 21-1)

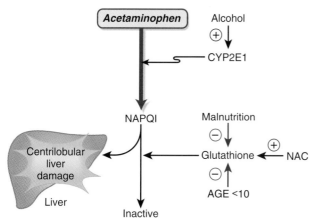

Figure 21-1.

- Acetaminophen is neither a narcotic nor a nonsteroidal antiinflammatory drug (NSAID). It is in a drug class of its own called **aniline** analgesics.
- Acetaminophen has analgesic and antipyretic effects similar to those of aspirin and NSAIDs and most likely exerts its effects through the inhibition of cyclooxygenase (COX).
- COX catalyzes the formation of prostaglandins (PGs) and other mediators that are important in the processing and signaling of pain and control of the thermoregulatory center in the brain.
- In contrast to NSAIDs and aspirin, acetaminophen is not an antiplatelet agent, nor does it possess antiinflammatory

properties; therefore there are differences in the mechanism of action compared with aspirin or NSAIDs:
- ▲ **Tissue selectivity**: Acetaminophen demonstrates variable COX inhibition in different tissues. Of primary importance, it inhibits prostaglandin E_2 (PGE_2) production in the central nervous system (CNS), which is probably the primary mediator of its analgesic and antipyretic properties.
- ▲ **COX site binding**: COX possesses two different catalytic sites: a COX site and a peroxidase site. Acetylsalicylic acid (ASA) and NSAIDs inhibit the COX site, whereas acetaminophen inhibits the peroxidase site.
- ▲ **Inhibition by hydroperoxide**: Hydroperoxide is produced by macrophages, which are important inflammatory cells; the hydroperoxide at the sites of inflammation displaces acetaminophen from the peroxidase site and thus dramatically limits the potential antiinflammatory action of acetaminophen. Furthermore, platelet 12-lipoxygenase produces hydroperoxide in platelets, which is likely the explanation for lack of antiplatelet effect by acetaminophen.

PHARMACOKINETICS
- Acetaminophen is metabolized in the liver by conjugation with sulfate or glucuronate (90%) and by CYP2E1 enzymes (5%), and the remainder is secreted unchanged in the urine (5%). The CYP2E1 enzyme pathway is particularly important because it is the basis for **acetaminophen toxicity**.

INDICATIONS
- Analgesia
- Antipyretic (reduces fever)

CONTRAINDICATIONS
- None of significance

SIDE EFFECTS
- Increased risk for asthma

IMPORTANT NOTES

■ Therapeutic doses of acetaminophen have no effect on the cardiovascular and respiratory systems or platelet function and do not produce gastric irritation, erosion, or bleeding.

Overdose

■ Acetaminophen exposure is the most commonly reported drug exposure reported to U.S. poison control centers.

■ The **therapeutic index** is about 10: the toxic dose is 10 times greater than the therapeutic dose (15 mg/kg versus 150 mg/kg). For example, if you weigh 100 kg, then an upper limit of a therapeutic dose would theoretically be 1500 mg and a toxic dose would be 15,000 mg. To put this in perspective, tablets and suppositories are usually in the range of 325 to 650 mg each. A U.S. Food and Drug Administration (FDA) panel of experts in 2009 recommended that the maximum single dose of acetaminophen in adults be lowered from 1000 to 650 mg.

■ Inadvertent co-ingestion of acetaminophen with other medications that also contain acetaminophen (such as cold remedies) is a cause of accidental overdose. Overdose can also occur with repeated *subtoxic* doses that, when combined over time, become toxic.

■ Because of hepatic metabolism, the liver is the predominant organ that is initially injured, and **fatal hepatic necrosis** can occur in severe and untreated overdoses. In less severe conditions, significant liver injury and dysfunction can occur, resulting in an increase in transaminases (aspartate transaminase [AST], alanine transaminase [ALT]) and abnormalities in coagulation because of abnormal production of hepatic coagulation proteins.

■ The mechanism of injury is as follows:
  ▲ Acetaminophen is metabolized in the liver via CYP2E1 to *N*-acetyl-*p*-benzoquinone imine (**NAPQI**). NAPQI is highly reactive, electrophilic, and toxic.
  ▲ NAPQI is quickly reduced by the natural antioxidant glutathione (**GSH**), a process that consumes GSH.
  ▲ When GSH stores become depleted, then NAPQI accumulates in the liver and starts to react with hepatocytes and proteins, causing permanent cellular damage. Injury is most prevalent where CYP2E1 activity is highest, which is in a centrilobular distribution.
  ▲ Less commonly, the same process can also occur in the kidney (see Figure 21-1).

■ Treatment is specifically targeted at replenishing GSH stores. This is accomplished through the administration of a GSH precursor called **N-acetylcysteine** (**NAC**).

■ NAC has been proposed to function as an antidote to acetaminophen via two *additional* mechanisms in addition to replenishment of GSH:
  ▲ NAC can substitute directly for GSH because it has antioxidant properties and directly reduces NAPQI.
  ▲ NAC provides sulfur to enhance the nontoxic conjugation pathway of acetaminophen metabolism.

■ Side effects of NAC include severe anaphylactoid reactions.

■ Acetaminophen is commonly marketed in combination with other medications. Common combinations include the following:
  ▲ Antihistamines and decongestants in common cold remedies
  ▲ Narcotic (codeine and oxycodone) combinations for added analgesia

Advanced

■ Factors that could increase the probability of acetaminophen toxicity include:
  ▲ Differences in CYP2E1 activity: increased activity would generate NAPQI faster and have a higher probability of toxicity.
    • Chronic alcohol consumption: increased activity
    • Genetic differences: variable activity
  ▲ Preexisting low GSH stores
    • Malnutrition
    • Age <10 years old
  ▲ Reduced capacity for hepatic conjugation (which would result in a great percentage of ingested drug to be metabolized by CYP2E1)

EVIDENCE

Analgesia

Acetaminophen versus Placebo for Treatment of Osteoarthritis

■ A Cochrane review in 2005 (seven studies) demonstrated that acetaminophen was superior to placebo in five of the seven randomized controlled trials (RCTs). A pooled analysis demonstrated a statistically significant but minimal difference that is of questionable clinical significance. The relative percent improvement in pain score from baseline was 5%, with an absolute change of 4 points on a 0-to-100 scale.

Acetaminophen versus Nonsteroidal Antiinflammatory Drugs for Treatment of Osteoarthritis

■ The same Cochrane review in 2005 (10 studies) demonstrated that acetaminophen was less effective overall than NSAIDs in terms of pain reduction, global assessments, and improvements in functional status. Patients taking traditional NSAIDS were more likely to experience an adverse GI event (relative risk [RR] 1.47). However, the median trial duration was only 6 weeks, which is too short to adequately assess adverse outcomes.

Acetaminophen plus Codeine versus Placebo

■ A Cochrane review in 2008 (26 studies, N = 2295 patients) of *postoperative patients* demonstrated significant differences for obtaining at least 50% pain relief over 4 to 6 hours, with a number needed to treat (NNT) of 2.2 for high doses (800 to 1000 mg acetaminophen plus 60 mg codeine) and smaller effect sizes for medium and smaller doses (as low as 325 mg acetaminophen with 30 mg codeine).

Acetaminophen Plus Codeine versus Acetaminophen Alone

■ A Cochrane review in 2008 (14 studies, N = 926 patients) of *postoperative patients* demonstrated that addition of codeine increased the proportion of participants achieving at least 50% pain relief over 4 to 6 hours by 10% to 15% and reduced the proportion of patients needing rescue medication by about 15%.

Safety
Risk of Asthma

■ A meta-analysis in 2009 (19 studies, N = 425,140 patients) demonstrated a pooled odds ratio (OR) of 1.63 for asthma among users of acetaminophen; that is, acetaminophen increased the risk of asthma by 60%. This risk was also present in children. Included studies were observational (no RCTs).

FYI

■ Nomenclature: By selective letter choosing, the drug names have been created as follows:
  ▲ Acetaminophen: para-**acetyl**amin**ophen**ol
  ▲ Paracetamol: **para**-**acet**yl**am**inophenol
  ▲ Tylenol: para-ace**tyl**aminoph**enol**
■ Para-acetaminophenol is probably one of very few drugs with two true generic names.
■ An *aniline* is a benzene ring with an attached NH_2.

Opioids

DESCRIPTION

Opioids bind opioid receptors and are primarily used for analgesia.

COMMON DRUGS

■ Morphine
■ Codeine
■ Semisynthetic:
  ▲ Oxy**codone**, hydro**codone**
  ▲ Diacetyl**morph**ine (heroin), hydro**morph**one, oxy**morphone**
■ Synthetic:
  ▲ **Fentanyl**, su**fentanil**, remi**fentanil**
  ▲ Loperamide, methadone
  ▲ Meperidine (pethidine)
■ Partial agonists:
  ▲ Nalbuphine, butorphanol, buprenorphine, pentazocine, tramadol
■ Antagonists:
  ▲ **Nal**oxone
  ▲ **Nal**trexone
    • Methylnaltrexone

MOA (MECHANISM OF ACTION)

■ The pain pathways in the body are very complex and only briefly summarized here. In short, opioids reduce the signaling and processing of pain pathways through a variety of receptor types, receptor locations, and complex interactions.
■ **Endogenous** opioids (endorphins, enkephalins, and dynorphins) stimulate the opioid receptors.
■ Exogenous opioids also bind multiple opioid receptors (Table 21-1). Opioid receptors are present in both the brain and the spinal cord, specifically:
  ▲ **Spinal cord:** dorsal horn
  ▲ **Brain:**

TABLE 21-1. Main Classes of Opioid Receptors

Receptor	Action
Mu (μ)	Sedation and euphoria Inhibition of respiration Slowed gastrointestinal transit (receptors in the bowel) Modulation of hormone and neurotransmitter release
Kappa (κ)	Dysphoria (through inhibition of dopamine release) Modulation of hormone and neurotransmitter release
Delta (δ)	Psychotomimetic (hallucinogenic) effects Slowed gastrointestinal transit

  • Thalamus (specifically the ventral caudal thalamus)
  • Descending inhibitory pathways (to the dorsal horn):
    ○ Periaqueductal gray area medulla (specifically the rostral ventral medulla)
    ○ Locus ceruleus
■ The **descending pathways** in the spinal cord decrease the pain processing that occurs in the spinal cord.
■ The opioid receptors are G protein coupled to the inhibitory G protein (G_i), but the downstream effects of each receptor are dependent on the cell type where it is located.

PHARMACOKINETICS (Table 21-2)

■ For equivalency, note that:
  ▲ Oral doses are less potent because of first-pass effect; oral doses are larger.
    • Codeine and oxycodone have a lower first-pass metabolism effect and therefore are effective when given orally.
  ▲ Fentanyl and sufentanil doses are measured in micrograms and are therefore much more potent than all other narcotics listed; remember that potency and efficacy are not the same.

TABLE 21-2. Important Characteristics of Some Commonly Used Opioids

Opioid	Equivalent Dose	Duration (h)	Efficacy
Codeine, oral	60 mg	3-4	Low
Oxycodone, oral	5 mg	3-4	Moderate
Hydrocodone	10 mg		Moderate
Hydromorphone, **oral**	2-3 mg	4-6	High
Hydromorphone, **intravenous**	0.2-0.3 mg	3-4	High
Morphine, **oral**	10 mg	3-4	High
Morphine, **intravenous**	2-3 mg	2-3	High
Methadone, oral	10 mg	6-8	High
Fentanyl, intravenous	50 mcg	1	High
Sufentanil, intravenous	10 mcg	1	High
Remifentanil, intravenous	Infusion	Minutes	High

▲ Lower-efficacy drugs (codeine, oxycodone, and hydrocodone) cannot produce as much analgesia as the high-efficacy narcotics.

■ Routes of administration:
  ▲ Oral and parenteral (intravenous, intramuscular, and subcutaneous) routes are the most common.
  ▲ Neuraxial (injected into the epidural or intrathecal spaces) administration by anesthesiologists is common as an adjunct to spinal or epidural anesthesia.
  ▲ Transdermal, rectal, and mucosal (oral lozenges) dosage forms also exist.

■ Important metabolites:
  ▲ Most opioids are metabolized by CYP3A4 and renally eliminated (except where the following information states otherwise).
  ▲ Morphine → morphine-3-glucuronide (90%), morphine-6-glucuronide (10%).
    • Morphine is metabolized by the liver (CYP3A4) and excreted by the kidneys.
    • The glucuronides (being water soluble) are eliminated by the kidneys; renal disease can prolong and increase the effects of morphine.
    • The glucuronides are water soluble; thus they do not *readily* cross the blood-brain barrier, but with high concentrations of drug, brain levels will increase.
    • Morphine-6-glucuronide is more potent and longer acting than the parent compound morphine. Its accumulation can result in an increased and prolonged opioid effect
    • Morphine-3-glucuronide is a neuroexcitant. It can cause seizures if it accumulates.
  ▲ Codeine → morphine (via CYP2D6)
    • Genetic variation in CYP2D6 has been implicated in the varying efficacy of codeine in different patients. Conversion of codeine to morphine is required for its efficacy.
  ▲ Meperidine → normeperidine
    • Normeperidine is a neuroexcitant. Accumulation (after repeated doses or in patients with renal failure) can cause seizures.

  ▲ Remifentanil is an ester and is metabolized within minutes by pseudocholinesterase. Its metabolites are essentially inactive.
  ▲ Diacetylmorphine (heroin) → morphine
    • Heroin, an ester, is converted to morphine via an esterase reaction, which is a fast reaction.
    • Heroin therefore has a very fast onset. Speed of onset is associated with the addictive profile of drugs. Faster-onset drugs are more addictive.

INDICATIONS
■ Analgesia
■ Antitussive (cough medication)
■ Antidiarrheal
■ Dyspnea (sensation of difficulty breathing)

CONTRAINDICATIONS
■ History of **addiction**: Caution must be used.
■ Decreased **level of consciousness**: There is an increased risk of further decreased level of consciousness and resultant respiratory compromise.
■ Coadministration of **sedatives** will greatly increase the risk of respiratory depression; caution must be used.

SIDE EFFECTS
■ **Respiratory depression**: All narcotics are powerful respiratory depressants. They can cause hypoventilation, hypoxia, and apnea. The effect is dose dependent. Low-efficacy opioids (codeine) are less likely to result in profound respiratory depression.
■ **Nausea and vomiting**: Some patients are exquisitely sensitive. This is a very common side effect. The mechanism involves stimulation of the chemoreceptor trigger zone, the area of the brain responsible for vomiting.
■ **Pruritus (itching)**: This effect is not mediated by histamine (the most common mediator for itchy skin) but is rather a centrally (in the brain) mediated effect. Patients will often scratch their nose about 45 seconds after receiving intravenous fentanyl. For some patients the itching can be very uncomfortable and distressing and could

mandate changing to a different opioid or stopping opioids completely.

- **Addiction:** Opioids are among the most commonly abused medications.
- **Urinary retention:** Difficulty emptying the bladder may develop.
- **Constipation:** This effect can be extremely severe. Codeine even in low doses can produce profound constipation. Mu receptors in the bowel are responsible for this side effect.
- **Miosis:** Constriction of pupils is common.
- **Truncal rigidity:** The thorax and abdomen can exhibit increased muscular tone. This effect is more common in patients administered high doses of the synthetic opioid fentanyl and related opioids. It usually does not occur with typical doses of morphine or codeine.
- **Sphincter of Oddi spasm:** Constriction of the sphincter of Oddi can occur; this causes very significant abdominal pain. It can be reversed with naloxone or glucagon.

IMPORTANT NOTES

- The cardinal signs of narcotic overadministration (or abuse) include the following:
  - ▲ Low respiratory rate (or apnea), hypoventilation (elevated PCO_2), and hypoxia
  - ▲ Miosis (constricted pupils)
  - ▲ Decreased level of consciousness
  - ▲ Needle puncture lesions and phlebitis (inflammation of veins); sometimes called *track marks*
- The cardinal signs of opioid withdrawal include rhinorrhea, lacrimation, yawning, chills, piloerection (goose bumps), hyperventilation, hyperthermia, mydriasis, muscular aches, vomiting, diarrhea, anxiety, and hostility.
- A new antagonist called **methylnaltrexone** is a methylated version of naltrexone. It is special because it does not cross the blood-brain barrier. Therefore it has the ability to antagonize all the *peripherally mediated* side effects of narcotics (mostly constipation) without reducing the analgesic effects (which are mediated within the CNS). The most common indication for methylnaltrexone is treatment of constipation.
- **Loperamide** is an antidiarrheal opioid. It is absorbed very poorly from the gastrointestinal tract and therefore, when given orally, acts on mu receptors in the stomach, intestine, and colon only, reducing motility.
- **Methadone** is most commonly used to control withdrawal symptoms in patients who are recovering from narcotic addiction (usually heroin) because it has a long half-life. Furthermore, methadone is also an N-methyl-D-aspartate (NMDA) receptor antagonist, and this property has been implicated in a role of preventing tolerance to methadone. NMDA antagonists are also analgesics. Methadone also has monoamine oxidase inhibitor (MAOI) properties. MAOIs are antidepressants.
- **Tramadol** is a very weak mu agonist whose mechanism of action is predominantly based on blockade of serotonin reuptake. It does not cause respiratory depression. It can

cause seizures, as can meperidine, which is in the same chemical class.

- **The partial agonists** all have kappa receptor activity and only limited mu receptor activity. This is significant because the mu receptor mediates analgesia, so partial agonists are less effective analgesics than full agonists.
  - ▲ **Partial agonists** should never be mixed with **full agonists.** The results are unpredictable.
- **Opioid antagonists** can precipitate severe withdrawal in patients who are physically dependent on opioids. They should be administered carefully.
- **Tolerance:** Opioid receptor down-regulation occurs with chronic administration of opioids. The result is that higher and higher doses are required to achieve the same effect. *Neuromodulation* is another term for tolerance.
- Although respiratory depression is a side effect of opioids, the same mechanism is responsible for **reducing the ventilatory drive** in patients who are short of breath; therefore opioids can reduce the unpleasant sensation of breathlessness and can be effective at relieving discomfort related to breathing in selected patients.

Advanced

- Patients of Asian descent (e.g., Chinese) are often more sensitive to opioids and usually require smaller doses.
- Patients who consume narcotics on a daily basis can have very significant levels of tolerance and require doses that are many times higher than narcotic naïve patients.
- **Meperidine** is the only opioid with local anesthetic properties.

EVIDENCE
Opioids versus Nonsteroidal Antiinflammatory Drugs for Treatment of Renal Colic

- A systematic review in 2004 (20 trials, 1613 participants) found that both NSAIDs and opioids led to clinically important reductions in patient-reported pain scores. Pooled analysis of six trials showed a greater reduction in pain scores for patients treated with NSAIDs than with opioids. Patients treated with NSAIDs were significantly less likely to require rescue analgesia (RR 0.75). Most trials showed a higher incidence of adverse events in patients treated with opioids. Compared with patients treated with opioids, those treated with NSAIDs had significantly less vomiting (0.35).

Opioids for Treatment of Chronic Back Pain

- A systematic review in 2007 examined multiple questions pertaining to opioid treatment of chronic low back pain. 11 studies showed that there was significant variation in how opioids are prescribed for chronic low back pain. A meta-analysis of the four studies assessing the efficacy of opioids compared with placebo or a nonopioid control did not show reduced pain with opioids. A meta-analysis of the five studies directly comparing the efficacy of different opioids demonstrated a nonsignificant reduction in pain from baseline.

▲ With respect to risk of addiction, the prevalence of lifetime substance use disorders ranged from 36% to 56%; the prevalence of current substance use disorders was as high as 43%; and aberrant medication-taking behaviors ("drug seeking") ranged from 5% to 24%. The authors found that the study was limited by retrieval and publication biases and poor study quality. No trial evaluating the efficacy of opioids was longer than 16 weeks.

■ A Cochrane review in 2007 (3 studies, 908 patients) found tramadol (a weak opioid) to be superior to placebo for decreasing pain and improving activities of daily living in patients with chronic back pain.

Opioids for Treatment of Dyspnea in Cancer Patients

■ A systematic review in 2008 found clinical and statistical significant benefit for dyspnea with systemic opioids administered orally or parenterally (average improvement was not quantified). Nebulized (inhaled) opioids were not effective at treating dyspnea.

FYI

■ The term *opioid* refers broadly to all compounds related to opium, although only morphine and codeine are actually produced by the opium poppy, *Papaver somniferum.*

■ The name *morphine* is from Morpheus, the Greek god of dreams. Morphine was first isolated in 1803 by Sertürner.

■ The word *opium* is derived from the Greek word *opos* meaning juice.

■ The word *narcotic* is derived from the Greek word meaning stupor. The term *narcotic* is often used in a legal context to refer to a variety of illegal substances; the term in medical vocabulary refers only to opioids.

■ Etorphine is an opioid with about 2000 times the potency of morphine. It is used as a large animal immobilizer (for veterinary use). One drop on the skin of a human would be fatal because of the profound respiratory depression. Carfentanil, another veterinary opioid, is 10,000 times more potent than morphine (and 10 times more potent than sufentanil, the most potent opioid for humans). Nonhuman mammals do not experience the same degree of respiratory depression as humans do, and so these drugs are suitable as immobilizing agents in large animals.

■ Mint and cannabis (in marijuana) are weak κ opioid receptor agonists.

■ Some opioid category names include the following:
  ▲ Phenanthrenes (naturally occurring): morphine, codeine
  ▲ Phenylpiperidines: meperidine, tramadol
  ▲ Anilidopiperidines: fentanyl, sufentanil, remifentanil
  ▲ Morphinans: butorphanol, nalbuphine

α_2 Agonists

DESCRIPTION

α_2 Agonists stimulate α_2 receptors with varying degrees of specificity.

PROTOTYPE AND COMMON DRUGS

■ Prototype: clonidine
■ Others: dexmedetomidine, apraclonidine, brimonidine

MOA (MECHANISM OF ACTION)

■ Glaucoma is characterized by increased intraocular pressure (IOP). Strategies to reduce intraocular pressure include reducing the production and secretion of aqueous humor and facilitating its drainage.

■ The exact mechanism by which α_2 agonists reduce IOP has not been established, but is likely multifactorial, employing several strategies:
  ▲ Reducing aqueous humor production:
    • α_2 Receptors in the ciliary body are stimulated.
    • Stimulation of α_2 receptors leads to feedback inhibition of norepinephrine release, leading to reduced stimulation of β receptors and reduced aqueous humor production.
  ▲ Enhancing aqueous humor outflow
■ Through a secondary mechanism, brimonidine may also have a neuroprotective role, mitigating the damage to the optic nerve caused by the elevated IOP.

■ The antihypertensive effect of α_2 agonists is a result of inhibition of presynaptic release of vasoconstrictors such as norepinephrine. Recall that the α_2 receptor is an autoreceptor (see Chapter 3). An autoreceptor is a receptor that when stimulated by an agonist, reduces release of transmitter into the synaptic cleft.

■ The sedative effect of α_2 agonists is caused by central inhibition of neurotransmitter release.

PHARMACOKINETICS

■ Brimonidine and apraclonidine are administered topically to the eye, and only a small amount reaches the systemic circulation.

■ Clonidine, on the other hand, is administered orally and is also available as a transdermal patch. Dexmedetomidine is administered intravenously.

INDICATIONS
Clonidine, Dexmedetomidine (Systemically Administered)

■ Hypertension (not first line)
■ Sedation

Brimonidine, Apraclonidine (Eye Drops Only)
- Glaucoma (open angle)
- Increased intraocular pressure

CONTRAINDICATIONS
- **Concomitant MAOIs:** MAOIs prevent the breakdown of norepinephrine, and this could lead to elevated blood pressure.

Clonidine, Dexmedetomidine
- **Patients with severe bradyarrhythmia:** Clonidine can induce marked bradycardia in some individuals.
- **Hypotension:** These agents lower blood pressure, so giving them to a patient with hypotension may drop the pressure to dangerously low levels.

SIDE EFFECTS
Oral Use
- **Dry mouth** is likely a centrally mediated effect, although the mechanism has not been confirmed.
- **Sedation:** Stimulation of central α_2 receptors has an inhibitory effect on neurotransmitter release. This is the desired effect when used for sedation.
- **Bradycardia,** likely caused by inhibition of catecholamine release, can be significant in some individuals.
- **Hypotension:** This is the desired effect when the drug is used as an antihypertensive but becomes a side effect in the sedation of patients who have normal (or low) blood pressure.

Topical Use (Brimonidine, Apraclonidine)
- **Ocular hyperemia, burning, stinging, and blurring** may occur.
- **Serious, rare** side effects have been observed in infants <3 months old, such as hypotension, bradycardia, hypothermia, apnea, dyspnea, and lethargy.

IMPORTANT NOTES
- The ability of clonidine to modulate neurotransmitter release has also led to its increasing use in attention-deficit/hyperactivity disorder (ADHD).
- Dexmedetomidine is an intravenous formulation that is available in some countries.

Advanced
- Although clonidine has been in use for several decades, the exact mechanism by which it exerts its antihypertensive effects is still in question.
- Clonidine is an imidazoline and binds to imidazoline (I) receptors.

EVIDENCE
In Primary Open Angle Glaucoma and Ocular Hypertension
- A 2007 Cochrane review of all medical interventions for glaucoma and ocular hypertension found three trials comparing brimonidine to timolol. There were no differences in visual field progression (glaucoma) or visual field defects (ocular hypertension) within 1 year. Timolol was better tolerated than brimonidine, as measured by the incidence of dropouts from drug-related adverse events (OR 0.21). There were no trials comparing brimonidine with placebo.

FYI
- Other antihypertensives target imidazoline receptors, including moxonidine, which like clonidine also targets α_2 receptors. Unlike clonidine, moxonidine primarily targets imidazoline receptors and has a secondary effect at α_2, whereas the reverse is true for clonidine.

Inhaled Anesthetics

DESCRIPTION
Used by anesthesiologists, these drugs are one component of a general anesthetic.

COMMON DRUGS
- Halogenated agents: halothane, isoflurane, sevoflurane, desflurane (older agents not listed)
- Other: nitrous oxide

MOA (MECHANISM OF ACTION) (Figure 21-2)
- The primary site of action in causing CNS depression is most likely the γ-aminobutyric acid A (**GABA$_A$**) **receptor.** Inhaled anesthetics activate these receptors.
- The GABA$_A$ receptor is linked to a **chloride** channel; this is important because one way to *turn off* a neuron is to **hyperpolarize** it so that it cannot be *depolarized* enough to trigger an action potential. Opening a chloride channel will allow the negatively charged chloride ion to enter the cell and will reduce the electrical charge inside the cell (thereby hyperpolarizing it) and effectively render the neuron unresponsive to incoming stimuli that would otherwise depolarize the cell.

PHARMACOKINETICS
- As their name suggests, these drugs are administered only via inhalation. They are supplied in liquid form and then

Inhaled anesthetics

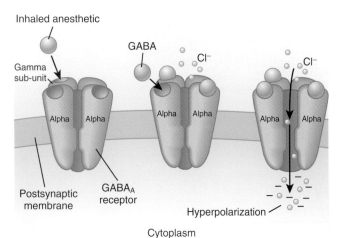

Figure 21-2.

vaporized using very precise vaporizers that are part of the anesthetic machine, the anesthetic oxygen and air mixture is combined with calculated doses of the inhaled anesthetic.

- Very small amounts of the drug are metabolized. For example, desflurane undergoes <0.02% metabolism, which is clinically insignificant. Older drugs had higher rates of metabolism, with halothane as high as 40%.
- The route of elimination is exhalation.
- Inhaled anesthetics move through the body by dissolving in the blood and distributing into tissues; the important tissue interfaces include the following:
  ▲ Lung ⇔ blood
  ▲ Blood ⇔ brain (and other *vessel-rich* tissues such as liver, kidney)
  ▲ Blood ⇔ fat (and other *vessel-poor* tissues)
    • When inhaled anesthetics are administered, the drug must enter the lungs, then the blood, then the brain.
    • For inhaled anesthetics to be eliminated, drug must exit the brain and other tissues, be carried to the lungs, and then exhaled.
    • Vessel-poor tissues are slow to take up and release drug. Therefore vessel-poor tissues can act as a *sink* and slowly absorb drug at the *early* parts of an anesthetic procedure (lowering the drug levels) but then at the *end* of a long anesthetic procedure can release drug, prolonging elimination of the drug.
  ▲ The **solubility** of an inhaled anesthetic affects the speed at which it is taken up by the body and exerts its action (speed of onset). The key point is that the **partial pressure** is the measure of the drug's *active form*. If a drug has a **high solubility,** then a lot of drug needs to be absorbed into blood and tissues before the partial pressure starts to rise; **this impedes the onset** of action of the drug. If the

solubility is low, then the partial pressure will rise quickly. Conversely, eliminating the drug follows the same rules, and high solubility correlates with slower elimination because more drug had to be dissolved into the body initially to achieve the desired partial pressure.
- Solubility is described for the blood and is called the **blood/gas coefficient.** The smaller the number, the less soluble the drug is in blood and therefore the faster it can change its partial pressure (because only a small amount of drug actually needs to be dissolved into the blood). The agents are ranked from *fastest to slowest* (lowest to highest solubility coefficient) as follows:
  ○ Desflurane < sevoflurane < isoflurane < halothane

INDICATIONS
- General anesthesia
- Severe refractory status asthmaticus (rare indication)

CONTRAINDICATION
- **Malignant hyperthermia (MH):** Inhaled anesthetics are one of the two triggers for MH. The other trigger is succinylcholine. A family history or personal history of MH is an **absolute** contraindication for the administration of these drugs.

SIDE EFFECTS
- **Hypotension** may occur.
- **Respiratory depression:** The respiratory drive in response to carbon dioxide is blunted, and blood CO_2 levels rise. The tidal volume is reduced, but the respiratory rate is actually increased (the reverse occurs with opioid respiratory depression).
- **Hepatic damage:** Very rare cases (1 in 30,000) have possibly been associated with **halothane,** but clearly defined cause and effect have not been established
- **Kidney damage** is a theoretical concern with **sevoflurane** in that it can produce a degradation byproduct from the carbon dioxide absorbents in the anesthetic machine called **compound A.** This has never clinically translated into renal damage in humans, however.

IMPORTANT NOTES
- The potency of inhaled anesthetics is measured by the **minimum anesthetic concentration (MAC),** which is strictly defined as the dose of inhaled anesthetic required to *prevent movement* in *50% of the population* in response to a *surgical stimulus* when *no other drugs* are administered. For example, the MAC of desflurane is 6%. Note that this definition is not the same as *the dose required to keep someone asleep.* Drugs such as opioids decrease the MAC requirements of a drug and are called *MAC-sparing agents.*
- Inhaled anesthetics cause hypotension. The primary mechanism is through vasodilation, although older agents (e.g., halothane) produced cardiac depression (decreased contractility and decreased heart rate), which caused hypotension.

- ▲ One indicator of anesthetic overdose is hypotension, although many different causes of hypotension can occur in the operating room.
- In addition to being vascular smooth muscle relaxants, inhaled anesthetics also relax bronchial smooth muscle and through this mechanism can help to relieve bronchospasm in rare cases of life-threatening refractory status asthmaticus.
- MH is a rare condition that is precipitated by **inhaled anesthetics** or **succinylcholine** (a paralyzing agent). It is caused by a *channelopathy*, which is a mutation in an ion channel in muscle. It is a life-threatening condition that occurs as a result of pathologically high levels of skeletal muscle contraction from **increased intracellular calcium** that occurs in the *absence* of neuromuscular stimulation. Because of the muscular contraction, the following effects occur:
  - ▲ Muscle rigidity leading to hyperthermia (similar to overheating in exercise)
  - ▲ Increased CO_2 production, heart rate, and blood pressure
  - ▲ Muscle breakdown leading to elevated potassium, creatine kinase (CK), and myoglobin in the blood
  - ▲ Renal failure caused by myoglobin
  - ▲ Metabolic acidosis caused by imbalance of oxygen supply/demand ratio in muscles, resulting in lactate production
- MH is treated with **dantrolene**, a drug that reduces intracellular calcium through binding the **ryanodine** receptor, which mediates calcium release from the sarcoplasmic reticulum.

Advanced

- **Nitrous oxide** has a MAC value of 104%. Therefore, it is not potent enough to be a solo anesthetic agent, because delivering a mixture of 100% nitrous oxide would mean that no oxygen could be delivered and the patient would die of asphyxiation. The greatest concentration that is administered is about 60% to 70%—a MAC value of 0.6 or 0.7. For this reason, nitrous is used only as an *adjuvant* drug for general anesthesia and is added to one of the other volatile anesthetics.
  - ▲ An oxygen–nitrous oxide mixture is often offered to women in labor as an analgesic drug to reduce the pain of contractions. It is inhaled through a mask at the start of and during contractions only.
- Xenon is a chemical that is also used as an inhaled anesthetic and in fact would be a very good inhaled anesthetic with few side effects. However, production costs are very high, and it is not commercially available.

FYI

- Ether was the first inhaled anesthetic. Most inhaled anesthetics (not including nitrous oxide or xenon) are fluorinated (fluorine is a halogen, thus the name "halogenated") derivatives of ether:
  - ▲ Ether: C-O-C backbone
  - ▲ Desflurane: C-C-O-C backbone with six fluorine atoms
  - ▲ Sevoflurane: C_2-C-O-C backbone with seven fluorine atoms
  - ▲ Isoflurane: C-C-O-C backbone with five fluorine atoms and one chlorine atom
- Earlier inhaled anesthetics such as chloroform and cyclopropane were flammable. They were mixed with oxygen, and the risk of explosion and fires resulted in their replacement.
- Nitrous oxide ("laughing gas") should not be confused with *nitric* oxide, a vasodilator that is also available as an inhaled drug.

Intravenous Anesthetics

DESCRIPTION

Intravenous anesthetics are also referred to as *general anesthetics* or *sedative-hypnotics*. The sedative effect is reduction of excitement (e.g., agitation or anxiety), whereas the hypnotic effect is production of sleep and unconsciousness.

PROTOTYPES AND COMMON DRUGS
GABA Mimetics

- Prototype: thiopental (pentothal)
- Others: propofol, etomidate, methohexital

NMDA Antagonists

- Prototype: Ketamine

MOA (MECHANISM OF ACTION)
γ-Aminobutyric Acid (GABA) (Figure 21-3)

- GABA is the major **inhibitory neurotransmitter** in the CNS. GABA binds to three different types of receptors: $GABA_A$, $GABA_B$, and $GABA_C$.
  - ▲ Binding of GABA to $GABA_A$ receptors leads to the opening of the chloride (Cl^-) channel, facilitating Cl^- influx and cellular hyperpolarization (making the inside more negative).
  - ▲ Hyperpolarization of a cell decreases the probability that the cell can be subsequently *de*polarized by other incoming excitatory signals; this will have a net inhibitory effect.

GABA acting IV anesthetics

Synaptic cleft

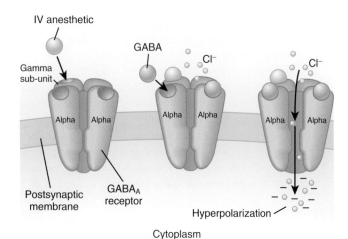

Figure 21-3.

■ Thiopental, propofol, and etomidate all bind to GABA$_A$ receptors and increase the influx of Cl$^-$ into the neuron, resulting in decreased neuronal activity.

N-Methyl-D-aspartate (NMDA)

■ Glutamate is an **excitatory neurotransmitter**, and NMDA receptors are one type of glutamate receptor.
■ Binding of glutamate to NMDA receptors results in opening of Ca^{2+} channels, leading to cellular depolarization and increased neuronal activity.
■ Blockade of glutamate at NMDA receptors therefore results in reduced excitation of neurons in the brain.

PHARMACOKINETICS

■ Intravenous anesthetics work within one *arm to brain* circulation time; that is, if the drug is administered through an intravenous line in the arm, it is the time required to circulate back to the heart and then up to the brain (usually less than 1 minute).
■ Compartmental distribution is a very important factor for intravenous anesthetics. When the drug is administered into the blood, it rapidly is taken up by the brain (inducing its effect), but very quickly the drug is also taken up by the *vessel-rich* organs (liver, muscle, kidney, heart), and this uptake quickly reduces the levels in the blood and therefore the brain in a matter of minutes. Therefore when the drug is given as a single bolus, the termination of action of the drug is primarily a result of redistribution of the drug and not metabolism or elimination of the drug. When the drug is given as an infusion, metabolism and elimination become important because all compartments would be equilibrated.

■ All drugs are hepatically metabolized and renally excreted. Chronic alcoholism induces hepatic enzymes and increases metabolism of all intravenous anesthetics.

INDICATIONS

■ In environments that include healthcare workers **skilled in resuscitation** and where **resuscitation equipment** is immediately available, indications include:
  ▲ Induction and/or maintenance of general anesthesia
  ▲ Sedation for procedures
  ▲ Intubation (placement of tube into trachea for mechanical ventilation)

CONTRAINDICATIONS

■ Lack of resuscitation knowledge, skill, or equipment
■ Lack of standard monitoring devices for vital signs

SIDE EFFECTS

■ **Respiratory depression:** The respiratory center is depressed with GABA agonists. It is typical for a patient who is administered a dose large enough to induce unconsciousness to develop apnea (to completely stop breathing). For this reason, administration of intravenous anesthetics (regardless of dose) must always be performed in the presence of healthcare workers who are skilled in respiratory resuscitation and who have respiratory resuscitation equipment immediately available.
■ **Hypotension:** Intravenous anesthetics, especially propofol, are myocardial depressants. They decrease contractility and often also reduce sympathetic nervous system activity.
■ **Addiction:** All drugs in this category both are psychologically addicting and induce physiologic dependence, tolerance, and withdrawal.
■ **Pain on injection** occurs with propofol and etomidate.
■ **Adrenal suppression** occurs with etomidate. For this reason, etomidate is not used as an infusion and is commonly used only as a single bolus.

IMPORTANT NOTES

■ All intravenous anesthetics have the potential for drug addiction.
■ **Dosage:** Some general concepts should be applied when choosing the dose of intravenous anesthetic. Administering a larger-than-required dose virtually guarantees significant hypotension:
  ▲ Elderly patients require *lower* doses compared with nonelderly adults, and children require higher doses (on a milligram-per-kilogram scale) compared with adults.
  ▲ Patients who are quite sick require *lower* doses.
  ▲ Chronic alcohol consumers require *higher* doses because alcohol also works on GABA receptors and results in GABA agonist tolerance owing to receptor downregulation. In fact, consumption of one alcoholic drink per day is enough to change responsiveness to GABA drugs.
    • The receptor tolerance in alcoholism is a stronger factor for requiring larger doses than is the increased

hepatic metabolism also induced by chronic alcohol abuse.

▲ Coadministration of other drugs (usually opioids) results in *lower* required doses.

■ **GABA-mimetics:**

▲ Do not have analgesic properties

▲ Cause apnea

▲ Lower cerebral blood flow and intracranial pressure (ICP)

■ **Ketamine:**

▲ In *contrast* to GABA-mimetic drugs, ketamine:

• Possesses **strong analgesic** properties

• Does **not cause apnea** when administered as a sole agent and given in typical therapeutic doses

• Is **dysphoric**: It produces very unpleasant sensations, hallucinations, and bad dreams. A benzodiazepine can be quite effective in reducing the dysphoria and is commonly coadministered with ketamine

• **Increases cerebral blood flow** (and potentially raises ICP), which is relevant in patients with brain injury or elevated ICP

▲ Causes **sympathetic nervous system activation** (resulting in increased heart rate and blood pressure) and therefore is the *least likely* to induce hypotension. However, it is still a direct myocardial depressant (reduces contractility), and in states in which the sympathetic nervous system is already highly activated (e.g., cardiogenic shock), ketamine retains potential for inducing hypotension.

▲ Causes **bronchodilation** (via sympathetic nervous system activation) and is therefore useful for intubation of patients with severe bronchospasm (asthmatic patients).

▲ Causes a **dissociative** state: Patients appear to be disconnected to what is happening around them and are unresponsive to stimuli; however, their eyes remain open, limbs may move involuntarily, and breathing is maintained.

■ **Propofol:**

▲ Is a strong **myocardial depressant** and should be given very cautiously, if at all, in patients with a weak heart (low systolic function).

▲ Is lipophilic and does not dissolve in water; therefore a lipid-containing, milk-colored emulsion is the vehicle in which it is administered. The emulsion **stings veins** when it is injected. It is often mixed with lidocaine, a local anesthetic, to reduce the stinging. A newer formulation called *fospropofol* is water soluble.

▲ Is now the intravenous general anesthetic most commonly used in North America. It has replaced thiopental, but thiopental is still used.

■ **Etomidate:**

▲ Has a much lower potential for lowering blood pressure compared with propofol or thiopental. It should be considered the drug of choice for patients at high risk for hypotension (e.g., those with severe cardiac disease or acute trauma with massive blood loss).

Advanced

■ Etomidate and propofol preferentially act at $GABA_A$ receptors that contain β_1 and β_2 *subunits* (not to be confused with the autonomic receptors with similar names). The β_2 subunit is probably the more important for mediating hypnotic and muscle-relaxing actions.

■ Barbiturates also facilitate the actions of GABA at multiple sites in the CNS, but in contrast to benzodiazepines they appear to increase the *duration* of the GABA-gated chloride channel openings. At high concentrations the barbiturates may also be GABA-mimetic, directly activating chloride channels.

■ Another type of excitatory glutamate receptor is the AMPA receptor. Barbiturates might also block the AMPA receptor, but this is not their primary mode of action.

FYI

■ Propofol was implicated in the death of Michael Jackson in 2009.

■ Dextromethorphan, an NMDA antagonist, is a commonly used cough suppressant and is found in many over-the-counter cough remedies.

■ Phencyclidine (street names are *PCP* or *angel dust*) is an NMDA agonist.

■ The flavor-enhancing chemical *MSG* is monosodium glutamate; it has the potential to increase neuronal activation via increased glutamate. Seizures can be induced in animal models with MSG.

■ Scenes from television shows that depict a person losing consciousness a couple of seconds (<5 seconds) after an injection would be realistic only if the injection were performed in the carotid artery.

Local Anesthetics

DESCRIPTION
Local anesthetics block neuron signal transmission.

PROTOTYPES AND COMMON DRUGS
Esters
- Prototype: cocaine
- Others: procaine, tetracaine, procaine, 2-chloroprocaine

Amides
- Prototype: lidocaine (lignocaine)
- Others: bupivacaine, ropivacaine, benzocaine, mepivacaine

MOA (MECHANISM OF ACTION)
- Neuronal transmission requires that an action potential be propagated from one end of a neuron to the other. Voltage-gated sodium channels open up as the wave of depolarization travels from one end of the neuron to the other. The opening of these ion channels permits sodium to enter the cell, causing depolarization, and is the primary method by which the wave of depolarization occurs.
- Local anesthetics bind these voltage-gated sodium channels. The ion channels can exist in three states: resting, activated (open), and inactivated. The local anesthetic binds them in the **inactivated state** and prevents them from transitioning to the open state; thus the ion channel remains closed and unresponsive to incoming depolarizing currents (Figure 21-4).
  - ▲ One factor for speed of onset of action of a local anesthetic is the frequency of firing of a nerve. Nerves that fire more frequently will be blocked earlier. Sensory nerves fire more frequently than motor nerves and therefore will be blocked earlier.
- The local anesthetic works on the intracellular side of the ion channel. Therefore the drug must first **cross the lipid cell membrane** before it can exert its action.
- Neurons that are covered in **myelin** are more difficult to block because the myelin impedes entry of the drug into the cell.
- Larger-**diameter** nerves are more difficult to block than are smaller-diameter nerves. They require higher doses and are blocked for shorter durations.
- There are three major classes of nerve function: sensory, motor, and autonomic. All types of nerves are susceptible to blockade by local anesthetic, but to varying degrees because of myelination and diameter:
  - ▲ **Autonomic** nerves are nonmyelinated and small; they are the easiest to block.
  - ▲ **Motor** nerves are large and myelinated; they are the hardest to block (and first to recover from blockade).
  - ▲ **Sensory** nerves are intermediate.
- Voltage-gated sodium channels are the primary ion channels in phase 0 of the **cardiac** action potential. Therefore,

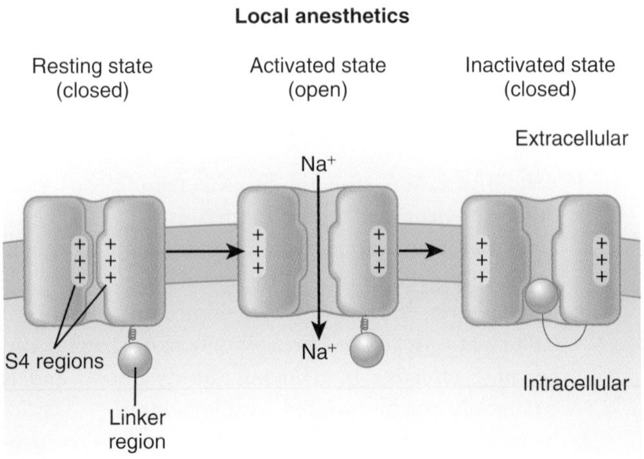

Local anesthetics

Figure 21-4.

local anesthetics are also classified as antiarrhythmics, specifically type 1b. This mechanism of action is discussed in more detail in the discussion of Na^+ channel blockers in Chapter 11 and is also responsible for cardiac toxicity of local anesthetics.

PHARMACOKINETICS
- Local anesthetics are most commonly injected, but other routes of administration include topical application: oral sprays, creams, and vaporized forms (for airways).
- There are important factors that dictate the potency, speed of onset, and duration of a local anesthetic:
  - ▲ **Lipid solubility:** Increased lipid solubility results in more drug being able to cross the cell membrane and bind the ion channel. The property of *increased* lipid solubility influences:
    - **Onset time** (shorter)
    - **Duration** (longer)
    - **Potency** (higher)
  - ▲ **pH:** Local anesthetics are weak bases. Therefore when the environment is acidic, the following reaction occurs: $B + H^+ \rightarrow BH^+$ (where B = base and represents the local anesthetic). From this equation, it can be seen that local anesthetics will be *ionized* (BH^+) and therefore *hydrophilic* (not lipid soluble) in an acid environment. Therefore, acidic tissues (such as an abscess or any infection) are very difficult to anesthetize with local anesthetic. An acid pH will **decrease** potency, speed of onset, and duration.
- Ester local anesthetics are predominantly metabolized via ester hydrolysis by **pseudocholinesterase**. Ester hydrolysis

TABLE 21-3. Local Anesthetic Durations		
Agent	**Duration Plain (minutes)**	**Duration with Epinephrine (minutes)**
2-Chloroprocaine	20-30	30-45
Procaine	15-30	30
Lidocaine	30-60	120
Mepivacaine	45-90	120
Prilocaine	30-90	120
Bupivacaine	120-240	180-240
Ropivacaine	120-240	180-240

is a fast reaction, and therefore ester local anesthetics have a shorter duration of action.

- Amide local anesthetics are metabolized (*N*-dealkylation and hydroxylation) by microsomal P-450 enzymes in the liver (Table 21-3).

INDICATIONS
- To provide local anesthesia
- Cardiac arrhythmias

CONTRAINDICATIONS
- Previous hypersensitivity to local anesthetic

SIDE EFFECTS
- Side effects more commonly occur when the toxic dose is approached or exceeded or if any dose is accidently injected into a blood vessel.
- CNS toxicity: The action of local anesthetic will also influence the neurons in the brain and gives rise to the following signs and symptoms:
  - ▲ Numbness or tingling around the lips and tongue (circumoral distribution)
  - ▲ Tinnitus (ringing in the ears)
  - ▲ Blurred vision
  - ▲ Agitation, disorientation, altered behavior or speech
  - ▲ Seizure
  - ▲ Coma
- **Cardiovascular toxicity** occurs at usually about 3 times the dose that is required to produce CNS toxicity, although this ratio is variable for different anesthetics. Bupivacaine is the most cardiotoxic. Electrical disturbances of the heart, including heart block, ventricular tachycardia, and ventricular fibrillation can occur, and these complications are life-threatening. Bupivacaine-induced ventricular fibrillation can be very resistant to treatment (defibrillation and antiarrhythmic treatment).
- **Consequences of unintentional intravascular injection:** Toxicity can occur very suddenly and with low doses of anesthetic if the anesthetic is injected directly into an artery or vein. If the anesthetic also contains epinephrine, the patient will experience symptoms related to tachycardia and hypertension as well.
- **Intraneural injection:** If a regional block is intended, injection of local anesthetic directly into the nerve can cause

nerve damage. This is not a concern for very small nerves branches.

IMPORTANT NOTES
- Onset time and duration are both dose dependent. Higher doses and higher concentrations of solution of local anesthetic will result in faster onset times and longer durations of action. The addition of low-dose epinephrine to the local anesthetic also prolongs the duration of action because it causes vasoconstriction and reduces blood flow, which slows the washout of the drug from the site of action.
- The location of injection strongly determines the effect of the local anesthetic. Only a segment of a neuron needs to be bound with local anesthetic to completely block its function (compared with blocking the entire length of the neuron). Therefore if local anesthetic is administered *upstream* to a large nerve, a very large *downstream* distribution of sensation can be blocked. This is the principle behind **spinal anesthetics**, in which a small dose (usually 1 to 3 mL) of a local anesthetic is administered to the cerebral spinal fluid in the lumbar spine and the result is often complete loss of all sensation and motor activity from the chest down to the toes!
  - ▲ Because sympathetic nerves are also blocked with this technique, a chemical **sympatholysis** occurs, resulting in vasodilation in the part of the body that is anesthetized; **hypotension** occurs commonly and is *usually* easily treated with a vasoconstrictor (usually an α_1 agonist) and intravenous fluid.
  - ▲ Other variants of this technique are called **regional blocks**, whereby local anesthetic is administered to large nerves (e.g., the brachial plexus) resulting in anesthesia to an entire limb.
- Small doses of epinephrine are often added to local anesthetic to prolong the duration of anesthesia. The epinephrine acts as a vasoconstrictor and thus reduces blood flow to the site of injection and reduces metabolism of the local anesthetic.
  - ▲ Inadvertent injection of these epinephrine-containing solutions into a blood vessel results in very significant tachycardia and hypertension, which are usually symptomatic for the patient.
  - ▲ Epinephrine also results in less bleeding because of the vasoconstriction and is useful for procedures in which bleeding is common (e.g., dental procedures).
- Injection of local anesthetic is painful (in addition to the pain of the needle). This is because the local anesthetic initially activates Na^+ channels, triggering initial depolarization before rendering the neurons inactive.

Advanced
- Structure: Local anesthetics contain a benzene (lipophilic) section connected to a hydrophilic section (often an amide). The connection between them is via either an ester or an amide bond, which is how the two categories of local anesthetics are designated.
- Benzocaine and prilocaine can cause **methemoglobinemia**, which is a condition in which hemoglobin iron is in the

- oxidized Fe^{3+} state instead of the normal Fe^{2+} state; this results in abnormal binding to oxygen. It is treated with **methylene blue.**
- True hypersensitivity reactions to local anesthetic agents—as distinct from systemic toxicity caused by excessive plasma concentration—are quite uncommon. Esters are more likely to induce an allergic reaction because they are derivatives of *p*-aminobenzoic acid, a known allergen.

FYI

- Amide local anesthetics have an *-i-* in the first part of the generic drug name (lidocaine, prilocaine, bupivacaine), whereas esters (tetracaine, procaine, cocaine) do not.

- Because ester hydrolysis is a fast reaction, drugs have been created specifically with an ester bond to deliberately produce a short duration of action. Some of these drugs include:
  - ▲ Succinylcholine (paralyzing drug)
  - ▲ Mivacurium (paralyzing drug)
  - ▲ Esmolol (β-blocker)
  - ▲ Remifentanil (an opioid)
  - ▲ Clevidipine (a dihydropyridine calcium channel blocker)

Baclofen

DESCRIPTION

Baclofen is a muscle relaxant (but not a paralytic).

PROTOTYPE

- Baclofen

MOA (MECHANISM OF ACTION)
γ-Aminobutyric Acid (GABA)

- GABA is the major **inhibitory neurotransmitter** in the CNS. GABA binds to three different types of receptors: $GABA_A$, $GABA_B$, and $GABA_C$.
  - ▲ Binding of GABA to $GABA_B$ receptors leads to the opening of the potassium (K^+) channel, facilitating K^+ efflux (leaving the cell) and thus cellular hyperpolarization (making the inside more negative).
  - ▲ Hyperpolarization of a cell decreases the probability that the cell can be subsequently *de*polarized by other incoming excitatory signals; this will have a net inhibitory effect.
  - ▲ Activation of these receptors also inhibits the influx of calcium ions into presynaptic terminals, further preventing depolarization.
- Note that most other GABA-mimetic drugs (benzodiazepines and intravenous anesthetics) are $GABA_A$ receptor modifiers, whereas baclofen increases GABA activity at $GABA_B$ receptors (Figure 21-5).
- Spasticity occurs because of increased activity of reflex circuits in the spinal cord. Normally there is descending inhibition of these circuits coming from the brain. The interruption or absence of this inhibition results in increased activity of the reflex circuit, resulting in increased muscle tone, clonus (repeated involuntary tremorlike contractions), and spasticity. Increased $GABA_B$ activity in the spinal cord decreases this reflex activity.

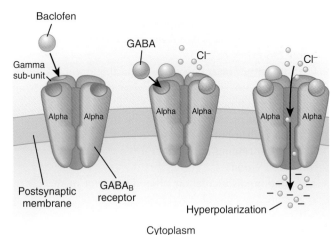

Baclofen

Synaptic cleft

Figure 21-5.

PHARMACOKINETICS

- Baclofen has poor lipid solubility, which results in low cerebrospinal levels when administered orally. Therefore baclofen is sometimes administered into the cerebral spinal fluid directly (intrathecal administration) via an implanted pump and catheter (which are implanted surgically).

INDICATIONS

- Muscle spasticity
  - ▲ Multiple sclerosis

▲ Spinal cord lesions
▲ Cerebral palsy

CONTRAINDICATIONS

■ None of special significance

SIDE EFFECTS

■ The GABA$_B$ receptor is an important component of both spinal cord and brain neurotransmission; therefore the side effects are primarily related to brain and spinal cord dysfunction
■ **CNS**: drowsiness, vertigo (dizziness), slurred speech, ataxia
■ **Neuromuscular**: weakness, hypotonia (decreased muscle tone)
■ **Cardiac**: chest pain, dyspnea, palpitation, syncope
■ **Urinary**: dysuria (pain on urination), enuresis (incontinence), hematuria (blood in urine), nocturia (night urination), urinary retention (inability to empty bladder), impotence, and inability to ejaculate. Bladder function is abnormal in patients with spinal cord injuries; the urinary tract is under control of the autonomic nervous system

(ANS), which is usually impaired in patients with spinal cord dysfunction.

IMPORTANT NOTES

■ **Avoid abrupt withdrawal** of the drug; abrupt withdrawal of intrathecal baclofen has resulted in severe spasticity:
  ▲ Muscle rigidity
  ▲ Rhabdomyolysis (muscle cellular breakdown from severe contractions)
  ▲ Fever (from increased muscle contraction, as in sustained exercise)
■ Severe reactions can be life-threatening.
■ Severe overdose of baclofen can **mimic brain death**: loss of brainstem reflexes (pupillary changes in response to light, corneal reflexes, gag reflex, cough reflex), apnea, loss of motor responses to painful stimuli.
■ Baclofen has been recently investigated for treatment of addiction, including cigarettes, alcohol, and cocaine. The basis for use in this indication is that GABA$_B$ can blunt the dopamine surge in the ventral striatum, which is an important mediator of the reward pathways, and can thus blunt the experienced reward that occurs with drug use.

Nondepolarizing Neuromuscular Blockers

DESCRIPTION

Nondepolarizing neuromuscular blockers are paralyzing drugs, also known as *muscle relaxants* or *paralytics*.

PROTOTYPE AND COMMON DRUGS

■ Prototype: Ve**curonium**
■ Others: Ro**curonium**, pan**curonium**, atra**curium**, cisatra**curium**, miva**curium**
■ Reversal agents (anti-cholinesterases):
  ▲ Neostigmine, edrophonium

MOA (MECHANISM OF ACTION)

■ Voluntary skeletal muscle contraction occurs when a motor neuron is depolarized. The distal end of the motor neuron is part of the **NMJ**, which is the anatomic connection between the neuron and muscle. The presynaptic membrane is the motor nerve, and the postsynaptic membrane is the **motor end plate** of the muscle cell.
■ The depolarizing motor neuron releases **acetylcholine**, and the ACh crosses the synapse and binds to **nicotinic ACh receptors** on the muscle cell. The binding of ACh to the motor end plate induces small mini-depolarizations. When enough mini-depolarizations occur, a full action potential is created in the muscle cell, which results in an increase in intracellular calcium levels and subsequent actin-myosin interactions, resulting in contraction (Figure 21-6).
■ NMJ blockers bind the nicotinic ACh receptor and competitively antagonize ACh, thereby preventing the signal

from the neuron to be communicated to the muscle. These drugs **do not** cause any depolarization of the muscle when they bind; therefore they are referred to as *nondepolarizing*. This is in contrast to the other class of paralytics, which are depolarizing.
■ Neuromuscular blockade can be partial or complete. If partial, then the strength of muscle contraction is reduced.
■ All **skeletal muscles** become paralyzed, including muscles for breathing, speech, and eyelid movement and all other skeletal muscle. Smooth muscles and cardiac muscle are **not** paralyzed because contraction is not dependent on the same neuromuscular transmission. Therefore the heart does not stop beating and smooth muscle function such as pupillary reflexes to light and gastrointestinal motility are not affected.
■ Paralytics *do not* affect level of consciousness; it is very difficult to know the exact level of consciousness of a person who is paralyzed, and therefore unconsciousness must be achieved before a patient is paralyzed.

Reversal of Blockade

■ If the patient remains paralyzed for longer than desired, then reversal medication can be administered to facilitate return of muscle strength.
■ Because these drugs are all **competitive** antagonists of ACh, increasing the concentration of ACh in the synaptic cleft will result in more ACh binding to ACh receptors on the motor end plate, and thus strength will be restored.

TABLE 21-4. Nondepolarizing Neuromuscular Junction Blockers			
Agent	**Duration**	**Metabolism and Elimination**	**Comments**
Mivacurium	Short	Pseudocholinesterase	Causes histamine release (hypotension)
Atracurium	Intermediate	Hoffman degradation	Duration not affected by liver or renal disease
Cisatracurium	Intermediate	Hoffman degradation	Duration not affected by liver or renal disease
Vecuronium	Intermediate	Biliary	
Rocuronium	Intermediate	Biliary	
Pancuronium	Long	Renal	Is vagolytic (causes increased heart rate)

Duration is based on *intubating* dose: short = 15 to 20 minutes, intermediate = 30 to 45 minutes, long = 2 to 3 hours.

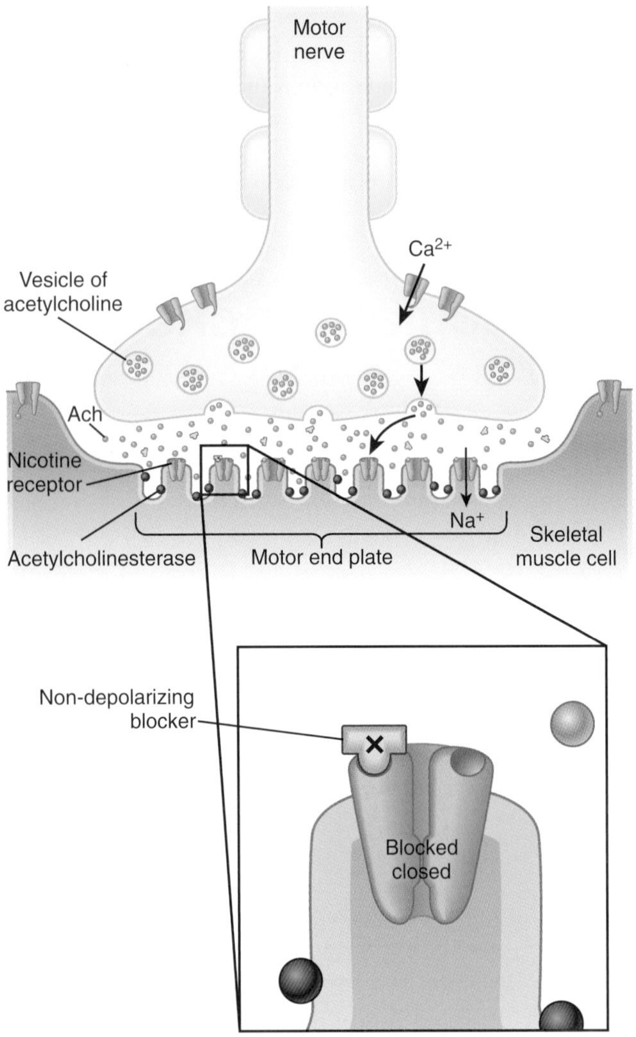

The neuromuscular junction

Figure 21-6.

■ **Cholinesterase** is the enzyme that breaks down ACh. **Anticholinesterases** are the drugs that inhibit cholinesterase, resulting in increased levels of ACh everywhere in the body.
  ▲ Increased ACh is desirable only in the motor end plate. ACh, however, will stimulate all **muscarinic and nicotinic** receptors in the body and can lead to the following

cholinergic side effects (mediated by muscarinic receptors):
  • Bradycardia
  • Salivation
  • Bronchospasm and increased airway secretions
  • Nausea, vomiting, and diarrhea
  • Urination
  ▲ Blocking the muscarinic receptors with an **anticholinergic** drug such as **atropine** or **glycopyrrolate** will reduce the incidence of these muscarinic side effects without influencing the effects on nicotinic receptors. Anticholinergic drugs are therefore routinely administered with anticholinesterase drugs.

PHARMACOKINETICS

■ There are important differences in duration of action and method of metabolism among the different drugs in this class. See Table 21-4.
  ▲ **Hoffman degradation** is simply spontaneous breakdown of the molecule at physiologic pH and temperature. This process occurs despite renal or hepatic failure, and therefore the duration of action of atracurium and cisatracurium is essentially unchanged in patients with renal or hepatic impairment.
  ▲ **Decreased metabolism or elimination** results in prolonged duration of action for the drug. This is undesirable when the drug is being used for surgery and the surgery is finished but the patient is still paralyzed; the anesthesiologist must then wait before waking the patient. Reversal medications can be given, but if the degree of paralysis is too high, then full reversal cannot be achieved.

INDICATIONS

■ Paralysis
  ▲ For surgery
  ▲ For intubation

CONTRAINDICATIONS

■ A conscious patient
■ Lack of skill or equipment to provide respiratory resuscitation:
  ▲ Bag-mask ventilation
  ▲ Intubation (insertion of breathing tube into trachea)

SIDE EFFECTS

■ Side effects are drug specific:
▲ Mivacurium: hypotension from histamine release (causes vasodilation)
▲ Pancuronium: tachycardia from the vagolytic effect

IMPORTANT NOTES

■ **Potency** and **time to onset**: Onset time is determined by the dose administered. For a given drug, giving a larger dose will result in a faster onset of paralysis. For drugs that are more potent (e.g., pancuronium is the most potent), a smaller dose is required for paralysis, but because a smaller dose is required, more potent drugs have a slower onset of action.

■ Potency of muscle relaxants is measured using the *effective dose* in 95% of the population (**ED$_{95}$**). For each drug, the ED$_{95}$ dose is different. As a general rule, an **intubating dose** (probably the most common indication for paralyzing drugs) is **twice the ED$_{95}$**.

■ The **degree of paralysis** can be measured with a small battery-powered device called a **nerve stimulator**. It essentially delivers a small electric shock. Electrodes (usually just electrocardiographic patches) are applied on top of the motor nerve of interest (usually the **ulnar nerve** at the wrist or the **facial nerve** at the temple). When the electrical shock is applied, a muscle that is not paralyzed will vigorously contract; a partially paralyzed muscle will demonstrate a small twitch, and a fully paralyzed muscle will not contract at all.

▲ If four electrical shocks are applied in succession, the test is called a **train of four**. This is important because each successive shock will release a slightly smaller amount of ACh from the presynaptic nerve; because the drugs are competitive antagonists, the **partially blocked muscle** will demonstrate *progressively smaller contractions*, a phenomenon called **fade**. A patient can have zero fade when as many as 50% of the nicotinic receptors are still occupied; therefore four full contractions with the nerve stimulator TOF test does *not guarantee* that the patient will have 100% strength.

▲ If a patient has *zero contractions* with the TOF test, he or she is *not likely* to respond to **reversal medication**. The only way to reverse paralysis in this patient is to wait until there are 1 to 2 twitches (the more the better) and then administer the reversal medication.

▲ Administering an *excessive dose* (in an attempt to overcome one's own impatience) of the reversal anticholinesterase will result in muscarinic side effects and can also *paradoxically reparalyze* the patient!

Advanced

■ Nondepolarizing muscle relaxant blockade is prolonged by inhaled anesthetics. This is relevant for anesthesiologists because inhaled anesthetics are very commonly coadministered with muscle relaxants.

■ During a long surgery a long-acting muscle relaxant might be used. However, near the end of surgery the anesthesiologist might want a shorter-acting, more titratable drug. However, mixing drugs has an unexpected synergistic effect: one would expect that converting from a long-duration to a short-duration drug would result in a shorter duration of action, but, in fact, in combination the two drugs frequently potentiate each other and the result can be a much longer duration of block than would have been expected from either drug. Mixing nondepolarizing drugs is not recommended.

■ Reversal drugs are used for other indications:
▲ **Myasthenia gravis** is a condition whereby antibodies to nicotinic receptors exist. The antibodies function like paralyzing drugs and cause weakness. Anticholinergic drugs are given to help antagonize the weakness effects of the antibodies.

■ A new reversal drug called **sugammadex** is in clinical trials. It works by binding (essentially removing from circulation) rocuronium. It appears to be safe and effective even when the patient is fully paralyzed with even a very large dose of rocuronium.

FYI

■ Curare is the historical prototype of nondepolarization neuromuscular blockers, but it is no longer used clinically. Curare (also called *D-tubocurare*) was the first paralytic used in anesthesia, but it has been replaced by newer agents. It was introduced to anesthesia around 1940. It was discovered in South America and was first used in poison arrows for hunting. It is harvested from the plant *Strychnos toxifera*. The toxin strychnine is also from this genus of plant (but from a different species).

■ SLUDGE is an acronym to help you remember the signs of **cholinergic syndrome**:
▲ Salivation
▲ Lacrimation
▲ Urination
▲ Diarrhea
▲ Gastrointestinal upset
▲ Emesis (vomiting)
▲ Unfortunately, the important bronchial signs (bronchospasm and secretions) are not included in the acronym.

■ Take care not to confuse the following terms, which are polar opposites of each other: *anticholinergic* and *anticholinesterase*. The former *blocks* muscarinic activity, whereas the latter *increases* both muscarinic and nicotinic receptor activity.

■ Drugs that are GABA-mimetic (they increase the action of the inhibitory neurotransmitter GABA) are also **muscle relaxants**. However, these drugs are not paralytic drugs. They act in the brain or spinal cord and reduce afferent transmission to the muscle. Examples of these drugs include benzodiazepines (GABA$_A$ enhancers), baclofen (GABA$_B$ enhancers), cyclobenzaprine, and methocarbamol.

■ The last nondepolarizing drug to come to market was rapacuronium. It had a very short time of onset and duration but was withdrawn from clinical practice in 2001 because of the risk of fatal bronchospasm.

Depolarizing Neuromuscular Blockers

DESCRIPTION

Depolarizing neuromuscular blockers are paralyzing drugs also known as *muscle relaxants.*

PROTOTYPE

■ Succinylcholine (suxamethonium)

MOA (MECHANISM OF ACTION)

■ Voluntary skeletal muscle contraction occurs when a motor neuron is depolarized. The distal end of the motor neuron is part of the **neuromuscular junction (NMJ)**, which is the anatomic connection between the neuron and muscle. The presynaptic membrane is the motor nerve, and the postsynaptic membrane is the **motor end plate** of the muscle cell.

■ The depolarizing motor neuron releases **acetylcholine** **(ACh)**, which crosses the synapse and binds to **nicotinic ACh receptors** on the muscle cell. The binding of ACh to the motor end plate induces small mini-depolarizations via opening sodium channels. When enough mini-depolarizations occur, a full action potential is created in the muscle cell, which results in an increase in intracellular calcium levels and subsequent actin-myosin interactions, resulting in contraction (Figure 21-7).

■ Succinylcholine **irreversibly** binds the nicotinic ACh receptor. Succinylcholine causes **opening** of the sodium channel controlled by the ACh receptor and a subsequent short-lived myofibril contraction (**fasciculation**); therefore it is referred to as *depolarizing.* However, because succinylcholine is not metabolized by cholinesterase, it remains bound to the nicotinic receptor for a longer duration. The sodium channel is locked in the open position, and the muscle stays in a **depolarized** state. However, the intracellular calcium is taken back up by the sarcoplasmic reticulum after its initial release, lowering the intracellular calcium level, and the actin-myosin coupling dissociates. For as long as the myocyte remains *de*polarized by the open sodium channel, it cannot accept a new action potential, and the intracellular calcium levels remain low.

  ▲ This depolarization also results in release of intracellular potassium into the blood; the typical rise in potassium is 0.5 to 1.0 mEq/L (the normal range of potassium is 3.5 to 5.0 mEq/L).

■ Neuromuscular blockade can be partial or complete. If partial, then the strength of muscle contraction is reduced.

■ All **skeletal muscles** become paralyzed; this includes muscles for breathing, speech, and eyelid movement and all other skeletal muscles. Smooth muscles and cardiac muscle are not paralyzed. Therefore the heart does not stop beating and smooth muscle function such as pupillary reflexes to light and gastrointestinal motility are not affected.

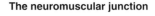

The neuromuscular junction

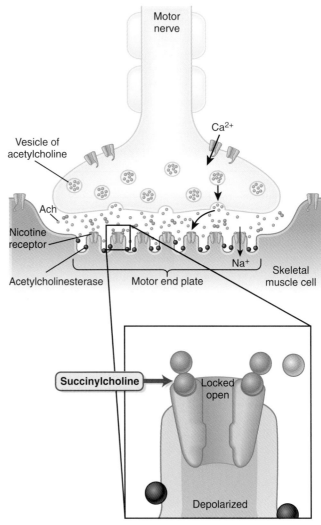

Figure 21-7.

■ Paralytics (drugs that cause paralysis) *do not* affect level of consciousness; it is very difficult to know the exact level of consciousness of a person who is paralyzed, and therefore unconsciousness must be achieved before a patient is paralyzed.

PHARMACOKINETICS

■ Succinylcholine is metabolized by **pseudocholinesterase**. This enzyme is similar to but not identical to acetylcholinesterase.

  ▲ Rarely, some individuals have a pseudocholinesterase deficiency. In these patients the duration of succinylcholine can be as long as 12 hours or more, depending on the dose given!

- Succinylcholine has a very short time to onset (45 seconds) and a very short duration of action (4 to 5 minutes). It is the shortest-acting paralytic drug currently available.

INDICATIONS
- **Intubation**
- **Electroconvulsive therapy (ECT):** With this treatment, an electric shock is administered to the brain, which induces a seizure. The paralytic is of benefit so that the limbs do not demonstrate vigorous tonic-clonic activity, which could cause injury. The patient is given a short-acting anesthetic before both the paralysis and the electric shock.

CONTRAINDICATIONS
- A conscious patient
- Lack of skill or equipment to provide respiratory resuscitation:
  - Bag-mask ventilation
  - Intubation (insertion of breathing tube into trachea)
- Risk of hyperkalemia:
  - **Hyperresponders:** In some patients there are *extrajunctional* (outside the NMJ) nicotinic receptors on the muscle that ACh can bind to; this binding can cause a greater-than-normal release of potassium.
    - **Burn patients:** from 1 day until 1 year after their burn
    - **Spinal cord paralysis patients:** from 1 day until 1 year after the injury. The higher on the spinal cord the injury is, the greater the risk
    - Muscular **dystrophy patients:** always at risk for hyperkalemia
  - **Preexisting hyperkalemia:** In patients with renal failure, potassium levels are often elevated (and would be further elevated 0.5 to 1.0 mEq/L with succinylcholine). However, if the potassium level is normal, patients with renal failure are normal responders and therefore it is safe to administer succinylcholine.
- Myotonic **dystrophy:** In these patients the depolarizing effect of succinylcholine is dramatically prolonged and results in widespread increased tone in all muscles. Patients who have this reaction have muscles of respiration also contracted, and therefore it is very difficult to ventilate these patients. Succinylcholine is absolutely contraindicated in these patients.
- **MH:** Succinylcholine is one of the two triggers for MH. The other trigger is inhaled (volatile) anesthetics.

SIDE EFFECTS
- **Hyperkalemia:** Intracellular potassium is released from muscle cells on depolarization, leading to a small rise in serum potassium.
- **Muscle pain** results from the transient fasciculations induced.
- **Bradycardia:** Because the chemical structure of succinylcholine is essentially two ACh molecules bound together end to end, it is not surprising that it can mimic ACh at muscarinic receptors. Although it does not produce a widespread muscarinic response, bradycardia and asystole have

occurred. This effect is more pronounced in children, and **atropine** is sometimes coadministered before succinylcholine to prevent bradycardia.

IMPORTANT NOTES
- Because succinylcholine binds irreversibly, there are important differences between it and the nondepolarizing drugs, which bind competitively:
  - Increasing the ACh concentration in the synaptic cleft via administration of **anticholinesterase drugs is not effective** in reversing the block.
  - The **train-of-four (TOF)** test (see the discussion of nondepolarizing NMJ blockers) exhibits different results with succinylcholine versus nondepolarizers:
    - With each stimulation, the amount of ACh released is slightly less than with the previous stimulation; because succinylcholine is *not* competitively bound, the concentration of ACh in the synaptic cleft *does not* influence the strength of contraction. The strength of contraction is **solely dependent on nicotinic receptor occupancy.** Therefore there is **no fade** when there is partial blockade by succinylcholine, which is in contrast to nondepolarizers.
- **Anticholinesterase drugs also inhibit pseudocholinesterase,** the enzyme that breaks down succinylcholine, so in fact both ACh and succinylcholine levels would be increased in the synaptic cleft. This is a second reason why paralytic reversal drugs are not effective with succinylcholine.
  - **Mivacurium,** a nondepolarizing paralytic, is also metabolized by pseudocholinesterase, so anticholinesterase drugs are not recommended for reversal for mivacurium either.
- **Phase 1 versus phase 2 blockade:** Phase 1 blockade is the TOF stimulation test result whereby no fade (all contractions are equal in size) is demonstrated. Phase 2 blockade occurs when **repeated doses or infusions** of succinylcholine are administered. **Phase 2 blockade does demonstrate fade** (the 4 contractions get smaller and smaller) just like nondepolarizing paralytics. However, it is no longer clinically common to administer repeated doses or infusions of succinylcholine, so phase 2 blockade with succinylcholine is not commonly seen.
- Potency of muscle relaxants is measured using the *effective dose* in 95% of the population (**ED$_{95}$**). For each drug, the ED$_{95}$ dose is different. As a general rule, an **intubating dose** (probably the most common indication for paralyzing drugs) is **twice the ED$_{95}$.**

Advanced
- In attempts to reduce muscle pain after succinylcholine-induced fasciculations, a *defasciculating* dose of a nondepolarizing paralytic (such as rocuronium or vecuronium) is given 5 minutes beforehand. This is only a very small dose so as not to produce paralysis in the awake patient; usually about 5% to 10% of the ED$_{95}$ is used ($\frac{1}{20}$ to $\frac{1}{10}$ of the intubating dose). Lidocaine has also been used to reduce postsuccinylcholine muscle pain.

- The **paradoxic paralysis** seen with an overdose of reversal (anticholinesterase) drugs results from the myocytes being continuously saturated with too much ACh, resulting in the sodium channels remaining in the open state, mimicking the action of succinylcholine. **Organophosphates** (insecticides and chemical warfare agents such as sarin) are anticholinesterases, and organophosphate poisoning results in a cholinergic syndrome (muscarinic side effects) and, in addition, paralysis.
- Probably the only reasons that succinylcholine remains in clinical practice despite the prominent side effects that are not present in nondepolarizing paralytics are its short onset of action and short duration of action. Rapacuronium, a fast-acting and ultra-short–duration nondepolarizing paralytic threatened to put an end to succinylcholine use, but it was withdrawn from the market in 2001 because of risk of bronchospasm.
- A new reversal drug called *sugammadex* binds (and rapidly reverses) rocuronium and vecuronium and could enable ultra-short–duration paralysis with nondepolarizers.

FYI

- Pseudocholinesterase is also called butyrylcholinesterase or plasma cholinesterase.
- Other drugs that are metabolized by pseudocholinesterase include:
  - ▲ Mivacurium (a nondepolarizing paralytic)
  - ▲ Procaine (an ester-type local anesthetic)

Nicotine

DESCRIPTION

Nicotine is a chemical with significant and varied pharmacologic properties; it is found in cigarette smoke and in products designed to assist in abstaining from smoking.

PROTOTYPES AND COMMON DRUGS
Full Agonists

- Prototype: nicotine

Partial Agonists

- Prototype: varenicline
- Others: cytisine

MOA (MECHANISM OF ACTION)

- There are several nicotine receptors, composed of alpha (α) and beta (β) subunits. The various α subunits and β subunits all appear in different combinations throughout the body. The most common subunits are $\alpha_4\beta_2$, $\alpha_3\beta_4$, and α_7.
- The $\alpha_4\beta_2$ **subunit** is the most common nicotinic receptor in the brain and is believed to be the subunit most responsible for nicotine addiction.
- Nicotine binds to presynaptic nicotinic $\alpha_4\beta_2$ receptors, which in turn leads to the **release of dopamine** into the **nucleus accumbens,** the "reward" pathway of the brain (Figure 21-8).
- In addition to dopamine, binding of nicotine to $\alpha_4\beta_2$ receptors leads to release of a variety of other neurotransmitters such as acetylcholine, norepinephrine, serotonin, GABA, endorphins, and glutamate. Many of these neurotransmitters are associated with mood, whereas others (GABA, endorphins) tend to have a calming or euphoric effect. Chronic cigarette smoking also appears to reduce levels of enzymes such as monoamine oxidase (MAO) that break down many of these neurotransmitters, including dopamine.

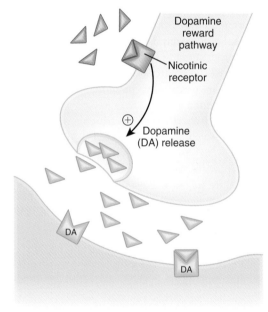

Nicotinic receptor agonists

Dopamine reward pathway

Nicotinic receptor

Dopamine (DA) release

DA

DA

Figure 21-8.

- Chronic nicotine use leads to **up-regulation** of $\alpha_4\beta_2$ receptors. Although this may seem counterintuitive, the up-regulation appears to be in response to **receptor desensitization.**
- Aside from stimulation of the reward pathway, nicotine acts on other nicotinic receptors in other areas of the body. For example the $\alpha_3\beta_4$ subunit likely mediates the cardiovascular effects of nicotine. Nicotine acts as a vasoconstrictor, increases heart rate and contractility, and may cause endothelial dysfunction.

■ The binding of a partial agonist to these receptors does two things:
1. It provides a low-level stimulation of nicotinic receptors and thus a low level release of dopamine when nicotine is not present (i.e., during periods of abstinence).
2. By binding to the nicotinic receptor, it prevents nicotine from binding when the patient is smoking. Therefore the *reward* the patient receives from smoking is blunted. In theory there is less reason to smoke and therefore less disincentive to remain abstinent once the patient has quit smoking.

PHARMACOKINETICS

■ Nicotine is rapidly absorbed, has a rapid onset of action when delivered by the inhalational route (cigarette smoking), and has a short elimination half-life (1 to 2 hours). The quick onset of action and the short half-life both contribute to the addictive properties of smoking.
■ Oral absorption of nicotine is poor, and nicotine acts as a gastric irritant, so nicotine is not currently available for oral administration.
■ The various nicotine replacement products all try to replace nicotine without replicating the rapid onset and offset of nicotine inhaled through cigarette smoke.
■ Varenicline undergoes minimal metabolism and is primarily (>92%) excreted unchanged, relying on renal elimination via filtration and secretion. Levels therefore accumulate in patients with moderate to severe renal impairment, and closer monitoring of these patients may be necessary.

INDICATION

■ Smoking cessation

CONTRAINDICATIONS

■ None of major significance

SIDE EFFECTS
Full Agonists
Local Effects
■ Irritation: Nicotine is an **irritant**, so the side effects of nicotine tend to reflect this, varying only by the site of application:
  ▲ **Patch:** Redness, itching, and burning can be mitigated somewhat by rotating the site of application of the patch.
  ▲ **Gum, inhaler, spray:** Irritation to oral mucosa and throat may occur.

Systemic Effects
■ The systemic effects of nicotine replacement are difficult to separate from the effects of smoking cessation itself, including nicotine withdrawal.
■ **Insomnia, vivid dreams:** These are likely mediated by dopamine release in the CNS. This effect might be more common with the patch, as it is often worn continuously. Sixteen-hour patches that can be removed at night are available.

Partial Agonists
■ **Nausea:** The mechanism has not been described; however, other agents that elevate dopamine levels in the CNS also promote nausea.

Serious
■ **Neuropsychiatric:** Events such as depression, agitation, hostility, and suicidality have been observed in the postmarketing period (see Important Notes for further details). The mechanism is unknown; however, agents that elevate dopamine levels in the CNS have been known to produce some of the same side effects.

IMPORTANT NOTES

■ Despite the acute effects of nicotine on the cardiovascular system (see Mechanism of Action), there is no clear evidence that nicotine itself increases risk of cardiovascular events. Recent concerns have arisen about an increased risk of mortality after coronary artery bypass surgery; however, these findings need to be confirmed by well-designed prospective studies. Currently the risk-to-benefit ratio of nicotine replacement in patients with cardiovascular disease is unknown.
■ Nicotine also inhibits apoptosis and promotes angiogenesis, both of which would be expected to promote tumor growth. However, there is also no clear evidence that chronic use of nicotine replacement medication has a carcinogenic effect.
■ A common dilemma is what to do with pregnant patients who wish to use nicotine replacement therapies to quit smoking and maintain abstinence. This is once again a risk-to-benefit assessment. Ideally a patient would abstain from smoking without any medical interventions during pregnancy, but if this is not possible the potential effects of multiple toxins in cigarette smoke must be weighed against the risk posed by nicotine itself.
■ High doses of nicotine are toxic, and this is particularly evident in children. Used transdermal patches typically contain significant amounts of nicotine, and patients are advised to dispose of them carefully so they are not accidently accessible to children and pets.
■ Reports of serious neuropsychiatric events with **varenicline** have emerged in the postmarketing period. These include depression, agitation, hostility, and suicidal thoughts or attempts. The interpretation of these findings is complicated by their similarity to the classic side effects of nicotine withdrawal.
■ Given their respective mechanisms, it is not expected that the combination of varenicline along with nicotine replacement therapies would provide any additional advantages over using either agent alone. Providing additional nicotine would simply increase competition for nicotinic receptors, reducing the effects of varenicline.

Advanced
Pharmacogenetics
■ The rate of nicotine metabolism is determined in part by polymorphisms in the genes for CYP2A6 as well as uridine

5'-diphosphate (UDP)–glucuronosyltransferases (UGTs), a secondary pathway of elimination. These differences are believed to explain why women metabolize nicotine more rapidly than men and why patients of Caucasian and Hispanic descent metabolize nicotine more rapidly than patients of Asian and Black descent.

EVIDENCE
Nicotine Replacement Therapies for Smoking Cessation
- A 2008 Cochrane review (111 trials, N > 40,000 participants) compared nicotine replacement therapies to other interventions and placebo as an aid to smoking cessation. Overall, nicotine replacement therapies performed better than control for improving abstinence rates (relative risk [RR] 1.58). Abstinence rates for individual interventions varied slightly: gum, RR 1.43; patch, RR 1.66; inhaler, RR 1.90; nasal spray, RR 2.02; and tablets or lozenges, RR 2.00. Only one study compared quit rates between nicotine replacement and other active comparators (bupropion), and quit rates were lower for the nicotine patch in this study, compared with bupropion.

Partial Agonists versus Placebo or Active Comparators for Smoking Cessation and Relapse Prevention
- A 2008 Cochrane review (nine trials, 7267 participants) compared varenicline with either placebo or bupropion for smoking cessation and relapse prevention. The pooled RR for continuous abstinence after 6 months versus placebo was 2.3. Varenicline also performed better than bupropion (RR 1.5) and nicotine replacement therapy (RR 1.3) for continuous abstinence at 12 months.
  - ▲ One cytisine trial was included; the reported results were that more cytisine-treated participants had stopped smoking after 2 years when compared with placebo-treated participants (1.6).

FYI
- Nicotine vaccines are currently in development. The vaccines would stimulate antibodies to nicotine, which would then form complexes with nicotine and prevent absorption of nicotine across the blood-brain barrier. Early results are promising, although positive responses are typically seen in those with sufficient antibody production.
- A metabolite of nicotine, cotinine, can be used as a test to determine whether someone has quit smoking.
- Varenicline was developed through modification of cytisine, a naturally occurring plant alkaloid that has been used in Europe as a treatment for tobacco dependence since the 1960s.

Dopamine and Dopamine Agonists

DESCRIPTION
Dopamine and dopamine agonists form a class of drugs consisting of dopamine itself and agents that mimic the actions of dopamine as agonists at dopamine receptors.

PROTOTYPE AND COMMON DRUGS
- **Dopamine:** levodopa (L-dopa)
- **Dopamine agonists:**
  - ▲ **Ergot derivatives:** bromocriptine
    - • **Others:** cabergoline, pergolide
  - ▲ **Nonergot:** pramipexole
    - • **Others:** ropinirole

MOA (MECHANISM OF ACTION)
- **Parkinson's disease** is characterized by the **progressive loss** of **dopaminergic neurons** in the **substantia nigra.** Dopamine is a catecholamine that is synthesized in these dopaminergic neurons and is released onto two pathways in the striatum that regulate coordinated movement.
  - ▲ The direct pathway, via the **D1** receptor, enables movement.
  - ▲ The indirect pathway, via the **D2** receptor, inhibits movement.
- The level of activity of the cells of the globus pallidus interna (GPi) and substantia nigra pars reticulata (SNpr) depends on the balance of input between excitatory glutamate (Glu) (+) and inhibitory GABA (−) (Figure 21-9).
- When the cells of the GPi and SNpr become more active, this increases release of inhibitory GABA (−) onto the thalamus, which in turn inhibits the release of excitatory Glu (+) onto the cerebral cortex.
- This reduction in release of Glu (+) onto the cerebral cortex is what leads to inhibition of movement.
- Because the level of activity of the GPi and SNpr depends on the input of GABA and Glu from the direct and indirect pathways, these pathways must be in balance for normal movement to be maintained.

Dopamine

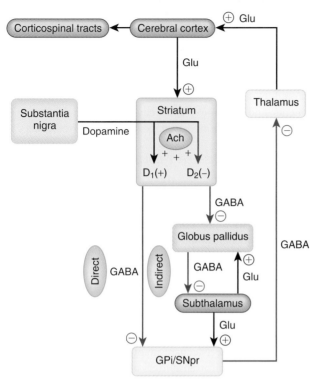

Figure 21-9.

- The balance between these direct and indirect pathways is disrupted in Parkinson's disease. **Low levels** of dopamine released onto these receptors leads to greater activation of D2 than D1 receptors, which results in a **net inhibitory** effect on movement.
- A balance also exists between dopamine and acetylcholine in the striatum. When dopamine levels are reduced, this leads to a relative excess of acetylcholine, an imbalance that also interferes with proper movement. That is why some patients are treated with anticholinergics in the early stages of Parkinson's disease.
- Dopamine also **inhibits prolactin release**, so dopamine agonists are also used to suppress lactation or to shrink prolactin-secreting tumors. Dopamine also **suppresses growth hormone release** in patients with acromegaly.

PHARMACOKINETICS
- Levodopa is the precursor of dopamine and is readily and completely converted to dopamine by the enzyme dopa decarboxylase (DDC). Levodopa is rapidly absorbed when administered orally, with a short plasma half-life of 1 to 3 hours. Dietary amino acids may compete for absorption sites in the small intestine; therefore administration with meals may delay absorption and reduce peak plasma concentrations.
- Once converted, dopamine is then metabolized and inactivated by catechol-O-methyltransferase (COMT) and monoamine oxidase (MAO). Another approach to enhancing dopaminergic transmission is to inhibit these enzymes,

thereby increasing dopamine levels. These agents, COMT inhibitors and MAO inhibitors, are discussed in Chapters 21 and 23.
- The dopamine agonists used in Parkinson's disease have longer durations of action than L-dopa. Cabergoline, an agent not used for Parkinson's disease, has an exceptionally long elimination half-life (approximately 100 hours).
- The absorption and extent of first-pass metabolism of bromocriptine is highly variable, leading to wide fluctuations in plasma concentrations and variability in dose response.

INDICATIONS
- Parkinson's disease (L-dopa, ropinirole, pergolide, pramipexole)
- Restless legs syndrome (pramipexole)
- Endocrine (bromocriptine, cabergoline):
  ▲ Acromegaly
  ▲ Amenorrhea-galactorrhea
  ▲ Prevention of lactation
  ▲ Prolactin-secreting adenoma

CONTRAINDICATIONS
Pramipexole, Ropinirole
- *Caution* should be exercised when driving or engaging in other activities that require alertness, because of the potential for sudden onset of sleep (see Side Effects).

SIDE EFFECTS
- Numerous side effects related to dopamine agonism:
  ▲ Nausea
  ▲ Peripheral edema
  ▲ Hypotension
  ▲ Hallucinations, vivid dreams

Serious
- **Sudden sleep onset** has occurred without warning and poses a potential risk for activities requiring attention, such as driving. This may be a class effect but has been confirmed with ropinirole and pramipexole.

IMPORTANT NOTES
- L-Dopa is almost always administered with a **peripheral decarboxylase inhibitor.** The reason for this is that L-dopa is readily converted to dopamine by decarboxylases before it even reaches the CNS. This dopamine is then converted to inactive metabolites and eliminated, or it acts on peripheral dopamine receptors, resulting in a number of side effects.
- Decarboxylase inhibitors such as **carbidopa** are not able to cross into the CNS; they therefore allow L-dopa to be converted to dopamine in the CNS but prevent this from occurring before L-dopa reaches the CNS.
- Initially, the therapeutic effects of dopamine appear to extend beyond its relatively short half-life. This is likely a result of the remaining ability of dopaminergic neurons in the substantia nigra to store and release dopamine. However, after this ability is inevitably lost through progression of Parkinson's disease, doses of L-dopa begin to

wear off quickly, in keeping with its short plasma half-life.

- A longstanding debate with L-dopa therapy is over the potential for dopamine itself to accelerate the cell death in the substantia nigra. The metabolism of dopamine produces free radicals, and free radical damage is considered to play a key role in the pathogenesis of Parkinson's disease. However, a definitive link has yet to be established, and until it is, L-dopa will likely remain the standard of care for management of Parkinson's disease symptoms.
- Dopamine agonists have theoretical advantages over L-dopa in Parkinson's disease in that they:
  1. Do not require enzymatic conversion for activity
  2. Have a longer duration of action
  3. Avoid the potential neurodegeneration associated with the conversion of L-dopa to free radicals
- The main differences between the ergot and nonergot dopamine agonists are in speed of titration and tolerability. Ergots can cause profound hypotension as well as nausea and fatigue initially; therefore they require slow upward adjustment.
- Pergolide has been discontinued in some jurisdictions over concerns about damage to heart valves.

EVIDENCE
Parkinson's Disease
Ropinirole versus Bromocriptine

- A 2001 Cochrane review (three trials, N = 482 patients) found that ropinirole and bromocriptine had similar effects in improving off-time and reducing L-dopa dose, without increasing adverse events such as dyskinesia. The authors noted that the three included studies might not have enough power to distinguish between agents. *Off-time* refers to wearing off of the effects of the drug, severely limiting the mobility of the patient.

Pramipexole versus Placebo

- A 2000 Cochrane review (four trials, N = 669 patients) compared pramipexole with placebo in patients with Parkinson's disease and long-term complications from L-dopa. Pramipexole reduced off-time, improved motor impairments and disability, and reduced L-dopa dose requirements, but it also increased dyskinetic adverse events.

Early Parkinson's Disease: L-Dopa versus Bromocriptine

- A 2007 Cochrane review examined six trials (N = 850 patients), but the studies were too heterogeneous for a meta-analysis to be conducted. The authors arrived at a qualitative conclusion that bromocriptine may be beneficial in delaying motor complications and dyskinesias, with comparable effects on impairment and disability.

FYI

- In the future we will likely discover that the pathophysiology of Parkinson's disease is much more complicated than described in the Mechanism of Action section and that several other neurotransmitters may be involved, including substance P and dynorphin. The significance of these transmitters in the pathophysiology of Parkinson's disease is an active area of research.
- For example, the previously described model would suggest that ideally, dopamine agonists should nonselectively stimulate both D1 and D2 receptors. However, most of the clinically useful dopamine agonists stimulate D2 receptors more than D1 receptors, and some are even considered to be D2 selective agonists.

Catechol-*O*-Methyl Transferase (COMT) Inhibitors

DESCRIPTION
COMT inhibitors are agents that inhibit the enzyme COMT. COMT breaks down levodopa.

PROTOTYPE AND COMMON DRUGS
- Prototype: enta**capone**
- Others: tol**capone**

MOA (MECHANISM OF ACTION)
- Parkinson's disease is characterized by the progressive loss of dopaminergic neurons in the substantia nigra. Dopamine is a catecholamine that is synthesized in these dopaminergic neurons and is released onto two pathways in the striatum that regulate coordinated movement.

- ▲ The direct pathway, via the D1 receptor, enables movement.
- ▲ The indirect pathway, via the D2 receptor, inhibits movement.
- The balance between these direct and indirect pathways is disrupted in Parkinson's disease. Low levels of dopamine released onto these receptors lead to greater activation of D2 than D1 receptors, which results in a net inhibitory effect on movement.
- COMT inhibitors **increase the amount of dopamine** available to the CNS. **COMT** is one of the two major enzymes involved in the metabolism of catecholamines (epinephrine, norepinephrine, and dopamine). Thus one of the ways COMT inhibitors increase dopamine is by inhibiting its breakdown (Figure 21-10).

COMT inhibitors

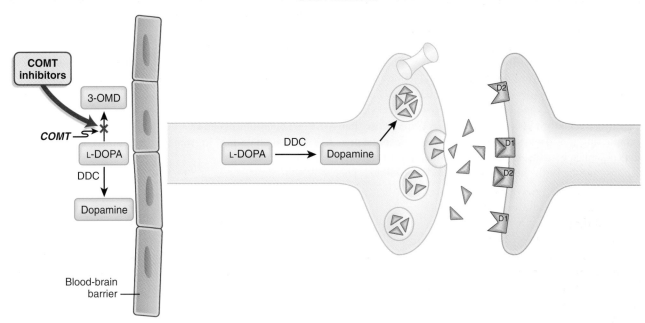

Figure 21-10.

- The COMT inhibitors also free up transporters for levodopa:
  - ▲ Dopa decarboxylase (DDC) is another enzyme that breaks down levodopa. When a DDC inhibitor such as carbidopa is used to inhibit the breakdown of levodopa, this leads to compensatory pathways of dopamine metabolism, including the COMT pathway.
  - ▲ The product of this pathway, 3-O-methyldopa (3-OMD), competes with levodopa for transporters, reducing the amount of dopamine available to the CNS. Inhibiting this pathway frees up transporters for levodopa.
- Therefore in order to have an effect, COMT inhibitors and DDC inhibitors are coadministered with levodopa.

PHARMACOKINETICS

- The elimination half-life of entacapone corresponds very closely with that of levodopa; therefore these two agents are administered simultaneously.
- A single dose of entacapone prolongs the half-life of L-dopa by 25% to 75%.

INDICATION

- Parkinson's disease
  - ▲ As an adjunct to levodopa-carbidopa or levodopa-benserazide in patients who experience "wearing off." Wearing-off is a phenomenon whereby the effect of drug wears off, resulting in immobility.

CONTRAINDICATIONS

- Concomitant use with **nonselective MAOIs**: This includes the use of an MAO-A and an MAO-B inhibitor in combina-tion. The MAO pathway becomes the key metabolic route for epinephrine and norepinephrine in the presence of COMT blockade. There should be at least a 2-week washout before initiation of treatment with a COMT inhib-itor. Caution should also be exercised in patients on MAO-B selective inhibitors, as these become nonselective at higher doses.
- History of neuroleptic malignant syndrome and/or non-traumatic rhabdomyolysis is a contraindication.
- **Liver impairment** is a contraindication because of hepato-toxicity seen with tolcapone.
- **Pheochromocytoma** is a contraindication because of increased risk of hypertensive crisis.

SIDE EFFECTS

- **Dopamine-related** effects include dyskinesia (peak dose), vivid dreams, hallucinations, nausea, hypotension.
- **Abdominal pain** may occur.
- **Diarrhea** may occur.
- **Discoloration of urine** is caused by the chemical structure of the drug and occurs only in alkaline urine. The side effect is harmless, but patients should be warned of the dark yellow or reddish brown tinge.

Serious

- **Hepatotoxicity**: observed only with tolcapone so far

IMPORTANT NOTES

- Entacapone does not cross the blood-brain barrier and is therefore a *peripheral* COMT inhibitor, whereas tolcapone is both a *central and peripheral* inhibitor.

EVIDENCE
COMT Inhibitors versus Dopamine Therapy in Parkinson's Disease Patients with Motor Complications on L-Dopa
- A 2004 Cochrane review compared COMT inhibitors (tolcapone) with pergolide (one trial, N = 203 over 12 weeks) and bromocriptine (one trial, N = 146 over 8 weeks). Tolcapone allowed for a greater reduction in L-dopa dose than bromocriptine and was similar to pergolide. Tolcapone produced similar benefits in motor impairment and disability ratings versus both bromocriptine and pergolide. The studies were underpowered to detect statistical differences for these efficacy outcomes, and there were no studies involving entacapone.
- Nausea, constipation, and orthostatic complaints were more common with bromocriptine and pergolide than with tolcapone.

FYI
- DDC inhibitors and COMT inhibitors are now being used in combination in some jurisdictions, in a tablet with levodopa.

Cholinesterase Inhibitors

DESCRIPTION
Cholinesterase inhibitors are a collection of agents that increase acetylcholine levels.

PROTOTYPE AND COMMON DRUGS
Reversible
- Prototype: donepezil
- Others: riva**stigmine**, pyrido**stigmine**, neo**stigmine**, galantamine, physo**stigmine**, edrophonium

MOA (MECHANISM OF ACTION)
- Acetylcholine is the main neurotransmitter in the parasympathetic arm of the ANS and a major neurotransmitter in the CNS.
- Acetylcholinesterase is the key enzyme involved in the **breakdown of acetylcholine** in the synapse.
- Acetylcholinesterase inhibitors bind to this enzyme, inhibiting its activity and leading to **an increase in acetylcholine in the synapse**, thus enhancing cholinergic transmission (Figure 21-11).
- Alzheimer's disease is characterized by profound cell death in the brain, with a progressive decline in cognitive function. The death of neurons leads to a reduction in the amount of acetylcholine released into the synapse as well as the amount of postsynaptic receptors on which acetylcholine acts.
- The efficacy of acetylcholinesterase inhibitors in Alzheimer's disease is believed to be a result of the enhanced cholinergic neurotransmission. Essentially, cholinesterase inhibitors maximize the remaining pool of acetylcholine by inhibiting its breakdown, thus reducing the decline in cognition.
- Cholinesterase inhibitors are not believed to be disease-modifying agents, and once cell death has reached a certain threshold, their effects begin to wane as there are too few remaining synapses for cognition to be significantly affected.

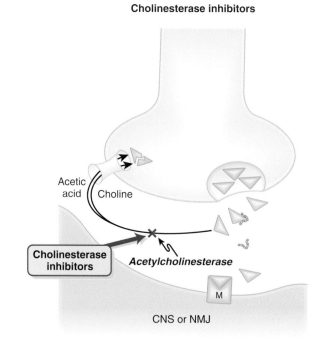

Cholinesterase inhibitors

Acetic acid

Choline

Cholinesterase inhibitors

Acetylcholinesterase

M

CNS or NMJ

Figure 21-11.

- Cholinesterase inhibitors are also used to enhance acetylcholine levels at the neuromuscular junction (NMJ), facilitating transmission and movement. They can therefore be used in patients with disorders of the NMJ, such as myasthenia gravis, a condition characterized by a reduction in the number of acetylcholine receptors at the NMJ. Cholinesterase inhibitors increase the amount of acetylcholine available to bind to these receptors, thus increasing the probability of binding.
- Cholinesterase inhibitors can also be used to reverse the effects of competitive NMJ blockers used in anesthesia (see also Nondepolarizing Neuromuscular Blockers).

- Pseudocholinesterase (butyrylcholinesterase) is another enzyme that breaks down acetylcholine. Rivastigmine inhibits both acetylcholinesterase and pseudocholinesterase and is therefore known as a *dual cholinesterase inhibitor.*

PHARMACOKINETICS

- Neostigmine and pyridostigmine are largely eliminated by the kidney. The elimination half-lives are 1 to 2 hours.
- Rivastigmine is available as a transdermal patch. The patch is intended to improve patient compliance.

INDICATIONS

- Alzheimer's disease
- Myasthenia gravis
- Reversal of nondepolarizing neuromuscular blockers
- Postoperative intestinal ileus
- Urinary retention

CONTRAINDICATIONS
Neostigmine, Pyridostigmine, Physostigmine, Edrophonium

- **Bronchial asthma:** Cholinergic stimulation would be expected to cause bronchoconstriction as well as an increase in bronchial secretions, both of which could exacerbate the symptoms of asthma and potentially promote an asthma attack.
- **Urinary or gastrointestinal obstruction:** Cholinergic stimulation promotes peristalsis of the gastrointestinal tract, which will exacerbate symptoms associated with obstruction. The same is true for urinary obstruction, as contraction of the bladder will worsen symptoms.

SIDE EFFECTS

- Consequences of enhanced cholinergic transmission:
  - Nausea, vomiting
  - Increased urination
  - Intestinal cramping, diarrhea
  - Increased secretions (bronchial, salivary)

IMPORTANT NOTES

- The cholinesterase inhibitors used to treat Alzheimer's disease are reversible inhibitors. Irreversible cholinesterase inhibitors lead to a profound increase in cholinergic neurotransmission, which in turn leads to convulsions, thick secretions that obstruct the airways, cardiac arrhythmias, and death. Irreversible cholinesterase inhibitors have been used as nerve gases in warfare (sarin gas) for decades and are also used in many pesticides.

EVIDENCE
Donepezil for Treatment of Alzheimer's Disease

- A 2006 Cochrane review (24 trials, N = 5796 participants) assessed whether donepezil improves the well-being of patients with dementia from Alzheimer's disease. Most of the participants had mild to moderate disease, and most studies were less than 6 months in duration. Donepezil improved cognition versus placebo. Some improvement was seen in global clinical scale, and improvements were also seen in activities of daily living and behavior but not in quality of life. Withdrawals were more frequent with donepezil 10 mg versus placebo. Results were similar for all severities of disease. Health resource use was reported in only two studies, and there were no differences versus placebo.
  - The incidences of nausea, vomiting, diarrhea, muscle cramping, dizziness, fatigue, and anorexia were higher in the 10-mg/day group than in the placebo group.

Galantamine for Mild Cognitive Impairment or Alzheimer's Disease

- A 2006 Cochrane review (10 trials, N = 6805 participants) assessed the clinical effects of galantamine in patients with mild cognitive impairment or probable or possible Alzheimer's disease. In Alzheimer's disease the authors found that galantamine was more effective than placebo in improving cognitive function, as well as some evidence of improvement on measures of activity of daily living and behavioral symptoms. In mild cognitive impairment, data from two trials suggest marginal clinical benefit but an increased incidence of death with galantamine.

Rivastigmine for Treatment of Alzheimer's Disease

- A 2009 Cochrane review (9 trials, N = 4775 participants) determined the efficacy and safety of rivastigmine for patients with dementia of the Alzheimer's type. High-dose rivastigmine (6 to 12 mg daily) improved measures of cognition and activities of daily living versus placebo. These differences were statistically significant for cognition only when lower doses of rivastigmine were used. The incidence of side effects such as nausea, vomiting, diarrhea, anorexia, headache, syncope, abdominal pain, and dizziness was higher than with placebo. One trial compared patches with capsules, finding no differences in efficacy but a lower incidence of side effects with the lower dose patch versus capsules.

FYI

- Metrifonate was an irreversible cholinesterase inhibitor whose development was halted after reports of life-threatening respiratory failure and death during the clinical trial process.
- An acronym to remember the effects of cholinergic overload is **SLUDGE:** salivation, lacrimation, urination, defecation, GI distress, emesis.

Ergot Alkaloids

DESCRIPTION

Ergots are naturally derived agents that are primarily vasoconstrictors, although they do possess other properties.

PROTOTYPE AND COMMON DRUGS

- Prototype: **ergo**tamine
- Others: dihydro**ergo**tamine, **ergo**novine, methyl**ergo**novine

MOA (MECHANISM OF ACTION)

- Migraines are believed to be caused by **cerebral vasodilation** and subsequent activation of pain fibers.
- The activation of pain fibers may be mediated by the release of transmitters such as vasoactive intestinal peptide (VIP), substance P, and calcitonin gene-related peptide (CGRP).
- Many ergots are agonists at serotonin 1B and 1D (5-HT$_{1B}$ and 5-HT$_{1D}$) receptors and thus possess similar properties to those of the triptans, serotonin agonists used in the treatment of acute migraine. Stimulation of these receptors leads to **vasoconstriction** of cerebral blood vessels (Figure 21-12).
- The 5-HT$_{1B}$ and 5-HT$_{1D}$ receptors are also presynaptic autoreceptors. Autoreceptors are receptors that when stimulated inhibit release of transmitters into the synaptic cleft. Thus the ergots inhibit the release of VIP, substance P, and CGRP, although a definitive link between these actions and the drugs' efficacy in migraine has not been confirmed.
- In addition, the ergots are **partial agonists at α$_1$-adrenergic receptors.** Stimulation of these receptors leads to **vasoconstriction of cerebral vessels.** It is believed that this vasoconstriction contributes to the efficacy of these agents in acute migraine, although a definitive link has not been established.
- Ergots also stimulate **uterine contractions,** and it is believed that this effect is mediated by 5-HT$_2$ receptors. This stimulation of contractions, coupled with vasoconstriction, is used to control bleeding in postpartum hemorrhage.

PHARMACOKINETICS

- Ergotamine undergoes extensive first-pass metabolism and has a very low oral bioavailability. In contrast, ergonovine and methylergonovine are rapidly absorbed and reach peak plasma levels in under 90 minutes, with plasma levels 10 times those of ergotamine.
- The biologic activity (vasoconstriction) of ergotamine (24 hours or more) extends well beyond its elimination half-life of 2 hours. The elimination half-life of ergonovine is even shorter than that of ergotamine.
- Ergotamine (oral, sublingual, rectal) and dihydroergotamine (injectable, nasal spray) are available in several dosage forms. The availability of nonoral dosage forms is important because patients with migraine also often have nausea and vomiting.
- For postpartum hemorrhage, ergotamine should never be administered intravenously, because of concerns over excessive vasoconstriction leading to hypertension.
- Ergotamine derivatives are metabolized via CYP3A4. Given the dangers associated with excessive ergotamine levels (see Side Effects), the concomitant use of strong CYP3A4 inhibitors should be avoided.

INDICATIONS

- Migraine
  - ▲ Acute: ergotamine, dihydroergotamine
  - ▲ Prophylaxis: methysergide
- Postpartum hemorrhage

CONTRAINDICATIONS

- **Coronary artery disease**: Vasoconstriction or spasm of coronary arteries may exacerbate symptoms and lead to myocardial ischemia.
- **Hypertension**: The pressor effects of the ergots may raise blood pressure, exacerbating hypertension.
- **Peripheral vascular disease** may lead to limb ischemia because of vasoconstriction of stenotic arteries.

Ergots

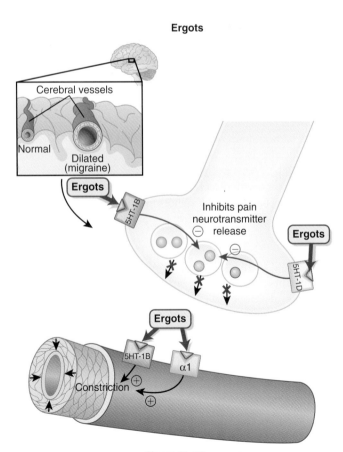

Figure 21-12.

- **Avoid using within 24 hours of triptans or other vaso-constrictors** because of additive vasoconstrictive effects.
- **Pregnancy:** Ergots may cause fetal distress, or miscarriage. Although not used during pregnancy, ergots can be used during labor to control hemorrhage (see later).

SIDE EFFECTS
- **Nausea and vomiting:** are likely a direct effect on the vomiting center in the brain.
- **Diarrhea:** Activation of serotonin receptors in the gut can enhance GI motility.
- **Numbness and tingling of extremities** are likely caused by vasoconstriction of microvessels feeding nerves.
- **Angina** is likely caused by vasoconstriction or vasospasm of coronary arteries.
- **Hypertension** is caused by vasoconstriction.

IMPORTANT NOTES
- The first use of ergots was to promote uterine contractions (an oxytocic) in childbirth in the 1500s. However, widespread use for this indication in the early 1800s was accompanied by an increase in the number of stillbirths. Excessive uterine contraction reduces blood flow to the fetus, and this is the likely reason for the stillbirths. In an early version of adverse drug reaction surveillance, ergot was no longer recommended for induction of labor but instead for postpartum hemorrhage, an indication that exists to this day.
- Caffeine is added to some ergot preparations (ergotamine oral and rectal) to both facilitate absorption and potentiate the analgesic effects. However, this also means that patients who are sensitive to caffeine may want to avoid these preparations. Caffeine (or caffeine withdrawal) can also be a precipitating factor with some migraine sufferers.
- There are strict administration guidelines for the use of ergotamine, because as a treatment for acute migraine it is used on an as-needed basis and because serious adverse effects can occur when toxic levels are reached.

- Dihydroergotamine also has strict administration guidelines.

FYI
- Ergot is derived from the fungus *Claviceps purpurea*.
- Ergot has been written about for centuries, although much of its history has been associated with its poisonous effects. Ergot is derived from a fungus found in grain; therefore there have been many instances throughout history in which mass ergot poisonings have occurred because of contaminated grain. Signs of ergot poisoning (*ergotism* or *St. Anthony's fire*) include gangrene of the limbs, with some limbs *falling off* without loss of blood, and spontaneous abortion. These situations occur because of extreme vasoconstriction of vessels.
- The most notorious ergot alkaloid is lysergic acid diethylamide (LSD). The *unique* properties of LSD were discovered accidentally in 1943 by Dr. Albert Hoffman of Sandoz Pharmaceuticals. After accidentally ingesting LSD during an experiment, Dr. Hoffman experienced the full hallucinogenic effects of this compound. The onset of action of LSD occurs in within 30 to 60 minutes, with effects peaking in 1 to 6 hours and dissipating in 8 to 12 hours.
- Ergonovine goes by a number of different names (ergometrine, ergotocine, ergosterine, ergobasine), owing to the fact that it was discovered in four different laboratories almost simultaneously. In Europe, the names *ergometrine* and *ergobasine* have persisted, whereas *ergonovine* was adopted in the United States.
- Bromocriptine, a dopamine agonist sometimes used in the treatment of Parkinson's disease, is actually a semisynthetic ergot (2-bromo-α-ergocriptine).
- Methysergide, a drug with similar (but not identical) mechanisms of action to the ergots, was withdrawn from the market in many jurisdictions because of safety concerns (heart valve damage).

Triptans

DESCRIPTION
Triptans are serotonin (5-HT) agonists used for treating and preventing migraines.

PROTOTYPE AND COMMON DRUGS
- Prototype: suma**triptan**
- Others: almo**triptan**, ele**triptan**, nara**triptan**, riza**triptan**, zolmi**triptan**

MOA (MECHANISM OF ACTION)
- Two major types of factors contribute to the development of migraine: **vascular** and **neurological.**

- Migraines are believed to be caused by **cerebral vasodilation** and subsequent activation of pain fibers. The activation of pain fibers may be mediated by the release of transmitters such as VIP, substance P, and CGRP (Figure 21-13).
- Triptans are agonists at 5-HT_{1B} and 5-HT_{1D} receptors, leading to **vasoconstriction** of cerebral vessels. It is believed that this vasoconstriction contributes to the efficacy of these agents in acute migraine, although a definitive link has not been established.
- The 5H-T_{1B} and 5H-T_{1D} receptors are also presynaptic autoreceptors. Autoreceptors are receptors that when stimulated inhibit release of transmitters into the synaptic cleft.

Triptans

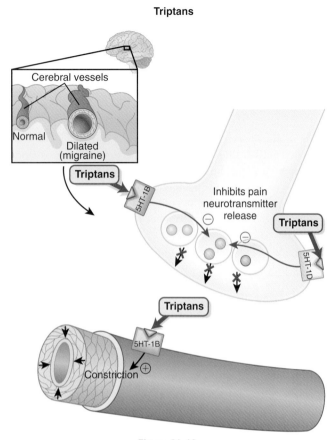

Figure 21-13.

Drug	Peak Plasma Concentration	Elimination Half-Life
Sumatriptan	PO: 1-2 h SC: 12 min	1-2 h
Zolmitriptan	PO: 1.5-2 h	2-3 h
Rizatriptan	PO: 1-1.5 h	1.6-2.5 h
Naratriptan	PO: 2-3 h	6 h
Almotriptan	PO: 1-3 h	3-4 h
Eletriptan	PO: 1.5 h	4 h

TABLE 21-5. Pharmacokinetic Characteristics of Triptans

PO, Orally; *SC,* subcutaneously.

Thus the triptans inhibit the release of VIP, substance P, and CGRP, although a definitive link between these actions and their efficacy in migraine has not been confirmed.

PHARMACOKINETICS

- The triptans are intended to be used acutely and are characterized by a rapid onset and short half-life. Their time to peak plasma concentration and elimination half-lives are summarized in Table 21-5.
- Sumatriptan is available in several different dosage forms: tablet, nasal spray, and subcutaneous injection. Zolmitriptan is also available as a nasal spray. Zolmitriptan and rizatriptan are available in quick-dissolve formulations.

- Sumatriptan and rizatriptan are primarily metabolized by MAO-A.
- Many migraine attacks are accompanied by nausea and vomiting; the oral route might not be practical in affected patients.

INDICATION

- Acute migraine

CONTRAINDICATIONS

- **Ischemic or vasospastic coronary artery disease:** The triptans work by inducing vasoconstriction, and this may worsen existing ischemia or vasospasm.
- **Uncontrolled hypertension:** Vasoconstriction may lead to transient elevations in blood pressure.
- **MAOIs:** The MAOIs inhibit the breakdown of serotonin and norepinephrine and are thus capable of inducing both serotonin syndrome and hypertensive crisis through a pressor effect. Pressor effects are also a concern with the triptans.
- **Severe hepatic or renal impairment** is a contraindication for naratriptan only.

SIDE EFFECTS

- **Cardiac events—rare but serious:**
  - Coronary artery vasospasm
  - Transient myocardial ischemia
  - Atrial or ventricular arrhythmias
  - Myocardial infarction
- **Pressure, tightness, or pain in chest, neck, or jaw:** likely caused by vasoconstriction and could indicate myocardial ischemia

IMPORTANT NOTES

- Triptans should be administered as close as possible to the onset of a migraine attack.
- Repeat doses of triptans can be administered if the headache returns. The interval between doses is based on the half-lives, with the shorter half-life oral agents allowing for repeat doses after 2 hours, and the longer-acting naratriptan allowing a repeat after 4 hours. Subcutaneous sumatriptan can be repeated only once in 24 hours (i.e., maximum 2 doses in 24 hours). All agents have a maximum dose allowed per 24 hours.

EVIDENCE

Sumatriptan versus Other Therapies or Placebo

- A 2003 Cochrane review (25 trials, N = 16,200 patients) found that sumatriptan elicited significantly more pain-free responses at 2 hours at the 25-mg (NNT 5) and 100-mg (NNT 7.5) doses but not the 50-mg dose, compared with placebo. All doses were statistically different from placebo for pain relief. Adverse events were more common with sumatriptan 100 mg versus placebo (number needed to harm [NNH] 7).
- Comparisons among various triptans did not yield any clear differences in either efficacy or safety and tolerability.
- Compared with ergotamine and caffeine, sumatriptan performed better for pain-free response at 2 hours (NNT 4.5)

and relief at 2 hours (NNT 6). Adverse events did not differ between agents.

FYI

■ A different class of serotonin receptor, the 5-HT₃ subtype, is an important receptor that mediates nausea and vomiting and has resulted in very effective antinausea medications (see Chapter 15).

■ Despite some lingering safety concerns, some jurisdictions have now approved over-the-counter sale of low-dose triptans.

Topiramate

DESCRIPTION

Topiramate is a unique antiseizure drug with multiple mechanisms of action.

PROTOTYPE

■ Topiramate

MOA (MECHANISM OF ACTION)

■ Topiramate is thought to work via multiple mechanisms:
  ▲ **Potentiation of GABA**
    • GABA is the major **inhibitory** neurotransmitter in the CNS, so enhancing its actions should have an inhibitory effect.
  ▲ **Na⁺ channel blockade**
    • Na⁺ channels exist in several conformations—activated, inactivated, and resting.
    • The rapid cycling through these states is implicated in the cause of seizures, and Na⁺ channel blockers inhibit this rapid cycling.
  ▲ **Glutamate antagonist**
    • Glutamate is a major **excitatory** neurotransmitter, so blocking its actions should have an antiexcitatory effect. The NMDA receptor is a glutamate receptor, and it is blocked by topiramate.
  ▲ **Ca⁺² channel blockade**
    • Several antiseizure drugs block voltage-sensitive Ca^{+2} channels, and dysfunction of Ca^{+2} channels has been implicated in several neurologic disorders (Figure 21-14).

■ Topiramate also inhibits several carbonic anhydrase isozymes. At present it does not appear that this contributes to its antiseizure effect.

■ The mechanism of action of topiramate in migraine has not been established. Current theories are that antagonism of glutamate receptors plays a role, as well as Ca^{+2} channel blockade.

PHARMACOKINETICS

■ Topiramate is rapidly and well absorbed and has an elimination half-life of approximately 20 hours.

■ It is not extensively metabolized. Its metabolism can be affected by enzyme inducers, including other antiseizure agents such as phenytoin and carbamazepine.

■ Topiramate may reduce levels of the estrogen component of oral contraceptives.

Topiramate

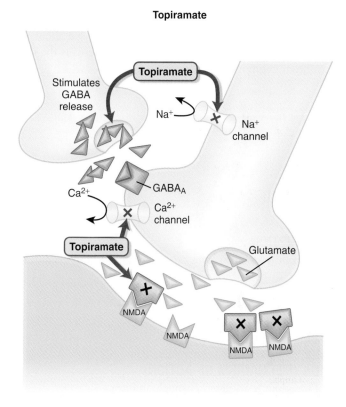

Figure 21-14.

INDICATIONS

■ Seizure disorders
■ Migraine

CONTRAINDICATIONS

■ None of major significance

SIDE EFFECTS
Serious

■ **Cognitive impairment:** This is relatively common with antiseizure drugs and may also be related to seizure disorders in general. Specific parameters affected include verbal memory and speed.

■ **Renal calculi:** Formation of kidney stones is likely related to the drug's effects on carbonic anhydrase.

Other

- **Paresthesia** is likely a result of carbonic anhydrase inhibition, although the mechanism has not been established. One theory is that carbonic anhydrase may help in clearing lactic acid from sensory nerves.
- **Fatigue and sedation** are possible effects.
- **Dizziness** may occur.
- **Weight loss** is a side effect of therapy but is also being exploited as a therapeutic effect in obese patients.

IMPORTANT NOTES

- Topiramate is being tried in a variety of off-label indications, with varying degrees of success. The diversity of this agent is likely a reflection of its multiple mechanisms of action, although concerns have also been raised about its overuse and misuse. One of the major concerns is the significant cognitive effects associated with its use.

- As with other antiseizure drugs, the dose of topiramate should be tapered gradually when therapy is discontinued in patients with seizure disorders.

EVIDENCE
Migraine Prophylaxis

- A 2004 Cochrane review (six studies, N = 900 patients) compared topiramate with placebo. Topiramate significantly reduced the frequency of migraine, with an NNT of 4 for reducing frequency of attacks by 50%.
- The same review included one study that found no difference in efficacy between topiramate and propranolol, and one study that reported a slight improvement in headache frequency with topiramate versus valproate.

Phenytoin

DESCRIPTION

Phenytoin is an antiseizure drug belonging to the hydantoin family.

PROTOTYPE AND COMMON DRUGS

- Prototype: phenytoin
- Other: fosphenytoin

MOA (MECHANISM OF ACTION)

- Phenytoin is a sodium channel inhibitor.
- Sodium channels exist in three conformations:
  - ▲ Closed—before activation
  - ▲ Open—during depolarization
  - ▲ Inactivated—shortly after the peak of depolarization (Figure 21-15)
- The probability of a channel existing in each state depends on the membrane potential.
- Phenytoin slows the rate of channel recovery from the inactivated state. This increases the threshold for action potentials and prevents repetitive firing.
- In secondarily generalized seizures, phenytoin prevents the rapid spread of seizure activity to other neurons.
- A key feature of the efficacy of phenytoin is that it selectively targets channels that are opening and closing at high frequency. This is referred to as targeting in a *use-dependent* manner. This allows phenytoin to target rapidly firing neurons, typical of those seen in partial seizures, while minimizing its effects on spontaneous neuronal activity.
- Phenytoin may also enhance the release of GABA and inhibit the release of glutamate from presynaptic neurons.

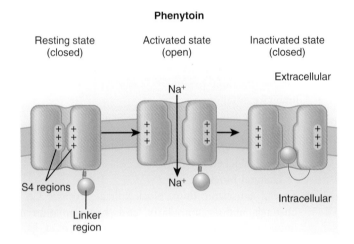

Phenytoin

Resting state (closed) Activated state (open) Inactivated state (closed)

Figure 21-15.

GABA is a key inhibitory and glutamate a key excitatory neurotransmitter; hence the net effect would be inhibitory and would also contribute to reducing neuronal activity. It is not clear whether these effects on GABA and glutamate are related to sodium channel blockade.

PHARMACOKINETICS

- Phenytoin is metabolized by CYP2C9/10 and to a lesser extent by CYP2C19.

- It exhibits **saturation kinetics**, meaning that at lower doses, metabolism is first order, then at higher doses the enzymes responsible for metabolizing phenytoin become saturated and metabolism switches to zero order. Toxicity can be reached *quickly* at higher doses.
- Phenytoin is a CYP450 enzyme inducer and is therefore capable of interacting with other agents. Because its metabolism is saturable, phenytoin may also inhibit the metabolism of coadministered drugs that use the same CYP enzymes for elimination.
- The elimination half-life of phenytoin is 22 hours on average but ranges from 7 to 42 hours.
- Phenytoin can be administered intravenously, but the rate of administration must not exceed 50 mg/min in adults and 1 to 3 mg/kg/min in neonates. This is because of the risk of hypotension.
- Fosphenytoin is a prodrug of phenytoin and was developed to overcome the low aqueous solubility of phenytoin, thus facilitating intravenous use.

INDICATIONS
- Seizure prophylaxis in patients with head injuries
- Partial seizures
- Generalized tonic-clonic seizures

CONTRAINDICATIONS
- **Cardiac conduction abnormalities (intravenous phenytoin)**: Intravenous phenytoin, being a Na^+ channel blocker, affects ventricular automaticity and is therefore contraindicated in patients at risk for being dependant on a ventricular escape rhythm, including those with sinus bradycardia, sinoatrial block, and second- and third-degree block.

SIDE EFFECTS
- **CNS: Diplopia, ataxia, and nystagmus** may occur. These types of sensory side effects may occur with agents that inhibit sodium channels, although a mechanism has not been established.
- **Gingival hyperplasia**: The mechanism is multifactorial, but phenytoin stimulates fibroblasts, enhances formation of granulation tissue, and promotes collagen deposition.
- **Hirsutism**: Excessive hair growth, typically facial hair, may occur in females. This can be a troubling and disfiguring side effect. The mechanism has not been established.
- **Bone deficiencies (rickets, osteomalacia)** may be caused by abnormal vitamin D metabolism induced by phenytoin, although the mechanism has not been established.

- **Decreased level of consciousness**: The mechanism for this effect has not been established.

With Intravenous Use
- Hypotension

IMPORTANT NOTES
- As is the case with a number of other antiepileptic drugs, phenytoin is teratogenic. This is particularly problematic because phenytoin also **induces the metabolism of oral contraceptives**, thus increasing the likelihood of an unexpected pregnancy.

EVIDENCE
Seizure Disorder
Phenytoin versus Oxcarbazepine
- A 2006 Cochrane review (two studies, N = 480 participants) found that oxcarbazepine improved the time to treatment withdrawal compared with phenytoin for patients with partial onset seizures. Otherwise the two drugs did not differ significantly from each other.

Status Epilepticus (Refractory Seizures)
- A 2005 Cochrane review compared various agents used in status epilepticus. In the only study (198 patients) that had a phenytoin arm, intravenous lorazepam was more effective at terminating seizures than intravenous phenytoin (RR of 0.62 for seizures continuing). There was no difference in adverse events between the two agents.

FYI
- Phenytoin was first synthesized in 1908, although it was not discovered to have anticonvulsant properties until 1938. Researchers at the time were looking for structural relatives of phenobarbital that lacked sedative properties and that were capable of suppressing electroshock convulsions in laboratory animals.
- The discovery of phenytoin as an effective antiseizure medication proved that antiseizure medications need not have sedating properties at therapeutic doses.
- Since the observation of gingival hyperplasia associated with phenytoin use over 70 years ago, researchers have periodically experimented with the use of topical phenytoin in wound healing.

Lamotrigine

DESCRIPTION
Lamotrigine is an antiseizure drug that works primarily by inhibiting sodium channels.

PROTOTYPE
- Lamotrigine

MOA (MECHANISM OF ACTION)
- Like many other antiseizure medications, lamotrigine is a sodium (Na^+) channel blocker.
- Sodium channels exist in three conformations:
  - **Closed**—before activation
  - **Open**—during depolarization
  - **Inactivated**—shortly after the peak of depolarization (Figure 21-16)

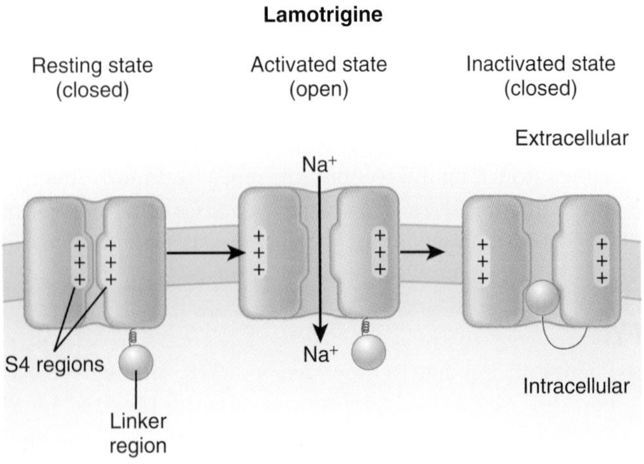

Lamotrigine

| Resting state (closed) | Activated state (open) | Inactivated state (closed) |

Figure 21-16.

- The probability of a channel existing in each state depends on the membrane potential.
- Lamotrigine slows the rate of channel recovery from the inactivated state. This increases the threshold for action potentials and prevents repetitive firing.
- The broad spectrum of action of lamotrigine, including its varied uses in psychiatry, suggest that it may also work through other mechanisms distinct from Na^+ channels. For example, lamotrigine may also **inhibit Ca^{2+} channels** and indirectly may also **inhibit glutamate release** from presynaptic nerve terminals, through its inhibition of either Na^+ or Ca^{2+} channels or both.
- Glutamate is an excitatory neurotransmitter that is believed to play a role in seizures as well as a number of psychiatric disorders, most notably bipolar disorder.

PHARMACOKINETICS
- Several of the commonly used antiseizure medications interact with lamotrigine. Phenytoin, carbamazepine, and phenobarbital are all CYP450 enzyme inducers and all reduce the half-life of lamotrigine, whereas valproate increases plasma levels of lamotrigine by inhibiting it metabolism.

INDICATIONS
- Seizure disorders
  - Partial seizures
  - Secondarily generalized seizures (these are seizures that precede a generalized tonic-clonic seizure)
- Bipolar disorder

CONTRAINDICATIONS
- None of major significance

SIDE EFFECTS
- **CNS** effects include dizziness, ataxia, blurred vision, and double vision. These types of sensory side effects occur with agents that inhibit sodium channels, although a mechanism has not been established.
- **Nausea and vomiting** may occur.

Serious
- **Rash**: Rashes can range from mild to severe, including **Stevens-Johnson syndrome** and **toxic epidermal necrolysis**. These rashes can be fatal in patients who are otherwise compromised, or if treatment is not discontinued and/or if the rash is not treated. The exact mechanism behind these severe reactions is not known.

IMPORTANT NOTES
- Lamotrigine is increasingly being used for psychiatric indications, including bipolar disorder. The idea to use lamotrigine in bipolar disorder first originated with the observation of its antiglutamatergic effects and the belief that this excitatory neurotransmitter may have a role in the pathogenesis of this illness.

EVIDENCE
Lamotrigine versus Carbamazepine Monotherapy for Seizure Disorders
- A 2006 Cochrane review (five trials, N = 1384 participants) compared lamotrigine to carbamazepine as monotherapy in partial-onset or generalized-onset tonic-clonic seizures. The authors found that time to treatment withdrawal was improved with lamotrigine over carbamazepine (hazard ratio 0.55), whereas time to first seizure and freedom from seizure were not statistically different between lamotrigine and carbamazepine.

FYI

- Lamotrigine was initially developed as an antifolate agent, at a time when folate was believed to play a role in seizure development. Although it proved to be only a weak inhibitor of dihydrofolate reductase, its other pharmacologic properties as an Na⁺ channel blocker led to its success as an antiseizure medication.

γ-Aminobutyric acid (GABA) Analogues

DESCRIPTION

GABA analogues are primarily used in the treatment of seizures and management of neuropathic pain.

PROTOTYPE AND COMMON DRUGS

- Prototype: **gaba**pentin
- Others: pre**gaba**lin

MOA (MECHANISM OF ACTION)

- Although gabapentin is a widely used drug, its exact mode of action is not fully understood.
- Seizures are characterized by an abnormal increase in neural activity in the brain. Two approaches to treating seizures are to reduce activity of excitatory neurotransmitters and to enhance activity of inhibitory neurotransmitters.
- Gabapentin's major mechanism in the treatment of seizure is via binding to the $\alpha_2\delta$ subunit of presynaptic voltage-gated Ca^{2+} channels in the brain. It is believed that by reducing the influx of Ca^{2+} at nerve terminals, the release of excitatory neurotransmitters such as glutamate is reduced, although the connection between the reduction of Ca^{2+} influx and inhibition of glutamate release has not been established (Figure 21-17).
- The structure of gabapentin is derived from GABA; therefore it has long been thought of as simply a GABA agonist. However, **gabapentin does not appear to bind to GABA receptors.** Instead, it may **promote the release of GABA.** As with other antiseizure medications that work through GABA, enhancement of the actions of this inhibitory neurotransmitter appears to counteract the excess excitatory neurotransmission that leads to seizures.

PHARMACOKINETICS

- Neither gabapentin nor pregabalin is metabolized to an appreciable extent. These agents do not appear to inhibit or induce other metabolizing enzymes, such as the CYP450 system; therefore pharmacokinetic drug interactions are not an issue.
- The clearance of pregabalin and gabapentin is reduced in patients with impaired renal function.

INDICATIONS

- Seizure disorders (adjunctive)
- Management of neuropathic pain

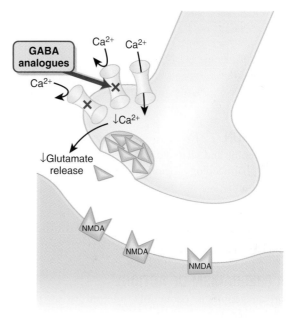

GABA analogues

Figure 21-17.

CONTRAINDICATIONS

- None of major significance

SIDE EFFECTS

- **Fatigue:** The mechanism has not been established, but these agents inhibit release of an excitatory neurotransmitter and enhance the release of an inhibitory neurotransmitter, resulting in a net inhibitory effect in the CNS.
- **Dizziness:** The mechanism has not been established.
- **Ataxia:** Lack of coordination in movement occurs because of disruption in central (cerebellar) function. The mechanism has not been established.

IMPORTANT NOTES

- Gabapentin has a very wide dosage range. The recommended dosage range begins at 300 mg and goes up to 1800 mg daily. However, patients have taken up to 3600 mg daily.

EVIDENCE
Pregabalin as Adjunctive Therapy in Drug-Resistant Partial Seizures

■ A 2008 Cochrane review (four trials, N = 1397 participants) compared a range of doses of pregabalin with placebo. The authors found that patients treated with pregabalin were more likely to experience a 50% reduction in seizures. However, pregabalin was not associated with freedom from seizures, and participants were significantly more likely to withdraw from treatment for any reason and for adverse events. Pregabalin elicited ataxia, dizziness, somnolence, and weight gain compared with placebo.

Gabapentin for Acute and Chronic Pain

■ A 2005 Cochrane review (15 studies, N = 1468 participants) examined RCTs assessing the analgesic effectiveness and adverse effects of gabapentin for pain management. Only one small study assessed acute pain, and it found no differences between gabapentin and placebo. In chronic pain, 42% of patients improved versus 19% on placebo.

FYI

■ Pregabalin was the first drug ever approved by the FDA for fibromyalgia.

Carbamazepine

DESCRIPTION

Carbamazepine and related drugs are agents related by chemistry and pharmacology, belonging to the *iminostilbene* class of anticonvulsants.

PROTOTYPE AND COMMON DRUGS

■ Prototype: carbamazepine
■ Others: oxcarbazepine

MOA (MECHANISM OF ACTION)

■ Carbamazepine is commonly referred to as a **sodium channel blocker.**
■ Seizures are caused by abnormal electrical discharges in the brain. These abnormal discharges propagate, spreading to other parts of the brain and producing abnormal movements, thoughts, or sensations. Antiseizures drugs work by inhibiting either the initiation or the propagation of these discharges.
■ Sodium channels play an important role in the generation and propagation of action potentials. They exist in three conformations:
  ▲ **Closed**—before activation
  ▲ **Open**—during depolarization
  ▲ **Inactivated**—shortly after the peak of depolarization (Figure 21-18)
■ The probability of a channel existing in each state depends on the membrane potential.
■ Carbamazepine **stabilizes the inactive form** of the Na$^+$ channel, which slows the rate of channel recovery from the inactivated state. This increases the threshold for action potentials and prevents repetitive firing.
■ Carbamazepine and other Na$^+$ channel blockers bind to the Na$^+$ channel when it is open. Because rapidly firing neurons, such as those found in seizure disorders are open a greater percentage of the time, these drugs tend to be selective for abnormal electrical activity found in a seizure focus and do

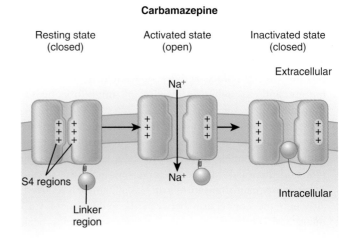

Carbamazepine

Resting state (closed) Activated state (open) Inactivated state (closed)

Na$^+$

S4 regions

Linker region

Extracellular

Intracellular

Na$^+$

Figure 21-18.

not suppress normal neuronal activity. This is referred to as **use-dependent** blockade and is essential for limiting the toxicity of these agents.
■ In addition to its effects on sodium channels, carbamazepine has several other actions, interacting with **adenosine receptors** and inhibiting the uptake and release of norepinephrine from brain synaptosomes; it may also potentiate the postsynaptic actions of GABA. Carbamazepine may also potentiate glutamatergic transmission. Whether any of these actions contribute to its clinical efficacy is unclear at present.

PHARMACOKINETICS

■ Carbamazepine is slowly and erratically absorbed, with peak plasma concentrations occurring anywhere from 4 to 24 hours after an oral dose.

- Carbamazepine (10,11-epoxide) and oxcarbazepine (10-monohydroxy; MHD) each have an active metabolite that contributes significantly to the activity of the drug. Oxcarbazepine is rapidly converted to its active metabolite and therefore acts more like a prodrug.
- Carbamazepine is metabolized by CYP3A4 and is an inducer of CYP3A and CYP2C. Oxcarbazepine induces CYP3A, although not to the same extent as carbamazepine.
- Carbamazepine is also an autoinducer, meaning that its half-life can decrease after prolonged therapy. Once its half-life becomes shorter, maintaining stable plasma levels can be a challenge; therefore the controlled-release (CR) formulation can be useful for obtaining stable levels.

INDICATIONS
- Partial seizures
- Generalized tonic-clonic (carbamazepine)
- Trigeminal neuralgia
  - ▲ Neuropathic pain, usually in the facial area, arising from the trigeminal nerves
- Bipolar disorder (carbamazepine)

CONTRAINDICATIONS
Carbamazepine
- **Hepatic disease**: See Side Effects.
- **Bone marrow suppression**: See Side Effects.
- **Atrioventricular heart block**: The mechanism has not been established, but likely is due to Na⁺ channel blockade.
- **MAOIs**: Carbamazepine also acts as a reuptake inhibitor; thus the same warnings against concomitant use with other reuptake inhibitors (or even having a washout when switching from one to the other) apply.

SIDE EFFECTS
- **Drowsiness**
- **Dizziness**
- **Ataxia**
- **Blurred vision**
- **Nausea, vomiting**

Serious
- **Dermatologic reactions** may occur, including **Stevens-Johnson syndrome** and **toxic epidermal necrolysis**, which are both very severe reactions with possible fatal outcomes.

- **Hematologic (carbamazepine)**: Infrequently, **agranulocytosis** and aplastic anemia, as well as leukopenia and thrombocytopenia, have been reported.
- **Hepatic (carbamazepine)**: **Hepatocellular** and **cholestatic jaundice** and **hepatitis** may occur.

IMPORTANT NOTES
- Generally, oxcarbazepine is considered to be better tolerated than carbamazepine.
- Perhaps because of its activity as a reuptake inhibitor, carbamazepine is increasingly being used in psychiatry, specifically as a mood stabilizer in acute mania and prophylaxis in bipolar disorder.

Advanced
Pharmacogenomics
- Asians appear to be at higher risk of developing the serious skin rashes associated with carbamazepine, including Stevens-Johnson syndrome and toxic epidermal necrolysis. A genetic screening test is available to identify a marker (HLA-B 1502) for increased risk.

EVIDENCE
Seizure Disorder
Carbamazepine versus Phenytoin
- A 2002 Cochrane review (three trials, N = 551 participants) compared these two agents in patients with partial-onset or generalized tonic-clonic seizures, using individual patient data from three trials (551 patients). The authors found no differences between carbamazepine and phenytoin for time to 6- or 12-month remission, time to first seizure, or time to withdrawal.

Carbamazepine versus Lamotrigine
- A 2006 Cochrane review (five trials, N = 1384 participants) compared these two agents in patients with partial-onset or generalized-onset tonic-clonic seizures, using individual patient data from five trials (1384 patients). The time to treatment withdrawal was significantly improved with lamotrigine compared with carbamazepine, whereas the time to first seizure and freedom from seizure at 6 months favored carbamazepine, although not by a statistically significant amount.

FYI
- Carbamazepine is chemically related to the tricyclic antidepressants (TCAs).

Barbiturates

DESCRIPTION
Barbiturates are CNS depressants.

PROTOTYPE AND COMMON DRUGS
- Prototype: Pheno**barbital**
- Others: Seco**barbital**, pento**barbital**, mepho**barbital**, but-a**barbital**, amo**barbital**

Anesthetics
- Thiopental, methohexital (covered in discussion of intravenous anesthetics)

MOA (MECHANISM OF ACTION)
- GABA is the major **inhibitory neurotransmitter** in the CNS. GABA binds to three different types of receptors: $GABA_A$, $GABA_B$, and $GABA_C$.
  - ▲ Binding of GABA to $GABA_A$ receptors leads to the opening of the chloride (Cl^-) channel, facilitating Cl^- influx and cellular hyperpolarization (making the inside more negative).
  - ▲ Hyperpolarization of a cell decreases the probability that the cell can be subsequently *de*polarized by other incoming excitatory signals; this will have a net inhibitory effect.
- Barbiturates increase the binding of GABA to $GABA_A$ receptors and increase the influx of Cl^- into the neuron, resulting in hyperpolarization and decreased neuronal activity.
- Barbiturates also potentiate the binding of benzodiazepines to $GABA_A$ receptors.
- The overall net effect of this binding is a global reduction in CNS activity; barbiturates are CNS depressants (Figure 21-19).
- Seizure activity is unwanted, increased neurologic activity. By suppressing all neural activity, the hope is to primarily suppress the neurons contributing to the seizure *before* depressing the neurons involved with normal function.
- The reticular activating system is one part of the brain that is important in the control of consciousness. It is also depressed with barbiturates.

PHARMACOKINETICS
- Barbiturates can be administered orally, intravenously, intramuscularly, and, less commonly, rectally.
- When administered via the intravenous route, a pronounced redistribution effect occurs: the drug levels in the blood are initially very high and equilibrate with the brain to have a strong effect. However, the drug also equilibrates with other tissues, and the concentration in the blood rapidly falls; the levels in the brain also rapidly fall in response to this, as the drug becomes redistributed to other tissues in the body.

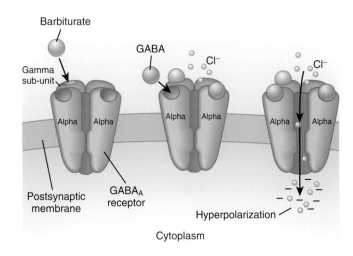

Barbiturate

Synaptic cleft

Figure 21-19.

- All barbiturates are liver enzyme inducers; they increase the activity of CYP2A and CYP3A enzymes, which results in faster metabolism (and thus reduced effect of) other, coadministered drugs that are also hepatically metabolized.
  - ▲ Barbiturates are an example of autoinducers: a drug that induces the same enzymes that metabolize it. This results in increased dose requirements over time, compared with initial dose requirements.

INDICATIONS
- **Seizure disorders**
- **Sedation:** Benzodiazepines have mostly replaced barbiturates for sedation and treatment of anxiety and sleep disorders.

CONTRAINDICATION
- **Porphyria** is a rare group of diseases caused by enzyme deficiencies resulting in accumulation of porphyrins, which are precursors to heme. Barbiturates can increase activity through these biochemical pathways and exacerbate accumulation of porphyrins.

SIDE EFFECTS
- **Sedation:** Antiseizure effects occur at a lower dose than sedation; however, some patients will need higher doses of treatment to suppress seizure activity, and the dose can approach a sedating dose. Therefore the **therapeutic index** between the antiseizure dose and the sedating dose is small.

- **Addiction:** Barbiturates are highly addictive.
- **Hypotension** may occur when barbiturates are given intravenously for anesthesia, especially in patients at risk (cardiac disease or trauma).

IMPORTANT NOTES

- Phenobarbital has more selective antiseizure properties relative to its sedative properties. As a result, it is the most commonly used barbiturate for treatment of seizures.
- Because of the **narrow therapeutic index** between antiseizure activity and sedation, most antiseizure medications are commonly measured in the blood to ensure that the target concentrations are appropriate. However, dosage should also be established on clinical grounds: the ultimate goal would be suppression of seizure activity and the absence of sedation. If both these goals are met, then the clinical outcome should out-prioritize the goal of meeting the blood levels. Some patients will require higher or lower blood levels (compared with the recommend range) to achieve these clinical endpoints.
- **Tolerance** occurs. Because of CNS receptor down-regulation and decreased sensitivity or responsiveness to continued agonism, progressively increasing doses are commonly required over time. Furthermore, the enzyme induction results in increased hepatic metabolism, a second factor that results in increased dose requirements over time.
- Chronically administered barbiturates over time will *virtually guarantee* **addiction and tolerance.** This type of administration should be avoided if used for sedation.
- Some medications include a combination of a barbiturate and an opioid. Because both medications are addictive, these drugs have *enormous* addiction potential.
- Barbiturate **toxicity** closely resembles *alcohol intoxication:*
  - ▲ Sedation may occur.
  - ▲ Slurred speech or dysarthria is caused by lack of coordination of the muscles required for speech.
  - ▲ Ataxia consists of a wide stance and unsteady gait resulting from uncoordinated movements and dizziness.
  - ▲ Nystagmus—jerky rhythmic movements of the eyes when the patient looks left or right—may occur.
  - ▲ A severely depressed level of consciousness (coma) may be present.
  - ▲ Hypotension may occur.
  - ▲ Respiratory depression (manifested by hypercarbia and/or hypoxia) can also be caused by airway obstruction: when a patient is very heavily sedated, the muscles supporting the airway are relaxed and the airway can be obstructed by the tongue.
- Barbiturate **withdrawal** closely resembles *alcohol withdrawal:*
  - ▲ Increased CNS activity:
    - • Agitation, sleep disturbances, hallucinations, seizures
    - • Increased sympathetic nervous system activity
      - ○ Tachycardia, hypertension, sweating

EVIDENCE
Phenobarbital versus Carbamazepine for Treatment of Seizures

- A 2003 Cochrane review (4 trials, N = 684 patients) demonstrated no difference in "time to first seizure" or "time to 12-month remission" between the two drugs. However, withdrawals were more common with phenobarbital, indicating more side effects with that drug.

FYI

- Barbiturates are derivatives of barbituric acid.
- The structure of barbiturates replaces the two hydrogen atoms at the C5 position with seven and nine carbon atoms. This side chain determines potency and degree of seizure activity.
- Replacing the =O at C2 with a sulfur creates a thiobarbiturate, which has greater lipid solubility and thus faster onset of action and shorter duration of activity. *Thio*barbiturates are therefore used as general anesthetics (Figure 21-20).

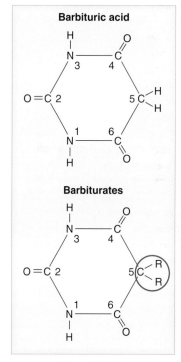

Figure 21-20.

- Ataxia (wide-stanced *dizzy* gait) is one hallmark of cerebellar dysfunction. Dysdiadokokinesis (difficulty placing your finger on an object when trying to point to an object in space) is another sign of cerebellar dysfunction.
- Amobarbital, also called sodium amytal, made guest appearances in the movies *True Lies* and *Meet the Fockers* as a truth serum. Through disinhibition and impairment of judgment, people may be more likely to be honest in situations in which they otherwise would not.

Valproate

DESCRIPTION

Valproates are drugs that reduce seizure frequency.

PROTOTYPE AND COMMON DRUGS

- Prototype: **val**proic acid
- Others: di**val**proex sodium

MOA (MECHANISM OF ACTION)

- Valproic acid works by several mechanisms. Its most established mechanism appears to be as a **sodium channel blocker**, with actions similar to those of carbamazepine and phenytoin.
- Sodium channels exist in three conformations (Figure 21-21):
  - ▲ **Closed**—before activation
  - ▲ **Open**—during depolarization
  - ▲ **Inactivated**—shortly after the peak of depolarization

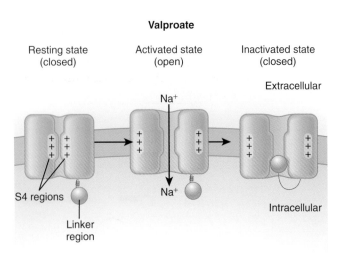

Valproate

Resting state (closed) Activated state (open) Inactivated state (closed)

Extracellular

Na⁺

S4 regions

Linker region

Na⁺

Intracellular

Figure 21-21.

- The probability of a channel existing in each state depends on the membrane potential.
- Valproate slows the rate of channel recovery from the inactivated state. This increases the threshold for action potentials and prevents repetitive firing.
- There is also increasing focus on the effects of valproate on GABA, the major **inhibitory neurotransmitter** in the CNS. Because seizures are characterized by abnormal excitation, enhancing the inhibitory effects of GABA is thought to be one way to control seizures.
- Valproate appears to enhance the effects of GABA by both **inhibiting its breakdown** by GABA transaminase and **pro-moting its synthesis** via the actions of glutamic acid decarboxylase, an enzyme responsible for GABA synthesis. The net increase in GABA levels may contribute significantly to the antiseizure efficacy of valproate.
- In addition to promoting the inhibitory effects of GABA, valproate may also block the excitatory effects of glutamate. Valproate also inhibits T-type calcium channels.

PHARMACOKINETICS

- Valproate is almost exclusively **eliminated by hepatic metabolism**, primarily by phase II enzymes rather than phase I (CYP450) enzymes.
- Valproate is, however, a **CYP2C9 enzyme inhibitor** and can interfere with the metabolism of other antiseizure medications such as phenytoin and phenobarbital.
- Valproate is more commonly used as a sustained release formulation, divalproex sodium.

INDICATIONS

- Absence seizures
- Partial seizures
- Generalized tonic-clonic seizures
- Bipolar disorder
- Migraine prophylaxis

CONTRAINDICATIONS

- **Significant hepatic disease or dysfunction.**
- **Pregnancy:** As is the case with a number of other antiseizure drugs, valproate is teratogenic, and its use in pregnancy should be considered only after a careful risk-benefit assessment.

SIDE EFFECTS

- Gastrointestinal (nausea, vomiting)

Serious, Rare

- **Hepatotoxicity:** Elevations in liver enzymes and bilirubin are relatively common; however, severe hepatotoxicity leading to liver failure and death is rare. Infants are at highest risk of developing severe hepatotoxicity. The mechanism has not been established; however, depletion of carnitine is believed to play a key role.

IMPORTANT NOTES

- The wide variety of mechanisms attributed to valproate may account for its use in a wide variety of indications. Even within seizure disorders, it is considered to have a **broad spectrum** of activity.
- Carnitine supplementation may play a role in mitigating the risk of hepatotoxicity with valproate. Carnitine is an amino acid derivative that plays an important role in the metabolism of fatty acids and in mitochondrial energy pro-

duction. Valproate depletes carnitine through several mechanisms: combining with it to increase renal excretion, inhibiting its reabsorption, and reducing carnitine synthesis.

Advanced

■ Valproate also inhibits histone deacetylase, an enzyme that is a target of newer anticancer therapies. It is not known whether histone deacetylase inhibition contributes to its antiseizure effects, but valproate is now being investigated as an anticancer drug.

EVIDENCE

Absence Seizures in Children and Adolescents

■ A 2005 Cochrane review (5 trials, N = 160 participants) found only a small number of low-quality trials with small sample sizes comparing valproate, ethosuximide, and lamotrigine with placebo in children or adolescents with absence seizures. The authors concluded that there was insufficient evidence to inform clinical practice and that larger trials were needed.

Versus Carbamazepine for Seizures

■ A 2000 Cochrane review (5 trials, N = 1265 participants), updated in 2007, compared valproate with carbamazepine for seizure disorder. There was no difference between these two agents for time to 12-month remission, time to first seizure, or time to treatment withdrawal in partial or generalized tonic-clonic seizures.

Versus Phenytoin for Generalized Tonic-Clonic Seizures

■ A 2003 Cochrane review (5 trials, N = 669 participants), updated in 2007, compared phenytoin with valproate for generalized tonic-clonic seizures. No differences between these two agents were found for time to 12-month remission, time to 6-month remission, time to first seizure, or time to treatment withdrawal.

Anticonvulsants for Migraine Prophylaxis

■ A 2004 Cochrane review (23 trials, N = 2927 participants), updated in 2006, assessed efficacy and tolerability of anticonvulsants for migraine prevention. Overall, anticonvulsants reduced migraine frequency by about 1.3 attacks per 28 days compared with placebo. More patients treated with anticonvulsants had a 50% or greater reduction in migraine frequency, compared with placebo (RR 2.25).

FYI

■ Several second-generation derivatives of valproic acid are in development, in hopes of minimizing its teratogenicity and hepatotoxicity.

■ Valproic acid was discovered over a century ago, although it gained wide acceptance as an anticonvulsant only in the past 50 years. It was originally used as an organic solvent, and its antiseizure properties were discovered by accident when a chemist was using it as a solvent when testing various agents for epilepsy.

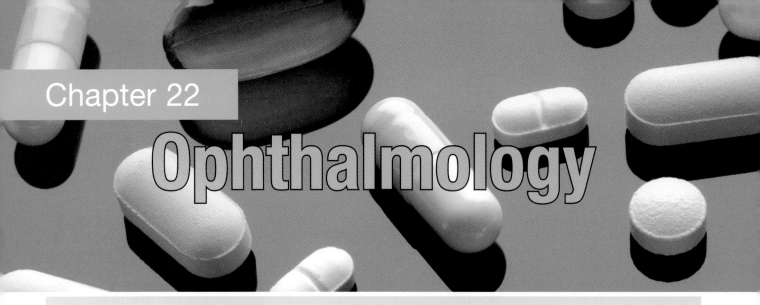

Chapter 22

Ophthalmology

Ophthalmic Prostaglandins

DESCRIPTION

Ophthalmic prostaglandins (PGs) are topically applied for treating glaucoma.

PROTOTYPE AND COMMON DRUGS

- Prototype: latano**prost** (all are $PGF_{2\alpha}$)
- Others: travo**prost**, bimato**prost**, uno**prost**one

MOA (MECHANISM OF ACTION)

- Glaucoma is characterized by increased intraocular pressure (IOP) and can lead to blindness if not treated. Strategies to reduce IOP include reducing the production and secretion of aqueous humor and facilitating its drainage.
- Drainage occurs via two main pathways
  - ▲ 80% to 90% via Schlemm's canal (the trabecular network)
  - ▲ 10% to 20% via the **uveoscleral** route (Figure 22-1)
- PGs bind prostaglandin F (FP) receptors that are located on the ciliary muscle and reduce IOP by **increasing outflow** of aqueous humor through the uveoscleral pathway. This is thought to be accomplished through the following mechanisms:
  - ▲ Relaxation of the ciliary muscle
  - ▲ Vasodilatation as a contributor to early effects
  - ▲ Remodeling or shrinking of the ciliary muscle, resulting in increased space for outflow as a mechanism for long-term control of glaucoma
- Administering exogenous PG-F (specifically $PGF_{2\alpha}$) stimulates the FP receptor and increases aqueous outflow through the mechanisms just described.

PHARMACOKINETICS

- These PGs are administered topically to the eye, and only a small amount reaches the systemic circulation.

INDICATION

- Glaucoma

CONTRAINDICATIONS

- Previous **cystoid macular edema** is a contraindication and previous incisional surgery on the eye is a risk factor; ocular PGs should be used with caution in these patients because of the increased risk of cystoid macular edema.

SIDE EFFECTS

- **Local irritation**: Conjunctival hyperemia (redness), itching, foreign body sensation, tearing, and eye pain are side effects.
- **Blurred vision** may occur.
- **Pigmentation of the iris**: This occurs in patients with mixed-color irises (green-brown or blue-brown) and is a result of increased deposition of melanin. Pigmentation of the palpebral skin (eyelids) also occurs.
- **Eyelash growth** occurs with unoprostone only.
- **Cystoid macular edema** involves accumulation of fluid in the macular area of the retina. This is a well-recognized complication of cataract surgery.
- **Punctate epithelial keratopathy** involves loss of superficial epithelial cells and associated defects on the cornea.

IMPORTANT NOTES

- Raised IOP eventually results in damage to the optic nerve and can result in blindness.
- Glaucoma is often asymptomatic in early stages of the disease, and when symptoms develop they are irreversible. Therefore patients with no special risk factors should be assessed every 2 years by an optometrist or ophthalmologist after the age of 40 for IOP changes. If present, glaucoma must be treated by an ophthalmologist.
- Other pharmacologic approaches to glaucoma include the following:
  - ▲ β-Blockers (decreased aqueous production)
  - ▲ α-Adrenergic agonists (increased aqueous outflow)
  - ▲ α_2 Agonists (decreased aqueous production)

Aqueous humor drainage

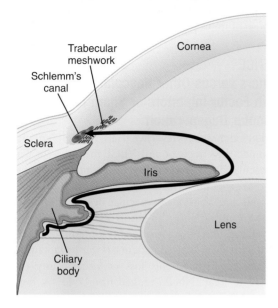

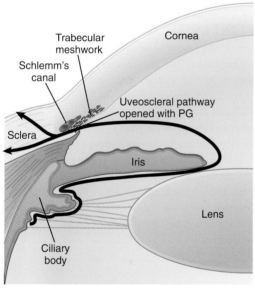

Figure 22-1.

▲ Parasympathomimetics (increased outflow)

▲ Carbonic anhydrase inhibitors (decreased aqueous production)

■ Most patients with glaucoma are treated with more than one medication simultaneously.

EVIDENCE

Prostaglandin versus Placebo

■ A Cochrane review in 2007 was unable to find any evidence comparing PGs with placebo for the treatment of glaucoma.

Prostaglandin versus Other Therapy for Glaucoma

■ A systematic review in 2008 (eight randomized controlled trials [RCTs], 1722 patients) did not find a significant reduction in the mean IOP in patients receiving latanoprost compared with those receiving brimonidine (α_2 agonist) but did find a significant reduction in mean IOP compared with the dorzolamide (carbonic anhydrase) group (WMD = 22.64). The number of ocular adverse events (excluding hyperemia) was significantly higher in the brimonidine group compared with the latanoprost group (relative risk [RR] = 0.66). The authors concluded that latanoprost was superior to dorzolamide but not brimonidine and those ocular adverse events were significantly fewer in latanoprost users than in brimonidine users. Neither travoprost nor bimatoprost was compared with dorzolamide or brimonidine in the present literature.

FYI

■ Iris bio-identification (photos of the iris used to identify people, analogous to a fingerprint) could be affected by pigment changes that result from the use of ocular PGs.

Aptamers

DESCRIPTION

Aptamers are a new approach to drug design that uses nucleotide sequences to bind to targets.

PROTOTYPE

■ Prototype: pegaptanib

MOA (MECHANISM OF ACTION)

■ Aptamers are **nucleotide sequences** that bind to biologic targets, typically proteins. Pegaptanib, the first aptamer

approved for human use, targets a protein called *vascular endothelial growth factor* (VEGF).

■ Age-related **macular degeneration** is characterized by an overgrowth of blood vessels in the macula of the eye. These vessels function poorly and also leak, which obscures vision and eventually leads to degeneration of the macula and blindness.

■ VEGF is an angiogenic growth factor whose function is to promote new blood vessel growth; it is believed to be largely responsible for this overgrowth of leaky, dysfunctional vessels in the macula. In addition to stimulating the growth of new blood vessels, VEGF also increases vascular permeability.

■ By binding to VEGF, pegaptanib prevents further growth of blood vessels and also reduces the leakage that promotes gradual loss of vision.

PHARMACOKINETICS

■ Pegaptanib is administered via intravitreal (directly into the vitreous of the eye) injection by an ophthalmologist. After injection, the drug slowly reaches the systemic circulation, although it is not believed to be widely distributed.

INDICATION

■ Age-related macular degeneration

CONTRAINDICATIONS

■ **Ocular infection:** Pegaptanib is administered via intravitreal injection; therefore the patient should be free of infection before this delicate procedure is performed.

SIDE EFFECTS

■ **Most of the side effects are caused by the local injection into the eye.**

■ **Increased IOP** is most likely a result simply of the administration of liquid into an enclosed space.

■ **Vitreous floaters** appear as floating objects in the patient's field of vision. These are simply the components of the injection, typically small air bubbles, and are thus considered harmless and temporary.

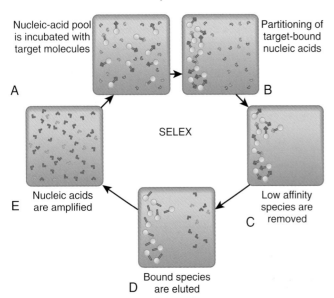

Aptamers

Nucleic-acid pool is incubated with target molecules

A

Partitioning of target-bound nucleic acids

B

SELEX

Low affinity species are removed

C

Bound species are eluted

D

Nucleic acids are amplified

E

Figure 22-2. (Modified from Bunka DHJ, Stockley PG: Aptamers come of age—at last, *Nat Rev Microb* 4:588, 2006. Reprinted by permission from Macmillan Publishers.)

Serious, Rare

■ **Endophthalmitis** results from infection of the eye, typically because of improper injection technique.

EVIDENCE

Aptamers versus Other Vascular Endothelial Growth Factor Inhibitors or Sham for Treatment of Macular Degeneration

■ A 2008 Cochrane review (five trials, N = 2500 participants) examined the effects of anti-VEGF therapies for neovascular macular degeneration. Two of the included studies compared pegaptanib versus sham treatment. A key outcome in assessing interventions in macular degeneration is deterioration of vision, with the cutoff for deterioration being a loss of ≥15 letters of visual acuity on an eye chart. Compared with sham-treated patients, fewer pegaptanib-treated patients experienced this loss of visual acuity (numbers needed to treat [NNTs] ranged from 7 to 14, depending on dose). Endophthalmitis occurred in 1.3% of pegaptanib-treated patients.

IMPORTANT NOTES

■ An important potential advantage of aptamers over monoclonal antibodies is that aptamers are unlikely to elicit an immune response, as they are not antibodies. Hypersensitivity reactions are an important limitation to the use of monoclonal antibodies in some patients.

■ Another advantage of aptamers over monoclonal antibodies is stability. Aptamers can withstand high temperatures and have a long shelf-life, making them more convenient in everyday use.

■ Another indication in which aptamers are being studied is cancer. Aptamers are smaller than monoclonal antibodies, and it is believed this may make it easier for them to penetrate tumors.

FYI

■ The term *aptamer* comes from the Latin *aptus*, meaning fitting.

■ Aptamers were first discovered in and continue their primary application in basic science research.

■ The SELEX process is an automated technique for manufacturing aptamers. It begins with a library of nucleotide sequences of varying lengths, which are then exposed to a ligand target. The sequences that do not bind to the ligand are then washed away. The remaining sequences are then amplified and subjected to another round of binding and removal. With each successive round, the techniques that are used to remove the less tightly bound sequences are intensified, such that with the end of each round, the remaining sequences have increased affinity for the ligand over those of the previous round (Figure 22-2).

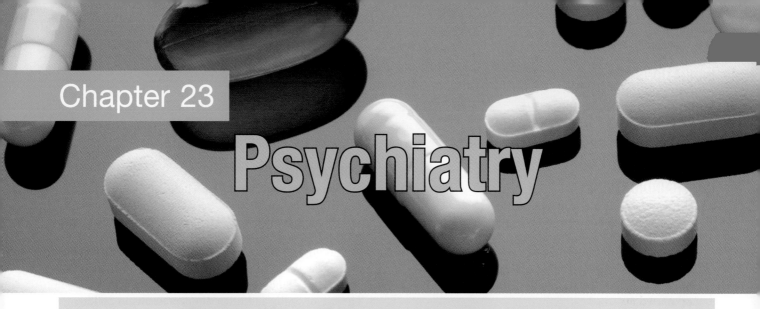

Chapter 23

Psychiatry

Selective Serotonin Reuptake Inhibitors (SSRIs)

DESCRIPTION
The selective serotonin reuptake inhibitors (SSRIs) inhibit the reuptake of serotonin in the synaptic cleft.

PROTOTYPE AND COMMON DRUGS
- Prototype: fluoxetine
- Others: paroxetine, fluvoxamine, sertraline, citalopram, escitalopram

MOA (MECHANISM OF ACTION)
- The monoamine hypothesis suggests that depression is caused by a **deficiency** of synaptic neurotransmitters such as serotonin (5-HT), norepinephrine, and dopamine. Serotonin, in particular, is associated with mood.
- Normally, 5-HT is released from presynaptic vesicles into the synaptic cleft, where it travels to postsynaptic receptors.
- Once released from these postsynaptic receptors, 5-HT is removed from the synaptic cleft by **reuptake transporters** located on the presynapse. Once it is taken up presynaptically, it is degraded (Figure 23-1).
- SSRIs **bind to this reuptake transporter**, preventing the removal of 5-HT and leading to increased 5-HT available to bind to postsynaptic receptors.
- The clinical efficacy of antidepressants is delayed a few weeks when compared with their pharmacological actions. It is therefore hypothesized that the efficacy of these agents in the treatment of depression is related to a downstream effect.
- There are a variety of theories as to what this downstream effect might be, although most involve either a change in receptor density or fundamental changes at the cellular level, including a reorganization of neurons.
- One of the examples of altered receptor density occurs with presynaptic 5-HT inhibitory autoreceptors. These autoreceptors reduce 5-HT release when bound by 5-HT. Excess 5-HT in the synapse because of SSRI therapy leads

SSRI

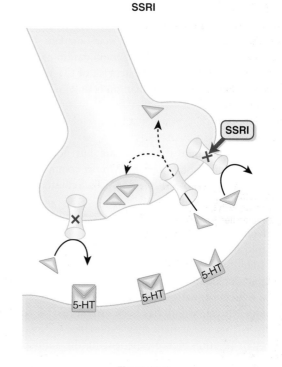

Figure 23-1.

to **down-regulation of this inhibitory autoreceptor** and enhanced release of 5-HT into the synapse.

PHARMACOKINETICS
- The SSRIs typically have long half-lives (24 hours or longer), allowing for once-daily administration.
- Fluoxetine has an active metabolite (norfluoxetine) and has the longest half-life (>100 hours) of all SSRIs. Fluoxetine is more prone to drug interactions, and more caution must be exercised to ensure a proper washout period after fluoxetine discontinuation.

INDICATIONS
- Major depressive disorder
- Obsessive compulsive disorder
- Generalized anxiety disorder
  - ▲ Including panic disorder
- Bulimia nervosa

CONTRAINDICATIONS
- **SSRIs and monoamine oxidase inhibitors (MAOIs):** SSRIs increase serotonin concentrations in the synapse, whereas MAOIs inhibit the breakdown of serotonin. Concomitant use can therefore lead to excessive serotonin (see details in Side Effects). When switching from an SSRI to an MAOI, or vice versa, allow for a washout period of at least 1 to 2 weeks.
- **SSRIs and thioridazine** (an antipsychotic): Thioridazine elicits QT interval prolongation, and fluoxetine in particular enhances this effect by inhibiting the metabolism of thioridazine. A washout period of at least 5 weeks should elapse before someone who was on fluoxetine should be started on thioridazine, and fluoxetine should not be initiated for at least 2 weeks after discontinuation of thioridazine. The seriousness of these drug interactions has led to the withdrawal of thioridazine in many markets.
- **Citalopram and pimozide:** The combination of these two agents is associated with a greater risk of QT interval prolongation, although the mechanism is unknown.

SIDE EFFECTS
Serious
- **Serotonin syndrome (SS)** is a rare but potentially life-threatening elevation in serotonin, most commonly caused by concomitant use of SSRIs and MAOIs. Symptoms include:
  - ▲ Hyperthermia
  - ▲ Muscle rigidity
  - ▲ Myoclonus
  - ▲ Rapid fluctuations in vital signs (because of autonomic instability)
  - ▲ Rapid fluctuations in mental status (confusion, irritability, extreme agitation, delirium, coma)
- **Suicide:** No causal link has been established. A common theory is that the patient may experience an increase in energy or ideation before experiencing the antidepressant effects, prompting suicidal acts instead of thoughts.

Non-Serious
- **Sexual dysfunction** may be both mechanical, as serotonin inhibits functions such as erections, ejaculation, lubrication, and orgasm, and central, as serotonin has an inhibitory effect on dopamine, a neurotransmitter believed to play an important role in arousal. *Note:* sexual dysfunction can also accompany depression.
- **Gastrointestinal (GI) distress:** Serotonin receptors are also found in the gut, and serotonin appears to have an effect on GI motility (cramping, diarrhea, nausea) that becomes intolerable in some patients. Nausea and vomiting are also likely mediated by activation of serotonin receptors in the CNS.
- **Agitation, insomnia:** These effects are likely via stimulation of central serotonin receptors. The intensity of this side effect can vary among the SSRI. In some cases, these side effects can be somewhat beneficial in patients who have fatigue or apathy and hypersomnia.

IMPORTANT NOTES
- As with other antidepressants, when an SSRI is being discontinued, the dose should be tapered gradually in order to avoid discontinuation symptoms, including dizziness, nausea, headache, and others. The incidence and severity appears to vary between SSRI, and longer half-life agents such as fluoxetine appear to be less likely to induce a discontinuation syndrome.
- The use of SSRIs and other antidepressants in children is currently under review. The focus of concern is the propensity to elicit behavioral and emotional changes, including an increased risk of self-harm and suicide. All antidepressants thus carry safety warnings for use in pediatrics.
- Although they all increase serotonin levels, the SSRIs are a heterogeneous class and should not be considered interchangeable. For example, citalopram is considered to be the most serotonin-selective of the SSRIs, although it does have affinity for H_1 receptors. Fluoxetine and sertraline have the highest affinity for dopamine D_2 receptors, whereas paroxetine has the most potent anticholinergic effects. The clinical consequences of this pharmacologic heterogeneity have yet to be fully characterized.
- SS and neuroleptic malignant syndrome (NMS), two rare but very serious complications of SSRIs or MAOIs and antipsychotics, respectively, share some common features including fever, increased muscle tone (more hyperreflexia with SS), and autonomic instability.

Advanced
Drug Interactions
- The SSRIs inhibit multiple CYP450 isozymes. Fluoxetine and paroxetine inhibit the CYP2D6 isoenzyme, and this can lead to clinically important drug interactions with drugs such as tricyclic antidepressants (TCAs), carbamazepine, or vinblastine. There is also a very serious interaction with thioridazine (see Contraindications).
- Other isozymes inhibited include:
  - ▲ CYP1A2 by fluvoxamine
  - ▲ CYP2C9, CYP2C19, and CYP3A4 by fluvoxamine and fluoxetine

EVIDENCE
Depression
- A 2005 Cochrane review (132 trials, N = 14,391 participants) compared fluoxetine with other antidepressants. The review found that among SSRIs, sertraline and paroxetine were more efficacious than fluoxetine in improving depression rating scores. Findings related to side effects were as follows:

▲ Sweating was more common with fluoxetine than with paroxetine.

▲ Nausea was more common with fluoxetine than with fluvoxamine.

▲ Weight loss was greater with fluoxetine than with SSRIs as a class.

■ The same review found fluoxetine to be less efficacious than venlafaxine or mirtazapine; fluoxetine caused less dry mouth, dizziness, sweating, and nausea compared with venlafaxine.

■ A 2007 Cochrane review (20 trials, N = 2000 patients) compared SSRIs with the TCA amitriptyline. The review found SSRIs and amitriptyline were equally efficacious but also found SSRIs to be more tolerable than amitriptyline.

Premenstrual Syndrome

■ A 2007 Cochrane review (31 trials, N = 844 participants) found that SSRIs were highly effective in the treatment of premenstrual symptoms, both physical and behavioral, compared with placebo. There were 2.5 times as many withdrawals because of adverse events among SSRI-treated subjects as among placebo-treated subjects.

Depression in Elderly People or Seniors

■ A 2006 Cochrane review (32 trials) compared various antidepressants to one another in depressed older adults. There were no statistically significant differences in efficacy between SSRIs and TCAs. There were fewer withdrawals because of side effects in the SSRI arms compared with TCAs.

FYI

■ The SSRIs were the first class of antidepressants that were discovered using "rational drug design." The strategy was based on the observation that TCAs inhibited noradrenaline (NA) or 5-HT reuptake to various extents. Scientists then discovered some nontricyclic compounds that were also reuptake inhibitors, acting on either NA or 5-HT to varying degrees. This led to the approval of the first such agent, zimeldine, which was withdrawn from the market after a few years.

Tricyclic Antidepressants (TCAs)

DESCRIPTION

TCAs are a class of antidepressants with a common chemical (tricyclic) structure and mode of action.

PROTOTYPE AND COMMON DRUGS

■ Prototype: amitriptyline

■ Others: desipramine, imipramine, nortriptyline, clomipramine, trimipramine, doxepin, maprotiline

MOA (MECHANISM OF ACTION)

■ The monoamine hypothesis suggests that depression is caused by a deficiency of synaptic neurotransmitters such as serotonin (5-HT), NA, and dopamine. Serotonin, in particular, is associated with mood.

■ Normally, 5-HT and NA are released from presynaptic vesicles into the synaptic cleft, where they travel to post-synaptic receptors.

■ Once released from these postsynaptic receptors, 5-HT and NA are removed from the synaptic cleft by reuptake transporters located on the presynapse.

■ The TCAs inhibit the reuptake of serotonin (5-HT) and NA into the presynaptic cell body, increasing the amount of 5-HT and NA available to bind to postsynaptic receptors (Figure 23-2).

■ TCAs antagonize other receptors: muscarinic, histamine (H₁), adrenergic (α₁) receptors. This accounts for their extensive list of side effects.

■ The clinical efficacy of antidepressants is delayed when compared with their pharmacologic actions. It is therefore

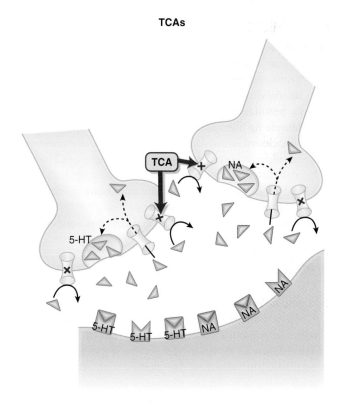

TCAs

Figure 23-2.

hypothesized that the efficacy of these agents in the treatment of depression is related to a downstream effect.
- A variety of theories exist regarding what this downstream effect might be, although most involve either a change in receptor density or fundamental changes at the cellular level, including a reorganization of neurons.

PHARMACOKINETICS
- Nortriptyline is a metabolite of amitriptyline.
- Desipramine is a metabolite of imipramine.
- TCAs are metabolized by CYP450 enzymes and are therefore prone to drug interactions with inhibitors or inducers of these enzymes.

INDICATIONS
- Depression
- Chronic pain (as an adjunct)

CONTRAINDICATIONS
- **Avoid concomitant use of TCAs and MAOIs:** TCAs increase serotonin concentrations in the synapse, whereas MAOIs inhibit the breakdown of serotonin. Concomitant use can therefore lead to excessive serotonin. When switching from a TCA to an MAOI, or vice versa, allow for a washout period of at least 2 weeks.

SIDE EFFECTS
- **Anticholinergic:**
  - Dry mouth
  - Confusion
  - Urinary retention
  - Constipation
  - Blurred vision
  - Increased intraocular pressure (IOP)
- **Sedation:** via blockade of histamine (H_1) receptors
- **Serious: Cardiovascular toxicities** are typically only seen when high doses are administered (see "Important Notes"). In high doses TCAs impair cardiac conduction, leading to a widening of the QRS complex and heart block, often accompanied by hypotension
- **Orthostatic hypotension:** related to blockade of α_1 receptors

IMPORTANT NOTES
- The TCAs are grouped as a class based on their chemical structure. Although as a class they are considered to be 5-HT or noradrenaline reuptake inhibitors, the degree of reuptake inhibition differs markedly among agents. See Table 23-1.
- Similarly, the affinities for blockade of receptors that mediate the side effects experienced by patients also differ markedly among agents. See Table 23-2.
- Because of their prominent antimuscarinic effects, TCAs should be used with caution in conditions that would be exacerbated by cholinergic antagonism: urinary retention, benign prostatic hyperplasia (BPH), glaucoma (closed angle), and increased IOP.

TABLE 23-1. Extent of Serotonin and Noradrenaline Reuptake Inhibition among TCAs

Agent	Serotonin (5HT)	Noradrenaline(NA)
Clomipramine	+++	+
Amitriptyline	++	±
Imipramine	+	+
Trimipramine	0	+
Doxepin	+	++
Nortriptyline	±	++
Desipramine	0	+++

+ symbols indicate extent of reuptake inhibition, with +++ exhibiting the greatest reuptake inhibition + exhibiting the least. 0 indicates no inhibition of the reuptake transporter for that neurotransmitter.

TABLE 23-2. Extent of Antagonism of Muscarinic, Histamine (H1), and α-1 Adrenergic Receptors among TCAs

Agent	Muscarinic	Histamine (H_1)	α_1
Amitriptyline	++++	++++	+++
Trimipramine	++	+++	++
Doxepin	++	+++	++
Imipramine	++	+	++
Clomipramine	++	+	++
Nortriptyline	++	+	+
Maprotiline	+	++	+
Desipramine	+	0	+

+ symbols indicate extent of receptor antagonism, with ++++ exhibiting the greatest antagonism + exhibiting the least. 0 indicates no antagonism at that receptor.

- TCAs are potentially fatal in overdose situations and have one of the highest mortality rates associated with overdose. Cardiac arrhythmias, hypotension, and central nervous system (CNS) involvement are the most common events associated with TCA overdose. TCAs undergo slow absorption; therefore a patient may arrive on his or her own at an emergency department with a fatal dose of TCAs that has not yet been absorbed. This propensity of TCAs to be fatal in overdose is particularly concerning, given the general FDA warning about increased risk of suicidality with antidepressant use.

Advanced
Drug Interactions
- Most TCAs exhibit some degree of CP450 enzyme inhibition. The most prominent inhibitors are amitriptyline, imipramine, clomipramine, and doxepin, mainly at CYP2C19.

EVIDENCE
Depression
- A 2007 Cochrane review (20 trials, N = 2000 patients) of amitriptyline versus other antidepressants found it to be at least as efficacious as SSRIs but also found it to have more side effects.

■ Similar results were seen in comparisons of amitriptyline versus other TCAs or heterocyclic drugs. Amitriptyline was as efficacious as these agents but had more side effects.

FYI

■ TCAs have been around for 50 years. Imipramine was the first TCA synthesized, and it was based on the tricyclic structure of the antipsychotic chlorpromazine. A study in 1958 found imipramine lacked efficacy in psychosis, but, surprisingly, a subgroup of patients with depression improved on imipramine. TCAs became the drugs of choice for treating depression for the next 30 years.

■ Nomenclature note: TCAs with an amine (N-) group on the middle ring end with *-amine*, whereas agents with an oxygen (O-) on the middle ring have *-ox-* in their name.

Serotonin Noradrenaline Reuptake Inhibitors (SNRIs)

DESCRIPTION

The SNRIs are reuptake inhibitors that increase the concentration of both serotonin (5-HT) and noradrenaline (NA) in the synaptic cleft.

PROTOTYPE AND COMMON DRUGS

■ Prototype: venlafaxine
■ Others: desvenlafaxine, duloxetine, milnacipran

MOA (MECHANISM OF ACTION)

■ The monoamine hypothesis suggests that depression is caused by a deficiency of synaptic neurotransmitters such as serotonin (5-HT), NA, and dopamine. Serotonin, in particular, is associated with mood.

■ Normally, 5-HT and NA are released from presynaptic vesicles into the synaptic cleft, where they travel to post-synaptic receptors.

■ Once released from these postsynaptic receptors, 5-HT and NA are removed from the synaptic cleft by reuptake transporters located on the presynapse. Once they are taken up presynaptically, they are degraded (Figure 23-3).

■ SNRIs **bind to these reuptake transporters,** preventing the removal of 5-HT and NA and leading to increased availability to bind to postsynaptic receptors.

■ Venlafaxine has much **higher affinity for the serotonin** reuptake transporter, and at low doses acts more like an SSRI. It is not until higher doses are used that it also blocks noradrenaline reuptake.

■ Conversely, milnacipran blocks serotonin and noradrenaline reuptake equally, whereas the other agents in this class fall somewhere between these two.

■ The clinical efficacy of antidepressants is delayed when compared with their pharmacologic actions. It is therefore hypothesized that the efficacy of these agents in the treatment of depression is related to a downstream effect.

■ A variety of theories exist regarding what this downstream effect might be, although most involve either a change in receptor density or fundamental changes at the cellular level, including a reorganization of neurons.

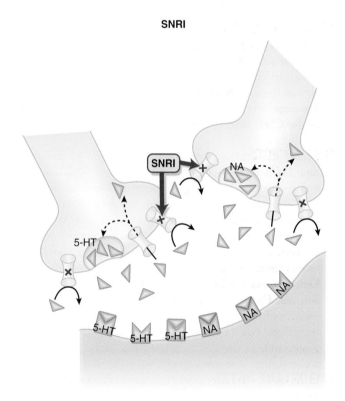

SNRI

Figure 23-3.

PHARMACOKINETICS

■ Compared with the SSRIs, the SNRIs have shorter elimination half-lives. Venlafaxine is available in an extended-release(ER) dosage form.

■ Venlafaxine has an active metabolite: O-desmethylvenlafaxine. The parent and its metabolites have lower clearance in patients with hepatic cirrhosis and severe renal disease, requiring a dose reduction.

■ Desvenlafaxine is primarily metabolized by glucuronidation, with only minor involvement from CYP3A4.

■ Milnacipran undergoes limited metabolism.

INDICATIONS

- Depression
- Generalized anxiety disorder (GAD)
- Social anxiety disorder
- Panic disorder

CONTRAINDICATIONS

- **SNRIs and MAOIs:** MAOIs inhibit the breakdown of serotonin. Concomitant use can therefore lead to excessive serotonin. When switching from an SNRI to an MAOI, or vice versa, allow for a washout period of at least 1 to 2 weeks.

SIDE EFFECTS

- **Gastrointestinal (GI) distress,** attributed to inhibition of serotonin reuptake, appears to be most common with venlafaxine. Stimulation of serotonin receptors in the brain likely mediates nausea. Serotonin receptors are also found in the gut, and serotonin appears to have an effect on GI motility that becomes intolerable in some patients, leading to cramping and diarrhea.
- **Dizziness** may occur although the mechanism is unknown.
- **Somnolence** may be secondary to sleep disturbances, although the mechanism is unknown.
- **Insomnia** may occur due to stimulation of 5-HT receptors in the CNS. Both the length and quality of sleep may be impaired.
- **Sexual dysfunction,** attributed to inhibition of serotonin reuptake, appears to be most common with venlafaxine. It may be both **mechanical,** as serotonin inhibits functions such as erections, ejaculation, lubrication, and orgasm, and **central,** as serotonin has an inhibitory effect on dopamine, a neurotransmitter believed to play an important role in arousal.
- **Sweating:** The mechanism for this effect has not been established.
- **Dry mouth** is likely caused by NA.
- **Sustained hypertension** is dose related. The elevation in blood pressure is likely caused by the pressor effects of increased NA. Patients should have blood pressure monitored.

IMPORTANT NOTES

- When an SNRI is being discontinued, the dose should be tapered gradually in order to avoid discontinuation symptoms, including aggression, agitation, convulsions, dysphoric mood, electric shock sensations, and others. These symptoms have been particularly evident with venlafaxine.
- The theory behind the development of the SNRIs was to try and increase the levels of two neurotransmitters (serotonin, noradrenaline) simultaneously, while avoiding many of the bothersome side effects of the TCAs, which also act as reuptake inhibitors of these two neurotransmitters. There is evidence to suggest that dual reuptake inhibition is more efficacious than selective inhibition (see Evidence section).
- Reboxetine was the first noradrenaline selective reuptake inhibitor, approved in Europe for treatment of depression.

It was rejected by the U.S. Food and Drug Administration (FDA) because of concerns over poor efficacy.

- All antidepressants carry an FDA warning about increased suicidality, particularly in younger (<25 years of age) patients. The mechanism has not been established and there is not enough data to determine whether a lower risk exists for some antidepressants compared with others. These concerns must also be balanced against the potential for increased risk of completed suicides in untreated depression.

Advanced
Pharmacogenetics

- Venlafaxine is extensively metabolized by CYP450, especially CYP2D6. CYP2D6 is subject to genetic polymorphisms; therefore metabolism varies among patients.

Drug Interactions

- Duloxetine and (to a lesser extent) venlafaxine are inhibitors of CYP2D6.

EVIDENCE
Venlafaxine versus Fluoxetine for Depression

- A 2005 Cochrane review (10 trials, N = 1831 participants) compared fluoxetine with venlafaxine. The authors found venlafaxine to be significantly better than fluoxetine (an SSRI) for improving depression rating scores. Some side effects were more common with venlafaxine than with fluoxetine, including dry mouth, dizziness, sweating, and nausea.

Venlafaxine for Generalized Anxiety Disorder

- A 2003 Cochrane review (8 trials, N = 2058 participants) examined the efficacy of various antidepressants for generalized anxiety disorder (GAD). Based on two trials, the authors found venlafaxine to be statistically better than placebo for treatment response, assessed by Clinical Global Impression (CGI) scores.

Milnacipran for Depression

- A 2009 Cochrane review (16 trials, N = 2277 participants) compared milnacipran with other antidepressants for depression. Milnacipran was associated with fewer withdrawals because of adverse events (a measure of tolerability) compared with the TCAs (odds ratio [OR] 0.55), and weak evidence suggested fewer adverse events of sleepiness or drowsiness, dry mouth, or constipation versus these agents.

FYI

- The next frontier in antidepressant drug design is the development of triple rather than dual reuptake inhibitors. The third neurotransmitter of interest is dopamine. These drugs are already in clinical trials.
- Serotonin (5-HT_3) antagonists are used to treat nausea and vomiting, and to treat irritable bowel syndrome.

Noradrenergic and Specific Serotonergic Antidepressants (NaSSAs)

DESCRIPTION

Noradrenergic and specific serotonergic antidepressants (NaSSAs) are antidepressants that increase the concentration of noradrenaline and serotonin in the synaptic cleft.

PROTOTYPE

- Mirtazapine

MOA (MECHANISM OF ACTION)

- NaSSAs have a **dual mechanism** of action:
  - ▲ Inhibition of α_2 autoreceptors and heteroreceptors
    - An **autoreceptor** is a receptor that when bound by ligand reduces release of that ligand into the synapse. The α_2 **receptor** is a classic example of an autoreceptor, as when it is bound by noradrenaline (NA) it inhibits NA release.
    - A **heteroreceptor** is like an autoreceptor, although when bound it can mediate the release of other neurotransmitters in addition to its own ligand.
    - Thus inhibition of these autoreceptors and heteroreceptors prevents the negative feedback of NA on **5-HT** and NA neurotransmission (Figure 23-4). Thus **neurotransmission is sustained**.
  - ▲ Antagonism of serotonin (5-HT$_2$) and 5-HT$_3$ **postsynaptic receptors**
    - This leads to **enhanced 5-HT$_1$** neurotransmission.
    - Blockade of 5-HT$_3$ receptors may lead to reduced incidence of gastrointestinal side effects.
- Mirtazapine has a low affinity for muscarinic and dopaminergic receptors. However, it has high affinity for histamine (H1) receptors. These receptors all mediate many of the side effects of antidepressants, although dopamine receptors play a role in mood disorders.

PHARMACOKINETICS

- Clearance is reduced in patients with liver disease (by 30%) or kidney disease (by 30% to 50%) and in the elderly. Dose reductions should therefore be considered in these populations.

SIDE EFFECTS

- **Sedation** occurs because of blockade of histamine receptors. It tends to predominate at lower doses, as increasing NA at higher doses counteracts this effect.
- **Increased appetite** may be due to H1 antagonism, although the mechanism is unclear. **Weight gain** may be due to H1 antagonism, although the mechanism is unclear.

Serious, Rare

- **Severe neutropenia** is rare.

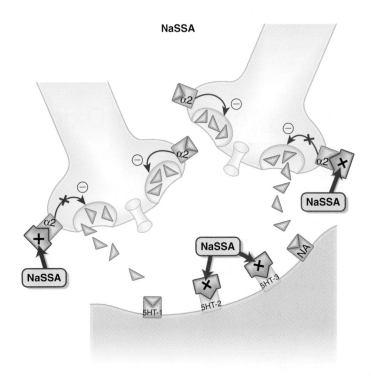

Figure 23-4.

IMPORTANT NOTES

- With its distinct mechanism, mirtazapine is seen as an alternative for patients intolerant to SSRIs. It has the advantage of lower incidence of sexual dysfunction, but it also has greater propensity for weight gain compared with SSRIs.
- Because of its sedative and appetite-stimulating effects, mirtazapine may theoretically be a more useful antidepressant in the elderly, as these patients often have depression accompanied by insomnia and weight loss.
- Although they are not thought of as being in the same class, the "atypical" antidepressants trazodone and nefazodone have some similarities to mirtazapine in their mechanisms of action. Both block 5-HT$_2$ postsynaptic receptors and promote serotonin neurotransmission, although trazodone and nefazodone enhance serotonin by inhibiting its reuptake.
- Nefazodone is also believed to inhibit the reuptake of noradrenaline. Nefazodone was withdrawn from North American markets in the early 2000s for hepatotoxicity, and trazodone, once a very popular antidepressant, has been supplanted by newer agents such as the SSRIs.
- All antidepressants carry an FDA warning about increased suicidality, particularly in younger (<25 years of age) patients. The mechanism has not been established and there is not enough data to determine whether a lower risk exists

for some antidepressants compared with others. These concerns must also be balanced against the potential for increased risk of completed suicides in untreated depression.

EVIDENCE
Versus Fluoxetine for Depression
■ A 2005 systematic review compared SSRIs with newer-generation antidepressants and included three studies of

mirtazapine. Mirtazapine had a better response rate than fluoxetine in two small studies (265 patients), and there were no differences between the two agents with respect to tolerability.

FYI
■ Mirtazapine is derived from mianserin, an antidepressant that has been available for many years in Europe.

Monoamine Oxidase Inhibitors (MAOIs)

DESCRIPTION
MAOIs are a heterogeneous group of agents that inhibit the monoamine oxidase (MAO) enzyme.

PROTOTYPES AND COMMON DRUGS
Selective (MAO-B)
■ Prototype: selegiline
■ Others: rasagiline

Selective (MAO-A), Reversible
■ Prototype: moclobemide

Nonselective, Irreversible
■ Prototype: phenelzine
■ Others: tranylcypromine

MOA (MECHANISM OF ACTION)
■ MAO degrades catecholamines, serotonin, and other endogenous amines in the CNS as well as in the periphery.
■ There are two key isoenzymes:
  ▲ MAO-A degrades epinephrine, norepinephrine, and serotonin.
  ▲ MAO-B degrades phenylethylamine.
  ▲ Both degrade dopamine.
■ The purpose of MAO inhibition is therefore to increase levels of these substances within the body, specifically the **CNS**. The efficacy of these agents is a result of their actions within the CNS, whereas the side effects are largely mediated by their actions outside of the CNS.
■ MAO inhibition can be either reversible or irreversible. Irreversible binding leads to a much more prolonged effect (Figure 23-5).
■ The benefits and adverse effects of MAOIs will therefore be determined by their **selectivity** for these isoenzymes and whether the inhibition is **reversible**.
■ Therefore **MAO-A inhibitors** are thought to work by increasing levels of amines such as **norepinephrine and serotonin**.
■ Because the MAO-B enzyme has no effect on epinephrine, norepinephrine, or serotonin, at normal doses **MAO-B inhibitors** increase **dopamine** levels in the CNS without

increasing levels of these other neurotransmitters. Parkinson's disease is characterized by a relative deficiency of dopamine in the CNS; therefore MAO-B inhibitors are used to treat Parkinson's disease.
■ At higher doses, MAO-B inhibitors begin to lose selectivity, and thus begin to inhibit MAO-A as well as MAO-B. Therefore in higher doses, MAO-B inhibitors can also be used to treat depression.
■ It is also believed that byproducts such as peroxide associated with dopamine degradation lead to further CNS damage in Parkinson's disease. Therefore an additional proposed mechanism of the MAO-B inhibitors is to inhibit the production of these toxic metabolites. There is also some work suggesting that these toxic byproducts may play a role in the pathophysiology of depression, suggesting a potential disease-modifying role for MAO inhibition in this condition, as well.

PHARMACOKINETICS
■ Moclobemide undergoes extensive hepatic metabolism by acetylation.
■ Selegiline is also metabolized in the liver, primarily by CYP2B6 and CYP1A2. Two metabolites have stimulant properties: L-amphetamine and L-methamphetamine. Selegiline is also available in a transdermal patch.
■ Rasagiline is metabolized primarily by CYP1A2.

INDICATIONS
■ Depression (atypical)

MAO-B Inhibitors
■ Parkinson's disease

CONTRAINDICATIONS
■ **Drug interaction: with sympathomimetics:** nonselective MAOIs may potentiate the hypertensive effects of sympathomimetics, leading to a hypertensive crisis that can be fatal. Methylphenidate, **dopamine, epinephrine, norepinephrine**, and similar agents (methyldopa, L-dopa, L-tryptophan, L-tyrosine, phenylalanine) should be avoided.
■ **Foods with tyramine:** See Side Effects.

MAOI

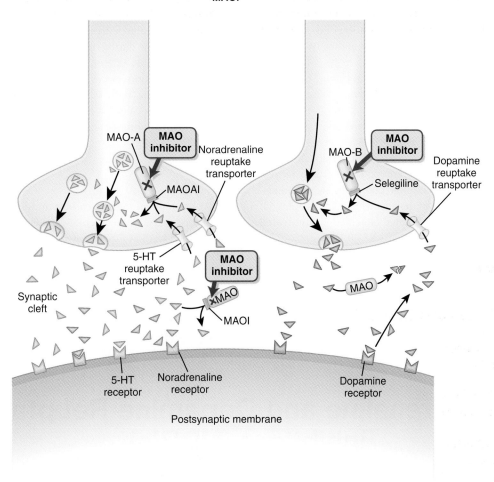

Figure 23-5.

SIDE EFFECTS

- **Sleep disturbances** include insomnia and reduction in rapid eye movement (REM) sleep. The insomnia is likely a central stimulatory effect from the increased monoamines, although a mechanism has not been established. Moclobemide, a reversible and selective MAO-A inhibitor, may cause fewer problems with sleep.
- **Weight gain** is a common side effect of antidepressants; likely, increased monoamines play a role, but the mechanism has not been established.
- **Postural hypotension:** The mechanism has not been established. This can be problematic in elderly patients, leading to falls. Note that this side effect is distinct from the hypertensive crisis, described later, which occurs because of an interaction with other agents and has a very specific mechanism.
- **Sexual disturbances:** The mechanism has not been established, although several antidepressants that affect monoamine levels have this side effect, and enhanced serotonin is believed to mediate sexual dysfunction with these agents.

Serious

- **Hypertensive crisis** occurs because of a drug-drug or drug-food interaction, leading to increased levels of norepinephrine and subsequent rapid elevation in blood pressure. Before the triggering factors (tyramine-rich foods) were identified, this interaction limited the utility of these agents.

IMPORTANT NOTES

- MAO-A in the gut breaks down tyramine, a chemical that stimulates the release of norepinephrine. Tyramine is typically found in aged foods such as cheese, wine, beer, yogurt, and yeast. Ingestion of these foods leads to increased tyramine, and because its breakdown is inhibited, there is increased norepinephrine release, leading to hypertensive crisis.
- Little MAO-B is found in the gut; therefore an MAO-B selective inhibitor will have minimal effect on the metabolism of dietary tyramine. Although MAO-B selectivity reduces the risk of hypertensive crisis, this selectivity is lost at higher doses.
- Reversible MAOIs lead to much less accumulation of tyramine and thus are considered to have minimal risk

for hypertensive crisis resulting from the wine-cheese reaction.

- A novel approach to avoiding accumulation of dietary tyramine is to bypass the GI MAO-A altogether by use of a patch.
- Linezolid, the first in a new class of antibiotics called the *oxazolidinones*, is also an MAOI. Concomitant use of these agents should therefore be avoided.
- All antidepressants carry an FDA warning about increased suicidality, particularly in younger (<25 years of age) patients. The mechanism has not been established and there is not enough data to determine whether a lower risk exists for some antidepressants compared with others. These concerns must also be balanced against the potential for increased risk of completed suicides in untreated depression.

EVIDENCE
MAO-B Inhibitors versus Dopaminergics for Early Parkinson's Disease

- A 2009 Cochrane review (two trials, N = 593 patients) compared MAO-B inhibitors with a dopamine agonist or levodopa in patients with early Parkinson's. No difference in deaths was found between selegiline and either agent, but patients treated with selegiline were more likely to need add-on therapy during follow-up than patients receiving levodopa (OR 12.02) or a dopamine agonist (OR 2.00). Motor fluctuations were reduced by MAO-B inhibitors versus levodopa (OR 0.55) but not dopamine agonists. Withdrawals because of adverse events were less common with MAO-B inhibitors compared with dopamine agonists (OR 0.11).

FYI

- MAOIs were among the earliest antidepressants, although their discovery was accidental. The first MAOI was actually developed to treat tuberculosis (TB). The drug was ineffective for TB but had "psychoenergizing" effects and was also discovered to be an MAOI.
- Phenylethylamine is a neurotransmitter believed to play a role in mood, although its exact role in the body has not been fully characterized. It is found in some "comfort foods," particularly chocolate, and is also sold as a supplement in some jurisdictions.

Noradrenaline and Dopamine Reuptake Inhibitors (NDRIs)

DESCRIPTION

Noradrenaline and dopamine reuptake inhibitors (NDRIs) are agents that inhibit the reuptake of both dopamine and norepinephrine. The NDRIs fall under a broader classification of atypical antidepressants, so named because they do not fit into any of the other antidepressant classes.

PROTOTYPE

- Bupropion

MOA (MECHANISM OF ACTION)

- Bupropion inhibits the presynaptic reuptake of both dopamine (DA) and noradrenaline (NA), leading to increased levels of both of these neurotransmitters in the synaptic cleft (Figure 23-6).
- The clinical efficacy of all antidepressants is delayed a few weeks when compared with their pharmacologic actions. It is therefore hypothesized that the efficacy of these agents in the treatment of depression is related to a downstream effect.
- A variety of theories exist regarding what this downstream effect might be, although most involve either a change in receptor density or fundamental changes at the cellular level, including a reorganization of neurons.
- With respect to smoking cessation, dopamine is believed to be the key neurotransmitter in the reward pathway

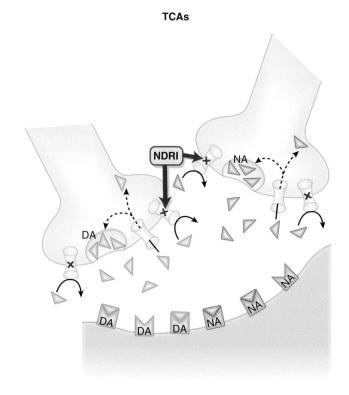

TCAs

Figure 23-6.

associated with addiction. It is believed that the increased levels of dopamine in the synapse help to mimic the reward associated with smoking, thus attenuating some of the withdrawal symptoms associated with abstinence.

- There is also some evidence that bupropion is a **nicotinic receptor antagonist.** By blocking the nicotinic receptor, bupropion prevents exogenously administered nicotine from binding to this receptor, attenuating the reward that smokers gain from nicotine.

PHARMACOKINETICS

- Bupropion is extensively metabolized, primarily through the CYP2B6 isozyme.

INDICATIONS

- Depression
- Smoking cessation

CONTRAINDICATIONS

- **Seizures:** Bupropion may lower the seizure threshold, so it must be avoided in individuals with a history of seizures or who are prone to seizures:
  - ▲ Patients undergoing drug or alcohol withdrawal
  - ▲ Prior diagnosis of bulimia or anorexia nervosa
- **MAOIs:** MAOIs inhibit the breakdown of neurotransmitters such as dopamine and norepinephrine. Simultaneous inhibition of the reuptake and breakdown of these neurotransmitters can lead to complications such as hypertensive crisis.
- **Thioridazine:** Bupropion may inhibit the metabolism of thioridazine, increasing the risk of ventricular arrhythmia and sudden cardiac death caused by elevated thioridazine levels.

SIDE EFFECTS

- **Dry mouth** may be caused by increased noradrenergic transmission.
- **Nausea** is a frequent side effect of dopaminergic agents, likely through a central effect.
- **Insomnia** may occur due to the stimulating effects of enhanced NA.

Rare, Serious

- **Seizures:** A small risk of seizures has been observed with the use of bupropion. The risk increases with higher doses.

IMPORTANT NOTES

- Bupropion is unique among antidepressants as an inhibitor of dopamine reuptake, leading to increased dopamine levels in the synapse. This has lead to its use as a smoking cessation therapy, the indication for which it is most commonly prescribed.
- Another unique feature of bupropion is its lack of serotonergic effects. Antidepressants are known for eliciting

sexual dysfunction, and this side effect has been attributed to their serotonergic properties. In clinical trials bupropion appears to have a lower propensity for sexual side effects compared with SSRIs and other serotonergic antidepressants.

- In many jurisdictions, bupropion is marketed under two separate names, Wellbutrin and Zyban. Wellbutrin is prescribed for depression, and Zyban is used for smoking cessation. Because of the risk of overdose signs and symptoms, specifically seizures, care must be taken to ensure that patients do not take Wellbutrin and Zyban concomitantly.
- Reboxetine is an antidepressant that selectively targets noradrenaline reuptake. It has received marketing approval in Europe but not in the United States because of concerns over poor efficacy.
- All antidepressants carry an FDA warning about increased suicidality, particularly in younger (<25 years of age) patients. The mechanism has not been established and there is not enough data to determine whether a lower risk exists for some antidepressants compared with others. These concerns must also be balanced against the potential for increased risk of completed suicides in untreated depression.

EVIDENCE
Smoking Cessation: Antidepressants versus Placebo

- A 2007 Cochrane review (53 trials) compared antidepressants to placebo or alternative pharmacotherapies for smoking cessation or relapse prevention. The review included 31 RCTs of bupropion versus placebo or no treatment for smoking cessation, finding that bupropion doubled the odds of cessation across these studies (OR 1.94). In four trials, nortriptyline also improved the odds of quitting smoking (OR 2.34).

Smoking Cessation: versus Varenicline (Partial Nicotine Agonist)

- A 2007 Cochrane review (7 trials, N = 7267 participants) assessed the efficacy and tolerability of varenicline versus other interventions and placebo for smoking cessation. The authors included three double-blind randomized controlled trials that compared bupropion with varenicline and when the data from these studies were combined, found that more varenicline subjects were abstinent or continuously abstinent from smoking at 12 months compared with bupropion (relative risk [RR] 1.52).

FYI

- Bupropion does not fit well into other drug classes; therefore it is often inappropriately lumped together with other agents. The simplest and most accurate classification is as an *atypical* agent.

Lithium

DESCRIPTION
Lithium is a chemical element used primarily in the treatment of bipolar disorder.

PROTOTYPE
- Lithium

MOA (MECHANISM OF ACTION)
- Decades after the discovery of lithium's utility in bipolar disorder, the mechanism behind its efficacy is still poorly understood.
- One thing that is clear is that lithium has multiple effects on second messengers (Figure 23-7):

Lithium

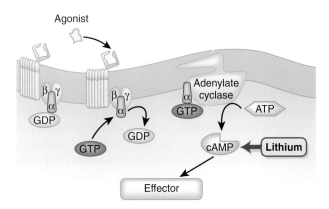

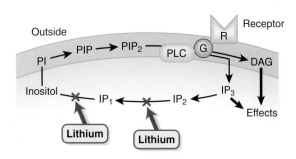

Figure 23-7.   *GDP*, Guanosine diphosphate; *GTP*, guanosine triphosphate; *ATP*, adenosine triphosphate; *IP1*, inositol monophosphate; *IP2*, inositol diphosphate; *IP3*, inositol triphosphate; *DAG*, diacylglycerol; *PLC*, phospholipase C; *PIP*, phosphoinositol phosphate; *PIP2*, phosphoinositol bisphosphate.

- Fine-tuning of cyclic adenosine monophosphate (cAMP)
  - Because lithium causes an increase in baseline cAMP and a decrease in stimulation of cAMP formation, lithium is able to fine-tune cAMP levels
- Depletion of inositol

- Inhibition of inositol monophosphatases, leading to a reduction in synaptic signaling through receptors that are coupled to phosphoinosital (PI) turnover
- Increasing evidence suggests that lithium may have a neuroprotective role in the CNS, although the connection between this and its efficacy in mania is unclear at present. Lithium has been reported to increase expression of the antiapoptotic protein bcl-2.
- Another neuroprotective factor thought to mediate the effects of lithium is the enzyme glycogen synthase kinase 3 (GSK-3). GSK-3 regulates numerous cellular processes such as gene transcription, synaptic plasticity, apoptosis, and circadian rhythms, among others. Lithium's inhibition of GSK-3 is believed to have a neuroprotective effect.

PHARMACOKINETICS
- Lithium has a narrow therapeutic index; therefore, small increases in lithium levels can lead to toxic effects. The effective plasma concentration is 0.6 to 1.25 mEq/L; moderate toxicity can occur starting at 1.5 mEq/L, and severe toxicity at 2 mEq/L.
- Lithium is almost exclusively excreted in the urine, with <1% in feces and smaller amounts excreted in sweat. Lithium is filtered freely, with 80% being reabsorbed in the nephron. In patients with normal renal function, 50% to 80% of a single dose is excreted in urine within 24 hours. Renal lithium excretion varies among individuals and is generally decreased in older patients and increased in younger patients.

INDICATIONS
- Bipolar disorder
- Treatment-refractory depression (adjunctive)

CONTRAINDICATIONS
- *In the presence of the following conditions, lithium should be used only with extreme caution, when other treatments have failed:*
  - **Significant renal or cardiovascular disease:** Lithium is cleared almost exclusively by the kidneys; therefore the risk of toxicity is high in those with compromised renal function. Lithium is also arrhythmogenic in some individuals (see later).
  - **Severe dehydration or sodium depletion:** Lithium toxicity can arise in cases in which the body tries to conserve sodium (see Pharmacokinetics for details).

SIDE EFFECTS
Serious
- **Acute lithium toxicity** causes nausea, vomiting, diarrhea, renal failure, neuromuscular dysfunction, ataxia, tremor, confusion, delirium, and seizures.
- **Arrhythmia:** Lithium inhibits K$^+$ entry into myocytes, which leads to abnormal repolarization and abnormal T-waves.

This can also lead to intracellular K⁺ depletion, and extracellular hyperkalemia, increasing the risk of sudden cardiac arrest from small changes in potassium levels.

- **Nephrotoxicity:** Nephrogenic **diabetes insipidus** (symptoms include polyuria and polydipsia) may occur after long-term therapy. The kidneys become insensitive to ADH. Irreversible kidney damage may also occur because of tubulo-interstitial nephropathy.
- **Weight gain:** The mechanism has not been established.
- **Nausea, GI irritation:** The mechanism has not been established.
- **Memory disturbances, cognitive dulling:** The mechanism has not been established.

IMPORTANT NOTES

- Lithium is unique among all psychotropic agents in that it lacks any sedative, euphoriant, or depressive effects in normal individuals who do not suffer from psychiatric illness.

Advanced
Drug Interactions

- A drug interaction between lithium and diuretics has a unique mechanism. In response to decreased volume secondary to diuretic use, the kidneys will try to retain Na⁺ in an effort to retain water. When the kidney reabsorbs Na⁺, it will also reabsorb Li⁺, as it has a hard time differentiating between these two monovalent cations.
- The clinical significance of this interaction is enhanced by the fact that lithium has a **narrow therapeutic index**, so only a small increase in Li⁺ levels can lead to toxicity. The same problem, enhanced Li⁺ reabsorption, can occur in patients with low Na⁺ levels or who are hypovolemic.

EVIDENCE
Bipolar Disorder

- A 2007 Health Technology Assessment (United Kingdom) review (45 trials) compared various mood stabilizers in preventing relapse in bipolar disorder. The authors found that lithium, valproate, lamotrigine, and olanzapine were more efficacious than placebo as maintenance therapy for relapse prevention. Lithium and olanzapine were effective for preventing manic relapses, but not for depressive relapses.

Lithium versus Placebo for Maintenance Treatment in Mood Disorders

- A 2001 Cochrane review (nine trials, N = 825 participants) compared lithium to placebo for treatment of mood disorder. Lithium was most beneficial at preventing relapse when used in bipolar disorder (OR 0.29). No significant benefit for relapse prevention was found in unipolar disorder. Because of low event rates, no conclusions could be drawn about the impact of lithium on suicide.

FYI

- The discovery of lithium, one of the most important drugs in psychiatry, is an example of serendipity and scientific acumen. In the late 1940s an Australian scientist was administering lithium salt to guinea pigs to increase the solubility of urates. After noting that lithium made the animals lethargic, he decided to give lithium carbonate to agitated or manic psychiatric patients. Lithium appeared to have a positive effect on mania, paving the way for its use for this indication.

First-Generation Antipsychotics

DESCRIPTION

Antipsychotics are agents used in the treatment of psychosis. First-generation antipsychotics are also referred to as *typical antipsychotics.*

PROTOTYPES AND COMMON DRUGS
Phenothiazines

- Prototype: chlorpromazine
- Others: thioridazine, fluphenazine, perphenazine, trifluoperazine, pipotiazine, pericyazine, prochlorperazine

Butyrophenones

- Prototype: Haloperidol
- Others: droperidol

Thioxanthenes

- Prototype: Flupenthixol
- Others: thiothixene, zuclopenthixol

MOA (MECHANISM OF ACTION)

- Dopamine is believed to play a key role in schizophrenia and thought disorders. Patients with schizophrenia experience hallucinations (visual, auditory, and tactile experiences in the absence of stimulation—for example, seeing something that is not there) and delusions (beliefs that are not true).
- There are several dopamine pathways in the CNS, but the following are key in both the efficacy and side effects of antipsychotic therapy:
  - ▲ Mesolimbic (behavior, mood)
  - ▲ Nigrostriatal (movement) Tuberoinfundibular (prolactin release) (Figure 23-8)
- All antipsychotics are **antagonists at dopamine D₂ receptors.** It is the antagonism of D₂ receptors in the mesolimbic pathway that is thought to alleviate the positive symptoms of schizophrenia. Blockade of D₂ receptors in other pathways is believed to result in many of the side effects of typical antipsychotics.

First and second generation antipsychotics

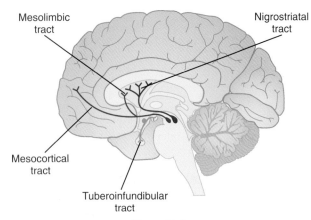

Figure 23-8.

- Recently, subtypes of the D_2 receptor have been identified: D_3, and D_4. Collectively, D_2, D_3, and D_4 receptors are often referred to as the "D_2-like receptors." These receptors all have different distributions in the brain and subtle differences in pharmacology that are still not fully understood.
- First-generation antipsychotics antagonize **numerous other receptors**, including adrenergic and cholinergic as well as histamine H_1 receptors. Although it is still unclear to what extent, if any, antagonism of these receptors contributes to the efficacy of antipsychotics, they have a clear role in mediating many of the **side effects** associated with these agents.

PHARMACOKINETICS

- Most antipsychotics are highly lipophilic (and therefore easily enter the brain) and accumulate in well-perfused tissues such as brain and lung. Because of their lipophilic nature, most antipsychotics have the potential to cross the placenta and to enter breast milk.
- A number of first-generation antipsychotics have active metabolites, including haloperidol, chlorpromazine, and thioridazine. The activity of these active metabolites may complicate the correlation of plasma drug monitoring with clinical efficacy.
- Elimination half-lives are typically in the 12- to 24-hour range, so all first-generation antipsychotics permit once-daily dosing.
- The elderly as well as the very young may have an impaired ability to metabolize antipsychotics.
- Several first-generation antipsychotics are available in parenteral formulations, both standard intravenous and intramuscular formulations to achieve faster onset, and depot formulations to achieve prolonged effects (Table 23-3).

INDICATIONS
Common

- Psychosis (from any cause, such as schizophrenia or drug use)
- Acute agitation, delirium, acute mania (haloperidol)
- Nausea and vomiting (droperidol, chlorpromazine, prochlorperazine)

TABLE 23-3. Onset and Duration of Action of Depot and Intramuscular Formulations of First-Generation Antipsychotics

	Onset	Duration
Depot		
Haloperidol decanoate		3 weeks
Fluphenazine decanoate		3-4 weeks
Pipotiazine palmitate		3-6 weeks
Intramuscular (IM)		
Haloperidol IM	30-45 minutes	
Chlorpromazine IM	15-30 minutes	
Fluphenazine IM	<1 hour	

Rare

- Tourette's syndrome (haloperidol)
- Intractable hiccups (chlorpromazine, haloperidol)

CONTRAINDICATION

- **Severe CNS depression:** Typical antipsychotics tend to have CNS depressant effects and should be avoided in conditions of decreased level of consciousness.

SIDE EFFECTS
Common

- **Anticholinergic** effects include dry mouth, constipation, difficulty urinating, and loss of accommodation.
- **α-Antagonism:** Orthostatic hypotension and ejaculatory failure may occur.
- **Sedation** is probably due to H1 receptor antagonism, and is more common with the phenothiazines.
- **Extrapyramidal syndrome (EPS):** Blockade of dopamine receptors in the basal ganglia leads to Parkinson-like symptoms such as slow movement (bradykinesia), stiffness, and tremor.
- **Tardive dyskinesia:** Slow-developing, *often permanent* dyskinesia typically appears well after initiation of therapy (months to years). This effect is characterized by repetitive, involuntary movements of the face, arms, and trunk. One theory is that D_2 receptors become hypersensitive after prolonged blockade. It can be very resistant to treatment.
- **Hyperprolactinemia:** Dopamine inhibits prolactin secretion. Antidopaminergic drugs will therefore have the potential to increase prolactin secretion, resulting in the following:
  - Amenorrhea (loss of menstrual period)
  - Galactorrhea (production of breast milk in women only, not in association with pregnancy)
  - Gynecomastia (feminization of men)
  - Decreased libido (sex drive)

Rare but Serious

- **Neuroleptic malignant syndrome (NMS)** is a rare but life-threatening side effect. The mechanism is not fully understood, but it is thought to be a result of inhibition of dopamine in the hypothalamus, an area responsible for temperature regulation.

▲ The condition is characterized by:
- Decreased or altered level of consciousness
- Increased muscle tone (rigidity)
- Fever
- Myoglobinemia and death, which occur in about 10% of these cases
- Autonomic instability (variable heart rates and blood pressures)

■ **Agranulocytosis**: A decreased white blood cell count can occur as a result of antipsychotics. This will result in undesired immunosuppression and requires discontinuation of the drug. This effect is observed with chlorpromazine and other phenothiazines (<0.1% of patients).

■ **Cardiac conduction abnormalities such as long QT (thioridazine, droperidol)** are a rare but serious side effect that has led to the market withdrawal of these agents in some jurisdictions. Antipsychotics appear to affect cardiac potassium channels, and these two agents are likely to have a greater impact on these channels than other agents.

IMPORTANT NOTES

■ There is increasing concern about the metabolic side effects associated with long-term use of antipsychotics. The risk of some of these side effects may be lower with first-generation antipsychotics compared with second generation antipsychotics (see Evidence section).

■ After many years of research, the exact causes of schizophrenia remain a mystery. There are several theories as to the neurochemical origins; most involve serotonin and dopamine playing a key role. Glutamate, an excitatory neurotransmitter, has also become a major focus of research, based on the observation that *N*-methyl-D-aspartate (NMDA) antagonists exacerbate cognitive impairment and psychosis in patients with schizophrenia. Glutamate receptor agonists are currently in development for schizophrenia.

Advanced
Drug Interactions
■ Chlorpromazine and haloperidol are metabolized through CYP2D6 and CYP3A4, fluphenazine through CYP2D6,

and trifluoperazine through CYP1A2; therefore caution should be exercised when using known inducers or inhibitors of these isozymes.

■ Haloperidol is an inhibitor of CYP3A4. Fluphenazine inhibits CYP2D6.

EVIDENCE
Risk of Diabetes in First- versus Second-Generation Antipsychotics

■ A 2008 systematic review (11 studies) compared diabetes risk among various antipsychotics. The majority of studies in this review were cross-sectional or retrospective cohort studies, which somewhat limits confidence in the analysis. The authors found an increased risk of diabetes in patients taking second-generation versus first-generation antipsychotics (RR 1.32). Data were insufficient to include aripiprazole, ziprasidone, and amisulpride in this analysis. Relative risks ranged from a low of 1.16 with risperidone to a high of 1.39 with clozapine. Differences in risk were statistically significant for all second-generation agents except risperidone.

FYI

■ Phenothiazines are among the earliest synthetic drugs, first synthesized in the late nineteenth century as a result of the development of aniline dyes. The first phenothiazines were antihistamines, and it was their sedative effects that led to their use in agitated psychiatric patients.

■ Chlorpromazine was developed in 1950 for use in anesthesia. Shortly after, it was used in psychiatry for agitation and anxiety. Initially its efficacy in these patients was attributed to its sedative properties, but it was later determined that chlorpromazine was effective in the treatment of a variety of psychoses.

■ The *extrapyramidal system* technically refers to the basal ganglia, but the term was coined in 1912 and originally referred to movement disorders in patients with liver disease.

Second-Generation Antipsychotics

DESCRIPTION
Antipsychotics are used to treat disorders of thought. Second-generation antipsychotics are also called *atypical antipsychotics*.

PROTOTYPE AND COMMON DRUGS
■ Prototype: cloz**apine**
■ Others: olanz**apine**, queti**apine**, risper**idone**, paliper**idone**, ziprasi**done**, aripiprazole

MOA (MECHANISM OF ACTION) (Figure 23-9)

■ Dopamine is believed to play a key role in schizophrenia and thought disorders. Patients with schizophrenia experience hallucinations (visual, auditory, and tactile experiences in the absence of stimulation—for example, seeing something that is not there) and delusions (beliefs that are not true).

■ The second-generation antipsychotics are believed to antagonize several different receptors, primarily **dopamine** and **serotonin** (5-HT).

First and second generation antipsychotics

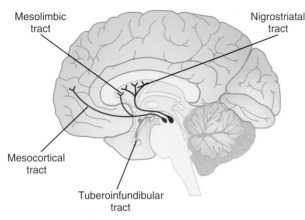

Figure 23-9.

- There are several dopamine pathways in the CNS, but the following are key in both the efficacy and side effects of antipsychotic therapy:
  - ▲ Mesolimbic (behavior)
  - ▲ Nigrostriatal (movement)
  - ▲ Tuberoinfundibular (prolactin release)
- All antipsychotic drugs are **D_2-receptor antagonists,** and it is believed that blockade of D_2 receptors in the **mesolimbic** pathway leads to an antipsychotic effect, addressing the positive symptoms of schizophrenia.
- Recently, subtypes of the D_2 receptor have been identified: D_3, and D_4. Collectively, D_2, D_3, and D_4 receptors are often referred to as the "D_2-like receptors." These receptors all have different distributions in the brain and subtle differences in pharmacology that are still not fully understood.
- The role of serotonin (specifically 5-HT_{2A}) antagonism in the efficacy of antipsychotics is less well understood. Unlike many of the first-generation agents, the second-generation agents are potent antagonists of 5-HT_{2A} receptors. Because second-generation agents are better at treating the negative symptoms of schizophrenia, it is believed that blockade of 5-HT_{2A} receptors may contribute to the improvement in negative symptoms.
- It is also thought that 5-HT_{2A} blockade might affect nigrostriatal dopamine release, leading to reduced extrapyramidal symptoms (EPS). Other theories accounting for the different propensities among antipsychotics to cause EPS include different D_2 binding affinities and anticholinergic activity.
- Second-generation antipsychotics, as first-generation antipsychotics, antagonize numerous other receptors, including adrenergic and cholinergic (particularly olanzapine and clozapine) as well as histamine H_1 receptors. Although it is still unclear to what extent, if any, antagonism of these receptors contributes to the efficacy of atypical antipsychotics, they have a clear role in mediating many of the side effects associated with these agents.

PHARMACOKINETICS
- The second-generation antipsychotics vary in bioavailability, elimination half-life, and metabolism.

- All are eliminated by hepatic metabolism, and all but one rely on the CYP450 system for their metabolism. Paliperidone is the active metabolite of risperidone and is not reliant on CYP450 for its metabolism.
- A long-acting intramuscular injection form of risperidone is available. It is administered every 2 weeks. Because of the delay in achieving therapeutic plasma concentrations, it is suggested that oral risperidone be given for the first 3 weeks after the initial IM injection.

INDICATIONS
- Schizophrenia
- Inappropriate behavior associated with dementia (risperidone)
- Acute mania associated with bipolar disorder (risperidone, olanzapine, quetiapine)

CONTRAINDICATIONS
All
- **History of neuroleptic malignant syndrome** (see Side Effects)

Clozapine
- **Myeloproliferative disorders** are a contraindication because of the risk of agranulocytosis with clozapine (see later).
- **Liver disease or failure** is a contraindication.
- **Severe renal or cardiac disease:** See the discussion of cardiovascular toxicity.
- **Paralytic ileus** is a contraindication because of significant anticholinergic effects.
- **Seizure disorders:** Clozapine appears to lower the seizure threshold, thus promoting seizures.

Ziprasidone
- **QT prolongation:** Ziprasidone may prolong the QT interval and therefore should be avoided in patients with a history of QT prolongation (see Side Effects). **Ziprasidone should also be avoided in patients with recent significant cardiac events for this reason.**

SIDE EFFECTS
- The side effect profile of atypical antipsychotics varies widely owing to their heterogeneous receptor binding profiles.

Serious
All Agents
- **Increased mortality in elderly patients:** These agents are associated with increased risk of death in elderly patients with dementia, from a variety of causes, largely cardiovascular or infectious. The mechanism is still unclear at this time.
- **Endocrine:**
  - ▲ **Weight gain** occurs because of suppression of satiety and other factors. The receptor responsible has not been established, although the focus is currently on H_1.
  - ▲ **Exacerbation of diabetes, hyperglycemia:** Diabetes (type 2) may simply be secondary to weight gain, but these agents might also affect glucose transporters.

▲ **Dyslipidemia** is probably secondary to weight gain.

▲ **Hyperprolactinemia:** Dopamine inhibits prolactin release, so dopamine blockade leads to increased prolactin release.

■ **Neuroleptic malignant syndrome (NMS)** is a rare but *critically life-threatening* effect seen with both first- and second-generation antipsychotics. The mechanism is not fully understood, but it is thought to be caused by inhibition of dopamine in the hypothalamus, an area responsible for temperature regulation. It is characterized by:

▲ Decreased or altered level of consciousness

▲ Fever

▲ Increased muscle tone (rigidity)

▲ Autonomic instability

▲ Myoglobinemia and death (in about 10% of cases)

Clozapine

■ **Agranulocytosis** can be fatal and necessitates weekly or biweekly blood monitoring of all patients taking clozapine. The risk is about 1% in the first 3 months and then decreases to about 0.01% after 1 year. Although agranulocytosis is a risk with all antipsychotics, it is much more common with clozapine compared to other agents.

■ **Seizures** may occur.

Quetiapine

■ **Cataracts:** No causal link has been established.

Ziprasidone

■ **QT interval prolongation:** As a class, the second-generation agents are considered to prolong the QT interval; however, ziprasidone is the only member of this class in which this adverse effect has lead to consistent clinically relevant events.

Nonserious Adverse Effects, Common to All Agents (to Varying Extents)

■ **Orthostatic hypotension** is most commonly observed with clozapine. This side effect is probably caused by α_1 blockade

■ **EPS** secondary to D_2 receptor blockade in the nigrostriatal region. The incidence of EPS is lower with second-generation compared with first-generation agents, and among the second-generation agents, is lowest with clozapine.

■ **Sedation** is probably caused by H1 antagonism. Among second-generation antipsychotics, clozapine is believed to cause the most sedation.

■ **Anticholinergic** effects are most commonly observed with clozapine. Exercise caution in patients with conditions exacerbated by cholinergic blockade, such as glaucoma (narrow angle), paralytic ileus, or enlarged prostate.

IMPORTANT NOTES

■ Clozapine is itself considered to be *atypical* among atypical antipsychotics, with a unique side effect profile and a greater degree of success in treatment-resistant patients. Thus many consider clozapine to be in a class of its own.

■ The second-generation antipsychotics are considered "atypical" because they do not cause EPS to the same extent as first-generation agents. It is important to note that EPS has still been observed with these agents, and the mechanistic rationale for why atypical agents are less likely to cause EPS has not been established.

■ The incidence of tardive dyskinesia tends to vary with age and drug class used. The incidence in children is low with second-generation antipsychotics, in adults it is lower with second-generation than first-generation agents, and first- and second-generation agents have the same annual incidence in the elderly.

■ The weight gain associated with antipsychotics can be significant and lead to long-term health issues such as type 2 diabetes and cardiovascular disease. It appears that olanzapine and clozapine may cause the greatest degree of weight gain among the second-generation agents.

■ Conversely, ziprasidone may be least associated with weight gain, and in fact has been associated with weight loss in some trials. The adverse lipid effects seen with other agents in this class are also not seen with ziprasidone. However, ziprasidone is associated with QT interval prolongation, a potentially fatal adverse effect. This creates an interesting dilemma—choosing between rare short-term side effects that are potentially fatal, and more common long-term side effects that have serious, but less readily identifiable consequences.

Advanced
Drug Interactions

■ Clozapine is metabolized by CYP1A2 and CYP3A4, and its metabolism is affected by notable inducers or inhibitors of these isozymes, such as the following:

▲ Inhibitors: erythromycin, cimetidine, azole antifungals, protease inhibitors, SSRIs

▲ Inducers: carbamazepine, phenytoin, rifampin, omeprazole, cigarette smoking

■ Olanzapine is a weak inhibitor of CYP1A2, CYP2D6, and CYP3A4, but it has not been shown to have significant effects on other drugs. The metabolism of olanzapine has been affected by the following:

▲ Inhibitor: fluvoxamine

■ Quetiapine is metabolized mainly by CYP3A4. Its metabolism is affected by the following:

▲ Inhibitor: azole antifungals, macrolide antibiotics

▲ Inducer: carbamazepine, phenytoin

■ Risperidone is metabolized by CYP2D6 and has a major active metabolite. The metabolism of risperidone is affected by the following:

▲ Inhibitors: fluoxetine, paroxetine

▲ Inducers: carbamazepine

EVIDENCE
Schizophrenia

■ A recent (2006) systematic review of atypical antipsychotics found differences in effectiveness among agents in this class:

386 Section II **Drug Classes**

- ▲ Clozapine reduced the risk of suicide in high-risk schizophrenic patients compared with olanzapine.
- ▲ Risperidone had a faster onset of effect, shorter length of hospitalization and lower rates of discontinuation than olanzapine. However, maintenance use of olanzapine was associated with a lower risk and longer time to treatment than risperidone or quetiapine.
- A 2010 Cochrane review (50 studies, N = 9476 participants) compared olanzapine with other second-generation agents. Fewer participants treated with olanzapine had to be rehospitalized compared with quetiapine (NNT 11, 2 RCTs) and ziprasidone (NNT 17, 2 RCTs) but not clozapine. Olanzapine improved symptoms more than aripiprazole (2 RCTs), quetiapine (10 RCTs), risperidone (15 RCTs) and ziprasidone (4 RCTs) but not amisulpride or clozapine. Olanzapine elicited more weight gain than all others except clozapine, and more EPS than quetiapine, but less EPS than risperidone and ziprasidone.

Psychosis and Aggression Associated with Alzheimer's Disease

- A 2006 Cochrane review (10 trials) found that although risperidone and olanzapine were useful in reducing aggression and risperidone was useful for psychosis, these agents also had serious harmful effects such as a higher incidence of stroke as well as EPS and other adverse events. There were insufficient data to assess cognitive function.

Safety in Patients with Alzheimer's Disease or Dementia

- A 2005 systematic review (15 trials, N = 5100 patients) examined the use of atypical antipsychotics versus placebo in patients with Alzheimer's disease or dementia. The risk of death was higher in patients taking atypicals (3.5% versus 2.3% of patients died) compared with placebo (OR 1.54).

FYI

- Clozapine is widely recognized as being the atypical antipsychotic with the greatest efficacy; however, its 50-year history has been tumultuous. From its early trials in the 1960s, clozapine was noted as being "atypical" because of its lack of disabling neurologic side effects. However, the lack of EPS was interpreted as an indication that it lacked antipsychotic efficacy as well, as at that time the two effects were considered to be connected.
- The first serious impediment to clozapine's widespread use was the discovery of orthostatic hypotension. After this hurdle was overcome, reports of deaths from severe blood disorders began to emerge from Finland in the mid-1970s. The incidence of agranulocytosis was much higher in the Finnish population, shedding light on a rare toxicity that had previously been overlooked. The manufacturer of clozapine dropped its request for approval by the FDA, and the drug became available only through a "compassionate use" program.
- Interest in clozapine reemerged in North America in the 1980s, because of both the rising health care costs of mental illness and the success the Europeans had had using a monitoring program to minimize harm. Clozapine was approved by the FDA in 1989 and continues to be a vital drug for those refractory to other therapies.

Benzodiazepines

DESCRIPTION

The benzodiazepines (BZDs) are a group of agents with primarily anxiolytic, sedative, and hypnotic effects.

PROTOTYPES AND COMMON DRUGS

- Prototype: lor**azepam**
- Others: alpr**azolam**, brom**azepam**, chlordiazepoxide, clon**azepam**, diaz**epam**, flur**azepam**, mid**azolam**, nitr**azepam**, oxa**zepam**, temaz**epam**, triaz**olam**

Antagonist

- Flumazenil

Atypical or Nonbenzodiazepines

- Prototype: zopiclone
- Others: zolpidem, eszopiclone, zaleplon

MOA (MECHANISM OF ACTION)

- γ-Aminobutyric acid (GABA) is the major inhibitory neurotransmitter in the CNS. GABA binds to three different types of receptors: $GABA_A$, $GABA_B$, and $GABA_C$.
  - ▲ Binding of GABA to $GABA_A$ receptors leads to the opening of the chloride (Cl^-) channel, facilitating Cl^- influx and cellular **hyperpolarization** (making the inside more negative).
  - ▲ Hyperpolarization of a cell decreases the probability that the cell can be subsequently *depolarized* by other incoming excitatory signals; this will have a net inhibitory effect Figure 23-10).
- BZDs also have their own receptor directly on the Cl^- channel. Binding of BZDs to this BZD receptor *enhances the effects of GABA* at the $GABA_A$ receptor.

Benzodiazapines

Synaptic cleft

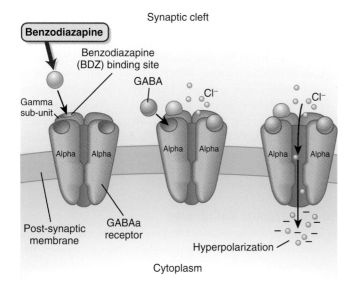

Figure 23-10.

- BZDs are unable to activate the GABA$_A$ receptor on their own; therefore BZDs have no pharmacologic effects on the Cl$^-$ channel when GABA is absent.
- Atypical BZDs also act as GABA enhancers but bind to a different subunit of the BZD receptor than typical BZDs.
- For example, the atypical BZDs zolpidem and zopiclone bind to the BZ1 (ω1) receptor subtype of the BZD receptor.

PHARMACOKINETICS

- The elimination half-lives of BZDs differ greatly (see Table 23-4).
- The elimination half-lives of BZDs play a key role in determining how they are used (see Important Notes for further discussion).
- Lorazepam, midazolam, and diazepam are all available for intravenous administration. Onset time is quite short (minutes) when these drugs are given intravenously.
- Patients who use alcohol regularly will have significant resistance to BZDs and require larger doses to achieve the same effect as would be achieved in an otherwise identical patient who does not use alcohol regularly.

INDICATIONS

- **Sedation for:**
  - ▲ Anxiety states (called *anxiolytics* when used this way)
  - ▲ Procedures
  - ▲ Acute agitation
- **Insomnia**
- **Acute seizure treatment**
- **Alcohol withdrawal**
  - ▲ BZDs are the first-line treatment for alcohol withdrawal and delirium tremens (DTs).

TABLE 23-4. Elimination Half-Lives of Various Benzodiazepines

Half-life Duration	Half-Life (Hours)
Short Half-Life Agents	
Triazolam	2-3
Intermediate Half-Life Agents	
Alprazolam	12-15
Lorazepam	10-20
Oxazepam	10-20
Temazepam	10-40
Chlordiazepoxide*	15-40
Long Half-Life Agents	
Diazepam*	20-80
Flurazepam*	40-100

*These agents have active metabolites

- **Muscle relaxation**
  - ▲ Useful for patients with restless leg syndrome and muscle spasms

CONTRAINDICATIONS

- Addiction to other drugs or past history of BZD addiction is a contraindication.
- **Sleep apnea:** Patients with central or obstructive sleep apnea have abnormal respiratory centers and may be at risk for exacerbations of sleep apnea if given sedatives of any type.

SIDE EFFECTS

- **Amnesia**—the impaired ability to remember—may be a *desired effect* for medical procedures.
- **Respiratory depression** may be seen at higher doses and can lead to respiratory acidosis, particularly in those with chronic obstructive pulmonary disease (COPD).
- **Decreased blood pressure, increased heart rate:** These cardiovascular effects are seen at higher doses and are likely mediated by a decrease in vascular resistance (midazolam) or cardiac output (diazepam).
- **Daytime sedation:** This is a continuation of the intended therapeutic effect of BZDs. The extent of sedation is largely a function of the half-life and frequency of use.
- **Disinhibition** may occur.

IMPORTANT NOTES

- BZDs are not analgesics. They do not reduce the perception of pain.
- The ability of BZDs to cause amnesia is advantageous in the performance of uncomfortable procedures, as the patient is still able to comply with instructions but does not retain memory of the procedure afterward.
- Although the clinical effects of the BZDs resemble and overlap with those of other sedative-hypnotics, BZDs are more effective as anxiolytics.
- Because BZDs are CNS depressants (inhibitors), and seizures are states of pathologically elevated electrical activity in the brain, BZDs are ideally suited for treating seizures.

- Tolerance, dependence, and withdrawal are all of major concern with BZDs. Discontinuation of BZDs can be particularly unpleasant for the patient and, typical of drug withdrawal, is characterized by side effects that are the opposite of those intended with therapy—that is, insomnia, anxiety, tremor, and (rarely) seizures.
- Longer half-life agents are less prone to cause withdrawal than agents with a short half-life, as the longer half-life agents allow time for receptor density to return to predrug levels before the drug is completely eliminated. However, for certain indications, particularly when used as hypnotics, shorter-acting agents are preferable because of their reduced propensity for a hangover effect (i.e., grogginess).
- Balancing the need to minimize withdrawal while avoiding BZD hangover is tricky, and it is strongly recommended that short-acting hypnotics such as triazolam be used sparingly.
- Flumazenil is a BZD antagonist that is used to reverse the sedative effects of BZDs.

Advanced

- BZDs can act as either agonists or inverse agonists at the BZD binding site on the $GABA_A$ receptor.
- $GABA_A$ and $GABA_C$ receptors are found on ion channels and are therefore said to be *ionotropic*. $GABA_B$ receptors are G protein coupled and are said to be *metabotropic*.

EVIDENCE
Generalized Anxiety Disorder

- A 2007 systematic review examined three commonly used BZDs—diazepam (12 trials), lorazepam (7 trials), and alprazolam (4 trials)—versus placebo. All included studies were DBRCTs. The authors chose withdrawal from study as their primary outcome measure, and fewer patients treated with BZD withdrew for any reason (RR 0.78) or for lack of efficacy (RR 0.29). However, more BZD-treated patients withdrew because of an adverse event compared with placebo (RR 1.54).

Older Adults with Insomnia

- A 2005 systematic review examined the risks and benefits of sedative use for insomnia in adults 60 years of age or older. The review included 20 DBRCTs, covering sleep quality, sleep time, awakenings, or latency of sleep onset. BZDs (830 participants) and non-BZDs (1099 participants) were the main interventions used, versus placebo (468 participants). Based on four studies, the authors calculated a number needed to treat (NNT) of 13 for improvement in sleep quality with sedatives. However, the number needed to harm (NNH) was six versus placebo. No difference in sleep quality was detected across three studies that compared BZDs with atypical BZDs. Sedatives increased sleep time by 25 minutes overall. Cognitive adverse effects were significantly more common with sedatives than with placebo (OR 4.78).

Benzodiazepine Withdrawal

- A 2006 Cochrane review (8 studies, 458 subjects). Although the studies could not be pooled, the authors concluded that progressive withdrawal from BZDs was preferred to abrupt withdrawal. Carbamazepine was identified as a potential adjunctive therapy to manage BZD withdrawal.

Alcohol Withdrawal

- A 2005 Cochrane review found that BZDs were significantly better for alcohol withdrawal seizures compared with placebo and had similar efficacy to other drugs, or anticonvulsants specifically. BZDs elicited similar changes in alcohol withdrawal scores compared with other drugs. The findings of the review are complicated by the heterogeneity among trials.

FYI

- The ability of BZDs and related GABA agonists to produce amnesia has led to their criminal use as *date rape* drugs.
- BZDs have their two nitrogen atoms at 1,4 positions. Other, *atypical* BZDs have their nitrogens at 1,5 positions. An example of this is clobazam, an anticonvulsant.
- Clozapine, an atypical antipsychotic, is a *di*benzodiazepine. It has two benzene rings attached to the seven-membered diazepine ring.

Central Nervous System Stimulants

DESCRIPTION

CNS stimulants are a heterogeneous class of compounds, structurally and pharmacologically related to amphetamine.

PROTOTYPES AND COMMON DRUGS
Amphetamines

- Prototype: amphetamine
- Others: dextro**amphetamine**, lisdex**amfetamine**, mixed **amphetamine** salts, meth**amphetamine**, MDMA (3,4-methylenedioxymeth**amphetamine**)

Nonamphetamines

- ▲ Prototype: **methylphenidate**
- ▲ Others: dex**methylphenidate**

MOA (MECHANISM OF ACTION)

- Methylphenidate and amphetamine work by increasing neurotransmitter levels in the synapse, specifically, levels of dopamine (DA) and noradrenaline (NA). They accomplish this through a variety of mechanisms.

- The primary mechanism is via stimulating the release of catecholamine from presynaptic vesicles.
- Methylphenidate and amphetamine **also inhibit the reuptake** of the monamines as well as inhibiting the activity of a key enzyme that breaks them down, MAO (Figure 23-11).

CNS stimulants

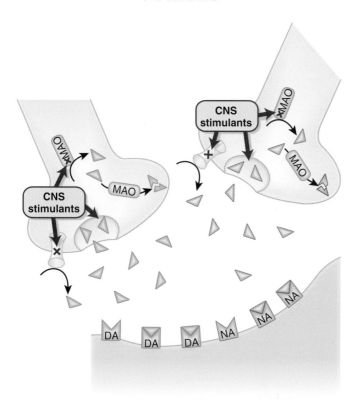

Figure 23-11.

- Methylphenidate and amphetamine increase dopamine levels in the prefrontal cortex, an area thought to play an important role in attention-deficit/hyperactivity disorder (ADHD). The connection between the increased dopamine and noradrenaline in the synapse and the behavioral improvements seen in ADHD is still unclear. Dopamine is thought to be the key neurotransmitter mediating the beneficial effects of these agents in ADHD.
- Increased dopamine levels in the nucleus accumbens elicits a euphoric effect and is likely most responsible for the use of these agents as drugs of abuse. Significant dopamine release in this area is typically seen only at higher doses.

PHARMACOKINETICS

- Wide variations in bioavailability of methylphenidate occur among individuals.
- The elimination half-life of methylphenidate is relatively short (approximately 2 hours); therefore it is also available in extended release (ER) forms. The main metabolite is

ritalinic acid, and the methylphenidate metabolites are mostly excreted in urine.

- Once-daily formulations are considered ideal for convenience. However, after evidence suggesting that the period immediately after a dose of methylphenidate provides the most benefit, manufacturers have tried to develop formulations that release the drug in a biphasic manner. These formulations have both an immediate-release (IR) and an ER component, in a variety of proportions. The agents with a large proportion of the IR component have greater efficacy early (2 hours) after administration, whereas the agents with a larger ER proportion have greater efficacy later (12 hours).
- Prodrugs such as lisdexamfetamine have been developed in an effort to reduce the abuse potential of these agents. Lisdexamfetamine is converted to dexamphetamine after oral administration, by the actions of the enzyme trypsin, which is found in the GI tract.
- A transdermal formulation of methylphenidate is also available. The patch is worn for 9 hours and provides continual release of methylphenidate over that time.

INDICATIONS

- ADHD
- Narcolepsy

CONTRAINDICATIONS

- Conditions in which CNS activation would create a problem: anxiety, tension, agitation, thyrotoxicosis
- **Conditions in which peripheral sympathetic stimulation would create a problem:** hypertension (moderate to severe), glaucoma, pheochromocytoma, symptomatic cardiovascular disease

SIDE EFFECTS

- **Central stimulant effects:**
  - ▲ Euphoria
  - ▲ Insomnia
  - ▲ Psychomotor stimulation
  - ▲ Anxiety
  - ▲ Hyperthermia
- **Peripheral sympathomimetic effects:** tachycardia, hypertension
- **Anorexia:** The reason for appetite suppression is unclear but is believed to be the result of the actions of these agents in the feeding center of the hypothalamus. This can be a particularly concerning side effect in children.

Serious

- **Sudden cardiac death:** Sudden deaths have been reported in adults and children who had a history of cardiac abnormalities. Stimulants therefore either are not recommended or should be used with extreme caution in these individuals.

IMPORTANT NOTES

- The short half-life of the IR formulations of methylphenidate means that doses are typically given early in the day in children (morning and noon), to maximize the effects of the drug while the child is in school and to hopefully minimize the insomnia and appetite suppressant side effects.

EVIDENCE
Safety of Methylphenidate in Adults

- A 2009 systematic review (26 trials, 811 participants) examined the safety of methylphenidate versus placebo for a variety of disorders, including ADHD, in adults. The trials were of relatively short duration (1 to 12 weeks) and therefore provide no information about chronic use. No serious (life-threatening or irreversible) adverse effects were reported in any studies. Dry mouth, anorexia, changes in mood, "jitteriness," depression or sadness, weight loss, and vertigo were the most common adverse events that occurred more frequently with methylphenidate than placebo. The five studies reporting cardiovascular changes found slight increases in blood pressure and pulse rate.

FYI

- Amphetamine was first introduced commercially in the 1930s as Benzedrine, for narcolepsy. The product was available without a prescription, and when word got out about its stimulant properties, sales soared until it reverted back to prescription-only status.

- Methylphenidate is an old drug that has seen a variety of indications over the years. First synthesized in 1944, it has been used for chronic fatigue, lethargy, and depression, among other indications.

- The behavioral effects of amphetamines in children were first noted 70 years ago. After observing positive responses in a small study of benzedrine, an amphetamine derivative, larger clinical trials demonstrated that "behavior disorders" in children responded to this agent.

- The CNS stimulants are a heterogeneous drug class, and that heterogeneity is seen in the wide variety of plant sources of agents in this class. Leaves of the shrub tree *Catha edulis*, native to Africa and the Middle East, contain norpseudoephedrine. Fresh leaves or stems are referred to as *Khat* and are an integral part of many social rituals in Middle Eastern countries such as Yemen. *Ephedra sinica* yields ephedra, an herb that dates back to first-century Chinese books of herbal medicine, used for asthma and upper respiratory tract infections.

- Ritalinic acid is the major metabolite of methylphenidate—hence the brand name, *Ritalin*.

- MDMA is also known as the street drug *ecstasy*.

- Dextroamphetamine is a stereoisomer of amphetamine and is considered to be approximately twice as potent as amphetamine.

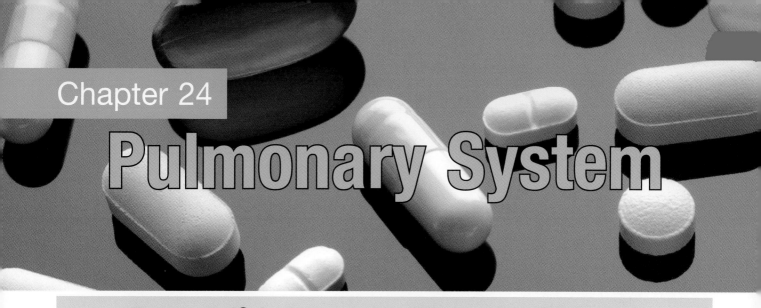

Chapter 24

Pulmonary System

Beta 2 (β₂) Agonists (Bronchodilators)

DESCRIPTION

β₂ Agonists are selective agonists for the β₂-adrenergic receptor. They are relatively selective and therefore also stimulate the β₁ receptor, but to a far lesser degree.

PROTOTYPE AND COMMON DRUGS
Short-Acting (Duration 3 to 4 Hours) β₂ Agonists (SABAs)

- Prototype: salbutamol (albuterol)
- Others: terbutaline, levalbuterol, pirbuterol

Long-Acting (Duration >12 Hours) β₂ Agonists (LABAs)

- Prototype: salme**terol**
- Others: formo**terol**

MOA (MECHANISM OF ACTION)

- Bronchoconstriction is one of the hallmarks of asthma.
- Stimulation of β₂ receptors in bronchial smooth muscle results in relaxation of bronchial smooth muscle. This results in a larger diameter airway, resulting in lower resistance to airflow in and out of the lungs (Figure 24-1).
- On a cellular level, the binding of an agonist to the β₂ receptors on bronchial smooth muscle activates an enzyme, adenylate cyclase, which converts adenosine triphosphate (ATP) to cyclic adenosine monophosphate (cAMP). It is these elevated levels of cAMP that lead to bronchodilation.
- β₂ Receptors are also found on other cells in the lung, including inflammatory cells.

PHARMACOKINETICS

- These drugs are all typically administered via inhalation: via metered dose inhaler (MDI), dry powder inhaler, or nebulizer (atomizes liquid drug into a mist). Inhalation delivers the drug to the lungs, where the highest concentra-tions are desired, thereby reducing the probability of side effects.
- Salbutamol is sometimes given as an intravenous infusion and is also available in oral form.
- Response to SABAs is rapid (response time 5 minutes) compared with inhaled anticholinergics (30 minutes).
- For LABAs, the response time of formoterol is similar to that of SABAs (5 minutes), but the onset of action of salmeterol is longer (15 to 20 minutes).
- Systemic uptake of inhaled drugs is significant, and sympathetic stimulation limits the maximum dose.
- Swallowing of drug that is deposited in the mouth and saliva will contribute to systemic absorption.

INDICATION

- Relief of **bronchospasm** from any cause:
  - Asthma
  - Emphysema (chronic obstructive pulmonary disease [COPD])
  - Anaphylaxis
  - Aspiration (inhalation of liquid or solid matter)

CONTRAINDICATIONS

- Severe bronchospasm is life-threatening. Therefore the indication for a β₂ agonist would outweigh most reasons not to give it.
- β₂ Agonists and (more accurately) β₁ agonists must be given with caution to patients in whom tachycardia is undesirable. These conditions include (but are not limited to) patients with severe coronary artery disease and aortic stenosis.

SIDE EFFECTS

- All side effects are related to overstimulation of β₂ and β₁ receptors and include primarily:
  - Tachycardia and palpitations
  - Tremor

Beta 2 agonists

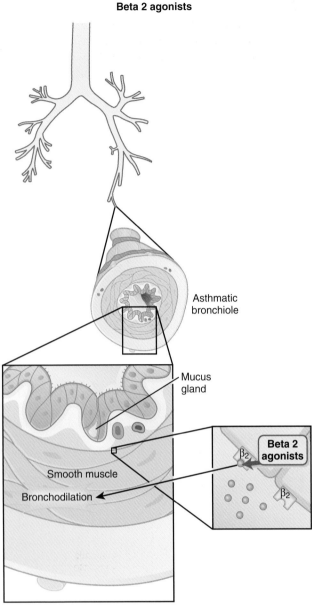

Figure 24-1.

▲ β Stimulation is involved with shifting K⁺ ions into cells. Therefore blood levels of K⁺ can be abnormally low (hypokalemia).

▲ β Stimulation is also involved with glucose metabolism, and excessive stimulation can result in **hyperglycemia**.

IMPORTANT NOTES

■ SABAs as required may be used as sole therapy in mild **episodic** asthma. Neither SABAs nor LABAs should be used as sole therapy in **persistent** asthma but should be combined with antiinflammatory therapy.

■ The combination of LABAs and ICSs has become standard therapy in the management of asthma. There are two reasons why this combination is believed to be so effective. First, the use of a bronchodilator is believed to open up the

TABLE 24-1. Fixed-Dose Combinations of Inhalers	
Salmeterol + fluticasone	Advair
Formoterol + budesonide	Symbicort
Salbutamol + ipratropium	Combivent

airways to improve distribution of the steroid. Second, it appears that chronic ICS use up-regulates β₂ receptors in the lungs. This is important because chronic use of β₂ agonists is believed to lead to a down-regulation of β₂ receptors in the lungs. Some available drugs are combinations of a bronchodilator and steroid together in one inhaler (Table 24-1).

■ Although use of ICS-LABA combinations is now a routine practice, the use of LABAs as monotherapy has prompted a lingering safety concern that has plagued these agents since their introduction into the market.

■ Pirbuterol is available in a breath-actuated MDI, meaning that the inhaler releases drug in response to patient inhalation.

EVIDENCE

Long-Acting β Agonists with or without Inhaled Corticosteroids in Adults or Children with Asthma

■ A 2007 Cochrane review (67 studies, 42,333 participants) examined the use of LABAs (salmeterol, 50 studies; formoterol, 17 studies) versus placebo. In these studies, patients were followed for 4 to 52 weeks. Patients were allowed to combine inhaled corticosteroids (ICSs) with LABAs in 40 studies, 24 studies did not permit ICSs, and three studies were unclear about ICS use. Use of LABAs, with or without ICSs, was associated with improvements in pulmonary function, symptoms, rescue medication use, and quality-of-life scores.

Formoterol Plus Inhaled Corticosteroids in Asthma

■ A 2009 Cochrane review (3 studies, N = 5905 patients) compared combinations of formoterol and ICSs with SABAs alone for relief of asthma symptoms. No clinically important advantages were found for the combination in patients with *mild* asthma. However, in more *severe* asthma, one study found that patients not well controlled on high-dose ICSs and who had had an exacerbation in the prior year had a reduced risk of exacerbations requiring oral steroids when using the combination versus terbutaline or formoterol monotherapy for relief. A study in children also found less serious adverse events with the combination of budesonide and formoterol for maintenance and relief.

Regular Formoterol versus Placebo or Short-Acting β Agonists in Chronic Asthma

■ A 2008 Cochrane review (22 studies, 8032 patients) compared serious adverse event rates for regular formoterol use with placebo or SABAs in chronic asthma. Nonfatal serious adverse events were increased versus placebo (odds ratio [OR] 1.57), but no increase was detected versus salbutamol or terbutaline. The increased risk over placebo was also seen in patients taking ICSs.

Inhaled Anticholinergics

DESCRIPTION

Inhaled anticholinergics antagonize the muscarinic receptor.

PROTOTYPE AND COMMON DRUGS

■ Prototype: Ipra**tropium**
■ Others: tio**tropium**

MOA (MECHANISM OF ACTION)

■ Parasympathetic stimulation of muscarinic receptors of the bronchioles results in bronchoconstriction and also increased bronchial secretions. These actions are largely mediated through M3 receptors, and to a lesser extent, M1 (Figure 24-2).
■ Antagonism of these muscarinic receptors **prevents bronchoconstriction and reduces secretions.** Tiotropium has greater selectivity for M3 receptors than ipratropium, which is considered to be relatively nonspecific for M1, M2, and M3 receptors. The clinical significance of this increased specificity has not been established.

PHARMACOKINETICS

■ Ipratropium and tiotropium are inhaled. They are quaternary compounds (therefore polarized and not apt to cross hydrophobic cell membranes). They do not readily cross the pulmonary membranes into the blood. Therefore, systemic absorption is low.
■ A lot of the drug ends up being swallowed. However, absorption from the gastrointestinal (GI) tract is also very low.
■ Compared with salbutamol, onset and duration of action are prolonged, likely because of minimal absorption from the lung.
■ Peak effect occurs at 30 to 90 minutes (slightly later than salbutamol). Duration is approximately 6 hours.
■ The duration of tiotropium is further prolonged (24 hours), because of its slow dissociation from receptors.

INDICATIONS

■ Acute asthma, but not as a first-line drug
■ COPD: both in acute exacerbations and also for chronic maintenance

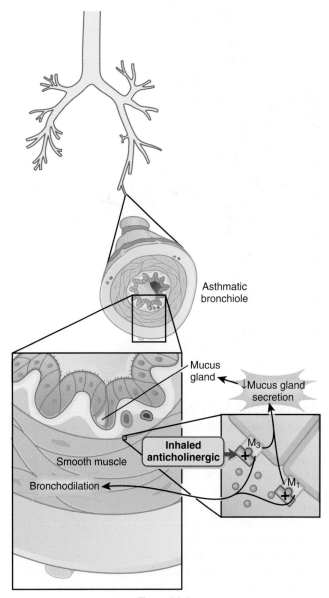

Asthmatic bronchiole

Asthmatic bronchiole

Mucus gland

↓Mucus gland secretion

Inhaled anticholinergic

Smooth muscle

Bronchodilation

M₃

M₁

Figure 24-2.

CONTRAINDICATIONS

- None of major significance
- When anticholinergics are used, caution should be exercised in patients who have conditions that would be exacerbated by cholinergic antagonism, such as glaucoma and urinary retention. However, because inhaled anticholinergics have low systemic absorption, this is typically not an issue in most patients.

SIDE EFFECTS

- Side effects are minimal because of minimal systemic absorption. Side effects would include the predictable effects of muscarinic antagonism in various organs.
- Local reactions such as dry mouth, nasal irritation, and nose bleeds are not uncommon.

IMPORTANT NOTES

- Ipratropium is slightly slower to act and possibly less effective than β_2 agonists for treatment of bronchial asthma.
- Tiotropium is administered once daily, therefore providing a potential convenience advantage over ipratropium.

EVIDENCE
Cardiovascular Safety

- A 2008 meta-analysis (17 trials, N = 14,783 patients) found an increased risk of the composite of cardiovascular death, myocardial infarction (MI), and stroke in patients on inhaled anticholinergics (1.8%) versus control therapy (1.2%). Specifically, risk of MI and cardiovascular death was increased, whereas risk of stroke was not.

Ipratropium versus Short-Acting β_2 Agonists in Chronic Obstructive Pulmonary Disease

- A 2006 Cochrane review (11 studies, N = 3912 patients) found small benefits of ipratropium over SABAs on measures of lung function, quality of life, and the requirement for oral steroids. The combination of ipratropium and SABAs was better than a β_2 agonist alone with respect to postbronchodilator lung function and a reduction in the need for oral steroids.

FYI

- Ipratropium (*Atrovent*) was derived from *atropine*.
- *Asthma cigarettes*, containing alkaloids from the belladonna plant, were an early and controversial treatment for asthma. These were the earliest inhaled anticholinergics and were used until the mid-twentieth century.

Leukotriene Receptor Antagonists

DESCRIPTION

Leukotriene receptor antagonists (LTRAs) are a newer class of drug used to treat bronchoconstriction. As the name implies, they antagonize leukotriene (LT) receptors. These drugs are taken orally (not inhaled).

PROTOTYPE AND COMMON DRUGS

- Prototype: monte**lukast**
- Others: zafir**lukast**

MOA (MECHANISM OF ACTION)

- Leukotrienes are biologically active fatty acids derived from the oxidative metabolism of **arachidonic acid**, via the enzyme 5-lipoxygenase.
- LT receptors such as LTC_4 and LTD_4 exert several effects that are commonly associated with asthma:
  - Bronchoconstriction
  - Hyperresponsive airways
  - Mucosal edema
  - Mucous hypersecretion
- Leukotriene receptor antagonists competitively and selectively block the LTD_4 receptor (Figure 24-3).

PHARMACOKINETICS

- Zafirlukast inhibits liver enzymes (CYP3A4) and therefore can increase the effects of warfarin.

INDICATIONS

- These drugs are **not** indicated for acute exacerbations of the disease. They are recommended for prophylaxis and chronic treatment of asthma.
- LTRAs can be tried when an inhaled steroid cannot be used, or if the inhaled steroid dose cannot be increased.

CONTRAINDICATIONS

- None of major significance

SIDE EFFECTS
Common and Not Serious

- Headache, vomiting, diarrhea

Rare and Serious

- Churg-Strauss syndrome (allergic granulomatosis) may occur. *Rare* in this case means 34.6 per million person-years. If 1 million people took the drug for 1 year, 35 patients would develop Churg-Strauss syndrome.

EVIDENCE
LRTAs versus Inhaled Corticosteroids (ICSs) for Chronic Asthma

- A 2000 Cochrane review (27 trials) compared the safety and efficacy of antileukotrienes to ICS in mild to moderate asthma. Patients treated with antileukotrienes were more

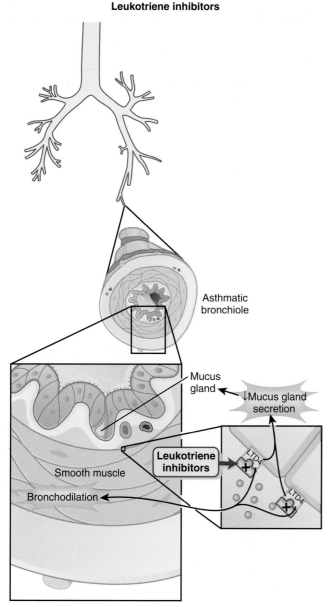

Leukotriene inhibitors

Asthmatic bronchiole

Mucus gland

↓Mucus gland secretion

Leukotriene inhibitors

LTD4

LTD4

Smooth muscle

Bronchodilation

Figure 24-3.

likely to have an exacerbation requiring systemic steroids (NNH = 26). ICS also improved pulmonary functions (FEV1), symptoms, nocturnal awakenings, rescue medication use, and quality of life to a greater extent than did antileukotrienes. More patients treated with antileukotrienes withdrew due to poor asthma control. The risk of side effects was no different between groups.

LTRAs Plus ICSs versus ICSs Alone for Chronic Asthma

■ A 2002 Cochrane review (27 studies) evaluated the effect of adding LTRAs to patients already treated with ICS for chronic asthma. The findings supported a modest improvement to lung function tests. There were statistically nonsignificant improvements in the need for rescue β_2 agonists.

LTRAs Plus ICSs versus Long-Acting β_2 Agonists (LABAs) Plus ICSs for Chronic Asthma

■ A 2006 Cochrane review (16 studies) evaluated the effect of adding LTRAs vs. LABAs to ICS in patients with chronic asthma. The findings showed a lower rate of requiring systemic steroids (RR = 0.83) with LABAs. Other endpoints including lung function tests, symptoms, and use of rescue β_2 agonists were also superior with LABAs. Withdrawals from treatment and side effects were similar in both groups.

FYI

■ Zileuton is a 5-lipoxygenase inhibitor approved for use in the United States but not in some other jurisdictions, due to safety concerns.
■ LTs were originally discovered in leukocytes, hence their prefix.
■ An *ene* bond is one in which there are two bonds between two carbon atoms (C=C). Leuktrienes have three of these bonds. The *ane* bond is a single bond (C–C).
■ Zafirlukast is administered twice a day. Montelukast is administered once a day.

Methylxanthines

DESCRIPTION

Xanthine is a purine base that can be found in both plants and animals. Methylxanthine is a methylated derivative of xanthine. A class of drug that has been around for a very long time, methylxanthines are administered orally but can have significant toxicities.

PROTOTYPE AND COMMON DRUGS

■ Prototype: Theophylline
■ Others: Aminophylline, caffeine

MOA (MECHANISM OF ACTION)

■ The mechanism of action of methylxanthines is not completely understood. There are three theories on how they work:
1. Inhibition of phosphodiesterase (PDE), the enzyme that degrades cAMP. Increased concentrations of cAMP cause bronchodilation.
2. Inhibition of the release of intracellular calcium, thereby decreasing smooth muscle contraction (bronchoconstriction)

3. Competitive antagonism of adenosine on the adenosine receptor

PHARMACOKINETICS
- Theophylline has a narrow therapeutic index.
- Many factors alter the rate of absorption of theophylline. Therefore serum levels can be difficult to predict. Toxicity may occur unexpectedly.

INDICATIONS
- As a second- or third-line drug for asthma and COPD
- Neonatal apnea (this is *not* the same as obstructive sleep apnea)

CONTRAINDICATION
- Active or symptomatic coronary heart disease is a contraindication. Methylxanthines increase cAMP, which will increase cardiac inotropy. Furthermore, the heart rate will be increased. Both these factors will impair the oxygen supply-demand ratio to the myocardium.

SIDE EFFECTS
- Side effects are common because of the unpredictability of serum levels and the narrow therapeutic index.
- **GI**: nausea, vomiting
- **Central nervous system (CNS)**: headache
- **Stimulatory effects**: insomnia, tremor, seizures, restlessness
- **Cardiovascular system (CVS)**: irregular heartbeat

EVIDENCE
Theophylline versus Long-Acting β Agonists for *Chronic Stable* Asthma
- A Cochrane review in 2007 (13 studies, N = 1344 patients) found that theophylline and LABAs are equally effective in improving symptoms and lung function (predicted FEV_1) in stable **asthma**. However, there are more side effects with theophylline (relative risk [RR], 2.27).

Theophylline versus Placebo for *Stable* COPD
- A Cochrane review in 2002 (20 studies, N = 873 patients) found that in patients with stable COPD, compared with placebo, theophylline caused a small increase of FEV_1 (weighted mean difference [WMD] 100 mL) and forced vital capacity (FVC) (WMD 195 mL/min) and slightly improved O_2 and CO_2 levels. There were no differences for the following endpoints: distance walked (exercise test), symptoms of breathlessness or wheeze, exacerbations, or dropouts. Patients who were surveyed preferred theophylline over placebo. All patients were receiving other medications for COPD in both the placebo and treatment arms.

Theophylline versus Placebo for Treatment of COPD *Exacerbations*
- A Cochrane review in 2003 (4 studies, N = 169 patients) found that the change in FEV_1 at 2 hours was similar in both groups but transiently increased with methylxanthines at 3 days (WMD 101 mL). Data on clinical outcomes were sparse. Trends toward improvements in hospitalization and length-of-stay were offset by a trend toward more relapses at 1 week. Changes in symptom scores were not significant. Methylxanthines caused more nausea and vomiting than placebo (OR 4.6) and trended toward more frequent tremor, palpitations, and arrhythmias.

FYI
- If you add a methyl (CH_3) group to xanthine, you get a methylxanthine. If you add a CH_3 group to theophylline, you get caffeine. The similarity to caffeine may explain the stimulatory side effects.
- Aminophylline is a combination mixture of theophylline and ethylenediamine (two amine groups connect by two carbons). It simply dissociates in the body to theophylline.

Inhaled Corticosteroids

DESCRIPTION
Inhaled corticosteroids (ICSs) are synthetically derived compounds based on cortisol, a steroid produced in the adrenal cortex. These compounds are also known as *glucocorticoids*.

PROTOTYPE AND COMMON DRUGS
- Prototype: budesonide
- Others: beclomethas**one**, triamcinol**one**, fluticas**one**

MOA (MECHANISM OF ACTION)
- Overall, steroids have a broad **antiinflammatory** effect. This counteracts the airway inflammation characteristic in asthma. A variety of mechanisms are believed to contribute to the antiinflammatory effects of corticosteroids:
  - ▲ Increased blood neutrophil counts: increase marrow release and decrease tissue margination
  - ▲ Decreased numbers of other white blood cells: lymphocytes, eosinophils, and macrophages

▲ Reduced function of lymphocytes and macrophages

▲ Reduced function of phospholipase A_2, resulting in reduced mediators of inflammation: prostaglandins (PGs) and leukotrienes (LTs)

■ Steroids exert their actions in a broad range of tissues, and therefore there are many effects of glucocorticoids.

■ Steroids also have a number of other effects, many of which are not beneficial but contribute to many of the harmful effects of these agents. Fortunately, the harmful effects are mitigated by the **minimal systemic absorption** associated with the inhalational route.

▲ Catabolism:

  • **Increased serum glucose:** increased gluconeogenesis, increased lipolysis, decreased uptake of glucose into tissues, and direct inhibition of insulin via cortisone (breakdown product of cortisol)

  • Mobilization of calcium from bones

  • Increased breakdown of muscle to liberate amino acids

▲ Antimitotic (decreased cell division)

▲ Water retention (because of mineralocorticoid effect)

■ Chronic ICS use may up-regulate β_2 receptors; β_2 receptors mediate bronchodilation.

PHARMACOKINETICS

■ Steroids are highly lipophilic: therefore they enter cells easily.

■ Available in a variety of delivery systems: aerosol, dry powder, and liquid (for nebulizers)

INDICATIONS

■ Asthma:

▲ To provide long-term control by reducing frequency and severity of exacerbations

▲ To enable less frequent use of bronchodilators

■ Chronic Obstructive Pulmonary Disease (COPD)

CONTRAINDICATIONS

■ No major contraindications

SIDE EFFECTS

■ Systemic side effects are uncommon because of low systemic absorption and low bioavailability

■ **Oral candidiasis** *(thrush)* occurs secondary to local immunosuppression.

■ **Dysphonia (hoarseness)** is a direct local effect on vocal chords.

■ **Sore throat** may occur.

■ At higher doses, side effects associated with systemic corticosteroids may develop, most notably **osteoporosis.** This is rare with inhaled steroids.

IMPORTANT NOTES

■ ICSs are typically used in combination with inhaled beta agonists, as these bronchodilators help to open the airways and facilitate deposition of the steroid.

■ Because of their potential for extensive systemic side effects, the use of systemic corticosteroids such as prednisone is typically reserved for severe asthma, preferably administered over short courses.

EVIDENCE

Long-Acting β_2 Agonists with or without ICSs in Adults or Children with Asthma

■ A 2007 Cochrane review (67 studies, N = 42,333 participants) examined the use of LABAs (salmeterol, 50 studies; formoterol, 17 studies) versus placebo. In these studies, patients were followed for 4 to 52 weeks. Patients were allowed to combine ICSs with LABA in 40 studies, whereas 24 studies did not permit ICS and three studies were unclear about ICS use. Use of LABAs with or without ICSs was associated with improvements in pulmonary function, symptoms, rescue medication use, and quality-of-life scores.

ICSs versus Nonsteroid Inhaled Therapy for Treatment of COPD

■ A 2008 systematic review (11 trials, N = 14,426 patients) compared ICS therapy for ≥6 months with nonsteroid inhaled therapy in patients with COPD. There was no difference in all-cause mortality, and a higher incidence of pneumonia was found with ICSs (RR 1.34).

FYI

■ The chronic use of corticosteroids in children has been a cause for concern owing to the growth-retarding effects of these agents. Determination of a causal relationship between chronic inhaled steroid use and stunted growth is complicated by the fact that asthma itself may also slow growth and development in children.

■ Nasally administered corticosteroids are used for chronic inflammatory problems of the nasal passages and sinuses.

Phosphodiesterase-5 Inhibitors

DESCRIPTION
Phosphodiesterase-5 (PDE5) inhibitors are vasodilators.

PROTOTYPE AND COMMON DRUGS
- Sildenafil
- Others: tadalafil, vardenafil, mirodenafil, udenafil

MOA (MECHANISM OF ACTION)
- PDE breaks down intracellular cyclic adenine monophosphate (cAMP) and cyclic guanosine monophosphate (cGMP).
- PDE inhibitors therefore result in **increased intracellular cAMP and cGMP.** The cell or tissue type affected will dictate the effect of the PDE inhibitor. Furthermore, different PDE subtypes have different selectivity for cAMP and cGMP. This is important because the two clinically important PDE inhibitors (types 3 and 5) are quite different from each other.
- PDE5 is distributed in the body primarily in vascular smooth muscle; thus, its effects primarily influence vascular tone.
- PDE5 is more selective for intracellular cGMP. cGMP interacts with nitric oxide (NO):
  - ▲ NO increases the conversion of guanosine triphosphate (GTP) to cGMP.
  - ▲ cGMP acts on protein kinases, specifically protein kinase G (PKG).
  - ▲ PKG acts on a variety of sites; the net effect is to lower intracellular Ca^{2+}, which results in uncoupling of actin and myosin, leading to smooth muscle relaxation and ultimately vasodilation (Figure 24-4).

Erectile Dysfunction
- Erections occur because the two corpora cavernosa and the single corpus spongiosum become filled with blood and then, under pressure, increase in size and impart resistance to bending. Filling the three corpora requires arterial vasodilation to increase blood flow.
- As the arterial vessels dilate, the corpora enlarge and become pressurized.

Pulmonary Hypertension
- *Pulmonary hypertension* refers to increased blood pressure in the pulmonary arterial system. There are many different causes, but a common component across many different causes is abnormally increased pulmonary vasoconstriction. Remember that blood pressure is proportional to resistance, and resistance to flow is greatly influenced by vascular tone.
- PDE5 inhibitors cause vasodilation in the pulmonary vessels and through this mechanism reduce pulmonary blood pressure.

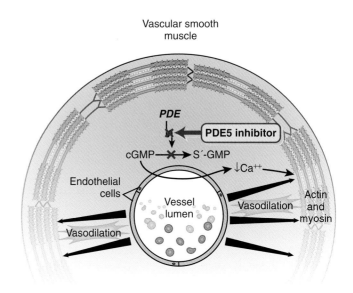

Figure 24-4.

TABLE 24-2. Onset and Elimination Half-Life of PDE-5 Inhibitors		
Drug	**Peak of Onset**	**Half-Life**
Sildenafil	60 minutes	4 hours
Vardenafil	60 minutes	4.7 hours
Tadalafil	120 minutes	17.5 hours

PHARMACOKINETICS
- Each of the drugs in this class have different onset times and half-lives and thus different durations of action (Table 24-2).
- Because PDE5 inhibitors are hepatically metabolized and eliminated by the kidney, they can accumulate and result in overdose when given to patients with renal dysfunction. This manifests as excessive vasodilation and hypotension.

INDICATIONS
- Erectile dysfunction
- Pulmonary hypertension

CONTRAINDICATIONS
- Renal failure is a relative contraindication because the steady state plasma levels can become dangerously elevated

when the drugs are administered by intravenous infusion for pulmonary hypertension.

- Nitroglycerin coadministration can cause severe and difficult-to-treat hypotension. **Coadministration of nitroglycerin is absolutely contraindicated.**

SIDE EFFECTS

- **Vasodilation** directly causes the following side effects:
  - ▲ Flushing
  - ▲ Headache
  - ▲ Hypotension
    - Presyncope (almost fainting) and syncope (fainting)
    - MI from decreased blood flow to the myocardium
    - Stroke from decreased blood flow to the brain
- **Priapism** (prolonged erection) can result in tissue *ischemia* of the penis. If an erection becomes painful or lasts for >2 hours, *emergency* medical attention should be obtained immediately.
- **Sudden hearing loss:** The mechanism of injury for this side effect has not yet been established. It is usually unilateral and can be reversible. Associated **vertigo** has also been documented.
- **Visual loss:** Nonarteritic anterior ischemic optic neuropathy (NAION) is a very rare condition that might be associated with increased risk.

IMPORTANT NOTES

- Coadministration of nitrates to patients with angina in the emergency room can result in **profound refractory hypotension.** Patients may not be completely forthcoming about the use of medications for erectile dysfunction, and therefore the risks of coadministration (if nitrates are about to be given) must be carefully explained to male patients.

Advanced

- PDE3 breaks down both cAMP and cGMP. The subtype of PDE determines the ratio of activity against cAMP versus cGMP. PDE3 preferentially acts on cAMP 10 times more than it does cGMP. The changes in cAMP and cGMP in different cells dictate the clinical effects seen in either the heart or the vasculature.
- PDEs are a superfamily. There are 11 subtypes. Currently, the other PDE inhibitor in clinical use is PDE3 (an example is milrinone), used in acute heart failure.

EVIDENCE
Erectile Dysfunction

- A systematic review in 2009 of 116 RCTs found that successful intercourse attempts were improved to 69% with sildenafil versus placebo (35%), with very similar findings for tadalafil, vardenafil, mirodenafil, and udenafil. Men with *severe* erectile dysfunction obtained more benefit than men with *mild* erectile dysfunction. Men with specific medical conditions (e.g., depression, diabetes, cardiovascular disease, prostate cancer) were also more likely to obtain benefit. Side effects, most commonly headache, flushing, rhinitis, and dyspepsia, were significantly more frequent. Risk of serious cardiovascular events was 0.2% to 0.5% with PDE5 inhibitors and 0.1% to 0.2% with placebo.

FYI

- Although popularized for the treatment of erectile dysfunction, PDE5 drugs were originally designed to treat pulmonary hypertension; a certain side effect led to the discovery of their more widely known use.
- Caffeine is a weak, nonspecific PDE inhibitor. This results in increased heart rate and, paradoxically (compared with PDE5 inhibitors), vasoconstriction.
- Theophylline, used in airway disease, is also a PDE inhibitor (see also the discussion of xanthines)

Endothelin Receptor Antagonists

DESCRIPTION
Endothelin (ET) receptor antagonists (ETRAs) are a class of agents related by their ability to antagonize ET receptors and dilate blood vessels.

PROTOTYPE AND COMMON DRUGS
Nonselective (ET$_A$ and ET$_B$)

- Prototype: Bo**sentan**
- Others: tezo**sentan**

Selective (ETA)

- Prototype: Sitax**sentan**
- Others: ambri**sentan**

MOA (MECHANISM OF ACTION)

- There are three isoforms of ET (ET-1, ET-2, ET-3) in humans, and two different receptors (ET$_A$ and ET$_B$). The ET-1 isoform is the focus of current drug development.
- ET-1 is activated by a family of ET-converting enzymes within vascular endothelial cells.

- ET_A receptors are found mainly on vascular **smooth muscle cells,** whereas ET_B receptors are found on vascular **endothelial cells** and to a lesser extent on smooth muscle cells.
- ET_A and ET_B are both G protein–coupled receptors. Binding of ET-1 to the ET_A or ET_B receptor on vascular smooth muscle cells leads to vasoconstriction, whereas binding to ET_B receptors on endothelial cells leads to release of nitric oxide, which then acts on vascular smooth muscle cells to induce a transient vasodilation (Figure 24-5).

Endothelin receptor antagonists

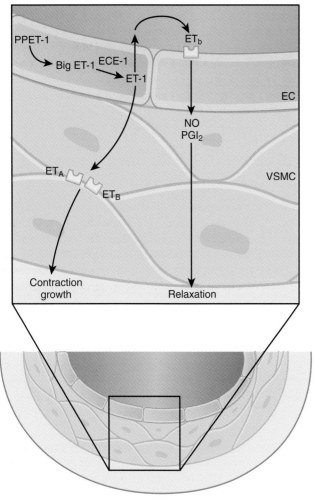

Figure 24-5.

- The vascular actions of ET_B receptors on smooth muscle (constriction) and endothelial cells (dilation) therefore oppose each other, meaning that the relative distribution of these receptors within a regional vascular bed will determine the response to nonselective ET antagonists.
- It is therefore believed that ET_A **selective antagonists may have greater ability to dilate blood vessels** than nonselective antagonists. However, the clinical impact of selective versus nonselective ET receptor antagonism has yet to be established in well-designed clinical trials.
- ET-1 also has several other effects, most notably in the kidney, and could play a potential role in promoting cell growth and remodeling and in carcinogenesis. Several cells in the kidney release ET-1, and the ET_B receptor appears to mediate both **natriuresis and diuresis.**

PHARMACOKINETICS
- These agents are metabolized by the liver.

INDICATIONS
- Pulmonary hypertension
- Essential hypertension

CONTRAINDICATIONS
- **Pregnancy:** ETs appear to play a role in the development of the embryo.
- **Liver impairment:** See Side Effects.

SIDE EFFECTS
- **Vasodilation,** resulting in the following effects:
  - ▲ Headache
  - ▲ Dizziness
  - ▲ Peripheral edema
  - ▲ Nasal congestion
  - ▲ Hypotension

Serious
- **Liver injury:** A reversible, asymptomatic increase in liver enzymes can progress to liver failure and death if the drug is not discontinued or the dose adjusted. This is thought to result from impaired transport and subsequent accumulation of toxic bile salts in hepatocytes. For a serious disorder this occurs relatively frequently; therefore liver enzymes should be monitored during therapy.

IMPORTANT NOTES
- ET is considered to be the most potent vasoconstrictor found in the human body, and therefore ET antagonists were thought to have great potential as leading antihypertensive agents. However, their major role has been seen in pulmonary hypertension, and they have not gained widespread use in hypertension.
- Given their propensity to cause liver injury, the future role of ETRAs in hypertension may be in treatment-resistant patients or in specific forms of hypertension that may benefit from ET antagonism.
- Patients with various forms of pulmonary hypertension, especially idiopathic, tend to have higher-than-normal ET-1 levels. This is the rationale for their use and success in the management of pulmonary hypertension.
- ETRAs are being investigated in a variety of other disorders in which remodeling and/or vasoconstriction play a role, including connective tissue disorders, Raynaud's disease, heart failure, erectile dysfunction, and various disorders of cerebral vasoconstriction.

Advanced
- ET_A has 10 times more binding affinity than does ET_B for ET-1.

- ET receptors are also located in the following organs: lung, heart, kidney, intestine, and adrenal gland. The receptors are especially dense in the heart and lungs.

Drug Interactions
- Bosentan is metabolized by hepatic CYP3A4 and CYP2C9 and is an inducer of both of these enzymes.

EVIDENCE
For Pulmonary Hypertension
- A 2009 Cochrane review (11 studies, N = 1457 participants) found that ETRAs (bosentan, sitaxsentan) did not improve mortality but did improve other measurements of pulmonary hypertension, including exercise capacity (improvement of 33.7 m on the 6-minute walk test), New York Heart Association/World Health Organization (NYHA/WHO) functional class, and dyspnea, as well as some measures of cardiopulmonary hemodynamics. These efficacy findings were largely in an idiopathic PH population. Hepatotoxicity was an uncommon side effect.

FYI
- The asp and scorpion venom toxins (sarafotoxins) are of the ET agonist family.
- The plasma half-life of ET-1 is 4 to 7 minutes.
- The ETRAs are unusually expensive for small molecule drugs (i.e., nonbiologics), typically priced at over $100 per day. Their high price may result in part from the fact that they are primarily used to treat a rare condition, pulmonary hypertension.
- Given that ET was just discovered in 1988, the development and approval of ETRAs such as bosentan (2001) occurred remarkably fast.

Vascular Prostaglandins

DESCRIPTION
Prostaglandins (PGs) are involved with many processes in the body; this section discusses cardiovascular uses of PGs.

PROTOTYPES AND COMMON DRUGS
PGI$_2$, Prostacyclin
- Prototype: Epo**prost**enol
- Others: Ilo**prost**, bera**prost**, t**prost**inil

PGE$_1$
- Prototype: Al**prost**adil

MOA (MECHANISM OF ACTION)
- PGs act on a family of receptors that are coupled to G proteins. Some G proteins are stimulatory, and some are inhibitory, depending on the specific receptor type; therefore, the physiologic effect of a given PG depends on the receptor and the tissue type.
- Prostacyclin (PGI$_2$) and its analogues are potent vasodilators and possess antithrombotic and antiproliferative properties.
- PGI$_2$ receptors are called *IP receptors*, and PGE receptors are called *EP receptors*.
- The endothelial cells are the major source of prostacyclin production. Therefore, endogenous prostacyclins are well positioned to exert their effects on blood cells, endothelial cells, and vascular smooth muscle cells.

Vasodilation
- The PGI receptor is expressed in endothelial cells, smooth muscle cells, leukocytes, and thrombocytes and is coupled with G$_s$ proteins, which then activate adenylate cyclase, leading to increased **cAMP**, which activates protein kinase A (PKA), finally leading to vasodilation (Figure 24-6).
- Prostacyclin also couples with G$_q$ proteins and activates vasoconstrictive pathways under certain circumstances in certain tissues, but this effect is overshadowed by the vasodilator effects.

Antiproliferation
- Endothelial damage, monocytes, fibroblasts, and the coagulation system all contribute to vascular fibrosis. Iloprost has been shown to inhibit the messenger RNA (mRNA) expression of important mediators of these processes, thereby demonstrating antiproliferative effects.
- Prostacyclin also activates peroxisome proliferator–activated receptors (PPARs) that are located in the **nucleus.** PPARs activate the apoptosis pathway, leading to accelerated programmed cell death.

Antiplatelet
- On the platelet, cyclooxygenase (COX)-1 catalyzes the prothrombotic mediator thromboxane, and COX-2 catalyzes the formation of prostacyclin, which is an antiaggregating agent.
- Prostacyclin increases intracellular cAMP in the platelet; thromboxane decreases cAMP.
- Manipulating the balance of thromboxane and prostacyclin in favor of prostacyclin results in an antiplatelet effect.

Pulmonary Hypertension
- Pulmonary hypertension is associated with vasoconstriction, thrombosis, and cellular proliferation. The three

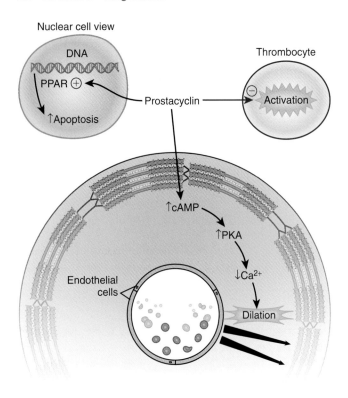

Figure 24-6.

actions of prostacyclins (vasodilation, antiproliferation, and antiplatelet) all potentially provide benefit to patients with pulmonary hypertension.

PHARMACOKINETICS

■ Routes of administration and half-lives are listed in Table 24-3.

■ A very important benefit of a drug with a short half-life, such as epoprostenol, is that when it is administered by intravenous infusion into the right side of the heart, the pulmonary circulation receives the highest dose of drug and the systemic circulation receives a lower exposure, reducing the probability of systemic side effects.

■ Furthermore, about 95% is inactivated after one circulation through the pulmonary circulation via enzymes that are specific for PGs.

INDICATIONS

■ **Pulmonary hypertension**: Prostacyclin is one of a few vasodilator treatments available.

■ Severe hypoxia with adult respiratory distress syndrome (**ARDS**): When inhaled, prostacyclin can selectively cause vasodilation of vessels that are adjacent to the few functioning alveoli (this is where the drug actually reaches the circulation) and helps to improve ventilation-perfusion matching.

Alprostadil Only

■ **Erectile dysfunction**: Although now usually treated with a PDE5 inhibitor, PGs can also be used for their vasodilation properties to treat erectile dysfunction.

■ Alprostadil can be used to maintain patency of the ductus arteriosus in a newborn who has a **duct-dependent congenital cardiac anomaly**.

CONTRAINDICATIONS

■ None of clinical significance

SIDE EFFECTS

■ Vasodilation:
  ▲ Flushing, headache, hypotension
■ Nausea and diarrhea

IMPORTANT NOTES

■ Pulmonary hypertension is a progressive disease. The right ventricle is not nearly as strong as the left ventricle, and its ability to work against high resistance is very limited. As the pulmonary resistance and pressures increase through progressive vasoconstriction and endothelial thickening and fibrosis, the right ventricle becomes less able to provide adequate cardiac output to the lungs.
  ▲ ET antagonists and PDE5 inhibitors are other vasodilators used in treatment of pulmonary hypertension.

■ Epoprostenol and iloprost, when administered long term, require an **implanted central venous catheter** (surgically placed, it goes into the right atrium via the subclavian or internal jugular vein) and a battery-powered infusion pump. Complications include catheter infections and pump problems; in addition, the route of administration requires much

TABLE 24-3. Pharmacokinetics of Prostaglandin Analogues Used in Pulmonary Hypertension			
Drug	**Route of Administration**	**Half-Life**	**Comments**
Epoprostenol	Intravenous (IV)	3-5 min	Permanent central IV catheter required
Iloprost	IV, inhaled	30 min	Permanent central IV catheter required
Beraprost	Oral	30 min	Four-times-a-day administration
Treprostinil	IV, subcutaneous	4.5 hours	Intermittent subcutaneous injections

more effort and maintenance than intermittent administration (subcutaneously or oral).

▲ Beraprost is orally administered. Treprostinil has a longer half-life and can be administered subcutaneously a few times a day. Neither of these drugs requires an infusion pump, so administration is much easier.

▲ In critically ill patients, the intravenous administration is more controlled and therefore preferred: doses can be quickly titrated according to the response of the patient.

■ **Effects on the airways** are different depending on the type of PG:

▲ PGI_2, PGE: bronchodilation

▲ $PGF_{2\alpha}$ (and thromboxane): bronchoconstriction

Advanced

■ Duct-dependent congenital cardiac abnormalities require an open communication (the ductus arteriosus) from the aorta to the pulmonary artery to allow flow between the pulmonary circulation and systemic circulation. Closure of the ductus in these patients (before urgent corrective surgery) is not compatible with life. One example is pulmonary atresia, a condition in which the pulmonary valve does not form and so there is no connection from the right ventricle to the pulmonary circulation; the only alternate route to the lungs is from the aorta through the ductus. Of course, some blood also continues down the aorta into the systemic circulation. Closure of the ductus would result in complete loss of blood flow to the lungs and death within minutes.

▲ In babies with a normal heart but persistently patent (open) ductus arteriosus (PDA), a **nonsteroidal antiinflammatory** (usually indomethacin) is given to inhibit endogenous PG–induced vasodilation of the ductus and increase the probability of spontaneous closure of the ductus.

EVIDENCE
Pulmonary Hypertension

■ A Cochrane meta-analysis in 2006 looked at the following:

▲ **Intravenous prostacyclin versus usual care** (3 studies, 101 patients): There were significant improvements in walking exercise capacity, cardiopulmonary hemodynamics, and NYHA functional class over a range of 3 days to 12 weeks.

▲ **Oral prostacyclin versus placebo** (two studies): Short-term data (3 to 6 months) indicated that there was a significant improvement in exercise capacity, but data from one study of 52 weeks reported no significant difference at 12 months. No significant differences were observed for any other outcome.

▲ **Subcutaneous treprostinil versus placebo** (two studies): One large study reported a significant median improve-

ment in exercise capacity of around 16 meters (over 8 to 12 weeks). Cardiopulmonary hemodynamics and symptom scores favored treprostinil. Infusion site pain and withdrawals because of adverse events were more frequent with treprostinil.

▲ **Inhaled prostacyclin versus placebo** (one study): There was a small but statistically significant increase in walking exercise capacity in patients treated with inhaled prostacyclin. Treatment led to better symptom scores and functional class status than with placebo. Side effects and adverse events were common in the studies.

FYI

■ In 1934 Dr. Ulf von Euler found that extracts of sheep vesicular gland dramatically lowered blood pressure when injected into animals. Human seminal fluid also seemed to possess similar qualities. Von Euler named it *prostaglandin*, believing that it originated in the prostate gland.

■ Nomenclature:

▲ *Eicosa* is Greek for 20. Eicosanoids have 20 carbon atoms. Eicosanoids include PGs, prostacyclins, LTs, and thromboxane. Arachidonic acid is the most abundant precursor.

▲ The letter after *PG* is a historical designation:

• Ether and phosphate buffer were first used to separate PGs in Sweden; the PGs that partitioned into ether were called *PGE*, and those in phosphate (spelled *fosfat* in Swedish) were called *PGF*.

• A further test, using acid and base, gave rise to *PGA* and *PGB*.

• The other letters have no significance and were simply filled in.

▲ The subscripted number refers to the number of double bonds (C=C).

• PGE_1 has a double bond at C5; PGE_3 has double bonds at C5, C13, and C17.

▲ The α or β designates the orientation (pointing in front of the molecule or pointing behind) of the second hydroxyl (-OH) group on the ring. Most PGs have only a single hydroxyl group on the ring; PGF has two.

• $PGF_{2\alpha}$ therefore was fractionated into phosphate, has two double bonds, and has a second hydroxyl group that is oriented behind the ring.

• Other uses of PGs include obstetric uses (see the discussion of reproductive prostaglandins in Chapter 14), ophthalmologic uses (see the discussion of ophthalmic prostaglandins in Chapter 22), and use as gastric protectants (see the discussion of gastrointestinal cytoprotectants in Chapter 15).

• COX-2 selective inhibitors have been associated with an increased rate of MI from thrombosis attributed to the balance of thromboxane over prostacyclin, making the platelets more likely to aggregate and become activated.

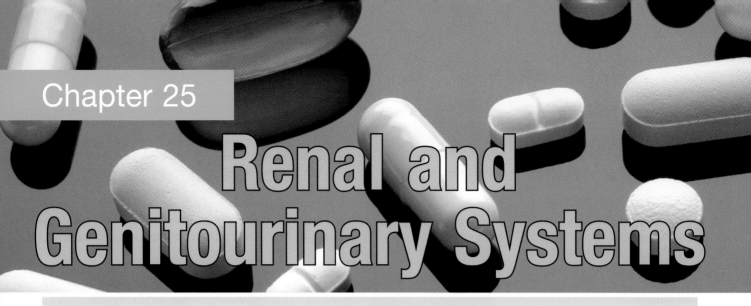

Chapter 25

Renal and Genitourinary Systems

Thiazide Diuretics

DESCRIPTION
Diuretics result in increased urine production and also lower blood pressure.

PROTOTYPE AND COMMON DRUGS
- Prototype: hydrochloro**thiazide**
- Others: chloro**thiazide**, chlorthalidone

MOA (MECHANISM OF ACTION)
- Generally speaking, diuretics manipulate a solute (usually Na^+), and water passively follows.
  - ▲ ↓ Na^+ reabsorbed in kidney → ↑ Na^+ lost in urine → ↑ water lost in urine
- Specifically, thiazide diuretics inhibit the **Na^+/Cl^- co-transporter channel** in the *distal tubule* of the nephron (Figure 25-1).
- Therefore Na^+, Cl^- (and water) remain in the lumen of the tubule: **natriuresis and diuresis**. In addition, the actions of the thiazides impact other ions.
- A passive **Na^+/H^+ exchange** occurs at a distal site in the tubule. Na^+ gradients drive this exchange. When the Na^+/Cl^- cotransporter is blocked, the Na^+ concentration in the lumen of the tubule is high, which facilitates Na^+ reabsorption in exchange for **excretion of H^+ ions** at this distal site. Therefore thiazides create alkalosis by H^+ ion loss through a secondary, passive exchange.
- Similarly, Na^+ is exchanged for K^+ at a distal site in the tubule. By enhancing delivery of Na^+ to distal sites of the nephron, Na^+ is exchanged for K^+, leading to **enhanced K^+ excretion**, in a similar manner to the K^+ depletion that occurs with loop diuretics.
- Thiazides also promote Ca^{+2} reabsorption through a poorly understood mechanism.
- Owing to the fact they act so distally in the nephron, after much of the Na^+ reabsorption has already occurred, thiazides are relatively weak diuretics when compared with loop diuretics.

Thiazide diuretics

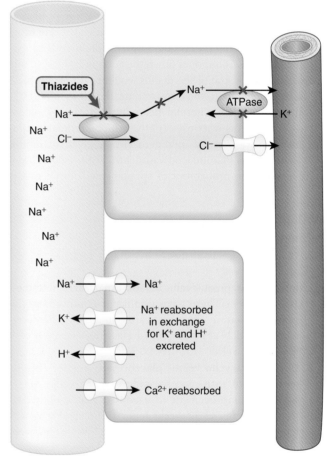

Figure 25-1.

- Thiazides are also vasodilators, an effect independent of their diuretic actions. Their antihypertensive effect is probably related mainly to this mechanism and not the diuretic mechanism.
- Effect on plasma ion concentrations:

▲ Decreased Na^+, Cl^-, K^+, Mg^{+2}

▲ Increased Ca^{+2}

▲ Increased HCO_3^-. (This creates a metabolic alkalosis.) This is a result of H^+ ion loss. Remember that the equation will shift left with a loss of H^+:

$$H^+ + HCO_3^- \rightleftharpoons H_2O + CO_2$$

PHARMACOKINETICS

■ Thiazide diuretics exert their pharmacologic actions from the luminal side; therefore they must be in the lumen of the tubule to achieve their effect.

■ Thiazides primarily enter the renal tubule through secretion in the proximal tubule (PT) via the organic acid co-transporter. In patients with renal impairment, higher doses of thiazides may be required to overcome impaired tubular secretion and maintain sufficient tubular concentrations to achieve a pharmacologic effect.

■ Most thiazides become ineffective once creatinine clearance gets too low (typically <30 to 50 mL/min).

INDICATIONS

■ First-line treatment for hypertension
■ Edema
■ Nephrogenic diabetes insipidus (DI) (rare)

CONTRAINDICATION

■ **Sulfa allergy:** Thiazide diuretics should be used with extreme caution (or not at all) in patients reporting hypersensitivity reactions to sulfa-containing drugs.

SIDE EFFECTS

■ Dehydration and decreased Na^+ occur.

■ **Hypokalemia or hypokalemic metabolic alkalosis:** Thiazide diuretics enhance excretion of both K^+ and H^+ because of increased distal tubule delivery of Na^+, and hence Na^+ reabsorption, in the distal nephron.

■ **Impaired glucose tolerance** is caused by impaired insulin release and diminished use of glucose.

■ **Hyperlipidemia:** Thiazide diuretics increase cholesterol and low-density lipoprotein (LDL); the mechanism has not been established.

■ **Hyperuricemia:** Thiazides compete with uric acid for secretion into the PT, reducing the excretion of uric acid. This can lead to attacks of gout.

■ **Impotency (rare)** is likely a result of reduced volume.

■ Renal dysfunction (increased serum creatinine) may occur secondary to hypovolemia and reduced blood pressure. This is typically only seen in patients with already reduced GFR.

IMPORTANT NOTES

■ Diuretics that act on the renal tubules require functioning kidneys to exert their effects. Patients with advanced renal dysfunction will not respond to these diuretics.

■ As noted, thiazides are weaker diuretics than loop diuretics (such as furosemide). This is because they act at a site distal to where loop diuretics act. The loop of Henle is positioned before the distal convoluted tubule, and 90% of Na^+ will have already been reabsorbed before the ultrafiltrate reaches the distal tubule.

■ Thiazides have what would appear to be a paradoxical role in the treatment of nephrogenic DI. Although the mechanism has not been confirmed, their efficacy likely stems from their ability to reduce intravascular volume, in turn stimulating Na^+ reabsorption and reducing the amount of fluid presented to the distal segments of the nephron.

■ By enhancing reabsorption of calcium and subsequent reduction in urinary calcium concentration, thiazides can be used to reduce formation of calcium-containing renal stones.

■ Hydrochlorothiazide has a relatively flat dose-response curve, and the effective dose range is 12.5 mg to 50 mg. Doses above 50 mg will only increase the incidence of side effects, without contributing to efficacy.

Advanced

■ Concomitant administration of thiazides with antiarrhythmic agents that prolong the QT interval (e.g., quinidine, sotalol) may predispose to *torsades de pointes*. The mechanism is unknown but may be related to hypokalemia induced by the thiazide.

EVIDENCE
As First-Line Agents in Hypertension

■ A 2009 Cochrane review (24 trials, N = 58,040 participants) compared benefits and harms of first-line antihypertensives with those of placebo or no treatment over a minimum of 1 year. Thiazides (19 trials) reduced mortality (relative risk [RR] 0.89), stroke (RR 0.63), and coronary heart disease (RR 0.84) versus placebo.

FYI

■ It is believed that thiazides also exert weak diuretic effects at the PT. Some thiazides inhibit carbonic anhydrase (CA) at this site, perhaps accounting for their diuretic effect at the PT.

■ Thiazides were derived from the CA inhibitor acetazolamide. It is therefore not surprising that some thiazides inhibit Na^+ reabsorption at the PT.

Loop Diuretics

DESCRIPTION

Diuretics result in increased urine production and also lower blood pressure.

PROTOTYPE AND COMMON DRUGS

- Prototype: furosemide
- Others: ethacrynic acid, torsemide, bumetanide

MOA (MECHANISM OF ACTION)

- Generally speaking, diuretics manipulate a solute (usually Na^+), and water passively follows:
  - ▲ ↓ Na^+ reabsorbed in kidney → ↑ Na^+ lost in urine → ↑ water lost in urine
- Loop diuretics inhibit the $Na^+/K^+/2Cl^-$ **co-transporter channel** in the *thick ascending limb (Henle's loop)* of the renal tubule. This results in less Na^+ being reabsorbed back into the body. Cl^- and K^+ also move in the same direction through this ion channel, as does Na^+ (Figure 25-2).

Loop diuretics

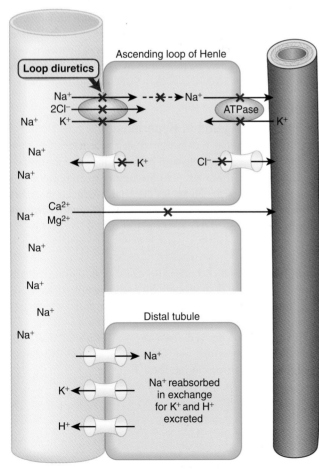

Figure 25-2.

- Therefore Na^+, Cl^-, **and** K^+ **are lost** in the urine: Natriuresis and diuresis. Blockade of the $Na^+/K^+/2Cl^-$ cotransporter has effects on other ions as well.
- Normally, the K^+ channel on the luminal membrane (cell membrane adjacent to the tubular lumen) and the Cl^- channel on the basolateral membrane (cell membrane opposite the tubular lumen) creates a potential difference between the tubular lumen (positive) and the interstitium (negative). Blockade of the $Na^+/K^+/2Cl^-$ cotransporter interferes with the ability of these channels to create this positive to negative gradient.
- Disruption of this electrochemical gradient facilitates excretion of Ca^{+2} and Mg^{+2}. Normally these divalent cations undergo paracellular reabsorption, repelled by the positively charged tubular lumen and attracted to the negatively charged interstitium. Attenuation of the positive to negative gradient reduces paracellular reabsorption of Ca^{+2} and Mg^{+2}, and they are excreted.
- A passive Na^+/H^+ **exchanger** is present at a distal site in the tubule. Na^+ gradients drive this exchange. When the $Na^+/K^+/2Cl^-$ channel is blocked, the Na^+ concentration in the lumen of the tubule is high, which facilitates the reabsorption of Na^+ and **excretion of** H^+ at this distal site. Therefore furosemide creates alkalosis by H^+ ion loss through a secondary, passive exchange.
- Similarly, by enhancing delivery of Na^+ to distal sites of the nephron, Na^+ is exchanged for K^+, leading to **enhanced** K^+ **excretion**, and this further depletes K^+.
- Like the thiazides, the loop diuretics are also believed to act as **vasodilators**, an effect independent of their diuretic actions. This may contribute to the anti-hypertensive effects of the loop diuretics.

Effect on Ions

- Decreased Na^+, K^+, Cl^-, Ca^{+2}, Mg^{+2}. Note the large number of cations excreted.
- Increased HCO_3^-. (This creates a metabolic alkalosis.) This is a result of H^+ ion loss. Remember that the equation will shift left with a loss of H^+:

$$H^+ + HCO_3^- \rightleftharpoons H_2O + CO_2$$

PHARMACOKINETICS

- Loop diuretics act on the apical (lumen) side of the tubule and therefore must be in the tubule in order to exert their effects.
- Most loop diuretics are bound extensively to plasma proteins, limiting delivery of these agents to the tubules by filtration. Therefore they rely on secretion by the organic acid transport system in the PT.

- The secretion of loop diuretics into the PT may be inhibited by agents that compete for weak acid secretion, such as nonsteroidal antiinflammatory drugs (NSAIDs) or probenecid.

INDICATIONS
- **Edema**
  - ▲ Heart failure
  - ▲ Nephrotic syndrome
  - ▲ Liver failure
- **Acute hypercalcemia**

CONTRAINDICATIONS
- Hypovolemia is a contraindication.
- Severe K^+ abnormalities are contraindications.
- **Sulfa allergy**: Furosemide, bumetanide, and torsemide may be cross-reactive in those who have an allergy to sulfonamides.

SIDE EFFECTS
- Dehydration may occur.
- **Hypokalemia** is caused by Na^+ reabsorption in exchange for K^+ excretion at the distal tubule.
- **Metabolic alkalosis** (increased HCO_3^-)
  - ▲ Increased exchange of Na^+ in the lumen for H^+ in the cell, resulting in H^+ loss.
  - ▲ Remember that $H_2O + CO_2 \rightleftharpoons H^+ + HCO_3^-$ and that decreased H^+ will drive the equation to the right and cause increased HCO_3^-.
- **Other electrolytes disturbances**: Given the large number of ions (Na^+, Cl^-, and so on) that are affected by these agents, electrolytes should be monitored.
- **Ototoxicity**: Reversible hearing loss occurs most often in those with reduced renal function or who are receiving other ototoxic agents such as aminoglycoside antibiotics. The mechanism has not been established, although the $Na^+/K^+/2Cl^-$ transporter is also found in the inner ear. High-dose furosemide can cause permanent **deafness**.
- **Hyperuricemia**: The reduction in volume induced by the potent actions of loops elicits a compensatory increase in uric acid reabsorption in the PT. Loop diuretics also compete with uric acid for secretion into the PT. Increased levels of uric acid may precipitate attacks of gout.

- Renal dysfunction (increased serum creatinine) may occur secondary to hypovolemia and reduced blood pressure. This is typically only seen when high doses are used in patients with already reduced GFR.

EVIDENCE
Diuretics versus Placebo or Other Interventions for Treatment of Heart Failure
- A 2006 Cochrane review (14 trials, N = 525 participants) compared diuretics with placebo (seven trials) and other interventions (seven trials) for treatment of heart failure. The diuretics included were a mixture of loop diuretics, potassium-sparing diuretics, and thiazides. Based on three trials (N = 202 participants), diuretic treatment reduced the odds of death versus placebo (OR 0.24), and in two trials (N = 169 participants) it reduced the odds of admission because of worsening heart failure (OR 0.07). Diuretics improved exercise capacity in four trials (N = 91 participants) versus active controls.

Blood-Pressure–Lowering Effect versus Placebo or No Treatment
- A 2009 Cochrane review (nine trials, N = 460 participants) compared the blood-pressure–lowering efficacy, tolerability, and biochemical effects of a variety of loop diuretics versus placebo or no treatment. The authors found a mean reduction (systolic/diastolic blood pressure) of −7.9/−4.4 mmHg and no differences between drugs in this class with respect to blood-pressure–lowering efficacy. This is considered to be a modest antihypertensive effect. Withdrawals because of adverse effects and biochemical changes were not significantly different from control.

IMPORTANT NOTES
- Diuretics that exert their effects by acting on the renal tubules require functioning kidneys to induce diuresis. Patients with advanced renal dysfunction will not respond to these diuretics.
- Loop diuretics are much stronger diuretics than thiazides. This is because they work in the loop of Henle, which is positioned before (proximal to) the distal convoluted tubule where the thiazides work.

Potassium-Sparing Diuretics

DESCRIPTION
Potassium-sparing diuretics are diuretics that result in increased urine production and also lower blood pressure while increasing serum levels of potassium.

PROTOTYPES AND COMMON DRUGS
Aldosterone Antagonist
- Prototypes: spironolact**one**
- Others: epleren**one**

Epithelial Na Channel (ENaC) Blockers

- Prototypes: Triamterene, amiloride

MOA (MECHANISM OF ACTION)

- Diuretics manipulate a solute (usually Na^+), and water passively follows:
  - ▲ ↓ Na^+ reabsorbed in kidney → ↑ Na^+ lost in urine → ↑ water lost in urine
- Thus most diuretics lead to enhanced Na^+ in the lumen of the tubule (i.e., the urine). High Na^+ concentrations in the tubule lead to a compensatory reabsorption of Na^+ in exchange for K^+ excretion in the distal nephron, leading to the hypokalemia associated with many diuretics.
- The goal of potassium-sparing diuretics is to prevent this reabsorption of Na^+ and subsequent loss of K^+ in the late distal tubule or collecting duct of the nephron.
- The exchange of Na^+ for K^+ in the distal nephron is mediated by the actions of the **epithelial Na^+ channel (ENaC)** on the luminal side of the membrane and the **Na^+/K^+-ATPase pump** on the basolateral membrane (side opposite the lumen of the tubule).
- The basolateral Na^+/K^+-ATPase pump creates a gradient for the entry of Na^+ into the cell from the ENaC on the luminal side of the membrane.
- The Na^+/K^+-ATPase pump actively pumps Na^+ out of the cell into the interstitium, in exchange for a K^+ ion.
  - ▲ The Na^+ that is lost from the cell is replaced by another Na^+ ion, which enters passively through ENaC.
  - ▲ The K^+ that entered the cell exits into the lumen of the tubule through a K^+ channel.
- The potassium-sparing diuretics inhibit this exchange of Na^+ for K^+ by inhibiting ENaC alone or both ENaC and the Na^+/K^+-ATPase pump.

Triamterene and Amiloride

- Amiloride and triamterene inhibit ENaC on the luminal membrane, preventing Na^+ from moving from the tubular lumen into the cell. This keeps Na^+ in the lumen of the tubule, therefore facilitating natriuresis.
- Reduced entry of Na^+ into the cell also reduces the amount of Na^+ that can be exchanged for K^+ at the ATPase pump. With the Na^+/K^+-ATPase pump unable to exchange Na^+ for K^+, the K^+ stays in the bloodstream.

Spironolactone and Eplerenone (Figure 25-3)

- **Spironolactone** and **eplerenone** directly antagonize aldosterone:
  - ▲ Normally, aldosterone binds to the **mineralocorticoid receptor** (MR).
  - ▲ The MR-aldosterone complex translocates to the nucleus, where it binds to specific DNA sequences to increase the number of ENaC channels and Na^+/K^+-ATPase pump.
  - ▲ Therefore, by blocking the MR, aldosterone antagonists inhibit the activity of ENaC and the Na^+/K^+-ATPase pump, reducing Na^+ reabsorption and producing mild natriuresis and diuresis.

Potassium-sparing diuretics

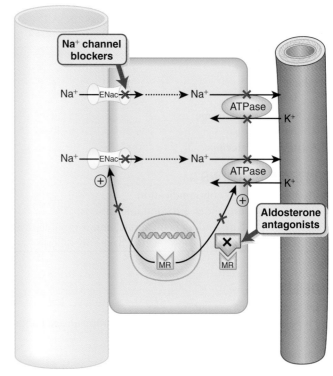

Figure 25-3.

  - ▲ Inhibiting the basolateral Na^+/K^+-ATPase pump reduces the excretion of K^+, increasing the amount of K^+ in blood.

Other Effects

- Spironolactone also binds to androgen and progesterone receptors. This is not by design but reflects the similarities in chemical structure between androgens (e.g., testosterone) progesterone, and aldosterone. Because these receptors are also similar in structure, spironolactone, which was designed before these receptors were mapped, binds to all three.
- Antagonism at these receptors leads to some of the side effects but has also led to some unique indications for spironolactone. Eplerenone was designed after the structure of the aldosterone receptor had been mapped and is therefore more specific for this receptor.

PHARMACOKINETICS

- Spironolactone has an active metabolite, canrenone, which is also marketed in some jurisdictions. Canrenone has a much longer elimination half-life (16 hours) than spironolactone (2 hours).

INDICATIONS

- As adjunct (add-on) therapy to a regular (potassium-depleting) diuretic such as a thiazide or loop diuretic, in the treatment of:
  - ▲ Hypertension
  - ▲ Congestive heart failure
- Primary hyperaldosteronism (spironolactone)

CONTRAINDICATION

- Severe K$^+$ abnormalities

SIDE EFFECTS

- **Hyperkalemia** can be exacerbated if the patient is taking another drug that raises potassium or is supplementing with potassium from the diet or from supplements. Patients with impaired renal function are also at higher risk for developing severe hyperkalemia.
- **Metabolic acidosis** occurs via decreased secretion of H$^+$ through the Na$^+$ channel.

Spironolactone Specific

- **Antiandrogenic actions:**
  - ▲ Gynecomastia
  - ▲ Menstrual disorders
  - ▲ Testicular atrophy

IMPORTANT NOTES

- K$^+$-sparing diuretics all produce a fairly modest diuresis and are typically given as adjunctive (add-on) therapy with more potent diuretics, with the intention of mitigating the hypokalemia associated with those agents.
- Antagonism of the aldosterone receptor might have beneficial effects beyond diuresis. The Randomized Aldactone Evaluation Study (RALES) found that treatment with spi-ronolactone significantly reduced mortality in a moderate-sized (approximately 800 subjects in each group) population, reducing the risk of death by about 30%. Risk of hospitalization was reduced by about 35%.
- The results of RALES suggested that in heart failure patients, spironolactone was not simply acting as a diuretic. There are many theories as to what this additional beneficial effect might be, but most focus around the link between elevated aldosterone and heart failure. A large trial, EPHESUS (N = 6000 patients), had similar results for eplerenone in patients who had developed heart failure after a myocardial infarction. However, in EPHESUS the magnitude of benefit was not as great as in RALES; therefore it is not clear whether aldosterone antagonism alone is contributing to benefit or whether there is some other factor involved.
- Drospirenone is a new progestogen that also antagonizes aldosterone receptors. It is used as a component in oral contraceptive regimens with estrogen, in the hope that the aldosterone antagonism will counteract the Na$^+$ and water retention from the estrogen.

FYI

- All three prototypical K$^+$-sparing diuretics (spironolactone, triamterene, and amiloride) are available in fixed-dose combinations (i.e., in the same pill) with hydrochlorothiazide.

Carbonic Anhydrase Inhibitors (CAIs)

DESCRIPTION

- Carbonic Anhydrase (CA) is classified as a diuretic, but its important *clinical* effects are related to its effect on acid-base balance and on intraocular fluid formation.

PROTOTYPE AND COMMON DRUGS

- Prototype: Aceta**zolamide**
- Others: Dor**zolamide**, brin**zolamide**, metha**zolamide**

MOA (MECHANISM OF ACTION)

- CA catalyzes the following reaction:

$$H_2CO_2 \rightleftharpoons H^+ + HCO_3^- \rightleftharpoons H_2O + CO_2$$

- CAIs inhibit this enzyme, which results in this reaction occurring at a *much* slower rate compared with the catalyzed rate, effectively stopping the reaction. The difference in reaction speed is over 1000-fold (Figure 25-4).
- CA is present at various sites throughout the nephron, but is mainly found on the luminal membrane of **proximal tubule** cells.
- CO$_2$ is highly lipophilic and easily crosses from the lumen into the tubule cell.

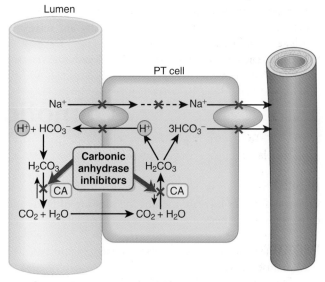

Carbonic anhydrase inhibitors

Figure 25-4.

- As seen in the diagram, this allows for the **recycling of H⁺** from the lumen into the cell and back to the lumen again.
- The Na^+ is transported across the basolateral membrane (the side opposite the tubular lumen) into the blood along with the HCO_3^-. The net effect of these movements is Na^+ and HCO_3^- reabsorption. Note that "H_2O" is embedded in HCO_3^-.
- The movement of these ions is largely driven by electrical and concentration gradients. Therefore inhibiting CA will effectively stop this entire cycle.
- Thus the effect of CAIs is to reduce the reabsorption of both Na^+ and HCO_3^-. The net effect is loss of Na^+ and HCO_3^- in the urine.
- The effect of CAIs on the acid-base status is that **loss of HCO_3^- lowers the pH.**

PHARMACOKINETICS
- Acetazolamide is cleared by the kidneys, whereas methazolamide is cleared primarily by the kidneys but also partially by the liver.
- Dorzolamide and brinzolamide are administered topically, as eye drops in the management of glaucoma.

INDICATIONS
- Glaucoma
- Metabolic alkalosis
- Acute mountain sickness (altitude sickness)

CONTRAINDICATIONS
- No major contraindications

SIDE EFFECTS
- **Hyperchloremic metabolic acidosis** occurs because of reduction in bicarbonate stores.
- **Renal stones**: Renal output of phosphates and calcium increases with CAI use. Chronic use of CAIs may also reduce excretion of solubilizing factors and, coupled with the alkalinization of the urine (Ca^{+2} salts are relatively insoluble at alkaline pH), creates an ideal environment for stone development.
- **Hypokalemia**: Additional $NaHCO_3$ in the collecting tubule stimulates the secretion of K^+ because of maintenance of the ion gradient.

IMPORTANT NOTES
- Acting early in the nephron, the diuretic actions of CAIs are countered by a number of sites for Na^+ reabsorption that appear distally in the tubule. That, coupled with the complication of metabolic acidosis, has limited the therapeutic usefulness of CAIs in the management of edema, and certainly in hypertension. In fact, CAIs are not even used for the treatment of edema or hypertension currently.
- The main use for CAIs at present is in the treatment of glaucoma (increased intraocular pressure [IOP]). The most popular agents are topical (dorzolamide, brinzolamide) drops administered to the eye. Locally administered agents are very low dose and therefore avoid the diuretic and systemic metabolic effects.
- The tendency toward metabolic acidosis helps to stimulate breathing, which, through a mechanism not entirely understood, helps a climber acclimatize more quickly to high altitude.

EVIDENCE
- One systematic review found that acetazolamide was more efficacious than placebo in preventing acute mountain sickness (number needed to treat [NNT], two to three). A lower dose was not found to be more effective than placebo.

FYI
- How do CAIs work in the treatment of glaucoma? Glaucoma is a condition of the eye characterized by increased intraocular pressure (IOP). CA located in the ciliary processes of the eye results in the formation of HCO_3^- in aqueous humor. By decreasing the rate of formation of aqueous humor, CAIs reduce IOP.

Osmotic Diuretics

DESCRIPTION
Osmotic diuretics increase the oncotic pressure of fluids and carry water with them.

PROTOTYPE
- Mannitol

MOA (MECHANISM OF ACTION)
- Osmotic agents increase the oncotic pressure of the blood; this pulls water from tissues and increases the volume of the blood acutely. The increased blood volume will inhibit renin release, thus increasing renal blood flow.
- Osmotic agents freely enter the glomerulus and Bowman's space and enter the nephron in the ultrafiltrate.
- Osmotic diuretics are not reabsorbed from the lumen of the nephron and create an osmotic force, pulling more fluid into the lumen. This is then carried out as urine.
- As a second primary mechanism for a diuretic, the increased renal blood flow effectively washes away solutes from the renal medulla, reducing tonicity in this region of the kidney.

The hypertonicity of the medulla is a major driving force for reabsorption of fluid from the renal tubule. Reducing this tonicity mitigates the forces that concentrate the urine in the ascending limb of Henle.

- Lowering the concentration of Na^+ in the ascending limb of Henle reduces the driving force for Na^+ reabsorption in this region, leading to diuresis.

PHARMACOKINETICS

- Osmotic diuretics are poorly absorbed, so they are given parenterally (intravenously).

INDICATIONS

- **Raised intracranial pressure (ICP) and cerebral edema.** The concept behind using osmotic manipulation for treating raised ICP is that water will get sucked out of the brain and into the blood (which has high osmotic pressure from the mannitol); this will reduce brain swelling and ICP.
- **Glaucoma** is an indication for use of these agents.
- **Disequilibrium syndrome in dialysis** (rare): Osmotic diuretics restore fluid to the extracellular compartment in patients who have been dialyzed and develop problems with the rapid shift in fluid and electrolytes that can sometimes accompany dialysis.

CONTRAINDICATIONS

- **Active cranial bleeding**: If bleeding is occurring into the brain, then the mannitol will be directly added to the brain and will raise the osmotic pressure in the brain and lead to water being *added* to the brain, which is the opposite of what the mannitol is being given for.
- **Continuous administration** of mannitol should not occur, because the drug will accumulate in the tissues and result in osmotic-induced tissue edema, including in the brain.

SIDE EFFECTS

- **Extracellular volume expansion**: Osmotic diuretics rapidly distribute to the extracellular compartment, extracting water from cells. Before onset of the diuresis, this can lead to expansion of the extracellular space. Frank pulmonary edema can arise in patients with heart failure or pulmonary congestion.
- **Dehydration and hypernatremia**: Excess use without fluid replacement can lead to dehydration. Composition of serum ions and fluid balance should be monitored.

IMPORTANT NOTES

- Osmotic diuretics increase the excretion of nearly all electrolytes (Na^+, K^+, Ca^{+2}, Mg^{+2}, Cl^-, HCO_3^-, and phosphate).
- Patients with uncontrolled diabetes mellitus will have an osmotic diuresis from elevated blood glucose. This is what causes polyuria (excessive urination), leading to thirst and excessive drinking of fluids (polydipsia).

EVIDENCE

Acute Traumatic Brain Injury

- A 2007 Cochrane review (four trials, N = 197 participants) compared different mannitol regimens with other interventions, including placebo and no treatment, in patients with acute traumatic brain injury. There was no difference in the incidence of death between mannitol and "standard care," pentobarbital, hypertonic saline, or placebo.

FYI

- Mannitol is a six-carbon sugar alcohol. It was first discovered in the sap of a plant and was thought to resemble biblical food; therefore the plant was called *manna ash*, after manna (biblical reference to food).

Antidiuretic Hormone (Vasopressin) Analogues

DESCRIPTION

Vasopressin analogues are analogues of the hormone vasopressin (also called *VP, antidiuretic hormone* [ADH] or *arginine vasopressin* [AVP]).

PROTOTYPE AND COMMON DRUGS

- Prototype: vaso**pressin** (identical to what the body produces)
- Others: desmo**pressin** (DDAVP), terli**pressin**

MOA (MECHANISM OF ACTION)

- Vasopressin is produced in the hypothalamus and stored in the posterior pituitary gland. Factors that stimulate its physiologic release include **increased serum osmolarity** and **hypotension**. Its primary actions are therefore to increase body water to control osmolality and to increase blood pressure. A third action that it exerts is to help stop bleeding through platelet stimulation.
- Vasopressin binds two types of receptors: V_1 and V_2. V_1 is subtyped into V_{1a} and V_{1b}. V_1 receptors are found in many locations of the body, including endothelium and many other sites. V_2 receptors are located in the collecting ducts of the nephron.
- At very low concentrations vasopressin acts on V_2 receptors. Only at higher doses are the V_1 receptors activated.

Vasoconstriction

- V_1 receptors are located on vascular smooth muscle and produce a **potent vasoconstrictor** effect when stimulated. This occurs only at higher serum levels of vasopressin.
- Activation of V_1 receptors results in increased intracellular calcium.
- The hemodynamic effects of vasopressin are similar to norepinephrine; the difference is that norepinephrine also possesses some β-agonist activity and therefore will increase heart rate and contractility, whereas vasopressin will not.

Antidiuresis

- Filtrate that reaches the collecting duct in the kidney has been diluted by previous tubules. Therefore filtrate that is reabsorbed in the collecting duct is quite dilute and low in sodium.
- V_2 receptors are located in the **collecting duct** of the nephron. When stimulated, they activate pores called *aquaporins* (e.g., **aquaporin 2**). These pores usually are stored in intracellular vesicles and when stimulated by vasopressin will fuse with the luminal membrane and **facilitate the reabsorption** of water from the nephron lumen back into the body. In the absence of the vasopressin and the aquaporins, the collecting duct is impermeable to water and will not absorb any water.
- Desmopressin is a synthetic compound; it is more specific for V_2 receptors and has a longer half-life than vasopressin. Compared with vasopressin, desmopressin (*DDAVP*) is **3000 times more selective for V_2 receptors.** Therefore desmopressin minimizes the potent vasoconstrictor effects associated with vasopressin.

Platelet Function

- Factor VIII and von Willebrand's factor (vWF) bind together and then bind platelets, which causes platelet activation. A deficiency in either of these two factors will result in decreased platelet function and bleeding disorders (hemophilia A and von Willebrand's disease).
- Desmopressin binds to V_2 receptors, which are instrumental in endothelial release of factor VIII.

PHARMACOKINETICS

- Both agents are poorly absorbed through the oral route.
- Vasopressin is administered by intravenous infusion. It has a short half-life and therefore is given by infusion.
- Desmopressin can be administered by the intravenous, subcutaneous injection, or intranasal routes. Intranasal is the preferred route of administration for desmopressin for patients not in the hospital.

INDICATIONS
Desmopressin

- To decrease urine production:
  - ▲ Central DI (deficiency of ADH secretion)
  - ▲ Nocturnal enuresis (bedwetting)
- To help reduce bleeding:

- ▲ von Willebrand's disease (vWF deficiency)
- ▲ Hemophilia A (factor VIII deficiency)

Vasopressin, Terlipressin

- To provide vasoconstriction:
  - ▲ Pathologic states of vasodilation:
    - Sepsis (vasopressin only)
    - Liver failure

CONTRAINDICATIONS

- **Desmopressin only:** patients at risk for unregulated water consumption (psychogenic polydipsia), because they can develop hyponatremia

SIDE EFFECTS
Vasopressin

- **Excessive vasoconstriction.** The use of vasopressin should be restricted to physicians trained in critical care.

Desmopressin

- **Water intoxication (hyponatremia):** This is caused by the antidiuretic action and results in water retention leading to dilution of electrolytes, specifically Na^+.
- **Hypotension** (paradoxical to other analogues): If administered by the intravenous route, desmopressin must be given slowly.

IMPORTANT NOTES

- DI can be classified as central (neurogenic) or nephrogenic.
  - ▲ Central DI is a condition of ADH deficiency caused by low or no production.
  - ▲ Nephrogenic DI is a condition of nonresponsiveness of the kidney to normal circulating levels of ADH.
- In DI there is too much water relative to Na^+ in the blood. Therefore, **hyponatremia** exists. Furthermore, there is very little water in the urine and so the **urine osmolality is very high.**
- Varices are abnormal blood veins: dilated, elongated, and tortuous. They are caused by abnormally high venous pressures. They are most commonly seen in the gastrointestinal (GI) tract (esophagus, anus) in patients with liver failure and portal hypertension and also in the legs when one-way valves in the upper leg fail to prevent backflow and pressure. Administration of vasopressin or other vasoconstricting analogues results in mesenteric vasoconstriction and reduced blood flow and thus reduced portal blood pressure. This is beneficial to patients with portal hypertension secondary to liver disease who have bleeding variceal vessels in the esophagus.
- There are many subtypes of von Willebrand's disease, depending on the levels of vWF in the body. Desmopressin is really effective in only the mild forms of the disease.
- V_2 *antagonists* are the newest class of diuretics. These agents are referred to as *aquaretics*, because by blocking V_2 receptors in the collecting duct they produce a water diuresis,

with minimal loss of electrolytes. The first aquaretic, tolvaptan, has been approved in most jurisdictions for patients with volume overload and electrolyte problems that would be exacerbated by conventional diuretics.

EVIDENCE
Desmopressin and Bedwetting (Enuresis) in Children

- A Cochrane review in 2002 (47 studies, 3448 children) demonstrated that desmopressin is effective at reducing bedwetting but that the effects do not persist when the drug is stopped. Using a wake-up alarm (the alarm goes off when the child gets wet) was just as effective as desmopressin but had better long-lasting effects.

Desmopressin and Surgical Blood Loss in Patients without Bleeding Disorders

- A Cochrane review in 2004 (19 studies, 1387 patients) demonstrated that bleeding with desmopressin was statistically less compared with placebo (mean difference = 241 mL less). However, there was no difference in blood transfusions, and the volume of blood loss reduction is not a *clinically* significant amount.

FYI

- From Latin:
  - ▲ *Diabetes:* to go through entirely (referring to water in the body)
  - ▲ *Insipid* means lack of flavor or taste. *Mellis* means honey.
  - ▲ The urine is bland in DI. The urine is sweet in diabetes mellitus.
  - ▲ *Varix* means twisted. Varicose veins are twisted.
- *DDAVP* stand for 1-desamino-8-D-arginine vasopressin.
- Aquaporin 1 is present in the *proximal tubule* and is responsible for water reabsorption in this part of the nephron. It is not responsive to AVP.
- Syndrome of inappropriate ADH (SIADH) is a condition of too much ADH. It is essentially the opposite of DI.
- Oxytocin and vasopressin are structurally very similar. Therefore oxytocin and vasopressin agonists or antagonists can interact with either receptor.

Anticholinergics: Bladder

DESCRIPTION

Bladder anticholinergics are agents that antagonize muscarinic receptors and are used to treat overactive bladder (OAB), a form of incontinence.

PROTOTYPE AND COMMON DRUGS
M3 Selective

- Prototype: darifenacin
- Others: solifenacin

Nonselective

- Prototype: oxybutynin
- Others: tolterodine, trospium

MOA (MECHANISM OF ACTION)

- The human bladder contains all five subtypes (M1 to M5) of muscarinic (M) receptors. Although M2 receptors are more abundant in this region, M3 receptors mediate contraction of the detrusor muscle in the bladder.

- Detrusor muscle contraction facilitates emptying of the bladder (micturition). Abnormal contractions of the detrusor, also known as *hyperreflexia*, can lead to incontinence, specifically **urge incontinence**. Urge incontinence is defined as the inability to reach the toilet in time following the urge to urinate (Figure 25-5).
- Anticholinergics that antagonize the **M3 receptor** inhibit these detrusor contractions, easing the symptoms of urge incontinence.
- Muscarinic receptors, both M3 and other subtypes, are also found throughout the human body.
  - ▲ M1 receptors are found in the central nervous system (CNS), on glands (enteric and salivary), and on enteric nerves.
  - ▲ M2 receptors are found in the CNS, heart, and smooth muscle, including the bladder.
  - ▲ M3 receptors are found in the CNS, heart, smooth muscle, and glands, in addition to the bladder.
- Because of the wide distribution of M receptors, anticholinergics for OAB have an extensive side effect profile, and

Anticholinergics for bladder

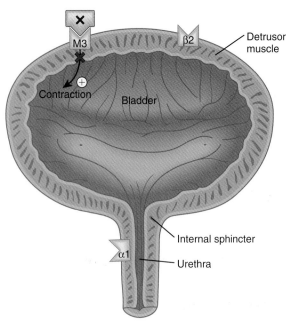

Figure 25-5.

considerable research is going into localizing the effects of these agents to the detrusor.

PHARMACOKINETICS

■ Most of the anticholinergics for OAB are lipophilic, meaning that they readily cross the blood-brain barrier. The exception is trospium, a polar molecule that does not cross into the brain.

■ The half-lives of these agents vary widely, and agents with short half-lives (oxybutynin, tolterodine) typically have extended-release (ER) preparations available.

■ Oxybutynin is also marketed as a transdermal patch. The patch is applied twice weekly and delivers 3.9 mg of oxybutynin per day.

INDICATION

■ OAB with symptoms of urge urinary incontinence, urgency, and frequency

CONTRAINDICATIONS

■ Conditions in which cholinergic blockade would exacerbate an already serious condition, or patients at risk for the following:
  ▲ Urinary retention
  ▲ Gastroparesis, gastric obstruction
  ▲ Narrow-angle glaucoma (uncontrolled)

SIDE EFFECTS

■ Typical anticholinergic side effects:

  ▲ Dry mouth
  ▲ Constipation
  ▲ Blurred vision
  ▲ Erythema
  ▲ Pruritus

IMPORTANT NOTES

■ CNS side effects are a concern with the use of anticholinergics, particularly in seniors and the elderly. Attempts have been made to develop compounds that either have limited penetration into the CNS (trospium) or that bind with lower affinity to M1 receptors (darifenacin), receptors that are thought to play an important role in cognition. However, although there is some evidence of reduced CNS side effects in older, otherwise-healthy patients, there is no definitive proof that these approaches are able to reduce the burden of CNS side effects in patients with OAB.

■ Some of the drugs used for treating irritable bowel syndrome also have anticholinergic properties, including dicyclomine. The antagonism of muscarinic receptors in the gut helps to reduce hypermotility and may also reduce spasms.

Advanced

■ All of the anticholinergics for OAB are metabolized by CYP3A4, with the exception of trospium, which is metabolized by non-CYP ester hydrolysis. Many of these agents are also metabolized by CYP2D6.

EVIDENCE
Anticholinergics for Overactive Bladder

■ A 2008 systematic review (83 trials) compared various anticholinergics in treating OAB. All the included anticholinergics (oxybutynin, tolterodine, fesoterodine, propiverine, solifenacin, darifenacin, and trospium) demonstrated efficacy in a variety of outcome measures related to incontinence (incontinence episodes, frequency, urgency) versus placebo.

■ Although there were no definitive conclusions with respect to comparisons among agents, there was some indication that newer agents (solifenacin) may have greater efficacy than slightly older agents (tolterodine) for some outcomes. Oxybutynin was the only agent with a higher risk of withdrawals versus placebo. Tolterodine consistently had the most favorable safety and tolerability data compared with other agents.

FYI

■ Controversy still exists over the relative benefit to risk of anticholinergics for OAB, particularly in seniors and the elderly. Although these agents have demonstrated improved symptoms versus placebo, the clinical significance of these benefits is constantly being weighed against a considerable list of side effects.

Alpha-1 (α_1) Antagonists

PROTOTYPE AND COMMON DRUGS
- Prototype: prazosin
- Others: terazosin, doxazosin, tamsulosin
- Nonurinary: phenoxybenzamine, phentolamine

MOA (MECHANISM OF ACTION)
- Antagonism of α_1 receptors on vascular smooth muscle induces vasodilation and decreases systemic vascular resistance (SVR).
- Both resistance (arterial) and capacitance (venous) vessels are dilated.
- α_1 Receptors are also found in the urinary sphincter (also smooth muscle) of the bladder. The sphincter controls the flow of urine out of the bladder (Figure 25-6).

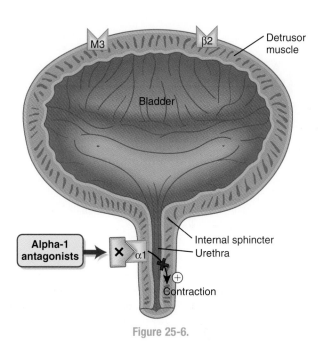

Alpha-1 antagonists

Figure 25-6.

- In patients with an enlarged prostate, pressure exerted by the prostate on the sphincter can interfere with normal urine flow. Therefore patients with an enlarged prostate experience hesitancy (difficulty starting urination) and typically do not urinate much at a time but experience urinary frequency.
- An α_1 antagonist can relax the urinary sphincter, which facilitates the flow of urine.
- Another rare use for α_1 antagonists is in the management of pheochromocytoma. This is a tumor of the adrenal medulla that secretes catecholamines such as epinephrine and norepinephrine. α_1 Antagonists such as phenoxyben-

zamine are used preoperatively and postoperatively to manage the symptoms of catecholamine excess.

PHARMACOKINETICS
- Prazosin has a short half-life and thus must be given twice daily. Longer-acting agents such as terazosin and doxazosin were developed to provide the advantage of once-daily administration.

INDICATIONS
- Benign prostatic hypertrophy (BPH)
- Hypertension (but not as first line)

Phentolamine and Phenoxybenzamine Only
- Management of patients with pheochromocytoma

CONTRAINDICATIONS
- No significant contraindications

SIDE EFFECTS
- **Orthostatic hypotension** is common and can be quite significant, usually occurring within 90 minutes of the first dose of the drug. It can lead to dizziness and falls.
- **Headache** might be caused by cerebral vasodilation.
- **Somnolence** may occur.
- **Nasal congestion** is caused by dilation of vessels in the nasal passages, causing mild swelling.
- **Palpitation** is a result of reflex tachycardia.
- **Cardiovascular events:** Although these agents are typically well tolerated, results of a recent study suggest that they may be associated with an increased risk, summarized in the Advanced section.

IMPORTANT NOTES
- Compensatory sympathetic nervous system responses such as renin release and tachycardia are significant in the short term. However, in many cases these reflex responses subside, leaving a vasodilatory effect that predominates in the long term.
- Tamsulosin was developed to selectively target α_{1A} receptors, which are found in the bladder sphincter and not in vascular smooth muscle. Therefore by antagonizing these α_{1A} receptors selectively, it is believed that tamsulosin will be less likely to cause orthostatic hypotension and therefore less likely to cause dizziness and falls.

Advanced
- The use of α antagonists in hypertension was dealt a severe blow after treatment in the doxazosin arm of the landmark ALLHAT study had to be halted prematurely after observations of a significantly increased incidence of congestive heart failure, angina, and stroke in subjects treated with this α antagonist.

EVIDENCE

Tamsulosin versus Placebo for Treatment of Benign Prostatic Hypertrophy

■ A 2002 Cochrane review (14 studies, N = 4122 participants) assessed tamsulosin for treatment of BPH. Tamsulosin improved symptoms and peak urine flow relative to placebo and was as effective as nonselective α antagonists. Men receiving a low dose of tamsulosin (0.2 mg) were less likely to discontinue treatment compared with men receiving terazosin. The adverse effects of terazosin increased markedly with increasing dose, compared with placebo. The most common adverse effects associated with tamsulosin were dizziness, rhinitis, and abnormal ejaculation.

Terazosin versus Other α-Blockers for Treatment of Benign Prostatic Obstruction

■ A 2000 Cochrane review (17 studies, N = 5151 participants) assessed terazosin versus placebo (10 trials), α-blockers (seven trials), or the 5α-reductase inhibitor finasteride (one trial) for benign prostatic obstruction. Terazosin improved symptom scores and urine flow rates more than placebo or finasteride and similarly to other α antagonists. The proportion of men discontinuing treatment was higher than the proportion of men receiving other α antagonists and was comparable to what was seen with placebo and finasteride. Adverse effects occurring more often than with placebo included dizziness, asthenia, headache, and postural hypotension.

FYI

■ Phenoxybenzamine is an irreversible antagonist of α_1 receptors, whereas other α_1 antagonists are reversible.
■ Phentolamine antagonizes both α_1 and α_2 receptors. Through antagonism of presynaptic α_2 receptors, it increases presynaptic noradrenaline release, which in turn stimulates the heart.
■ Yohimbine is an α_2 antagonist with limited antagonism of α_1 receptors. It is not widely used, but as with phentolamine, it can promote norepinephrine release and can be used in patients with orthostatic hypotension. It was also once used to treat erectile dysfunction, although it has been effectively replaced by the phosphodiesterase inhibitors (e.g., sildenafil).

5α-Reductase Inhibitors

DESCRIPTION

5α-Reductase inhibitors are a class of drugs that reduce the production of dihydrotestosterone (DHT), the active form of testosterone.

PROTOTYPE AND COMMON DRUGS

■ Prototype: finasteride
■ Others: dutasteride

MOA (MECHANISM OF ACTION)

■ The 5α-reductase enzyme is the last step in the synthesis of DHT, the active form of testosterone (Figure 25-7).
■ Prostate cells depend on stimulation by DHT for their growth. Reducing levels of DHT will therefore slow growth of the prostate.
■ The 5α-reductase type II isoform is highly expressed in prostate epithelial cells.
■ Selective or nonselective blockade of this enzyme results in decreased formation of DHT, inhibiting the growth-stimulating effects of this androgen.

PHARMACOKINETICS

■ No drug interactions of clinical significance have been detected with finasteride. Dutasteride is metabolized by CYP3A4; thus the potential for drug interactions with inhibitors or inducers of this isozyme does exist.

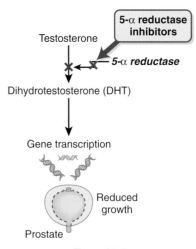

5-α reductase inhibitors

Testosterone → Dihydrotestosterone (DHT) → Gene transcription → Reduced growth

Prostate

Figure 25-7.

INDICATIONS

■ BPH
■ Male pattern baldness

CONTRAINDICATION

■ **Pregnancy:** Women of childbearing age should not use 5α-reductase inhibitors. They are strictly contraindicated in pregnancy. Testosterone is essential for development of genitalia in males; therefore these agents can lead to abnormal development. Pregnant women are advised not only to avoid taking the medication but also to avoid even handling the pills.

SIDE EFFECTS

- **Sexual dysfunction**: Decreased libido, ejaculation disorders, and erectile dysfunction are caused by the antiandrogenic effects.

EVIDENCE
Finasteride versus Placebo for Prevention of Prostate Cancer

- A 2008 Cochrane review (nine trials, N = 34,410 males) examined the effectiveness and harms of 5α-reductase inhibitors in preventing prostate cancer. Finasteride reduced the risk of prostate cancer by 2.9% (incidence of 6.3% in finasteride versus 9.2% in placebo). Impaired erectile function or endocrine effects were more common with finasteride than with placebo. However, the risk of high-grade disease may be increased with finasteride therapy. The authors recommended that future studies examine the impact of 5α-reductase inhibitors on mortality and also further examine the risk associated with development of high-grade cancers.

IMPORTANT NOTES

- Because of their lowering effects on prostate serum antigen (PSA), there is concern that 5α-reductase inhibitors may mask elevations in PSA associated with a malignancy of the prostate. This could lead to a delay in the diagnosis of prostate cancer because of false-negative screening test results.
- The 5α-reductase inhibitors have not performed well in comparative trials with α antagonists for treatment of BPH. This is thought to result from, at least in part, the fact that the beneficial effects of 5α-reductase inhibitors are more gradual, whereas symptomatic improvement with α antagonists occurs rapidly.
- As a means of overcoming the delayed effects of 5α-reductase inhibitors, consideration has been given to combining α antagonists with these agents. The Medical Therapy of Prostatic Symptoms (MTOPS) trial found that the combination of doxazosin and finasteride performed better than either agent alone in a variety of key clinical indicators of BPH progression, over the course of 4.5 years.
- The effects of finasteride in treating male pattern baldness are also delayed. Patients are typically advised to undergo a 3- to 6-month trial before expecting any noticeable results.

FYI

- The dose of finasteride used to treat male pattern baldness is lower than that used to treat BPH.

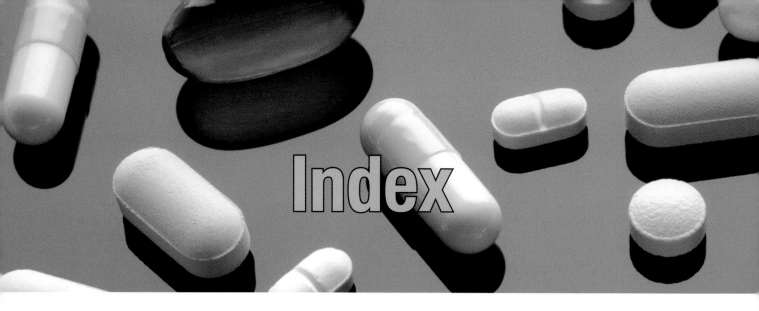

Index

Page numbers followed by f or t indicate figures and tables respectively.